The PHYSICIAN ASSISTANT EMERGENCY MEDICINE HANDBOOK

The PHYSICIAN ASSISTANT EMERGENCY MEDICINE HANDBOOK

Steven W. Salyer, PhD, PA-C

Program Director
Emergency Medicine
Physician Assistant
Specialty Training Program
Brooke Army Medical Center
Fort Sam Houston, Texas

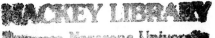
W.B. Saunders Company

A Division of Harcourt Brace & Company
Philadelphia London Toronto Montreal Sydney Tokyo

W.B. SAUNDERS COMPANY
A Division of Harcourt Brace & Company

The Curtis Center
Independence Square West
Philadelphia, Pennsylvania 19106

Library of Congress Cataloging-in-Publication Data

Salyer, Steven W.
The physician assistant emergency medicine handbook / Steven W. Salyer.

    p.   cm.

ISBN 0–7216–5869–5

1. Medical emergencies—Handbooks, manuals, etc.   2. Physicians'
  assistants—Handbooks, manuals, etc.   I. Title.   [DNLM:
  1. Emergencies—handbooks.   2. Emergency Medicine—
  methods—handbooks.   WP 39 S186p 1997]

RC86.8.S25 1997   616.02′5—dc20

DNLM/DLC

          96–7416

To my wife Sally and my children Laura Emilie and Warren Zachary, who gave up so much of their "daddy time" while I wrote this book.

And to the "Cavalry Troopers" of 3rd Squadron, 2nd Armored Cavalry Regiment, who lived, fought, and died during Desert Storm, February, 1991.

Preface

The specialty of Emergency Medicine and the concept of Physician Assistant (PA) are both about 25 years old. Their history and acceptance in the medical community have many parallels. They represent the newest type of practitioners in the medical community and are now both accepted specialties.

This book was written out of necessity, not brilliance. After practicing in a family practice–type setting in the United States Army for 5 years, I applied for and was accepted in the Emergency Medicine Physician Assistant Residency at Brooke Army Medical Hospital, San Antonio, Texas. I soon realized that I needed a simple and easily accessible knowledge base. As a PA, I found none. I then started my own "peripheral brain" — like so many of us did in PA school. Out of this peripheral brain material grew this book over the past 3 years.

Emergency medicine is one of the fastest growing segments of the PA profession and rightfully so. We are cost-effective staff in the emergency department. We deliver quality medicine to 90% of the patients a physician can see in either an "acute-care" or a "fast-track" environment. But let's not be fooled by the terms acute care and fast track. The patient who presents to the emergency department is not always a "fast tracker," and accurate diagnosis and intervention are often necessitated. Any PA who has spent any time in any ED knows that there are often "zebras" around every corner.

As emergency medicine expands, however, so will our profession as part of emergency medicine. Many physicians and hospitals have overcome the belief that PAs should see only the fast-track patients. As more and more residency-trained PAs enter the ED, so will the job description expand into the care of the trauma and cardiac patient. Emergency medicine PAs have already proved themselves competent to the medical community and to the patients served by them in rural emergency departments. Many rural hospital emergency departments are staffed solely by emergency medicine PAs at night and on weekends. We have met this challenge and have provided exceptional service in these communities.

I spent 4 years in the 3rd Squadron, 2nd Armored Cavalry Regiment in Amberg, Germany. The 2nd Cavalry is the longest continuous active-duty military organization in the United States Army. During World War I in France, they were given the regimental motto of *Toujours Pret*, which means always ready in French. This motto reminds me of what we do in emergency medicine. We are truly always ready for whatever comes into the ED. We are many patients' last resort, not only for their medical problems, but also for their hearts, minds, and souls. Just being a good listener is often all that is needed.

We who have chosen the ED as our home must understand that we have a tremendous power over and responsibility for those who enter our ED. We have the power to save and change the lives of these individuals. No matter how bad things get, no matter what time of day or night, no matter who the person is, we are truly always ready to fix, care for, or listen to any problems. We should not take this powerful responsibility we have chosen lightly. We have been blessed with this power to heal and to change lives.

This book was written by a PA for PA students, as they go through their ED rotation; for new PAs who have never practiced in the ED; and for experienced PAs who work in the ED and need a quick reference guide.

As managed care changes and expands, I can see a great future for the marriage of PAs and emergency medicine specialists. I offer this handbook to those who chose the marriage of the two greatest professions on earth — emergency medicine and physician assistant: *Toujours Pret.*

Steven W. Salyer

Acknowledgments

I would like to thank a few special people who helped me along my journey in life and as an emergency medicine physician assistant. To Major Peter Forsberg, PA-C, United States Army: thanks, Pete. You have done more for Physician Assistant Emergency Medicine than we will ever be able to thank you for.

A special thanks to Dr. David McMicken and the other physicians, PAs, and nurse practitioners in the ED at The Medical Center, Columbus, Georgia, during 1992–93. You gave me the love for emergency medicine: thanks, guys!

Thanks to the staff and residents at Brooke Army Medical Center, Fort Sam Houston, Texas, during my residency in 1993–94. You taught me the "art" of emergency medicine.

To those who were staff and residents at Darnall Army Community Hospital, Fort Hood, Texas, from 1994–1996, who put up with me the past 2 years while I wrote this book. Thanks!

And a very, very special thanks to Colonel Joseph L. Krawczyk Jr. (Ret.), the finest leader under whom I have ever served. You taught me fairness, frankness, understanding, compassion, and leadership and to never be too busy to listen to anyone. Rank not only has its privileges but also its responsibilities. Always trust in your people to do the job they are trained for. Thanks, Joe.

Steven W. Salyer

Contents

Chapter 1

Acute Surgical Abdominal Emergencies

ACUTE APPENDICITIS

Definition

Acute appendicitis is an acute inflammatory process of the appendix that is usually secondary to outflow obstruction of the appendix lymph tissue with secondary bacterial invasion.

Epidemiology

Acute appendicitis occurs in 1 in 1000 patients each year or 6% of the population of the United States. It is the most common abdominal surgical procedure in children and the most common nongynecologic surgical procedure in pregnant women. Acute appendicitis is most common in the 10- to 30-year-old age group but can occur at any age. Only 20 to 30% of appendices are ruptured at the time of surgery, with a slight predominance of males over females. Mortality rate is between 0.1% and 0.2% for unruptured appendix and from 3 to 5% for a ruptured appendix. The greater the delay in diagnosis, the greater are the morbidity and mortality rates.

Pathology

The role of the appendix is unknown. It is a small hollow, muscular tube that is 6 to 9 cm in size and is located about 2.5 cm from the ileocolic junction. The appendix has both vagus and sympathetic innervation. The most common cause of acute appendicitis is obstruction with bacterial invasion, with the two most common organisms being *Escherichia coli* and *Bacteroides*. An appendolith is the most common cause of appendix obstruction. With an obstruction the normal mucosal secretions continue until the appendix reaches capacity, resulting in distention. As swelling continues, cramping ensues and vascular congestion occurs. Arterial inflow continues without lymph outflow. At this point bacterial invasion occurs, and the risk of gangrene and necrosis is increased secondary to arterial stasis and infarction of the appendix. This usually occurs along the antimesenteric border of the appendix. Perforation and spillage of the infected contents of the appendix usually occur between 24 and 36 hours after onset of the obstruction. When spillage of the contents of the appendix occurs, peritonitis ensues.

Clinical Presentation/Examination

The average time between the onset of abdominal pain and the patient's presentation to the emergency department is 18 hours. The pain usually starts around the periumbilical area or in the lower epigastric region. Over about 18 hours the pain becomes more localized in the right lower quadrant at McBurney's point. The patient can present with anorexia, malaise, diarrhea, or constipation; however, no rules apply to the patient who has acute appendicitis. When the female patient is pregnant, the appendix rises in the abdomen as the uterus is displaced superiorly when it enlarges. A pregnant patient with acute appendicitis can present with flank pain or right upper quadrant pain. In a male patient, a retroileal appendix can cause testicular pain.

A patient will often describe the pain as dull in onset or crampy; however, as the appendix becomes more inflamed, the pain becomes more localized. The patient's level of pain will increase by a bump in the road on the way to the hospital, hip shake, jumping, or coughing. The elderly patient may complain of abdominal distention or bloating and often states that he or she needs a laxative. Fever is often present, and some patients present with urinary complaints.

All patients require a rectal examination to rule out a gastrointestinal (GI) bleed. There is often tenderness at the right lateral rectal wall. All female patients require a pelvic examination to assess for cervical os discharge or tenderness or adnexal fullness or tenderness. A pregnancy test should always be done on all female patients to rule out pregnancy (i.e., symptoms of ectopic pregnancy). Pelvic inflammatory disease (PID) or ectopic pregnancy can mimic acute appendicitis. The patient's stool should be checked for the presence of any blood or mucus. Crohn's disease or ulcerative colitis should always be considered in the differential diagnosis of acute appendicitis.

Rovsing's sign is referred pain in the right lower quadrant with palpation in the left lower quadrant. Diffuse tenderness can be a sign of peritonitis secondary to rupture of an acute appendicitis. Guarding and rebound tenderness are usually present—both are signs of peritonitis. If the right hip is extended passively or flexed against resistance, this position will irritate the iliopsoas muscle and cause pain—this is called the psoas sign. If the patient feels pain when the hip is passively rotated internally and the right ankle is placed on the left knee, this is a sign of inflammation around the obturator muscle and is called the obturator sign. These signs are not specific for acute appendicitis but indicate an inflammatory process in the right lower quadrant of the abdomen.

Diagnosis

The diagnosis of an acute appendicitis is based on the patient's clinical presentation, the duration of symptoms, and a white blood cell count with a shift to the left. Diagnostic laparoscopy is an invasive study that is now being used prior to laparotomy at some institutions.

Laboratory Findings

All patients who present with acute pain in the abdomen should have a complete blood count (CBC), electrolytes, amylase, lipase, liver function test (LFT), urinalysis, and pregnancy test (if female) drawn. The white blood cell count is usually between 14,000 and 16,000 with a shift to the left. All other laboratory findings are usually normal.

Radiography

All patients with acute pain in the abdomen should have a series of x-rays of the abdomen to include a chest x-ray to rule out small bowel obstruction, air in the gallbladder, kidney stones, gallstones, or pneumonia situated on the right diaphragm causing irritation to the diaphragm and thus abdominal pain. Pneumonia is a very common finding in children who present with abdominal pain. A plain film can detect a fecalith.

A barium enema is used by some institutions to diagnose acute appendicitis. If the appendix does not fill with barium, then it is obstructed. Barium enemas are rarely performed, secondary to the certainty of the patient's clinical presentation in regard to acute appendicitis.

Ultrasound is now being used on a limited basis to detect acute appendicitis. Ultrasound has a 75 to 90% sensitivity rate and a 86 to 100% specificity rate, respectively. Ultrasound is noninvasive and inexpensive and involves no exposure to radiation.

Treatment

A patient with acute pain in the abdomen who is suspected to have acute appendicitis should be treated with intravenous (IV) fluids (1 to 2 liters of normal saline) and antiemetics. Pain medication should not be given until the exact cause of the abdominal pain has been determined. Pain medications often confuse the results of physical examination. If the patient is in severe pain, pain medication should only be given after the surgeon has been consulted and has examined the patient.

The aforementioned laboratory and radiographic examinations should be performed. Again, a pelvic examination should always be done on a female patient, and a rectal examination should be performed on all patients. Early surgical consultation is always appropriate, especially when a ruptured appendix is suspected.

HERNIAS

Definition

A hernia is a protrusion of viscus through an acquired or congenital opening from one space into another space. There are several different kinds of hernias. The two most common types are internal and external hernias. Hernias are further described as reducible or incarcerated. Hernias secondary to previous surgery are called incisional hernias. A double hernia (or bilateral hernia) has both direct and indirect components. A sliding hernia involves one wall of the hernial sac. Richter's hernia is an incarcerated or strangulated hernia that involves only one wall of the viscus.

Epidemiology

Children and females are at the greatest risk of having femoral hernias. Obturator hernias occur more commonly in elderly women. Indirect hernias are most common in males and are also more common in the young. Direct hernias are more common in the older population and are rare in children. Umbilical hernias are common in newborn black children and in the obese elderly populations.

Pathology

There are many causes of hernias. Heredity and congenital malformations are the two most important factors involved in the development of a hernia. In congenital malformations, a part of the abdominal wall fails to form properly. Enlarged inguinal rings may be hereditary. An indirect inguinal hernia is one that protrudes down the inguinal canal and is lateral to the inferior epigastric vessels. Indirect hernias often incarcerate. These hernias are more common in men than in women secondary to the embryologic descent of the male's testicle.

Direct inguinal hernias are ones that protrude through Hesselbach's triangle. Hesselbach's triangle is bordered by the inguinal ligament, the lateral border of the rectus abdominis muscle, and the inferior epigastric vessels. Direct hernias rarely incarcerate.

Obturator hernias occur more commonly in elderly women than in elderly men. The hernia protrudes through the obturator foramen, between the superior and inferior rami, and down into the medial thigh.

A femoral hernia is one that protrudes below the inguinal ligament into the femoral canal. Femoral hernias are more common in females than in males. If the femoral hernia occurs above the epigastric vessels in the linea semilunaris, it is called a spigelian hernia.

Umbilical hernias are caused by a defect in the umbilical area. These hernias usually close by the patient's second birthday. Umbilical hernias again recur in the aged obese patient and in patients with severe or chronic ascites. Umbilical hernias also occur with increased frequency in the pregnant patient.

Clinical Presentation

Most patients present with a nonpainful lump or knot around the groin. Some patients have a "dragging" sensation in the groin area. A patient who is in pain usually presents with an incarcerated hernia.

If the hernia is strangulated and necrotic, the patient can present in acute sepsis. Women with obturator hernias present with knee and thigh pain along the distribution of the the obturator nerve. Women with femoral hernias have ipsilateral inguinal pain.

Reducible hernias are ones that can be easily reduced with the patient in the supine position and by exerting direct pressure. If the hernia cannot be reduced, it must be considered incarcerated. Incarcerated hernias can lead to bowel obstruction. If the hernia is incarcerated, the patient can present with tachycardia, tachypnea, nausea, vomiting, fever, or sepsis.

Groin hernias can be easily confused with swollen lymph nodes. Lymph nodes are usually firm and mobile and are usually multiple in presentation. A single node is rare. Furthermore, incarcerated hernias do not transilluminate as hydroceles do.

Examination

All patients should be given a complete examination, including a rectal examination and a guaiac test. Female patients should receive a complete pelvic examination to rule out PID or ectopic pregnancy.

Diagnosis

The diagnosis of a hernia is made after taking a clinical history and a physical examination.

Laboratory Findings

If the hernia is believed to be incarcerated, a CBC, electrolytes, blood urea nitrogen (BUN), creatinine, and urinalysis should be performed. If the patient is female and in child-bearing years, a pregnancy test should be done. If the patient appears septic, secondary to incarceration, blood cultures should be drawn. If electrolyte levels infer acidosis or a high anion gap, an arterial blood gas should be taken.

Radiography

A two-view chest x-ray and supine and upright abdominal x-rays should be performed to rule out bowel obstruction, gallstones, or kidney stones that might cause referred pain in the groin.

Treatment

If the hernia is easily reducible, and the patient is taking fluid and food by mouth and is in less than moderate pain, then this patient can be referred routinely to a surgeon. If the hernia is incarcerated, an immediate surgical consultation is necessary.

If the hernia is incarcerated, an attempt can be made to reduce the hernia. The patient should be placed in the Trendelenburg position. A warm compress applied to the area can sometimes reduce edema and allow easier reduction. Gentle, steady compression should be applied to the hernia; however, the hernia should not be forced back in. If the hernia cannot be reduced, an infusion of normal saline or lactated Ringer's solution should be started IV. The aforementioned laboratory examinations should be performed. A nasogastric tube should be placed to decompress the bowel and decrease proximal pressure on the hernia. If sepsis or necrosis of the bowel is suspected, broad-spectrum antibiotics and vigorous fluid resuscitation should be administered. A surgeon should be consulted immediately.

INTESTINAL OBSTRUCTIONS

Definition

The term ileus is used to describe an intestinal obstruction. Intestinal bowel obstruction, or ileus, is divided into two types: (1) paralytic or (2) dynamic. Paralytic ileus is usually caused secondary to surgery. A failure of the inadequate contraction by the intestine slows or stops the intestinal contents from progressing through the bowel, thus the term paralytic ileus.

A dynamic ileus is a term used to describe a mechanical obstruction. Dynamic ileuses are further divided into intrinsic and extrinsic obstructions. Small bowel and large bowel obstructions are different entities, caused by different mechanisms, and have different presentations and treatments.

Epidemiology

The mortality rate for a small bowel obstruction is approximately 5%. Adhesions from previous abdominal surgeries account for 50% of all small bowel obstructions. Neoplasms cause 15% of all small bowel obstructions, and hernias cause another 15% of small bowel obstructions. In the pediatric population, most small bowel obstructions are caused by intussusception and congenital lesions. Large bowel obstruction or colonic obstruction is usually secondary to carcinoma, fecal impaction, diverticulitis, or volvulus.

Pathology

The cause of a small bowel obstruction can come from inside or outside the intestine. Tumors, polyps, congenital diaphragm, Meckel's diverticulum, bezoars, carcinoma, and impacted feces are common causes. Foreign bodies that are lodged in the bowel are also common forms of obstruction.

Crohn's disease, atresia, and stenosis are intrinsic causes of obstruction from the bowel wall itself. Bowel that has received radiation, chemical trauma, or blunt trauma can precipitate an obstruction. Endometriosis or carcinoma that comes through the bowel wall can cause an obstruction. Abscesses from other organs or the bowel itself can cause an obstruction.

The normal bowel secretes 5 to 6 liters of fluid a day. When an obstruction occurs, the intraluminal pressure increases and can reach 20 to 30 mm of water with continued peristalsis. When intraluminal pressure exceeds 20 mm of water, hypersecretion occurs. This hypersecretion causes increased pressure proximal to the lesion. This hypersecretion can reach 5 to 10 liters during a 24-hour period. The bowel continues to perform its peristaltic movement until the pressure is so great that retrograde peristalsis occurs and thus vomiting ensues.

As the intraluminal pressure increases and approaches 30 mm of water, the bowel swells thus causing lymphatic stasis. When the intraluminal pressure approaches 50 mm of water, venous flow of the bowel is occluded; capillary hemorrhage occurs; and bowel death ensues. Arterial blood flow does not diminish before 90 mm of water. When arterial flow is occluded, bowel necrosis or gangrene occurs. The more bowel that is involved, the greater is the area of necrosis. If the obstruction is a closed loop, at two points of obstruction, the greater will be the area of bowel death. As the contents of the bowel become more and more stagnant, bacteria in the bowel can cause the release of vasoactive toxins and secondary infection. If this process is not addressed as soon as bowel death occurs and necrosis ensues, bacterial peritonitis and sepsis will follow.

Clinical Presentation/Examination

The most common presenting complaint of intestinal obstruction is midline abdominal pain that localizes poorly. Pain will fluctuate, and the patient will feel or seem restless. The patient will often vomit and will give a history of narrowing stools or liquid stools or no flatus or possibly no stool at all. The cessation of all flatus signifies a complete obstruction. The pain is often described as dull and generalized and is usually more severe in small bowel obstructions than in large bowel obstructions. Vomiting is more prevalent in small bowel obstructions than in large bowel obstructions. Vomiting is often bilious in early small bowel obstruction; however, as the obstruction persists over time, the vomit may become fecalent. Patients with a small bowel obstruction secondary to a hernia often present with a complaint of a small "knot" in the groin area on previous occasions, which has now become tender and swollen. Infants often present with a history of a painful testicle, increased fussiness, or poor feeding. Always consider intussusception in an infant with abdominal pain, projectile vomiting, difficulty feeding, increased fussiness, or continuous crying.

An obturator hernia obstruction is usually found in elderly women who present with pain in one of their knees and along the medial side of one of their thighs, in the distribution of the obturator nerve. They usually have no prior history of abdominal surgery.

Patients with obstruction secondary to bezoars usually have a history of the loss of the pylorus secondary to a pyloroplasty or pyloric resection with gastric surgery. Always obtain a history of prior radiation therapy or abdominal surgery. Adhesions are still the primary cause of obstruction of the small bowel, secondary to prior surgery or radiation therapy. An acute obstruction caused by impaction can occur if the patient has used certain drugs (e.g., codeine) or if the patient has used laxatives on a chronic basis and has then stopped using them.

Colonic obstructions are almost always never secondary to adhesions or hernia. Fecal impaction in the debilitated patient is a common cause. The most common cause of obstruction of the colon is cancer. An obstruction usually presents with left-sided colon symptoms. Complications of diverticulitis are also a common cause of colon obstruction. As the colon swells secondary to the diverticular lesions, the colon lumen narrows. If complete swelling or impaction occurs, obstruction ensues. Chronic swelling from diverticular disease can also cause scarring of the colon. If the adhesions are in sufficient quantity, narrowing of the colon lumen occurs and an obstruction ensues. As the obstruction progresses, abdominal distention is a common feature in the course of the obstruction. Tympany is often present. Always perform a rectal examination on any patient with abdominal complaints to rule out a GI bleed. With an obstruction there may or may not be stool in the rectum. Blood may or may not be present secondary to the presence or absence of gangrene or necrosis. Always examine the patient for a hernia: inguinal, umbilical, femoral, incisional, or internal.

A volvulus is a section of the bowel that twists on itself and usually occurs in the sigmoid colon. It is common in patients in a nursing home or in patients with chronic constipation. Cecal volvulus can also occur but is less common than is sigmoid volvulus.

Diagnosis

A diagnosis is made by clinical presentation, physical examination, radiography studies, and laboratory studies.

Laboratory Findings

A CBC, amylase, lipase, electrolytes, BUN, creatinine, bilirubin, LFTs, and urinalysis are done. If the patient is septic and has abdominal pain, a blood culture should be taken. If a female is in child-bearing years, a pregnancy test should be performed. An arterial blood gas should be taken if the patient is severely ill to determine acidosis. Laboratory tests are nonspecific in the diagnosis of a bowel obstruction but can indicate the severity of the accompanying complications of the ileus. The electrolyte levels will indicate the severity of the electrolyte and acid-base disturbances. Leukocytosis is often present with a shift to the left. Amylase is often mildly elevated but is nonspecific. As the patient becomes more dehydrated, the BUN level will rise.

Radiography

Two-view abdominal radiography should be performed on all patients with acute abdominal pain. The results of the radiography will show a different finding in relationship to the time when the patient presents with an obstruction. At an early stage the results of the x-ray of the abdomen will be normal. As the obstruction progresses, air and fluid will accumulate and air-fluid levels will occur. Radiography can also show dilated loops of bowel or the string of beads sign.

In a small bowel obstruction, the transverse loops of bowel of the small intestine have moderate to severe gaseous distention. There will be little or no air in the colon. When air is trapped beneath a stretched valvula, a string of beads sign can be present. Absence of all gas in the colon is indicative of complete small bowel obstruction. The air-fluid levels are often step-like or resemble stacked coins.

If the colon is obstructed, the colon will be distended proximal to the lesion and no air will be present in the colon distal to the lesion.

Treatment

Patients with suspected bowel obstruction need fluid and electrolyte stabilization. The combination of a rising BUN, elevated white blood cell count, elevated temperature, tachypnea, tachycardia, and a decreasing blood pressure is a sign of toxicity or gangrenous or necrotic bowel. These patients need vigorous fluid resuscitation.

All patients need placement of a urinary catheter in order to monitor fluid output. They should be placed on a cardiac monitor and pulse oximetry. The aforementioned laboratory examinations should be performed. Patients with long-standing obstruction are usually hypokalemic and require potassium.

The first important treatment after fluid resuscitation is the insertion of a nasogastric tube to decompress the bowel. A nasogastric tube also prevents further distention of the bowel and often is the only treatment necessary to relieve a paralytic ileus. If conservative treatment is the only treatment initiated these patients must be afebrile and hemodynamically stable. Paralytic bowel obstruction can often be treated with only nasogastric suctioning, fluid therapy, and fecal impaction removal by digital evacuation. The patient's vital signs and fluid and electrolyte status must be monitored closely. This approach is controversial because some surgeons believe that all bowel obstructions require surgery. Antibiotics should be given if sepsis, gangrene, or necrotic bowel is suspected or is present.

Mechanical or dynamic bowel obstructions require early surgical treatment. If the patient is septic, early surgical consultation should be standard procedure after fluid and electrolyte resuscitation, nasogastric suctioning, and administration of antibiotics.

BIBLIOGRAPHY

Davis JH, Drucker WR, Foster RS (eds): Clinical Surgery. St Louis, CV Mosby, 1987

Hamilton GC, Sanders AB, Strange GR, et al (eds): Emergency Medicine: An Approach to Clinical Problem-Solving. Philadelphia, WB Saunders, 1991

Hardy JD, Kukora JS, Paass HI (eds): Hardy's Textbook of Surgery. Philadelphia, JB Lippincott, 1983

Kravis TC, Warner CG, Jacobs LM (eds): Emergency Medicine: A Comprehensive Review, 3rd ed. New York, Raven Press, 1993

May HL, Aghababian RV, Fleisher GR (eds): Emergency Medicine, 2nd ed. Boston, Little, Brown, 1992

Morris PJ, Malt RA (eds): Oxford Textbook of Surgery. New York, Oxford University Press, 1994

Pearson RD, Guerrant RL, Braunwald E, et al (eds): Harrison's Principles of Internal Medicine, 11th ed. New York, McGraw-Hill, 1987

Rosen P, Barkin RM (eds): Emergency Medicine: Concepts and Clinical Practice, 3rd ed. St Louis, Mosby-Year Book, 1992

Schwartz GR, Cayten CG, Mangelsen MA, et al (eds): Principles and Practice of Emergency Medicine. Philadelphia, Lea & Febiger, 1992

Schwartz SI, Shires GT, Spencer FC (eds): Principles of Surgery, 5th ed. New York, McGraw-Hill, 1989

Tierney LM, McPhee SJ, Papadakis MA (eds): Current Medical Diagnosis and Treatment, 33rd ed. Norwalk, CT, Appleton & Lange, 1994

Tintinalli JE, Krone RL, Ruiz E (eds): Emergency Medicine: A Comprehensive Study Guide, 4th ed. New York, McGraw-Hill, 1996

Chapter 2

Cardiology

ABDOMINAL AORTIC ANEURYSM

Abdominal aortic aneurysm (AAA) can be classified as ruptured, leaking, or intact. The aorta enters the abdomen at the 12th thoracic vertebra. It has three main anterior branches: the celiac artery, the superior mesenteric artery, and the inferior mesenteric artery. The aorta has three lateral branches: the suprarenal artery, the renal artery, and the testicular or ovarian artery. There are five lateral abdominal arteries and three terminal branches of the iliac arteries and the median sacral artery. There are three layers of the vessel wall: the intima, the media, and the adventitia. By definition, a true aneurysm is larger than 3 cm and localized and involves all three layers of the vessel wall. The intima consists of smooth-layered endothelial cells. The media consists of elastic fibers. The adventitia consists of elastic fibers, nerves fibers, and nutrient vessels. Most AAAs arise below the renal arteries and expand approximately 0.5 cm each year. Aortic aneurysms occur exclusively in the abdomen and never occur in the chest. Aortic dissections occur exclusively in the thorax. The pathophysiology of an aortic aneurysm is believed to be caused by the loss or failure of elastin in the media, causing stiffness of the vessel wall. With loss of elastin, there is a compensated mechanism involving collagen, giving the cell wall increased tensile strength. When the collagen compensation mechanism is overwhelmed, secondary to stiffness, an aneurysm ruptures. There is a sevenfold increase in the likelihood of having an AAA if a close relative has had one.

Types of Aneurysms

1. A true aneurysm involves all three layers.
2. A false aneurysm does not involve all three layers of the vessel but includes a perforation of the intima and the media, and the adventitia contain the contents of the vessel.
3. A dissecting aneurysm involves a longitudinal cleavage of the aortic media by a dissecting column of blood.

Risk Factors

1. Age—older than 60 years of age
2. Male sex
3. White race
4. Family history
5. Smoker
6. Hypertension
7. Coronary artery disease

Signs and Symptoms

1. Abdominal or back pain
2. Dull flank discomfort
3. Vomiting
4. Lower leg neurologic complaints
5. Lightheadedness or syncope
6. Tachycardia
7. Systolic hypertension
8. Orthostatic hypotension
9. Fever with inflammatory AAA and *Staphylococcus aureus* from contact with adjacent structures
10. Asymmetric or absent femoral pulses (big red flag!)
11. Pulsatile abdominal mass, usually palpated above the navel
12. Hypotension
13. Leaking aneurysms, which present with a tender mass in the lower left quadrant and a hematoma and can be mistaken for diverticulitis
14. Left-sided testicular pain in males, which may be mistaken for a urethral obstruction
15. Jaundice, secondary to compression of the bile duct by the aneurysm, which may be mistaken for choledocholithiasis

Treatment

1. Provide immediate surgical intervention if signs and symptoms of a true leaking or ruptured aneurysm present.
2. Place two 14-g or 16-g intravenous (IV) lines containing crystalloids.
3. Provide oxygen and a cardiac monitor and do an electrocardiogram (ECG).
4. Take x-rays of the abdomen; look for calcification of aneurysms, soft-tissue masses, complete loss of renal outlines or renal displacement, or peritoneal flank stripe changes.
5. Check laboratory values: a complete blood count (CBC); prothrombin time (PT), partial thromboplastin time (PTT), sodium, calcium, potassium, chloride, blood urea nitrogen (BUN), creatinine (BUN and creatinine levels will help you to determine if the renal artery is involved), CO_2, glucose, magnesium, blood typed and crossmatched (at least 4 to 6 units along with 4 units of fresh frozen plasma), cardiac enzymes if you know that the patient has cardiac problems or if you expect the patient may have an ischemic event.
6. Do an ultrasound because it is the best method of evaluation in the emergency department.
7. Take a computed tomography (CT) scan if the patient is stable.
8. Do angiography.
9. Do magnetic resonance imaging (MRI).
10. If the patient is unstable, get an immediate surgical consultation.

Guidelines for Repair for an Asymptomatic AAA

1. 4 cm or greater should be repaired as soon as possible.
2. 3 to 4 cm can be watched.

AORTIC DISSECTION

Aortic dissection occurs two to three times more often than a rupturing AAA. It occurs two to three times more in males than in females
and has a higher incidence in blacks. AAA has a familial incidence
and occurs in Marfan's syndrome, Ehlers-Danlos syndrome, Turner's
syndrome, congenital heart syndrome, and coarctation of the aorta. It
rarely occurs in persons younger than 40 years of age. Blunt trauma
(not dissection) is the major cause of aortic rupture. By definition,
aortic dissection is the longitudinal cleavage of the aortic media by a
dissecting column of blood. The repetitive swinging of the aorta
against the spine and the posterior heart causes flexion of the ascending and descending aorta as the heart beats. With limited space
anteriorly and posteriorly and with the repetitive swinging of the
aorta, medial degeneration will occur. This repetitive mechanical
force over time accompanied by systemic hypertension causes dissection. An enlarging hematoma, with dissection, will migrate in an
antegrade and retrograde direction and will create a false lumen in
the media. This outer false lumen is very thin and can rupture in the
presence of hypertension. Dissections involving the ascending aorta
are much more lethal than are those involving the distal aorta. Approximately 75% of patients with untreated aortic dissections die
within 2 weeks.

DeBakey's Classification of Aortic Dissection

Type I—involving the ascending aorta, the aortic arch, and the
descending aorta

Type II—confined to the ascending aorta

Type III—involving the descending aorta distal to the left
subclavian artery

Risk Factors

1. Male
2. Black race
3. Hypertension
4. Marfan's syndrome
5. Ehlers-Danlos syndrome
6. Turner's syndrome
7. Age of 50 to 60 years
8. Tobacco use

Signs and Symptoms

1. Pain as the most common presenting complaint (The pain is excruciating; has usually an abrupt onset; and is described as "tearing" or "ripping" or "knife-like.")
2. Pain in the anterior chest associated with ascending dissection
3. Pain in the neck and jaw associated with aortic arch dissection
4. Interscapular pain associated with aortic arch dissection
5. Pain in the lumbar or abdominal areas involving aortic dissection below the diaphragm
6. Pain often migrating as dissection increases
7. Tachycardia
8. Apprehensiveness
9. Hypotension, clammy skin, altered mental status, and decreased capillary refill
10. Often hypertensive at an early stage; hypotensive at a late stage
11. Pulse deficits and blood pressure differences in the extremities (the key to diagnosis) with unilaterally weakened or absent pulses
12. Aortic regurgitation or insufficiency with a musical, vibratory tone of variable intensity
13. Possibly cardiac tamponade, muffled heart sounds, jugular venous distention, pulsus paradoxus, tachycardia, and hypotension
14. Can present with hemiplegia or hemianesthesia
15. Horner's syndrome

Treatment

I. Immediate surgical consultation if aortic dissection is suspected
II. Two 14-g or 16-g IVs with crystalloids
III. Oxygen
IV. Laboratory values: CBC, PT, PTT, potassium, chloride, CO_2, magnesium, calcium, BUN, creatinine, glucose, creatine phosphokine (CPK), CPK-MB, aspartate aminotransferase (AST), alanine aminotransferase (ALT), lactic dehydrogenase (LDH), type and cross 6 to 10 units of blood and 4 units of fresh frozen plasma
V. On an ECG, look for:
  A. Left ventricular hypertrophy
  B. New heart block
VI. Chest x-ray
  A. Mediastinal widening
  B. Calcium sign—calcium deposit on the outermost portion of the aorta greater than 5 cm
VII. Echocardiography
VIII. CT

IX. Aortography—the "gold standard" for diagnosis of aortic dissection
X. MRI—excellent and very specific for aortic dissection
XI. Blood pressure control (the goal of systolic pressure being 100 to 120 mm Hg)
   A. Sodium nitroprusside, starting at 0.5 to 3 μg/min until the desired pressure is reached
   B. Propranolol (β-blocker) for heart rate control. (Start at 1 mg IV every 5 minutes to reduce heart rate to 60 to 80 beats/min, and give 3 to 6 mg every 4 to 6 hours for rate control.)
   C. Esmolol can be given as a continuous infusion (a loading dose of 500 μg/kg over 1 minute, then 50 μg/min over 4 minutes); if no response occurs, give another loading dose over 1 minute and then titrate the dose up to 200 μg/min to achieve the desired heart rate.
XII. Immediate surgical consultation

AUTOMATIC IMPLANTABLE CARDIOVERTER-DEFIBRILLATORS

Definition

Automatic implantable cardioverter-defibrillators (AICDs) are used in patients who are at high risk for fatal ventricular arrhythmias, which constitute a leading cause of sudden death. The device is placed surgically by left thoracostomy or median sternotomy or by subxiphoid, subcostal, and transdiaphragmatic approaches. The pericardium is opened; the ventricular patches are placed on the ventricles; and the sensing electrodes are placed in the ventricles. The cost of placement of an AICD is from $45,000 to $50,000 per unit. MRI will permanently damage an AICD and should not be performed on a patient without consultation with the patient's cardiologist.

Epidemiology

From 1985 to 1990 more than 10,000 AICDs were implanted in patients who were at risk for sudden death.

Biomechanical Issues

The pulse generator of the AICD is sealed in a titanium case that weighs approximately 250 to 300 g. Its size is approximately 10.8 × 2 × 7.6 cm. The power source lasts approximately 2 to 3 years, which allows the AICD to deliver approximately 100 shocks per lifetime. It takes approximately 5 to 15 seconds of sensing a ventricular arrhythmia before a shock of 25 joules (J) is delivered. A total of four shocks is delivered, after which no further shocks occur. However, if a change in the rhythm occurs, four more shocks are delivered. The cycle from the time of sensing to delivery of the shock is approximately 30 to 35 seconds.

Testing the AICD

To test the function of the AICD place a ring magnet over the upper right corner of the AICD, which is usually implanted in the abdomen. The AICD is either in the active or inactive mode. When the ring magnet is placed over the AICD, beeps will occur if the AICD is sensing the QRS complex and is in the active mode. When the magnet is left on for 30 seconds, a continuous tone is heard, which indicates that the device has been inactivated. To reactive the AICD, simply leave the ring magnet on the device until the beeping is heard, indicating that the device is sensing the QRS complex and, if in the active mode, is functioning.

There is also a telemetry interrogation device called AIDCHECK, which can noninvasively test the AICD. AIDCHECK can test the circuitry, the number of shocks delivered, and the capacitor charging cycle.

Complications

Intraoperative death rates are in the range of 1 to 30%. The most common long-term complication of the AICD is inadvertent shocks. The rate of inadvertent shocks ranges from 1.3 to 34.6%. Inadvertent shocks can be caused by false sensing of sinus tachycardia, atrial fibrillation, or rapid ventricular response. Shivering, diaphragmatic activity, or certain arm movements can also cause an electrical discharge. Inadvertent shocks can occur if the electrode fractures, migrates, or fails.

Rare causes of malfunction include pulmonary embolism, abdominal pocket infection, thrombosis, pericardial effusion, cardiac fibrosis, and ventricular or atrial perforations. Panic disorders, adjustment disorders, major depressive episodes, or falls can also cause inadvertent shocks.

Clinical Presentation

Patients who present to the emergency department (ED) with AICD fall into one of the four following categories:

1. Noncardiac complaints unrelated to the AICD are treated as if the patient does not have an AICD. The ED health care provider must remember that the AICD can be a source of infection, pulmonary embolism, or sepsis.
2. Cardiac complaints, chest pain, congestive heart failure (CHF), angina, and acute myocardial infarction are addressed the same as for a patient who does not have an AICD. The ED health care provider must also consider the complications of the AICD, which are cardiac fibrosis, atrial or ventricular perforation,

pericarditis, pericardial effusion, and infections of the electrode patch or lead wire.
3. AICD-related problems include complaints of one or more shocks from the AICD. The health care provider must search for the cause of the malfunction. Is the device in the active or inactive mode? Is muscle activity causing the electrical discharge? Is a cardiac rhythm causing the electrical discharge?
4. The patient with an AICD who presents in cardiac arrest is treated the same as any patient who presents in cardiac arrest.

EVALUATION OF AICD MALFUNCTION

History

1. What was the patient doing when the AICD discharged? Did the patient fall, or was the patient involved in a motor vehicle accident or have syncope or presyncope?
2. How long has the AICD been implanted? (The lifetime is 2 to 3 years.)
3. What kind of AICD is implanted?
4. How many shocks does the AICD deliver? (Remember that the device will only discharge four times for one type of cardiac arrhythmia and more than four times for more than one type of arrhythmia.)

Physical Examination

1. What are the patient's vital signs?
2. What are the readings from the ECG and cardiac monitor? Is the patient bradycardic or tachycardic? What cardiac rhythm is the patient in?
3. Is there redness or a break in the skin around the generator site or evidence of trauma or infection?

Evaluation

1. ECG
2. Chest x-ray
3. Electrolytes, cardiac enzymes, CBC, and urinalysis (UA). (Remember that if the AICD has discharged, the patient's urine may be positive for blood [urine myoglobin] and the CK and CK-MB will be elevated. If the patient is taking digoxin, check for toxicity.)

Hospital Admission Criteria

1. More than one shock in succession
2. More than two shocks in 1 week
3. Presence of ischemia, electrolyte imbalance, or drug toxicity

When in doubt, admit the patient to the hospital and consult with the patient's cardiologist.

CARDIAC ARRHYTHMIAS

SINUS ARRHYTHMIAS

Criteria

1. Normal P wave and PR intervals
2. Normal 1:1 atrioventricular (AV) conduction
3. At least 0.12 sec between the shortest and the longest PP intervals

History and Clinical Significance

1. Usually seen in children and young adults
2. Can be respiratory in nature (phasic), which will accelerate the heart rate during inspiration and decelerate the heart rate during expiration
3. Nonphasic arrhythmias can occur without inspiration or expiration, and both can occur when there is increased vagal tone.

Treatment

Usually no treatment is required for sinus arrhythmia, and the condition resolves in adulthood.

SINUS BRADYCARDIA

Criteria

1. Sinus node rate less than 60 beats/min
2. Normal P wave and PR intervals
3. Normal 1:1 AV conduction

History and Clinical Significance

I. Caused by suppression in sinoatrial (SA) node discharge
II. Can be seen in:
    Well-conditioned athletes
    Sleep
    Vagal stimulation
    Medications
      Digoxin
      β-Blockers
      Calcium channel blockers
      Narcotics
      Quinidine
      Reserpine
    Acute myocardial infarction
    Carotid sinus hypersensitivity
    Increased intracranial pressure
    Hypothyroidism

Treatment

1. Treat if the rate is less than 50 beats/min and the patient has symptomatic hypotension.
2. Use atropine 0.5 mg IV every 5 minutes until the desired rate is obtained.
3. If atropine fails to work, use isoproterenol with a starting dose of 0.5 μg/min followed by a constant infusion, titrating to a desired rate above 60 beats/min.

PREMATURE ATRIAL CONTRACTIONS

Criteria

1. The ectopic P wave has a different shape and direction.
2. P waves will appear sooner than the next expected beat.
3. P waves may or may not be conducted through the AV node.
4. The QRS complex will be normal if there is not a P wave during ventricular contraction.
5. The sinus node rate will reset after the premature atrial contraction (PAC), and the RR interval will be the same after resetting.

History and Clinical Significance

I. Can be seen at any age
II. Can be caused by (suspected):
     Coffee
     Fatigue
     Stress
     Alcohol
     Tobacco
     Chronic obstructive pulmonary disease (COPD)
     Ischemic heart disease
     Digitalis toxicity
III. PACs can possibly cause:
     Atrial fibrillation
     Atrial flutter
     Atrial tachycardia

Treatment

I. Stop any precipitating drugs or toxins.
II. Treat any underlying disorders.
III. Can use:
     Quinidine
       Oral dose, 200 to 400 mg four times a day (QID) (as a first choice)
       IV dose, 600 mg IV, then 400 mg every 2 hours (not to exceed 16 mg/min). Watch for hypotension.
     Procainamide
       IV dose, 100 mg IV over 5 minutes at 20 mg/min until the arrhythmia is controlled

β-Blockers
    Metoprolol (Lopressor), 5 mg IV push
    Esmolol (Brevibloc), 25 to 50 μg/min to a maximum dose of
        300 μg/kg/min
    Labetalol (Normodyne), 20 mg IV push, then double the
        dose every 10 minutes until the desired effect is achieved

ATRIAL FLUTTER

Criteria

1. Regular atrial rate, coming from the same focus, thus a
   "sawtooth" pattern
2. Atrial rate between 250 and 350 per minute
3. 2:1 AV block usually occurs, but it can be greater.
4. Normal QRS interval of less than 0.4 sec

History

I. Can occur in a normal heart
II. Seen most commonly in patients with ischemic heart disease or
    acute myocardial infarction
III. Can also be seen in:
    Digoxin toxicity
    Blunt chest trauma
    Pulmonary embolism (PE)
    CHF
    Myocarditis

Treatment

I. Cardioversion: 25 to 50 J will convert to normal sinus rhythm in
   most cases.
II. Verapamil, 5 to 10 mg IV push
III. Quinidine
    Oral dose, 200 to 400 mg QID (as a first choice)
    IV dose, 600 mg IV, then 400 mg every 2 hours, not to exceed
        16 mg/min; watch for hypotension
IV. Procainamide
    IV dose, 100 mg over 5 minutes at 20 mg/min until the
        arrhythmia is controlled; then a maintenance dose of 1 to 4
        mg/min
V. β-Blockers
    Metoprolol, 5 mg IV push
    Esmolol, a loading dose of 500 μg/kg over 1 minute, followed
        by an infusion starting at 50 μg/min over 4 minutes. If no
        response occurs, give another 500-μg/kg bolus, then 100 μg/
        kg/min over 4 minutes, up to a maximum dose of 300 μg/
        kg/min.
    Labetalol, 20 mg IV push then double the dose every 10
        minutes until the desired effect is achieved.

ATRIAL FIBRILLATION

Criteria

1. Multiple areas of atrial discharge, causing discharge and contraction and a "quivering" of the atrial wall
2. Atrial rate greater than 400 per minute
3. Irregular ventricular response (170 to 180 per minute)
4. QRS can be wide

History and Clinical Significance

I. Usually found in:
>   Rheumatic heart disease
>   Hypertension
>   Ischemic heart disease
>   Thyrotoxicosis
>   COPD
>   Acute alcoholic intoxication
>   Atrial septal defect
>   Pericarditis
>   Any process that increases vagal tone

II. Predisposes patients to atrial emboli, thus increasing the risk of a PE or systemic venous embolism

Treatment

I. Treat with cardioversion at 100 to 200 J in the unstable patient with hemodynamic deterioration.

II. In a more stable patient, treat with verapamil, 5 to 10 mg IV push, which will slow the ventricular rate to 60 to 70 beats/min. (The goal is to slow the ventricular rate.)

III. β-Blockers
>   Metoprolol, 5 mg IV
>   Esmolol, a loading dose of 500 μg/kg over 1 minute, followed by an infusion starting at 50 μg/min, over 4 minutes. If no response, give another bolus of 500 μg/kg, then 100 μg/kg/min over 4 minutes, to a maximum dose of 300 μg/kg/min
>   Labetalol, 20 mg IV push, then double the dose every 10 minutes until the desired effect is achieved

IV. After the ventricular rate is controlled, give procainamide, 100 mg IV every 5 minutes at 20 mg/min until the arrhythmia is controlled; then give a maintenance dose of 1 to 4 mg/min.

SUPRAVENTRICULAR TACHYCARDIA

Criteria

1. Regular, rapid rhythm
2. Usually a P wave before each QRS
3. Rate of 100 to 250 beats/min

History and Clinical Significance

I. Supraventricular tachycardia (SVT) is caused by a re-entry or ectopic pacemaker in the area above the bifurcation of the bundle of His

II. Re-entry causes symptomatic preventive supraventricular tachycardia (PSVT).

III. A 2:1 AV block can occur.

IV. SVT is often mistaken for atrial flutter with AV block

V. SVT is seen in:
    Acute myocardial infarction
    COPD
    Acute pericarditis
    Rheumatic heart disease
    Mitral valve prolapse
    Pneumonia
    Alcoholism
    Digoxin toxicity, coined paroxysmal atrial tachycardia (PAT) with AV block

VI. Causes dizziness, lightheadedness, and palpations

VII. Causes frank heart failure in patients with heart disease and PE in patients with ventricular failure

Treatment

Treatment of SVT if caused by digoxin toxicity:

1. If SVT is caused by digoxin toxicity, stop the digoxin therapy.
2. Correct hypokalemia.
3. Consider digoxin-specific antibody fragments (Fab) if the patient is deteriorating hemodynamically or is having ventricular arrhythmias.
4. Use phenytoin IV with a loading dose of 15 to 18 mg/kg.
5. Give magnesium sulfate, 1 g IV.
6. *Do not cardiovert*, since this is potentially hazardous.

Treatment of SVT if not caused by digoxin toxicity:

I. Adenosine, 6-mg IV bolus, works in seconds; if failure to convert in 2 minutes, give a second dose of 12 mg IV

II. Verapamil, 5 to 10 mg IV

III. β-Blockers
    Esmolol, loading dose of 500 μg/kg over 1 minute, followed by an infusion starting at 50 μg/min, over 4 minutes. If no response, give another 500-μg/kg bolus, then 100 μg/kg/min over 4 minutes, to a maximum dose of 300 μg/kg/min
    Propranolol 0.5 to 1 mg IV slowly over 60 seconds; can be repeated every 5 minutes to a maximum dose of 0.1 mg/kg

IV. Digoxin 0.5 mg IV; can be repeated at 0.25 mg in 30 to 60 minutes, until the desired response is obtained, or a maximum dose of 0.02 mg/kg

V. Synchronized cardioversion in any unstable patient with pulmonary edema, hypotension, or severe chest pain

MULTIFOCAL ATRIAL TACHYCARDIA

Criteria

1. Atrial rate greater than 100 beats/min
2. Three or more P waves or dissimilar configuration in a single electrocardiographic lead
3. Irregular PP and PR intervals

History and Clinical Significance

Multifocal atrial tachycardia (MAT) is often seen in theophylline toxicity, digitalis intoxication, severe pulmonary disease, or cardiac disease (major causes). MAT can also be seen but is less common in pulmonary edema, electrolyte or metabolic imbalance, septicemia, hypoxemia, and hypercapnia. The majority of patients with MAT will have COPD or acute decompensation of serious cardiorespiratory disease. Patients with MAT have a 50 to 60% mortality rate. Always check for theophylline toxicity when you see an arrhythmia looking like atrial fibrillation that meets MAT criteria, and the patient is on theophylline. MAT is usually confused with atrial fibrillation and occurs most commonly in the elderly.

Treatment

1. Attempt to correct any underlying causes (e.g., theophylline toxicity, CHF).
2. If the patient is not actively wheezing, you can use metoprolol, 5 to 10 mg IV or 2 to 3 mg IV in increments every 2 minutes until a response is noted.
3. Give an oral dose of metoprolol, 25 mg every 6 hours
4. Pre-treat possible hypotension, secondary to metoprolol, with 1 ampule of calcium gluconate (10 ml/ampule of 10% solution; 90 mg of elemental calcium).
5. Give verapamil, 5 to 10 mg IV, but this drug is not as effective as metoprolol. If verapamil is used, pre-treat with 1 ampule of calcium gluconate (10 ml/ampule of a 10% solution; 90 mg of elemental calcium).

AUTOMATIC ATRIAL TACHYCARDIA

Criteria

1. Looks like third-degree AV block
2. In automatic atrial tachycardia (AAT), the PP intervals are the same distance apart. The RR intervals are irregular and different lengths, but there is a P wave before each QRS complex.
3. In third-degree AV block, the PP intervals are equal and the RR intervals are equal.

History and Clinical Significance

AAT can be mistaken for atrial fibrillation or flutter.

Treatment

1. Use procainamide to slow the rate. Give an oral dose of 250 to 1000 mg every 3 hours. An IV dose of 100 mg can be given every 5 minutes (or 50 mg/min up to 1 g). The maintenance infusion is 2 to 6 mg/min. Serum procainamide levels of 8 to 12 μg/ml correlate with clinical efficacy.
2. After a therapeutic dose of procainamide, cardioversion should start at 50 to 100 J.

Contraindications to Cardioversion

1. Digitalis toxicity
2. Repeated short-lived tachycardias
3. MAT
4. Hemodynamically stable atrial fibrillation associated with rheumatic heart disease
5. Supraventricular arrhythmias and hypertension
6. Complete heart block
7. Recurrent supraventricular arrhythmias
8. Atrial fibrillation with a slow ventricular response in the absence of digitalis and in patients with evidence of sick sinus syndrome. Employ caution in the case of the elderly with coronary artery disease and disease of the conduction system.

PREMATURE VENTRICULAR CONTRACTIONS

Criteria

1. Premature wide QRS complex
2. No preceding P wave
3. ST segment and T wave are directed in the major QRS deflection
4. Usually do not affect the SA node
5. Can produce a retrograde P wave

History and Clinical Significance

1. Can be seen in patients without heart disease
2. Can be seen in patients with ischemic heart disease
3. Seen in patients with acute myocardial infarction

Axis Determination

Upright (positive, more above the baseline than below) QRS wave in leads I and aVF, with a normal axis (0 to +90)

QRS wave upright (positive) in lead I and negative in aVF, with a left-axis deviation (0 to −90)

QRS wave negative in lead I and upright (positive) lead aVF, with a right axis deviation ($+90$ to $+180$)

QRS wave negative in both leads I and aVF, with an extreme right axis deviation ($+180$ to -90 (360)).

Ventricular hypertrophy is a correlation that exists between the thickness of the ventricular muscle and the magnitude of its depolarization wave (the R wave). Features of ventricular hypertrophy on an ECG are:

1. An increase in height in the R wave
2. Prolongation of the QRS duration
3. Lenghtening of the activation time over the hypertrophied ventricle
4. ST segment depression
5. T wave abnormalities consisting typically of asymmetric inversion that is shallow or deep

LEFT VENTRICULAR HYPERTROPHY

1. Usually left axis deviation (0 to -30)
2. In lead aVL, a tall R wave greater than 11 mm, ST segment depression, and an inverted T wave
3. Tall R waves and depressed ST segments and inverted T waves in leads V_4, V_5, and V_6
4. QRS duration may exceed 0.10 sec
5. S wave in V_1 plus R wave in V_5 or V_6 over 35 mm (SV1 + RV5/6) (older than 35 years of age)

RIGHT VENTRICULAR HYPERTROPHY

1. Axis normal or may be deviated to the right ($+110$)
2. Tall R waves in leads II, III, and aVR
3. R wave gets progressively smaller from V_1 to V_6
4. R wave greater than S wave in V_1
5. Sometimes tall, peaked P waves in leads I, II, and aVF

LEFT ATRIAL ABNORMALITY (HYPERTROPHY)

1. Broad (>0.12 sec) notched P wave in leads I and II
2. A wide (1 mm $\times$ 0.04 sec) terminal negative deflection in lead V_1

RIGHT ATRIAL ABNORMALITY (HYPERTROPHY)

1. Tall peaked P waves in leads II, III and aVF (>2.5 mm in lead II).
2. Tall peaked diphasic P waves in V_1 with tall initial component.
3. Sometimes markedly inverted P waves in lead V_1.

RIGHT BUNDLE BRANCH BLOCK

1. Wide S wave in leads I and V_4, V_5, and V_6
2. Wide R and R′ in lead aVR
3. R and R′ in leads V_1 and V_2

LEFT BUNDLE BRANCH BLOCK

1. R and R' in leads V_5 and V_6
2. Wide S wave in V_1 and V_2
3. QRS less than 0.12 sec (3 blocks) in precordial leads

PULMONARY INFARCTION

1. "S1Q3" wide S wave in lead I and large Q wave in lead III
2. Inverted T waves in leads V_1, V_2, V_3, and V_4
3. ST depression in lead II
4. A transient right bundle branch block

EMPHYSEMA

Low voltage is seen in all leads.

ELECTROLYTE IMBALANCE

- Hyperkalemia (increased K^+): Wide flat P waves with wide QRS, with peaked T waves
- Hypokalemia (decreased K^+): Very flat T waves and can see U waves
- Hypercalcemia (increased Ca^{2+}): Short QT segment
- Hypocalcemia (decreased Ca^{2+}): Long QT segment

EVALUATION OF CARDIAC CHEST PAIN

Chest pain may be caused by either somatic or visceral nerves. Somatic pain is dermal in origin and can be well localized. Visceral pain is poorly localized pain of internal organ origin. The heart, gastrointestinal viscera, and lungs are of visceral origin. The pericardium and the diaphragm are innervated by the parasympathetic phrenic nerve.

Differential Diagnosis of Chest Pain

Acute myocardial infarction	Esophageal rupture
Unstable angina	Cardiac tamponade
PE	Herpes zoster
Aortic dissection	Cervical radicular pain
Pericarditis	Pleuritis
Pneumonia	Pneumothorax
Esophageal reflux	Tension pneumothorax
Hiatal hernia	Mitral valve prolapse
Costochondritis	Hyperventilation/stress

The etiology of myocardial ischemia is decreased oxygen supply caused by coronary artery obstruction, which is usually a fixed lesion caused by atherosclerosis. Arterial spasm can cause a non-fixed lesion. Systemic hypotension reduces preload and can cause ischemia. Severe anemia reduces oxygen supply to the coronary muscle and can also cause ischemia. Myocardial hypertrophy will increase myocardial oxygen demand, with decreased pump function, and this will cause ischemia. Tachycardia also increases myocardial oxygen demand, especially in CHF. Two major changes take place within the myocardial cells during ischemia: (1) electrical activity alterations occur, and (2) decreased contractions occur.

Pathophysiology of Acute Myocardial Ischemia

Acute myocardial ischemia is caused by acute intracoronary thrombosis with association of arterial spasm. Ischemia impairs ventricular contractility, hence a reduction in arterial pressure, leading to reduced intracoronary perfusion. This "stiff" ventricular wall causes loss if ventricular distensibility, leading to loss of systolic contraction, leading to hypokinetic or akinetic area of the heart. *Hypokinetic* refers to decreased wall motion, and *akinetic* refers to a prolonged postsystolic interval when the the heart is at rest.

Risk Factors

Age	Family history of myocardial infarction before 55
Male sex	years of age
Hypertension	Cigarette smoking
Diabetes mellitus	Hypercholesterolemia

Symptoms of Acute Myocardial Infarction

1. A dull pressure-like chest pain, located in the substernal, midsternal, or left peristernal area (The patient often states that the pain is like "a bear is squeezing my chest or an elephant is sitting on my chest." Ischemia is caused by decreased oxygen supply to the myocardial muscle.)
2. Burning epigastric pain or indigestion
3. Dyspnea
4. Radiating pain into the neck (throat angina)
5. Radiating pain into the shoulders, from the medial side of the left arm to the elbow
6. Jaw pain
7. Numbness or tingling around the lips and the mouth
8. Pain lasts longer than 15 to 30 minutes
9. Fear of impending doom or death

Physical Examination Findings

In general appearance, the patient is usually short of breath or in acute distress and feels "like something is going to happen." The patient will often ask, "Am I going to die?" Ask yourself, does this patient look like he is having a heart attack? Get a feel for the *entire* patient. The patient will often hold the middle of chest, placing a fist on the chest to identify the area of pain. The patient's skin is often flushed around the neck and chest, and the patient will feel better sitting up than lying down or leaning forward.

Heart Examination

Will sometimes have an S_4 heart sound due to a decrease in left ventricular compliance ("stiff ventricle"), and this sound is best heard with the patient in the left lateral decubitus position

S_1 may be decreased due to the decrease in left ventricular contraction impairment

S_2 can be split due to prolonged left ventricular ejection

S_3 usually cannot be heard, but if heard will be very soft, in an adult is always a sign of heart disease, usually structural

Listen for new systolic murmurs; they can indicate:

1. Mitral valve regurgitation due to papillary muscle rupture or systolic dysfunction
2. Septal rupture of ventricle
3. Friction rub of pericarditis, heard best by leaning the patient forward in sitting position
4. Is there a thrill or a rub?
5. Look at the internal jugular vein (IJV)
    Low IJV pressure (Look for hypotension in AMI.)
    High IJV, cardiogenic shock, pericardial tamponade (Consider a right ventricular infarct at an early stage with increased IJV and without a history of CHF.)
    Is there an A wave?

Palpate the anterior chest wall to detect if there is a thrill or ventricular septal rupture versus a ruptured papillary muscle. (A septal rupture will have a palpable thrill.)

Is there a murmur present?

1. Inspiration increases blood flow to the right ventricle, which will increase right-sided murmurs and gallops. Inspiration will increase the sound of tricuspid regurgitation and will decrease the sound of mitral regurgitation.
2. The Valsalva maneuver will increase systolic murmurs of mitral valve prolapse and hypertrophic cardiomyopathy.
3. The Valsalva maneuver will decrease the intensity of the systolic murmurs of aortic valve stenosis and mitral regurgitation.
4. An isometric hand grip increases peripheral vascular resistance; thus, the intensity of aortic regurgitation, ventricular septal defect, and mitral regurgitation will increase.
5. Following a premature ventricular contraction (PVC), there will be a pause.
    Listen to the beat after the PVC.
    Is there a decrease in the intensity of murmur, cardiomyopathy, or aortic stenosis?

Is there no change in intensity of murmur? (Consider mitral regurgitation if this is the case.)

Vital Signs

- May have mild fever to 39° C (103° F)
- Pulse rate less than 40 beats/min suggests a complete heart block (Take the patient's pulse yourself to check if it is regular or irregular. Check pulses in all extremities.)
- Blood pressure—hypotension versus hypertension. (If hypotension with bradycardia consider a right-sided myocardial infarction early; take the patient's blood pressure in both arms.)
- Respirations—tachypnea, heart wanting more oxygen versus a PE

ECG Changes in Acute Myocardial Infarction

ECG Interpretation: Myocardial Infarction		
Infarction Site	**ECG Leads Showing Infarction**	**Relative Incidence (%)**
Anteroseptal	V_1, V_2	9
Anteroapical	V_2, V_3	42
Anterolateral	I, aVL, V_4, V_5, V_6	9
Inferior	II, III, aVF	33
Posterior wall	V_1, V_2	3
Right ventricle	V_2, V_3, V_{4R}	
Anterior	Q waves in V_1, V_2, V_3, V_4	
Lateral	Q waves in I and aVL	
Posterior	Large R wave in V_1, V_2, and significant Q wave in V_6	
Inferior	Q wave in II, III, and aVF	

ST segment changes overlying myocardial injury will cause ST elevation in an acute infarction. Q waves are the most diagnostic finding on an ECG for myocardial infarction. They are abnormally wide (0.04 sec) and have a deep (25% to one third of the height of the R wave in a given lead) wave in the QRS complex.

1. The Q wave in leads III or aVL has no special significance alone.
2. Q wave infarcts tend to be larger than non–Q wave infarcts.

T Waves

1. T wave inversion is characteristic of ischemia (a decrease in oxygen supply to myocardium).

2. ST segment changes overlying myocardial injury will cause an ST elevation in an acute myocardial infarction.
3. A subendocardial infarction will have a flat ST wave depression.

Arteries of Infarction

■ Anterior infarction-occlusion of the anterior descending branch of the left coronary artery

Coronary Artery

■ Lateral infarction-occlusion of the circumflex branch of the left coronary artery
■ Posterior infarction-occlusion of the right coronary artery
■ Inferior infarction either the right or left coronary arteries, depending on which artery is the *dominant* artery

Acute Inferior Wall Infarction

■ Less impairment in left ventricular function
■ Best seen in inferior leads II, III, and aVF
■ Look for ST segment depression in leads V_1, V_2, V_3, and V_4. If there is an ST segment depression in any of these leads of 1 mm, consider involvement of the left anterior descending coronary artery along with inferior wall infarction.

Right Ventricular Infarction

Do an ECG with right-sided precordial leads; look at how lead V_{4R} overlies the right ventricle.
This is almost always associated with left ventricular damage.
Watch for severe right ventricular dysfunction.
1. Elevated right atrial pressure
2. Hypotension
3. Normal or decreased left pressure
4. Jugular venous distention
5. Clear lung fields
6. Kussmaul's sign—a rise in venous pressure with quiet inspirations
7. Patients with a right ventricular infarct are dependent on an elevated right ventricular filling pressure to maintain right cardiac output. These patients need fluid! Also use dobutamine, which is an inotropic agent, to maintain cardiac output. Dobutamine works better than dopamine, because dobutamine increases cardiac output. Use dopamine to increase blood pressure and to keep the kidneys perfused.

Anterior Infarction

- Q waves in leads V$_1$ and V$_2$
- Look for *Wellen's* T wave inversions (T waves are inverted and very large) in leads V$_2$ and V$_3$, late in the myocardial infarction process; almost pathologic for an occlusion of the left anterior descending artery; has a poor prognosis.
- Consider temporary pacing with new-onset left bundle branch block or third-degree AV block with an acute anterior infarction.

Cardiac Enzymes			
Enzyme	Earliest Rise (hr)	Peak (hr)	Days to Normalization
CK	6–9	24–30	3–4
CK-MB	3–4	18–24	2
AST (SGOT)	8–12	36–48	3–5
LDH	12–24	48–96	7–10

Treatment of Acute Myocardial Infarction

- Place the patient on a cardiac monitor.
- Provide oxygen per nasal cannula at a rate of 2 to 6 l/min, and remember that the patient might have COPD. However, if the heart needs oxygen, the patient needs oxygen! Oxygen corrects hypoxemia, which is often present in acute myocardial infarction.
- Establish two IVs—one with lactated Ringer's solution or normal saline and one saline lock to draw blood.
- Give sublingual nitroglycerin (NTG), 0.4 to 0.6 mg, and establish IV before giving NTG.
- Start an IV drip of NTG at 10 μg/min, increasing the rate by 5 μg/min until the patient is pain free, the patient's blood pressure falls, and the patient is hypotensive. The systolic blood pressure should be no less than 90 to 100 mm Hg. NTG dilates epicardial arteries, increases collateral flow, and decreases left ventricular aneurysms. NTG improves left ventricular compliance. Do not give NTG if the patient has marked bradycardia, tachycardia, or hypotension.
- Give 160 mg of aspirin (unless the patient is hypersensitive to aspirin). Aspirin inhibits platelet aggregation.
- Give morphine, 2 to 20 mg every 5 to 10 minutes, as needed for pain. Morphine also reduces afterload by venous and arterial dilatation. Do not give morphine with significant bradycardia, heart rate less than 50 per minute, or hypotension. With inferior infarctions consider meperidine when bradycardia is present because of its vagolytic properties.
- Heparin reduces the reocclusion of coronary arteries and prevents deep venous thrombosis of the lower extremities. Heparin reduces ventricular mural thrombosis in anterior wall infarctions and

reduces the risk of cerebrovascular accidents. Heparin catalyzes antithrombin III, which inactivates thrombin factors IIa and Xa. A dose of heparin is 5000 to 10,000 units in a bolus then 1000 units/hr to 1.5 to 2 times the control of the PTT. Contradictions are: prolonged cardiopulmonary resuscitation (CPR), a recent cerebrovascular accident (CVA), a active GI bleed, or hemorrhagic retinopathy.

- Magnesium is a cofactor of the sodium, potassium, adenosine triphosphatase, and calcium-adenosine triphosphatase cycles. Magnesium maintains membrane stability, which is important in arrhythmias such as ventricular tachycardia, ventricular fibrillation, and atrial tachycardia, which are all seen in acute myocardial infarction. With high intracellular sodium concentrations (seen with low magnesium), magnesium will cause an increase in the sodium-calcium countertransport mechanism, which leads to higher intracellular calcium levels and allows for increased depolarization, thus arrhythmias. Magnesium may prevent a coronary spasm. It also prevents sudden death, slows the sinoatrial node, lowers systemic resistance, dilates coronary arteries, decreases platelet aggregation catecholamine-induced myocardial necrosis, and reduces the size of a myocardial infarction. Dosing is 1 to 2 g over 5 to 60 minutes, then 0.5 to 1 g/hr for up to 24 hours.

- β-Blockers reduce long-term mortality by 20%. β-Blockers reduce the possibility of reinfarction and the size of the infarction and sudden death. β-Blockers also reduce the myocardial oxygen demand by reducing the heart rate and myocardial contractility. Diastole is prolonged, thus reducing myocardial wall tension and improving blood flow to the subendocardium in infarction. Do not use if the following are present: hypotension, bradycardia, severe left ventricular dysfunction, second-degree AV block types I and II, third-degree AV block, severe COPD, or asthma. Be careful when using concurrently with calcium channel blockers, poorly controlled insulin-dependent diabetes, or first-degree AV block. Give metoprolol at a dose of 5 to 10 mg via slow IV push to a pulse rate of less than 60/minute.

- Thrombolytic therapy salvages the ischemic myocardium but not the myocardium that has already necrosed. Streptokinase and human recombinant tissue plasminogen activator (rt-PA) are the two most commonly used thrombolytic agents. Anisoylated streptokinase-plasminogen activator complex (APSAC) is also available but is the most expensive. Streptokinase is produced by β-hemolytic streptococci, which form a 1:1 complex with plasminogen, which converts plasminogen to plasmin inactivation clotting factors V, VII, and XII. (All thrombolytics work in this way.) Plasmin lyses fibrin clots if ischemic. Streptokinase is given in a dose of 1.5 million units over 1 hour. APSAC is given as a 30-unit IV bolus over 5 minutes. rt-PA is given as a 15-mg bolus IV, then 0.75 mg/kg over 30 minutes, with a maximum dose of 50 mg in the first 30 minutes, then 35 mg over 60 minutes. If streptokinase has been used before, use rt-PA on second thrombolytic therapy.

APSAC: Heparinize 4 to 6 hours after a bolus of APSAC.

Streptokinase: Use heparin when the PTT has fallen to twice the control level.

rt-PA: Heparinize simultaneously when rt-PA is administered.

- Reperfusion arrhythmias are often seen with thrombolytics, and accelerated idioventricular rhythms and PVCs are often seen. They do not usually require therapy.

Eligibility

1. Longer than 6 hours from the onset of chest pain or symptoms (for best outcome)
2. 6 to 12 hours from the onset of symptoms and sometimes up to 24 hours
3. No upper age limit
4. ST segment elevation of greater than 1 mm in two contiguous leads
5. New bundle branch block in acute myocardial infarction

Absolute Contraindications

1. Active internal bleeding
2. Suspected aortic dissection
3. Prolonged or traumatic CPR (>10 minutes)
4. Recent head trauma or intracranial neoplasm
5. Hypertension not responsive to therapy
6. Previous allergy to streptokinase or APSAC
7. Recent streptococcal infection (This can predispose the patient to an allergic reaction; thus, in this case, rt-PA should be given instead of streptokinase.)
8. Pregnancy
9. Trauma or surgery in the past 2 weeks
10. CVA or stroke in the previous 2 months

Relative Contraindications

1. Hemorrhagic retinopathy
2. Active peptic ulcer disease
3. History of CVA
4. Current use of anticoagulants

rt-PA Protocol

A separate IV line must be placed for rt-PA.
A lidocaine bolus (50 to 100 mg) followed by 2 mg/min

Two protocols:
1. 100 mg of rt-PA is given in 200 ml of D5W (0.5 mg/ml). rt-PA is given as a 15-mg IV bolus; then 0.75 mg/kg over 30 minutes. A maximum dose of 50 mg is given in the first 30 minutes; then 35 mg over 60 minutes

OR

2. 100 mg rt-PA is given in 200 ml of D5W or normal saline (0.5 mg/ml). During the first hour, 60 mg is given: a 10-mg bolus (0.1 mg/kg) or 20 ml over 2 to 10 minutes via an IVAC pump set at 120 ml/hr, then 50 mg (the remainder which is 100 ml) over the rest of the hour. During the second hour 20 mg (40 ml) is given via an IVAC at 40 ml/hr. During the third hour 20 mg (40 ml) is given via an IVAC pump set at 40 ml/hr.

Streptokinase Protocol

- Dedicated IV line for streptokinase
- Hydrocortisone 100 mg IV
- Benadryl, 50 mg IV
- Streptokinase, 1.5 million units in 100 ml of D5W or 0.9% normal saline over 1 hour

APSAC Protocol

A total dose of 30 units is given as a 5-ml bolus over 5 minutes.

Hemodynamic Management

In symptomatic hypotension caused by pump failure, cardiogenic shock (systolic blood pressure less than 80 mm Hg), hypotension should be treated with dopamine 5 to 10 $\mu g/kg/min$.

Dysrhythmias are treated per ACLS protocols.

Laboratory Studies

Levels are checked for the following: CBC, PT, PTT, calcium, magnesium, BUN, creatinine, chloride, CO_2, glucose, sodium, potassium, and cardiac enzymes (CK, CK-MB, LDH, and AST).

Procedures

- Chest x-ray (Look for a wide mediastinum, greater than 8 cm, and be careful when giving thrombolytics.)
- Foley catheterization for measurement of input and output
- Pulse oximetry (Keep above 95%.)

Quick Reference for Acute Myocardial Infarction

- Two IVs with normal saline 0.9% or D5W to keep open the heparin or saline lock.

- Draw laboratory measures when starting IVs, CBC, SMA-8, calcium, magnesium, PT, PTT, cardiac enzymes: CK, CK-MB, LDH, AST.

- Give oxygen via nasal cannula at 2 to 6 l/min.

- Place the patient on a monitor.

- Determine the level of chest pain on a scale of 1 to 10. Write the level of pain on serial ECGs, and notice ECG changes with changes in pain.

- Is this an acute myocardial infarction on the ECG? Anterior, inferior, lateral or right ventricular, will determine therapy. Remember that a right ventricular infarct is fluid dependent on right-ventricular filling pressure, so encourage fluids.

- Give sublingual NTG 0.4 or 0.6 mg to relieve pain, after IV access.

- Give morphine sulfate 2 to 20 mg for pain relief. (The goal is to have a pain-free patient as soon as possible with morphine and NTG.)

- Start an NTG drip at 10 μg and titrate the rate up until the patient is free of pain. Watch for hypotension.

- Take a portable chest x-ray, and look at the mediastinum (if >8 cm, look for aortic dissection or an aneurysm). Look for CHF and COPD.

- Determine the patient's coagulation status by checking his or her history.

- Assess the risk factors.

- Determine if the patient is a candidate for heparin or thrombolytics.

- β-Blockers should be given if the patient is not bradycardic or hypotensive, give metoprolol, 5 to 10 mg slow IV push.

- Consult a cardiologist early to determine if the patient is a candidate for an emergency angioplasty.

CARDIAC TAMPONADE

Cardiac tamponade can be either constrictive or restrictive. Both can cause decreased filling of the ventricles, decreased ventricular volumes, reduced ventricular compliance, and impaired cardiac output. As little as 20 ml of fluid in a traumatic or iatrogenic patient can cause significant impairment of cardiac filling.

Nontraumatic Causes (Constrictive)

1. Constrictive pericarditis
2. Tuberculosis
3. Viral or idiopathic
4. Uremic pericarditis
5. Malignant ideologies
6. Rheumatoid disease

Signs and Symptoms

1. Jugular venous distention (JVD), can be above the angle of the jaw, thus you might not see the top of the JVD
2. Pulsus paradoxus in excess of 10 mm Hg is the hallmark of advanced cardiac tamponade. (Pulsus paradoxus is performed by taking the blood pressure; as the patient breathes quietly, lower the cuff pressure to the systolic level. At that point note the pressure, then lower the pressure until the systolic sound can be heard throughout the respiratory cycle. There should be no difference in these two levels of sound greater than 3 or 4 mm Hg.)
3. Hypotension
4. Tachycardia
5. Muffled heart sounds
6. Anxiety
7. Sudden chest pain
8. Pericardial friction rub can often be heard
9. Electrical alternans: alternating patterns of high and low voltage on the ECG that affect the P, QRS, and T waves

Treatment

1. Oxygen
2. IV normal saline 0.9% to keep two IV lines open
3. Laboratory testing of CBC, PT, PTT, potassium, chloride, CO_2, magnesium, calcium, BUN, creatine, glucose, CPK, CPK-MB, AST, ALT, LDH, type and cross 6 to 10 units of blood, and 4 units of fresh frozen plasma
4. Chest x-ray (A large cardiac silhouette might be seen.)
5. Echography
6. Drainage of pericardial fluid by pericardiocentesis

CONGESTIVE HEART FAILURE

CHF is the failure of the heart to meet the circulatory demands of the body at normal filling pressure. This failure produces retention of fluids in the body. CHF is categorized as:

1. Acute or chronic
2. Failure of the right or left ventricles, or both
3. Cardiac output: low, normal, or high

Pathophysiology

In CHF, the fluid retention is caused by an increase in right ventricular volume and pressure. This increase in pressure causes vascular fluid to be moved interstitially. With a decrease in cardiac contractility and output, there is compensation of arteriolar vasoconstriction. This constriction ensures perfusion to the brain and heart, and blood is shunted away from the bowel, muscle, and kidneys. With less blood going to the kidneys, the renin-angiotensin-aldosterone system causes an increase in sodium retention, thus causing fluid retention. This fluid retention causes pulmonary vascular congestion and edema, secondary to increased left atrial pressure, which causes elevated capillary pressure. The increased fluid volume in the lungs causes a decrease in lung compliance, which causes dyspnea. Paroxysmal nocturnal dyspnea is caused by peripheral fluid (dependent edema) being redistributed back into the lungs secondary to the supine position. In the case of severe pulmonary edema, the edema irritates the bronchioles and causes bronchial spasm and wheezing. Preload is the filling pressure that the left ventricle must fill against in diastole. Preload is indirectly measured by pulmonary arterial wedge pressure (PAWP), and the normal PAWP is less than 8 to 15 mm Hg. Afterload is the pressure that the left ventricle must pump against in systole and is measured by the mean aortic pressure. The Frank-Starling law states that the myocardial cell will contract with greater force as its precontraction length increases. In CHF, the myocardial cells are stretched to their maximum length. Thus, output is decreased secondary to decreased contraction of the individual myocardial cells. The heart is unable to expel all the blood during systole, causing increased pulmonary edema. As the heart attempts to maintain cardiac output, it hypertrophies secondary to pressure and volume overload. A hypertrophied heart increases oxygen demand and reduces ventricular compliance, producing a "stiff ventricle." With decreased output, baroreceptors cause peripheral vasoconstriction, causing increased heart rate and myocardial contractility, thus increasing cardiac oxygen demand.

Common precipitating events include:

1. Artial fibrillation
2. Acute myocardial infarction or ischemia
3. Increased sodium intake
4. β-Blockers

5. Calcium channel antagonists
6. Physical overexertion
7. Discontinuation of digoxin

RIGHT-SIDED FAILURE

Right-sided failure is most commonly caused by left-sided heart failure. Isolated right-sided heart failure is caused by:

1. Congenital heart disease
2. Viral or idiopathic myocarditis
3. Pulmonary arterial hypertension
4. Mitral valve disease
5. Tricuspid valve disease
6. Restrictive cardiomyopathies
7. Infiltrative cardiomyopathies
8. Cirrhosis
9. Nephrotic syndrome

Right-sided failure is differentiated from left-sided failure by the following:

1. Edema occurs in dependent areas and not in the lungs.
2. Cardiac output is decreased.
3. Systemic blood pressure is usually decreased.
4. Left-sided failure causes pulmonary edema.
5. A positive hepatojugular reflux is a sign of right-sided heart failure.
6. Hepatic tenderness and enlargement occur, and PT interval is prolonged.
7. With severe right-sided heart failure, you will hear tricuspid regurgitation on examination.
8. Hyponatremia is common.

LEFT-SIDED FAILURE

Left-sided failure is usually caused by:

1. Coronary heart disease
2. Hypertension
3. Aortic valve disease
4. Mitral valve disease
5. Dilated cardiomyopathy

Signs and Symptoms

  I. Exertional dyspnea (occurs first)
  II. Paroxysmal nocturnal dyspnea (occurs second)
  III. Orthopnea (occurs third)
  IV. Dry to frothy cough or sputum
  V. Lung examination
      S_3 and S_4
      Rales or wheezing

VI. Pulsus alternans
VII. ECG:
>   Nonspecific ECG abnormalities
>   Hypertrophy
>   Subendocardial ischemia
>   Conduction disturbances
VIII. Chest x-ray to detect the three stages of CHF:
>   Stage 1: Pulmonary vasoconstriction and redistribution of blood to upper lung fields; PAWP of 12 to 18 mm Hg
>   Stage 2: Interstitial edema, with blurred edges of blood vessels, Kerley A and B lines, and PAWP of 18 to 25 mm Hg
>   Stage 3: Hazy perihilar infiltrates, "butterfly" looking perihilar areas, and PAWP of greater than 25 mm Hg

Treatment

- Laboratory values: CBC, calcium, magnesium, sodium, potassium, chloride, BUN, creatinine, glucose, CO_2, LDH, CPK, CPK-MB, AST, and ALT
- Give IV normal saline 0.9%, to keep IV lines open. A patient with a right-sided myocardial infarction needs fluid, not CHF.
- Place the patient on a cardiac monitor.
- Take an arterial blood gas, and look for respiratory acidosis or metabolic acidosis.
- Do an ECG, and look for acute myocardial infarction, right-sided myocardial infarction, and signs of PE.
- Chest x-ray, PE signs, wide mediastinum
- Give oxygen in high concentrations by mask or nasal cannula.
- Apply NTG paste to the anterior chest wall or give NTG IV or SL (0.4 mg). NTG reduces preload by dilating both the arteries and the veins. (Apply 1 inch of paste to the anterior chest wall, or start an IV at 10 μg/min.) Watch the patient's blood pressure for hypotension. Do not use NTG in the case of hypotension. If the patient is having chest pain, titrate the dose up until the patient is free of pain.
- With furosemide (Lasix), start with 1 mg/kg (the usual dose is 40 mg IV). If the patient is taking the oral form, double the oral dose or use bumetanide (Bumex) 1 mg/kg IV.
- Give morphine sulfate, 2 to 5 mg IV, which decreases anxiety, preload, and pulmonary congestion.
- Insert a Foley catheter and check the patient's urine input and output. Keep the patient urinating, but do not dry the patient out. Output should be 1 to 2 ml/kg/hr of urine.

Cardiogenic Shock

Watch for the following:

1. Pulmonary congestion
2. Hypotension

3. Decreased peripheral profusion

Patients in cardiogenic shock have lost 40% or more of their ventricular muscle mass. The preload must be decreased, and the blood pressure must be adequate to perfuse the heart, brain, and kidneys.

I. Preload is reduced by nitrates, morphine, and diuretics
II. In cardiogenic shock use dopamine, a direct inotropic agent, and vasopressor agent
      The starting dose of dopamine is 2 to 5 μg/kg/min renal dose. Titrate the dose from 5 to 15 μg/kg/min to the desired blood pressure.
III. With heart failure, add dobutamine, which has primary β_1-agonist effects with some β_2- and α-agonist effects. Dobutamine increases cardiac output and decreases PAWP in patients who are in heart failure. When severe pulmonary congestion is present, consider using a vasodilator concurrently. A dose of dobutamine starts at 5 μg/kg/min and should be titrated to effect.
IV. If the patient is hypertensive and in CHF, use nitroprusside at a rate of 1 μg/kg/min. Titrate to the desired blood pressure. Nitroprusside is a potent mixed venous and arteriolar dilator. This drug is effective in lowering blood pressure in heart failure patients who are in hypertensive crisis. Nitroprusside can be used in combination with dopamine in heart failure due to low cardiac output.

HYPERTENSIVE EMERGENCIES

There are four types of hypertensive emergencies:

1. Hypertensive emergencies
2. Hypertensive urgencies
3. Mild, uncomplicated hypertension
4. Transient hypertension

A true hypertensive emergency is an increase in blood pressure that shows signs and symptoms of end-organ damage. Organs at risk are the heart, brain, and kidneys. The level of blood pressure is not the diagnostic basis for a hypertensive emergency. Evidence of end-organ damage guides the therapy. The goal in hypertensive emergencies is to lower the pressure to "normal" for a particular patient. The goal is a 30% reduction in blood pressure in 30 minutes, without going below the level of the patient's autoregulation limit. In the chronic hypertensive patient, this limit is approximately 120 mm Hg diastolic. Hypertensive encephalopathy is the most devastating complication of a true hypertensive crisis. Encephalopathy is caused by hyperperfusion of the brain with loss of the integrity of the blood-brain barrier. The loss of integrity causes a change in the autoregulation of the cerebral blood flow. This causes an increased transportation of fluid into the brain. Prolonged increased pressure causes vascular necrosis in the brain. Signs and symptoms of hypertensive encephalopathy are:

Severe headache	Twitching and myoclonus
Altered mental status	Vomiting and nausea
Coma	Lethargy
Aphasia	Cranial nerve palsies
Blindness	Hemiparesis
Retinal hemorrhage, cotton wool spots	Confusion
	Papilledema and exudates

Hypertensive urgencies include:

1. No signs or symptoms of end-organ damage
2. Diastolic pressure usually greater than 115 mm Hg
3. Usually caused by noncompliance with medications
4. The goal is to reduce blood pressure slowly over 24 to 48 hours
5. Rapid lowering of blood pressure is potentially harmful

Mild, uncomplicated hypertension involves:

1. No signs or symptoms of end-organ damage
2. Diastolic pressure lower than 155 mm Hg
3. Should not be treated, but needs a 5-day check on blood pressure and follow-up within 7 days

TRANSIENT HYPERTENSION

1. Can be above or below diastolic pressure of 115 mm Hg.
2. Can be caused by:

Stroke	Dehydration
Alcohol withdrawal	Anxiety
Pancreatitis	Drug overdose

3. Treatment is to treat the underlying causes
4. Treat the patient's symptoms, not his or her blood pressure

HYPERTENSIVE EMERGENCIES

History

CVAs	Ischemic heart disease
Hypertension in the past	Is the patient taking his or her medications?
Alcohol use	
Blurred vision	Drug abuse (cocaine)
Diplopia	Hemiparesis
Head trauma	Seizure history
Tearing abdominal pain	Previous hypertensive crisis
History of aortic aneurysm	Acute onset of pain
Ask about new onset of chest pain or abdominal pain	

Physical Examination

Take blood pressure every 5 minutes

Do a tilt test

Perform a funduscopic examination: look for grade 3 or grade 4 changes

Check for carotid, renal, and abdominal bruits.

Check pulses in all extremities.

Perform a complete heart examination, and listen for new murmurs, rubs, and clicks

Perform a complete pulmonary examination, and listen for wheezing or rales.

Laboratory Tests

CBC, BUN, creatinine, glucose, sodium, potassium, chloride, CO_2, magnesium, calcium, UA

Look at UA for:
1. Proteinuria, red blood cells, or casts, a sign of end-organ renal damage
2. Proteinuria, hypertension, edema, hyperreflexia, eclampsia in pregnancy after 12 weeks

ECG: look for acute myocardial infarction or ischemia

Chest x-ray, cardiomegaly, signs of PE, pneumothorax, PE, or dissecting aortic aneurysm

Treatment

Upon initial presentation, do the following:

Place the patient on oxygen.

Place the patient on a cardiac monitor.

Give normal saline IV to keep the IV line open.

Take a blood pressure every 5 minutes, or sooner if needed.

Do a chest x-ray.

Take an ABG; look at the alveolar-arterial gradient; and rule out a PE.

Do an ECG.

In specific hypertensive situations:

CVA
1. Decrease blood pressure 20 to 30%, slowly, because a reduction that is too rapid will cause further ischemia in thrombolytic stroke. Use sodium nitroprusside or labetalol.

Eclampsia
1. Third trimester
2. Hyperreflexia
3. Confusion
4. Headache
5. Epigastric pain
6. Seizure
7. Young, primigravidas, multigravidas older than 35 years of age
8. Give magnesium sulfate in a bolus of 4 to 6 g IV, then 1 to 2 g/hr. Watch for toxic levels greater than 8 mEq/l, the therapeutic range is 6 to 8 mEq/l.)
9. Hydralazine, 10 to 20 mg IV for hypertension

Common Medications Used in Hypertensive Emergencies

Sodium nitroprusside (Nipride)
1. Rapidly acting arterial dilator and venodilator
2. Use in hypertensive encephalopathy, acute pulmonary edema, dissecting aneurysm, myocardial ischemia, aortic dissection.
3. 50 mg of nitroprusside in 500 ml of D5W gives you 10 μg/ml
4. Start IV drip at 0.5 mg/kg/min and titrate to effect. (The average effective dose is 3 μg/kg/min, with a dose range of 0.5 to 10 μg/kg/min.)
5. Prolonged use of sodium nitroprusside can cause thiocyanate toxicity and hepatic dysfunction.

Propranolol (Inderal)
1. Nonselective β-blocker that reduces cardiac output
2. Use as adjutant in dissecting aneurysm
3. Dose of 1 mg IV to a maximum dose of 3 mg IV

Labetalol (Normodyne, Trandate)
1. Selective α-blocker and nonselective β-blocker
2. Use in hypertensive emergencies when sodium nitroprusside has failed
3. Can be given as a 20- to 40-mg bolus every 30 to 60 minutes
4. If no response in 60 minutes, can double the dose to a maximum dose of 300 mg
5. Given IV, mix 200 mg in 200 ml of D5W to run at 2 mg/min (2 ml/min)

Nitroglycerin
1. Causes arterial dilatation and venodilation
2. Use in moderate hypertension, unstable angina, pulmonary edema, and acute myocardial infarction
3. Starting dose of 10 μg/min. Increase by 5 μg every 5 minutes. Watch for hypotension!

Diazoxide (Hyperstat)
1. Direct arterial dilator
2. Use in prehospital care
3. Can be given as a 50-mg bolus every 5 to 10 minutes

Nifedipine (Procardia)
1. Calcium channel blocker
2. Use in hypertensive urgencies
3. Dose of 10 to 20 mg sublingually (SL). Chew and swallow after a hole is placed in the capsule.

Hydralazine (Apresoline)
1. Direct arterial dilator
2. Use in eclampsia
3. Dose, 10 to 20 mg IV or 10 to 50 mg IV

Prazosin (Minipress)
1. Adrenergic blocker
2. Arterial and venous forms have an equally potent effect
3. Dose of 1 mg orally

Phentolamine (Regitine)
1. Completely blocks postsynaptic and presynaptic α-adrenergic receptors and vasodilates arterial and venous beds
2. Decreases renin secretion
3. Used in hypertensive urgencies
4. Dose of 0.2 mg as a loading dose orally. Give 0.1 mg every hour until the diastolic pressure is below 115 mm Hg.

Captopril (Capoten)
1. Angiotensin-converting enzyme inhibitor
2. Dose of 25 mg orally three times a day

PERICARDITIS

Signs and Symptoms

1. The characteristic pericardial friction rub sounds "scratchy or creaky." It is heard best at the lower left sternal border with the patient leaning forward. The examiner should use the diaphragm of the stethoscope and should listen to the patient's respirations. The rub is caused by friction between the inflamed visceral pericardium and the parietal pericardium.
2. Patients will complain of a substernal chest pain that is described as "sharp" but does not radiate to arms. The pain increases when the patient lies down and decreases when the patient leans forward. It often radiates to the left trapezius muscle, causing shoulder pain.
3. Breathing may be shallow secondary to pain.
4. Friction rubs will be intermittent.
5. Low-grade fever occurs in viral, high-grade bacterial pericarditis.

Types of Causes of Pericarditis

I. Viral or idiopathic
   A. Coxsackie virus B5, B6 (most common)
   B. Echovirus (second most common)

    C. Adenovirus
    D. Influenza
    E. Chickenpox
    F. AIDS
 II. Bacterial causes
    A. Staphylococci (most common)
    B. Pneumococci (secondary from pneumonia)
    C. Streptococci
    D. Meningococci
    E. Tuberculosis
    F. *Haemophilus influenzae*
    G. *Mycoplasma pneumoniae*
    H. Salmonella
    I. Psittacosis
 III. Trauma to the chest
 IV. Radiation therapy
  V. Fungal
    A. Coccidioidomycosis
    B. Histoplasmosis
    C. Aspergillosis
    D. Blastomycosis
 VI. Tumors
    A. Primary
    B. Metastatic
    C. Sarcoid
 VII. Amebiasis
VIII. Rickettsia
  IX. Myocardial infarction (Dressler's syndrome)
   X. Dissection aneurysm
  XI. Uremia
 XII. Rheumatoid arthritis

ECG Changes

  I. Four stages:
       Stage I: This stage will occur hours to days after the onset of
          pericarditis. Diffuse ST-segment elevation in leads I, II, aVL,
          aVF, and V_2 through V_6, with reciprocal ST depression in
          aVR and V_1. ST segments will concave upward. Some PR
          depression may occur.
       Stage II: ST and PR segments normalize, and the ECG looks
          normal.
       Stage III: There is characteristic deep symmetric T wave
          inversion throughout the ECG.
       Stage IV: The T waves normalize and the ECG is normal.
 II. To differentiate acute myocardial infarction from pericarditis,
     look at the ST segments. In pericarditis, the ST segments will
     concave upward, rather than convex upward in an acute

myocardial infarction. T wave inversions are not seen in pericarditis, as are seen in acute myocardial infarction.

III. To distinguish early repolarization from acute pericarditis, look at the PR interval. In early repolarization, the PR segment is not depressed as in pericarditis. Look at the ST segment and the T wave amplitude in V_5 and V_6. If the height of the T wave is greater than 0.25% of the ST segment, then the diagnosis is likely to be pericarditis. If the height of the T wave is less than 0.25% of the ST segment, then this is likely to be early repolarization.

Laboratory Studies

1. WBC is usually elevated
2. Erythocyte sedimentation rate is usually elevated
3. BUN and creatine are elevated in end-stage renal disease when the patient is on chronic hemodialysis; also seen in uremic pericarditis, calcium, magnesium, chloride, CO_2, sodium, potassium, glucose, phosphorus
4. Cardiac enzymes: CPK, CPK-MB, AST, ALT, LDH, GGT, CPK-MB will be elevated in 75% of patients with pericarditis
5. Streptococcal serology
6. Blood cultures
7. Thyroid function tests
8. Purified protein derivative (PPD)
9. Fungal cultures, if suspected or immunocompromised

Diagnosis

Echocardiography is the "gold standard" for diagnosis of pericarditis. A chest x-ray is not very helpful in pericarditis, unless you have an old chest x-ray to compare the size of the cardiac silhouette. The chest x-ray can be enlarged with pericarditis. Diagnosis is confirmed by pericardiocentesis.

Treatment

I. Viral or idiopathic
   A. Analgesia with aspirin or nonsteroidal anti-inflammatory drugs (NSAIDs)
   B. Corticosteroids if NSAID failure, low dose
   C. Admit the patient to the hospital for pain management if uncontrolled with NSAIDs
II. Uremic
   A. With hemodynamic compromise, daily dialysis is required
   B. Avoid NSAID and exacerbation of bleeding
   C. Hemodynamically compromised pericardial fluid must be drained immediately
III. Acute myocardial pericarditis
   A. NSAID, watch for hemodynamic instability, treat AMI

IV. Post myocardial pericarditis (Dressler's syndrome)
  A. Symptoms include, fever, pleuritis, leukocytosis, pericardial friction rub, chest x-ray evidence of pericardial pleural effusion
  B. Treatment includes NSAIDs and corticosteroids if refractory to NSAIDs
V. Neoplastic
  A. Therapeutic pericardiocentesis
  B. Pericardial fluid cytology for diagnostic management
VI. Bacterial
  A. Usually caused by *Staphylococcus* in adults or *Haemophilus influenzae* in children
  B. IV antibiotics should be started immediately.

Definitive surgical management is carried out by thoracotomy with pericardial resection with tube drainage of the pericardial cavity.

PROSTHETIC HEART VALVE DYSFUNCTION

Definition

There are over 40 different kinds of prosthetic heart valves. They are categorized by class, type, and model. The class of the valve is based on the type of material that the valve is made of—bioprosthetic or mechanical. A valve is classified as a bioprosthetic valve if it is made up of any type of animal tissue or human, homographic, xenographic (nonhuman), or heterographic tissue. Mechanical valves are made entirely of carbons, durable plastics, or metal alloys. Mechanical valves are subdivided into the mechanical valve type; ball-in-cage, single-tilting disk, or bileaflet. The model of the valve describes the particular design of the valve.

Prosthetic Heart Valves		
Class	**Type**	**Model**
Mechanical	Caged ball	Starr-Edwards
	Tilting disk	Omniscience/Omnicarbon Björk-Shiley Medtronic-Hall
	Bileaflet	Carbomedics St Jude Duromedics
Bioprosthetic	Pericardial	Mitroflow Ionescu-Shiley Carpentier-Edwards
	Porcine	Intact Hancock-I, II, MO

Physical Examination

1. An aortic valve prosthetic device will cause a mid-peaking systolic murmur and a louder closing sound. The opening sound may be inaudible.
2. A mitral valve prosthetic device can produce two types of murmurs. A low-frequency diastolic rumble will be heard in a smaller prosthetic valve, caused by turbulent inflow and mild mitral stenosis. The second type of murmur is caused by a partial obstruction of the left ventricular outflow track by the ring sewing procedure. A mid-peaking, diamond-shaped systolic murmur will radiate to the carotid arteries. Each model presents with a different kind of murmur.

Chest X-Ray

The chest x-ray allows the health care provider to determine the valve model and location in most patients. On a posteroanterior (PA) chest x-ray the heart valve location can be determined by:

1. The location of the aortic valve is in the center of the cardiac silhouette. It is superior and medial to the mitral valve. It is sometimes difficult to determine the difference between the locations of the aortic valve and the mitral valves. The aortic valve lies at a 20- to 30-degree angle. Struits, if present, lie superior and toward the patient's right side.
2. The mitral valve is in the center of the cardiac silhouette and is inferior and lateral to the aortic valve. It lies at a 20- to 30-degree angle. Struits (holding the valve in place), if present, lie inferior and to the patient's left side.
3. The tricuspid valve is the most vertical and inferior valve on the cardiac silhouette. It lies over the spine.
4. The pulmonary valve is the most superior of the four valves. It lies lateral to the spine and just above the AV groove. It lies horizontally.

Complications

Complications of prosthetic heart valves include systemic emboli (12.7%), fever and dizziness (3.9%), pulmonary edema (30.2%), congestive heart failure (39%), coronary ischemic syndrome, myocardial infarction, unstable angina (6.8%), and unknown etiology and no symptoms (7.4%).

Thromboembolism is the most common complication of prosthetic heart valves. There is no variability in thromboembolism rates in regard to particular valves. Mitral valves are believed to be more thrombogenic than aortic valves, secondary to an increased higher incidence of atrial fibrillation and poorer left ventricular systolic function, secondary to a larger left atrium.

Patients with thromboembolic valvular heart disease can present with numerous symptoms. Valvular stenosis causes regurgitation secondary to failure of complete valve closure by a thrombus. Patients can present with dyspnea (the most common presenting complaint), coronary ischemic syndrome, angina, or acute myocardial infarction. Most patients who present with thromboembolic valvular disease are not adequately anticoagulated. The diagnosis of thrombus valvular disease is based on the signs of dyspnea and pulmonary congestion and on a patient who is not adequately anticoagulated; who does not have a normal click; or who has new regurgitation or a louder stenotic murmur.

A transthoracic or transesophageal echocardiogram is used to confirm the diagnosis of a thrombus. Transesophageal echocardiography can best be utilized in the diagnosis of a thrombus on a bioprosthetic valve, which does not have radiopaque leaflets. Cinefluoroscopy can provide information on leaflet motion.

Treatment of a valvular thrombus consists of administration of heparin in a stable patient. Lytic therapy should not be given to patients with left-sided valvular thrombus, secondary to the increase risk of embolism. Lytic therapy can be considered in patients with right-sided valvular thrombosis.

In the hemodynamically unstable patient with valvular thrombus, the use of lytic therapy is often lifesaving. It should be administered immediately. Lytic therapy should be given in consultation with the patient's cardiologist and a surgeon. Thrombolytic therapy has not been approved by the Federal Drug Administration (FDA) for lysis of a clot in a thrombosed mechanical valve and is considered investigational.

Streptokinase is the most commonly used thrombolytic agent used to treat a thrombosed mechanical valve. Dosing of streptokinase involves a bolus of 250,000 to 500,000 units over 20 to 30 minutes, then 100,000 to 150,000 units/hr for a minimum of 10 hours and up to 72 hours or longer.

The use of urokinase is optional, and the recommended dosage is given as a bolus of 4400 units/kg over 10 to 15 minutes.

Tissue plasminogen activator (t-PA) is given as a bolus of 10 mg followed by 90 mg over 90 minutes.

ENDOCARDITIS OR PROSTHETIC VALVE ENDOCARDITIS

Prosthetic valve endocarditis (PVE) must be considered if the results of two or more blood cultures are positive, with or without signs of extracardiac infection, signs and symptoms of endocarditis, fever, petechiae, change in a murmur or a new murmur, splenomegaly, hematuria, peripheral emboli, or positive signs on echocardiography, microbiologic or histologic proof by biopsy or autopsy.

PVE is divided into two categories: (1) early, less than 60 days postoperatively, and (2) late, more than 60 days postoperatively. The mortality rate from PVE is in the range of 53 to 69%, and mortality from early PVE can reach 29 to 100%. Increased risk factors for mortality from PVE is new-onset CHF, new AV conduction abnormalities, valve dehiscence, aneurysm formation, emboli, nonstreptococcal PVE, and positive cultures after 2 to 3 days of antibiotic therapy.

Staphylococcus epidermidis is the most common organism that causes PVE. Streptococci are more commonly found in late PVE. *S. epidermidis*, gram-negative bacilli, and diphtheroids are found in early PVE. *Candida* and *Aspergillus* are rare causes of PVE.

Diagnosis

An echocardiogram is used to diagnose PVE. It is harder to diagnosis endocarditis by echocardiogram in prosthetic heart valves than in native valves. Diagnosis is made by noting positive vegetation growth on valves or abnormal valve movement on the echocardiogram and positive blood cultures. Blood cultures to test for fungal endocarditis can be negative.

Treatment

The choice of antibiotic therapy is based on culture and sensitivity results. Bactericidal drugs should be chosen over bacteriostatic drugs. Synergistic drugs should be chosen. Gentamicin and vancomycin should be used in the first 12 months after surgery based on the likelihood of the organism. After 12 to 18 months, the choices of antibiotics are penicillin or ampicillin with gentamicin. Anticoagulation should be continued during PVE unless an acute CVA or an intracranial hemorrhage occurs. If a CVA occurs, anticoagulation should be resumed after 48 to 72 hours if no signs of intracranial hemorrhage are present.

HEMOLYTIC ANEMIA

Hemolytic anemia is due to the mechanical trauma from the closing of the disk against the valve seat and from the leaking around the valve once the valve is closed. The leaking is a *static leak*, designed into the valve to wash off the leaflet surfaces and prevent the formation of a thrombus on the valve. Red blood cells are damaged when they are caught between the valve leaflets and the valve ring under pressure of the valve closing.

Diagnosis

The elevation of lactic dehydrogenase (LDH) correlates with the severity of the hemolysis of this process. Elevated bilirubin, reticulocytosis along with schistocytosis, and helmet cells are noted.

If severe hemolytic anemia is noted with mild decompensation, β-blockers can be used to reduce the shearing force.

Treatment

Synthetic erythropoietin can also be given to increase the rate of red blood cell production. If there is no improvement in the anemia, a pathologic paraprosthetic leak should be considered.

A primary structural failure is very rare but can occur. The bioprosthesis valve will fail more gradually than the mechanical valve, but rarely under 5 years of use. The failure rate of the mechanical valve is greater after 10 years of use.

Patients with structural failures will present with severe and new onset regurgitation, dyspnea, chest pain, loss of normal heart valve clicks, and altered mental status. If a prosthetic aortic valve fails, a sudden cardiac collapse will occur. The patient will usually live for less than 10 minutes. A patient with mitral valve failure can survive for several hours.

Patients with bioprosthetic valve failure will present with gradual and less dramatic failure. The valve will become stenotic and covered with a thin layer of fibrin, followed by leukocytes, and then by new endothelial cells. Perforation of the leaflet, calcium deposits, tears, valvular regurgitation, cuspal tears, or stenosis will occur. Bioprosthetic valves usually do not have regurgitant murmurs, thus a new onset of a regurgitant murmur with a bioprosthetic valve must be considered as a primary valve failure until proven otherwise.

Diagnosis

Echocardiography is used to determine a paraprosthetic leak from a primary valve failure. Blood cultures are taken to rule out PVE. Patients with stenotic lesions will have longer and louder murmurs.

Treatment

An immediate surgical and cardiologic consultation should be made. Oxygen should be given, and treatment of the hemodynamic unstable patient should be performed.

PULMONARY EMBOLISM

A PE is caused by the classic triad of venostasis, hypercoagulability, and vessel wall inflammation. Most PEs arise from the deep vein system of the lower extremities. Popliteal thromboses cause 50% of PEs, with femoral vein involvement morbidity reaching 70%. Calf vein involvement is seldom the cause of PEs. PEs are the third most common cause of death in the United States. PEs occur when a fragment of a thrombus breaks off and is carried via the vena cava to the right side of the heart. This fragment then lodges in the pulmonary artery tree, causing either complete or partial obstruction to the distal pulmonary tree. Of proven PEs, 70% will have a provable clot in the pelvis or lower extremity. The PE causes a ventilation-perfusion (V/Q) mismatch. Major causes of PE are:

1. Amniotic fluid PE in abortion or post partum period at the end of the first stage of labor

2. Pelvic or leg thrombus
3. Right-sided heart thrombus
4. IV drug use
5. Cardiac vegetations
6. Fat embolism in trauma patients
7. Fracture of large long bones, tibia, and femur
8. Orogenital sex

Signs and Symptoms

1. Chest pain is the most common presenting complaint and is often noted 3 to 4 days before the patient presents to the ED; 90% will present with chest pain.
2. Dyspnea occurs sometimes during the course of the presentation (80%).
3. Hypoxia produces anxiety and apprehension (60%).
4. A history of a syncopal episode may be present.
5. Tachypnea and respirations greater than 16 occur in 90% of presenting patients.
6. The patient may present with rales, wheezing, friction rubs, or rhonchi.

Risk Factors

1. Burns
2. Obesity
3. DVT
4. Trauma
5. Heart disease, CHF, atrial fibrillation
6. Postoperative period
7. Prolonged immobilization

Three Classical Types of Presentations

  I. Pulmonary infarction or hemorrhage
     A. Presents with pleuritic chest pain
     B. Will look like pleuritis or infectious pneumonitis
 II. Submassive embolism without infarction
     A. Presents with unexplained dyspnea on exertion or rest
     B. Will look like infection, CHF, asthma, hyperventilation
III. Massive embolism
     A. Presents with acute cor pulmonale (enlarged right ventricle secondary to malfunction of the lungs)
     B. Will look like an acute myocardial infarction, hypovolemia, or septic shock

Prognosis

1. 10% will die in 1 hour
2. When diagnosis is made, survivors have an 8% mortality rate

3. Death after 24 hours occurs in the chronically ill patients
4. High incidence of recurrence

Diagnosis

Diagnosis can be based on the following:

Arterial blood gas interpretation
  1. Alveolar-arterial gradient (room air at sea level) of 150-(measured PaO_2 + $PaCO_2/0.8$) or alveolar-arterial gradient of 140-(PO_2 + PCO_2)
  2. Normal less than 10 mm Hg in youth and 20 mm Hg in adults (A useful rule is that the alveolar-arterial gradient should never be greater than 10 plus one tenth of the patient's age.)
  3. A patient with a decreased PaO_2 and an increased alveolar-arterial gradient, in the setting of a suspected PE, is highly predictable if a PE

ECG changes:
  1. Right-heart strain, tall peaked P waves
  2. Right axis deviation
  3. New right bundle branch block
  4. S1-Q3-T3 pattern, large S wave in lead I, large Q wave in lead III, ST depression in lead II, with T wave inversion in lead III
  5. T wave inversion in V_1 to V_4
  6. Tachycardia
  7. Nonspecific ST-T wave changes
  8. Atrial fibrillation

Chest x-ray:
  1. Nonspecific and insensitive
  2. Hampton's hump, a triangular, plural-based, infiltrate, frequently located at the costophrenic junction apex toward the hilum
  3. Westermark's sign, dilated pulmonary vessels to the embolism, along with collapse of those distally, with a sharp cut-off
  4. Normal chest x-ray results will occur in 30%
  5. One half will have an elevated hemidiaphragm
  6. One third will develop transient parenchymal infiltrates

V/Q scan results based on Bayes' theorem, and a V/Q scan interpretation:
  1. Normal scan with no perfusion defects
     a. Sensitivity of 2% (2% of patients with this pattern will have a PE)
     b. Positive predictive value of 4% (4% do have a PE)
     c. 96% with this pattern do not have a PE
  2. Low probability, small perfusion defects
     a. Sensitivity of 16% (16% of patients with a PE will have this pattern)
     b. Positive predictive value of 14% (14% do have a PE)
     c. 86% with this pattern do not have a PE

3. Intermediate probability, any V/Q scan no classified as "high" or "low"
   a. Sensitivity of 41% (41% of patients with a PE will have this pattern)
   b. Positive predictive value of 30% (30% do have a PE)
   c. 70% with this pattern do not have a PE
4. High probability, two or more segmental or larger defects
   a. Sensitivity of 41% (41% of patients with a PE will have this pattern)
   b. Positive predicative value of 87% (87% will have a PE)
   c. 13% with this pattern will not have a PE

Pulmonary angiography (the "gold standard" of diagnosis of a PE)

Treatment

I. High dose of oxygen
II. Treat hypotension if present with IV crystalloids if CVP is low, dopamine 5 to 10 µg/kg/min is normal or high
III. Laboratory values: CBC, PT, PTT, sodium, potassium, chloride, CO_2, BUN, creatinine, glucose, CPK, CPK-MB, LDH, AST, and ALT
IV. ABG
V. Two 14- to 16-gauge IVs of crystalloids
VI. Placement of a Swan-Ganz catheter
VII. Heparin, started at 10,000-unit bolus, then 25 units/kg/hr; PTT to 1 1/2 to 2 times control values (In case of abnormal bleeding caused by heparin, use protamine sulfate. Each milligram of protamine sulfate neutralizes approximately 100 units of heparin.)
VIII. Thrombolytic therapy in PE
   A. Criteria
      1. A hemodynamically compromised patient who has not responded to stabilization procedures
      2. Pulmonary angiography has documented a massive PE
      3. Consultation with a pulmonary specialist
IX. Pulmonary embolectomy can be used in consultation with a thoracic surgeon

TRANSVENOUS PACEMAKERS

Definition

Transvenous pacemakers (TP) have been used since the 1950s. The complication rate of TP is as high as 6%.

Epidemiology

Approximately 300,000 TPs are placed or replaced in the United States each year. The North American Society of Pacing and

Electrophysiology/British Pacing and Electrophysiology Group Generic Pacemaker Code is the nomenclature used to describe the functions of the different kinds of pacemakers. The term "position" describes the code of the specific characteristic of a pacemaker.

Position I—Chamber paced; 0 = none; A = atrium;
   V = ventricle; D = dual

Position II—Chamber sensed; 0 = none; A = atrium;
   V = ventricle; D = dual

Position III—Response to sensing; 0 = none; I = inhibited;
   T = triggered; D = dual

Position IV—Rate of modulation and programmability; 0 = none;
   S = simple programmable; M = multiprogrammable;
   C = communicating; R = rate modulation

Positive V—Antitachycardia features; 0 = none;
   P = antitachycardiac pacing; S = shock; D = dual

Pacemaker Malfunction

When a lead is disrupted or a pacemaker has a generator failure, the pacemaker will fail. A pacemaker will malfunction for three main reasons:

1. Failure to pace
2. Failure to sense
3. Failure to capture

A lead can break, become dislodged from its site of attachment or fracture after trauma. Microwave radiation is seldom the cause of malfunction with new federal regulations governing the shielding of microwave components and the shielding of the TP leads proper. MRIs can cause any TP to function in a asynchronous mode. TP is also affected by transcutaneous electrical nerve stimulation (TENS), which should be avoided. Transthoracic defibrillation and lithotripsy can affect TP. Flight in an aircraft has no affect on TP.

A patient with a malfunctioning TP can present with a wide variety of symptoms, based on their underlying cardiac disease. Chest pain, hypotension, CHF, shortness of breath, syncope, dizziness, tachycardia, or bradycardia—all can occur with TP malfunction.

Complications of Malfunctioning Pacemakers

Pacemakers can cause anxiety in up to 27% of patients with pacemakers implanted. Depression, loss of independence, and denial can occur. The feeling of "going crazy" with choking, trembling, chest pain, numbness and tingling, dizziness and palpitations, nausea, and shortness of breath can occur. After it has been determined that the pacemaker is functioning properly, the patient can be treated with antidepressant medication and can be referred for psychiatric help.

Infections can occur after placement of a pacemaker. *Staphylococcus aureus* is the most common infection after placement of the pacemaker. *S. epidermidis* is the organism responsible for later infections. *Corynebacterium, Candida*, and group B *Streptococcus* are rare causes of infection. Treatment of infected pacemaker wires in the ED can be achieved by giving cefazolin or vancomycin and gentamicin. All patients with infected pacemaker wires should be admitted to the hospital and a consultation should be made with a cardiologist.

Swelling, redness, and localized eczema within 2 weeks to 2 years after placement of the pacemaker, after cellulitis has been ruled out, can be diagnosed as *pacemaker dermatitis*. It is caused by the material that the pacemaker is manufactured of.

Pacemaker-mediated tachycardia (PMT) is a common malfunction of dual-chambered pacemakers. PMT can be terminated by placing a pacemaker magnet on the pacemaker and eliminating the atrial sensing and blocking the anterograde pathway.

If a pacemaker magnet is not available, isometric exercises with 1 to 3 chest thumbs or external pacing at an output of 10 to 20 mA can be used to terminate PMT. In older models, a runaway pacemaker can be a sign of battery failure.

If the pacemaker is sensing at a rate greater than 200 beats/min, and the pacemaker magnet fails to terminate the tachycardia, the health care provider can make a sterile incision over the pacemaker pouch and disconnect the leads from the generator. If this causes the patient to become hemodynamically unstable secondary to bradycardia, the disconnected pacemaker leads can be attached to an external temporary pacemaker.

A **pacemaker twiddler's syndrome** (PTS) is a rare complication of pacemaker malfunction. In PTS the pacemaker generator is either purposefully or inadvertently manipulated, or "twiddling" of the generator causes the leads to be fractured, coiled around the generator, or dislodged from their implantation sites. This "twiddling" can present as a malfunction of the pacemaker.

Diagnosis of a Malfunctional Pacemaker

Karkal and Syverud have developed a four-step plan for evaluating a malfunctioning pacemaker:

1. *Assess the integrity of the battery.* A pacemaker magnet is placed over the TP. If the pacemaker is functioning correctly, then the pacemaker will function at the pacemaker magnet rate. If there is a decrease of 10% or more in the pacemaker magnet rate, then battery depletion is suggested.
2. *Assess the pacemaker rhythm.* Monitor the cardiac monitor, watching the pacemaker spikes. If the pacemaker spikes are faster than the programmed rate, then a runaway pacemaker, pacemaker-induced tachycardia, or external artifact must be considered. If pacemaker spikes are absent or at a slower rate than programmed, oversensing, failure to discharge, or hysteresis

must be considered. If the pacemaker is functioning properly, no pacemaker spikes will be seen if the intrinsic heart rate is higher than the programmed rate.

3. *Assess for capture.* Perform an ECG. The myocardium should depolarize within 300 msec after the pacemaker spike. Causes of failure to capture include ischemia, drugs, fibrosis, lead fracture, lead displacement, generator failure, or high myocardial stimulation threshold.

4. *Assess sensing function.* Monitor the ECG. Watch for competing native impulses and pacer spikes. If sensing is normal, there will be no discharges if native impulses and depolarizations are adequate. If sensing is adequate, consider a generator malfunction.

BIBLIOGRAPHY

Eagle KA, Harber E, DeSanctis E, Austen WG (eds): The Practice of Cardiology, 2nd ed. Boston, Little, Brown, 1989

Hurst JW, Logue RB, Rackley CE (eds): The Heart, 6th ed. New York, McGraw-Hill, 1994

Morgan JA, Stack LB (eds): Patients with indwelling devices: Automatic implantable cardioverter-defibrillators. Emerg Med Clin North Am, August, 1994

Pearson RD, Guerrant RL: Shigellosis. *In* Braunwald E, Isselbacher KJ, Petersdorf RG, et al (eds): Harrison's Principles of Internal Medicine, 11th ed. New York, McGraw-Hill, 1987

Rosen P, Barkin RM (eds): Emergency Medicine: Concepts and Clinical Practice, 3rd ed. St Louis, Mosby-Year Book, 1992

Tintinalli JE, Krone RL, Ruiz E (eds): Emergency Medicine: A Comprehensive Study Guide, 3rd ed. New York, McGraw-Hill, 1992

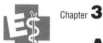

Chapter 3

Acute Dermatologic Emergencies

ERYTHEMA MULTIFORME

Definition

Erythema multiforme is a spectrum of disease, which is an acute self-limiting disease that is precipitated by a variety of factors. It presents with a sudden onset of erythematous or violaceous papules, macules, vesicles, or bullae. The hallmark of erythema multiforme is a target lesion that presents prior to the involvement of the soles, palms, and backs of the hands and feet. *Stevens-Johnson syndrome* is a severe life-threatening form of erythema multiforme.

Epidemiology

Erythema multiforme affects males twice as often as females and is seen more in the spring and fall than in the winter or summer. Malignancies and drugs are the common causes of this disease in the older population. In children, infections are often the precipitating event. Fifty percent of all cases will have an identifiable cause that is usually secondary to adenovirus, histoplasmosis, herpesvirus, or an atypical pneumonia. If Stevens-Johnson syndrome is present, there is a 5 to 10% mortality rate.

Pathology

Erythema multiforme is secondary to a hypersensitivity reaction precipitated by a number of conditions, chemicals, or drugs. Common infectious diseases that can cause erythema multiforme are cat-scratch fever, thyroid disease, mumps, diphtheria, histoplasmosis, *Mycoplasma* pneumonia, herpes simplex virus types I and II, cholera, and lymphogranuloma venereum. Common drugs that can cause an acute exacerbation of erythema multiforme include: the barbiturates, penicillins, sulfonamides, carbamazepine, phenylbutazone, oxyphenbutazone, chlorpropamide, and phenytoin. Any malignancy can cause erythema multiforme, with or without radiation therapy.

Clinical Presentation

Patients can present with a wide variety of presentations, including macular, papular, vesicular, or bullous lesions. The erythematous macules can present as urticarial plaques, but erythema multiforme usually lacks the pruritus of urticaria. This fact can help to differentiate it from true urticarial lesions. When vesiculobullous lesions do occur, they usually develop where the pre-existing macules, wheels, or papules were located. The oral mucous membranes can also be affected in bullous lesions and can resemble herpes lesions.

Almost all exacerbations of erythema multiforme initially present with a target lesion. This lesion has a bright red erythematous border with a dusky center that resembles a bull's eye or halo.

All erythema multiforme lesions can take up to 2 to 4 weeks to appear. These lesions usually occur in crops and heal in 7 to 10 days after their appearance. The patient's skin can become hypopigmented or hyperpigmented after the lesions resolve.

The severe form of erythema multiforme is *Stevens-Johnson syndrome*. It presents with fever, myalgias, malaise, and arthralgias. There is usually severe mucocutaneous involvement of the cheeks, lips, eyes, vagina, palate, anus, and nose and severe stomatitis often occurs. With eye involvement, purulent conjunctivitis may be present. If Stevens-Johnson syndrome is present, the eyes can develop corneal ulcerations, panophthalmitis, anterior uveitis, corneal opacities, and blindness. The esophagus, tracheobronchial tree, and pharynx can also be involved. The lesions begin as blisters that rupture and become grayish-white epithelial lesions with blood-crusted denuded bases. If the penis is involved, severe balanitis can be present. If the vagina is involved, severe vulvovaginitis can develop into stenosis of the vagina. There is marked multisystem involvement with Stevens-Johnson syndrome. Acute renal tubular necrosis, which can progress to acute renal failure, can occur.

Examination

The patient should be given a complete examination, including a rectal examination. If the patient is female, a complete pelvic examination should include a visual examination of the vagina. The oral mucosa should be examined for lesions.

Diagnosis

A diagnosis is made by clinical presentation, history or presence of a target lesion, and presence of causative factors. If the presentation is questionable, a skin biopsy should be performed. Appropriate studies should be done to rule in or out underlying causes based on a history of new or chronic illnesses or medications such as phenytoin.

Laboratory Findings

On histopathologic examination, the bullae are subepidermal, and the epidermal cells are necrotic. There is lymphocytic infiltrate above the capillaries and venules in the upper dermis. In mild cases, no laboratory examinations are required. In the presence of Stevens-Johnson syndrome, appropriate laboratory examinations should be performed to rule out acute renal failure or other multisystem organ involvement.

Treatment

Patients with mild forms of erythema multiforme can be treated as outpatients with mild topical corticosteroids. If severe mucous membrane involvement is present or if large amounts of skin are involved, the patient should be hospitalized in a burn unit with good fluid and electrolyte therapy. Secondary infections should be treated with antibiotics. The use of systemic corticosteroids is somewhat controversial. Some authors believe that corticosteroids will worsen the course of the disease and are contraindicated in the treatment of Stevens-Johnson syndrome. Corticosteroids probably should not be used in any form of erythema multiforme.

If the patient has mild painful oral lesions, the pain can be treated with diphenhydramine hydrochloride elixir or viscous lidocaine oral swishes. If bullous lesions are present, they can be treated with wet compresses of 1:16,000 potassium permanganate or 0.05% silver nitrate solution several times a day. If the eye is involved, the patient should be referred to an ophthalmologist for an evaluation.

EXFOLIATIVE DERMATITIS

Definition

Exfoliative dermatitis is an acute or chronic skin condition that involves most of the skin's surface. It presents as a scaly erythematous dermatitis, and it can be abrupt or insidious in onset.

Epidemiology

Exfoliative dermatitis is seen in males twice as often as in females, and 75% of these patients are older than 40 years of age. There is often multisystem organ involvement. True exfoliative dermatitis is usually a chronic condition with a mean duration of 5 years and a median duration of 10 months. Exfoliative dermatitis can last up to 20 years and have no underlying discernible cause.

Pathology

Exfoliative dermatitis is secondary to a response to a chemical, idiopathic, underlying systemic disease or drug reaction. Exfoliative dermatitis can be secondary to pityriasis rubra pilaris, lichen planus, seborrheic dermatitis, psoriasis, atopic dermatitis, or contact dermatitis. Malignancies including leukemia, lymphoma, or solid tumors can also cause exfoliative dermatitis. Idiopathic causes can account for up to 15 to 45% of all flares.

Drug- or medication-induced exfoliative dermatitis is secondary to an excessive number of drug-sensitized suppressor-cytoxic T lymphocytes and may be secondary to a true T cell immunoregulatory disorder.

Clinical Presentation

Exfoliative dermatitis can be secondary to contact allergens, malignancy, or medications. Flares secondary to underlying disorders usually present slowly, and a malignancy should be considered.

Patients can present with a scaling or flaking epidermatitis that is erythematous and is warm to touch. The patient will often complain of pruritus, a low-grade fever, a chilly sensation of the skin, or a tightness of the skin. In patients with chronic exfoliative dermatitis, their presenting complaint can be loss of body or scalp hair or dystrophic nails. A diffuse or patchy postinflammatory hyperpigmentation or even hypopigmentation can also occur in chronic cases. In chronic cases, chronic lymphadenopathy or gynecomastia can be present. Widespread vasodilation can also be present, leading to the patient complaining of "always" being cold secondary to excessive heat loss and impairment of temperature regulation caused by large areas of exfoliative dermatitis. In severe cases, hypothermia can be present. The vasodilation can lead to increased cardiac output and thus place stress on the heart, leading to high-output cardiac failure, dyspnea, and dependent edema.

If splenomegaly is present, leukemia or lymphoma should be considered. Steatorrhea can also be present. There can also be excessive water loss secondary to transepidermal water loss, which can lead to a negative nitrogen balance and protein loss.

Examination

The patient should be given a complete examination. A good dermatologic examination should be performed along with a good cardiac examination.

Diagnosis

A diagnosis is made by history, physical examination, and clinical presentation in regard to the underlying disease.

Laboratory Findings

All patients should have a complete blood count (CBC), electrolytes, blood urea nitrogen (BUN), creatinine, erythrocyte sedimentation rate, and urinalysis to rule out underlying disease. Serum albumin can be decreased in the presence of steatorrhea. If cardiac failure is considered, cardiac enzymes should be drawn. A chest x-ray should also be performed.

Treatment

Treatment is directed at discovering an underlying cause. The patient is often diagnosed as having idiopathic exfoliative dermatitis. Any patient with an acute, new onset of exfoliative dermatitis should be admitted to the hospital for evaluation of underlying causes. Solid tumor, leukemia, or lymphoma should be considered in a new onset of exfoliative dermatitis. If lymphadenopathy is present, a lymph node should be biopsied to rule out a malignancy. A history of current, new, or chronic medication or chemical exposure should be obtained. The patient should also be evaluated for cardiac failure.

Mild cases of idiopathic dermatitis can be treated with topical corticosteroid creams or lotions. Oral antihistamines can be given to treat pruritus. If severe dermatitis is present, oral corticosteroids can be given. Prednisone should be given in a dose of 40 to 60 mg/day and should be increased by 20 mg/day until positive results are obtained. Once a positive response is obtained, the dose should be tapered over several weeks or months until the drug is discontinued. All patients with exfoliative dermatitis should be referred to a dermatologist or an internal medicine physician.

TOXIC EPIDERMAL NECROLYSIS

Definition

Toxic epidermal necrolysis is secondary to a staphylococcal infection or a chemical or drug reaction. It is also called *scalded skin syndrome*.

Epidemiology

Toxic epidermal necrolysis is caused by a staphylococcal infection, called *staphylococcal scalded skin syndrome*, which is usually seen in children younger than 5 years of age. There is a 5% mortality rate for widespread exfoliation secondary to staphylococcal infection.

Toxic epidermal necrolysis secondary to chemical or drug reactions is seen mainly in adults. It carries a 5 to 50% mortality rate secondary to fluid loss and severe secondary infections.

Pathology

Toxic epidermal necrolysis secondary to a staphylococcal infection is caused by a staphylococcal toxin, which cleaves the epidermis beneath the stratum granulosum and separates the dermis from the epidermis. There may be a specific receptor-toxin interaction that causes the denudation. The danger of this type of denudation is when a large area of skin is involved, and thus severe fluid loss and hypothermia can occur.

Clinical Presentation/Examination

Patients often present with a history of an upper respiratory infection or purulent conjunctivitis. Patients present with lesions of the periorificial areas of the face, neck, axillae, and groin. These areas appear suddenly as tender erythematous patches of skin that become loosened and denuded and have a glistening base after skin loss. Patients can present with mild cases of bullous impetigo or almost a complete skin exfoliation. If pressure is applied laterally to the lesions, the skin will separate from the epidermis (a positive Nikolsky sign). The mucous membranes are usually not involved in staphylococcal infections. In about 24 to 48 hours after the initial presentation, flaccid bullae can sometimes develop and will separate spontaneously into what is described as rumpled sheets, with a moist erythematous base. The denudation resolves in 5 to 7 days.

In adults, toxic epidermal necrolysis secondary to chemicals or drugs presents as a separation of the skin at the dermoepidermal junction and is usually widespread, involving the mucous membranes. The skin is necrotic; however, little infiltration is noted upon examination. The lesions, which are often confused with erythema multiforme, heal slowly in 1 to 3 weeks.

Diagnosis

A diagnosis is made by a history of staphylococcal infection, exposure to drugs or chemicals, and clinical presentation. Several techniques are used to determine if the scalded skin syndrome is secondary to staphylococcal infection. Take a No. 15 blade scalpel and scrape the denuded base of the involved skin, then place this sample on a slide. If acantholytic keratinocytes are present, then the infection is secondary to staphylococcal infection. If a nonstaphylococcal type of toxic epidermal necrolysis (with drug or chemical causes) is present, then cellular debris, inflammatory cells, or basal cell keratinocytes will be present on examination.

A frozen section of peeled skin from a fresh lesion should be acquired. Look at the dermoepidermal junction. If only stratum corneum and a few granular cells are present, then the necrolysis is secondary to a staphylococcal infection. If the junction has a full-thickness split, then the necrolysis is secondary to drugs or chemicals. A definitive diagnosis is made by a skin biopsy.

Laboratory Findings

A CBC, electrolytes, blood culture, and urine culture should be obtained on every patient with toxic epidermal necrolysis. Cultures for *Staphylococcus aureus* should be obtained from the skin, throat, nose, perineum, and conjunctiva.

Treatment

The mainstay of treatment for toxic epidermal necrolysis is fluid, electrolyte, and temperature (body heat loss) support. The lesions are treated as second-degree burns. The patient has lost the protective barrier (skin). Adults can lose 2 to 6 liters of fluid a day, depending on the amount of skin involved. There is usually a greater loss of fluid in the first few days than in the latter days of the illness. Hypothermia should be treated aggressively.

Penicillinase-resistant penicillin IV should be administered to patients who have a staphylococcal infection. Corticosteroids should not be given. If the area of denudation is large, the patient should be treated in a burn unit. Sulfadiazine silver and mafenide acetate creams should be avoided since these drugs are often toxic to a patient with toxic epidermal necrolysis, and these drugs also delay epithelialization.

In patients with drug- or chemical-induced toxic epidermal necrolysis, antibiotics should not be given prophylactically unless an infection has been identified. If the patient's eye is involved, an ophthalmology consultation should be made. All patients should be admitted to the hospital for evaluation and for fluid and electrolyte treatment.

TOXICODENDRON DERMATITIS

Definition

Toxicodendron dermatitis or contact dermatitis is caused by poison ivy, oak, or sumac in the United States.

Epidemiology

Seventy percent of the population of the United States is susceptible to contact dermatitis. Dark-skinned persons are less susceptible to contact dermatitis than are fair-skinned persons. Poison ivy is found throughout the United States. Poison oak is more common on the west coast of the United States. Poison oak consists of two species: *Toxicodendron diversilobum* western poison oak and *T. diversilobum* eastern poison oak. Poison ivy also has two species: *T. rydergii* and *T. radicans*. *T. rydergii* is a nonclimbing shrub form, and *T. radicans* can either be a shrub form or a climbing vine form. Both poison ivy and poison oak have three leaflets and can be identified by their U- or V-shaped leaf scars and by their typical lenticels, flowers, and fruits that grow from the angle between the leaf and the branch. The fruit arises from a *panicle* that bears an off-white fruit.

There is only one form of poison sumac—*T. vernix*—which is a shrub or tree that grows in wooded swampy areas of the United States. Poison sumac has 7 to 13 leaflets per leaf. Sumac bears the same kind of fruit as poison oak and ivy.

All types of *Toxicodendrons* bear flowers, roots, seeds, berries, and stems that contain a milky sap that darkens when exposed to air. This black lacquer-like sap appears where the plant has been broken and can help to provide a clue to whether the plant belongs to the *Toxicodendron* species.

Pathology

All of the *Toxicodendron* species produce an antigenic oleoresin. When the oleoresin evaporates, a solvent, urushiol, is left. This solvent produces pentadecylcatechol, which causes dermatitis. There is cross-sensitivity to all resins of poison ivy, oak, and sumac. There is more resin in young plants than in old plants. Urushiol oxidizes faster when exposed to heat and moisture of the body. It can be destroyed rapidly by soaking the affected area in water.

Clinical Presentation

Patients with contact dermatitis present with clinical symptoms in as little as 30 minutes after exposure. The first signs usually appear in about 2 days after exposure. Patients can develop erythema, papules, vesicles, bullae, pruritus, and redness. The dermatitis is not spread by ruptured vesicles. The fluid in the vesicles contains no antigen, thus the dermatitis cannot be spread by rupturing of vesicles. The lesions often present in crusty, weeping linear configurations with streaks of erythema and papulovesicles. The dermatitis usually disappears without complications, but leukoderma and hyperpigmentation can occur along with erythema multiforme.

Diagnosis

A diagnosis is made by history of contact and by clinical presentation.

Laboratory Findings

Leukocytosis and eosinophils of 5 to 10% can occur in patients who have severe cases of poison ivy.

Treatment

Treatment is based on the level of severity and on the location of the eruption. Mild, limited cases can be treated with calamine lotion and steroids, creams, lotions, or sprays. A hot water soak can relieve mild pruritus. Antihistamines can also be given to control mild pruritus.

Domeboro's soaks (aluminum sulfate) diluted to a 10:1 mixture can also be applied every 30 to 60 minutes to relieve pruritus. Potassium permanganate baths can be utilized for large areas. Colloidal oatmeal (Aveeno) can also be used to treat pruritus.

Systemic corticosteroids such as prednisone (40 to 60 mg tapered over 2 to 3 weeks) should be used in every instance except mild cases. Dexamethasone acetate (Decadron) 8 mg intramuscularly (IM) with triamcinolone (Aristocort) or 40 mg IM as a one-dose injection can also be used. Prednisone is not given orally if the injection is given. A shorter course of less than 2 weeks should not be used secondary to rebound exacerbations. The patient should be examined for signs of secondary infection, which, if present, should be treated with antibiotics.

In the case of a patient with a severe reaction, or if the patient's profession chronically exposes him or her to *Toxicodendron*, the patient can be referred to an allergist for desensitization. The patient will be required to take high doses of urushiol orally for 4 to 8 months for the purpose of desensitization.

URTICARIA

Definition

Urticaria is also known as the hives, cnidosis, and nettle rash. Urticaria is a vascular reaction of the skin to many different antigens and chemical substances. Urticaria can be classified as acute or chronic. If urticaria lasts longer than 4 to 6 weeks, it is considered chronic.

Angioedema (Quincke's edema) is a form of subcutaneous urticaria. Some of the other types of urticaria include vibratory, dermatographia, pressure, aquagenic, cholinergic, adrenergic, cold, solar, heat, exercise, and papular urticaria.

Epidemiology

Of the population, 15 to 20% will experience urticaria in their lifetimes. Chronic urticaria is found more often in women in their 40s and 50s.

Pathology

The wheals are caused by localized edema secondary to transvascular fluid extravasation. Urticaria can involve many mediators, including bradykinin, histamine, acetylcholine, and kallikrein. The urticarial response to a substance can be immunologic or nonimmunologic. Nonimmunologic-mediated urticaria is usually secondary to the degranulation of mast cells, which is secondary to ingestion of aspirin, foods, drugs, or narcotics. Numerous etiologies include fungal infections; inhalants such as dusts, molds, animal danders, pollen, aerosols; insect stings; malignancy; parasitic infections; hyperthyroidism; sinusitis; pregnancy; contact chemicals such as cosmetics; textiles; marine animals; physical agents such as cold, heat, sunlight, and pressure; viral infections such as mononucleosis and coxsackievirus; and antibiotics—all can cause urticaria. Food additives, physical or emotional stress, menthol, and serum sickness can also cause urticaria.

Clinical Presentation

Patients present with a severe stinging, itching, or prickling sensation. Often those who are having an urticarial reaction to penicillin will have urticaria on the palms and soles. Patients can also present with tissue involvement other than the skin, including the lungs, bowel, and vascular system, which can lead to anaphylaxis. Patients can present with asthma, coryza, diarrhea, shortness of breath, and abdominal pain. Severe life-threatening laryngeal edema can occur with severe urticaria.

Angioedema usually affects the genitals, eyelids, lips, lobes of the ears, and mucous membranes, including the tongue, larynx, and mouth. The affected area is usually not ecchymotic and is only slightly tender. There will be diffuse edema of the hands and feet. Angioedema often occurs at night during sleep. Headaches, seizure, urticaria, and angioedema have been found in encephalopathy. Angioedema is believed to be caused by the same factors as urticaria. There is also a hereditary form of angioedema.

Examination

On examination the skin will have the appearance of wheals, which are elevated, white, or red evanescent plaques that are usually surrounded by a red halo or flare. There may be subcutaneous swelling (angioedema) of the eyelids or lips.

Diagnosis

A diagnosis is made by clinical presentation of transitory urticarial wheals.

Laboratory Findings

On histologic examination, the dermis will reveal capillary and venous vasodilation. On a CBC differential examination, eosinophilia may be present.

Treatment

Whatever the offending agent (e.g., foods, drugs, chemicals, soaps, or detergent) that caused the acute urticarial exacerbation, the reaction should be stopped. If urticaria is secondary to an environmental exposure, the patient should be protected from this exposure as much as possible. If severe urticaria is present with possible onset of anaphylaxis, the patient should receive diphenhydramine (Benadryl), 50 mg IV; methylprednisolone sodium succinate (Solu-Medrol), 2 mg/kg IV; and epinephrine 1:1000 subcutaneously (SQ) 0.3 to 1 ml; or epinephrine suspension (Sus-Phrine) 0.1 to 0.3 ml SQ. The patient should be placed on oxygen and have at least one large-gauge IV of normal saline 0.9% placed. In severe attacks, terbutaline (Brethine), a β_2-adrenergic agent, can be given 1.25 mg orally three times a day (TID). Terbutaline can also be given SQ or IV if the patient is in anaphylaxis. Cimetidine (Tagamet), 300 mg IV, can also be used for severe attacks of urticaria. An oral β-agonist (albuterol) should be given if wheezing is present.

In a mild case in which the patient has no respiratory problems, diarrhea, shortness of breath, nausea, or vomiting, the patient can be given hydroxyzine (Atarax), 25 mg by mouth as needed every 4 to 6 hours or diphenhydramine, 50 mg every 4 to 6 hours as needed for pruritus. Terfenadine (Seldane), 60 mg orally twice a day, can also be given; however, this drug has a much less sedating effect for pruritus. Patients can also be given a short 5-day course of prednisone 1 mg/kg for 5 days for treatment of urticaria. If urticaria is severe or chronic, a 3-week tapered course of prednisone should be given.

Any patient with respiratory problems, wheezing, nausea, vomiting, or diarrhea or who has a history of an anaphylactic reaction should be admitted to the hospital.

BIBLIOGRAPHY

Arnold HL, Odom RB, James WD (eds): Andrews' Diseases of the Skin: Clinical Dermatology, 8th ed. Philadelphia, WB Saunders, 1990

Braunwald E, Isselbacher KJ, Petersdorf RG, et al (eds): Harrison's Principles of Internal Medicine, 11th ed. New York, McGraw-Hill, 1987

Hamilton GC, Sanders AB, Strange GR, et al (eds): Emergency Medicine: An Approach to Clinical Problem-Solving. Philadelphia, WB Saunders, 1991

Kravis TC, Warner CG, Jacobs LM (eds): Emergency Medicine: A Comprehensive Review, 3rd ed. New York, Raven Press, 1993

May HL, Aghababian RV, Fleisher GR (eds): Emergency Medicine, 2nd ed. Boston, Little, Brown, 1992

Rosen P, Barkin RM (eds): Emergency Medicine: Concepts and Clinical Practice, 3rd ed. St Louis, Mosby-Year Book, 1992

Schwartz GR, Cayten CG, Mangelsen MA, et al (eds): Principles and Practice of Emergency Medicine. Philadelphia, Lea & Febiger, 1992

Tierney LM, McPhee SJ, Papadakis MA (eds): Current Medical Diagnosis and Treatment, 33rd ed. Norwalk, CT, Appleton & Lange, 1993

Tintinalli JE, Krone RL, Ruiz E (eds): Emergency Medicine: A Comprehensive Study Guide, 4th ed. New York, McGraw-Hill, 1996

Wilkins EW, Dineen JJ, Gross PL (eds): Emergency Medicine Scientific Foundations and Current Practices, 3rd ed. Baltimore, Williams & Wilkins, 1989

Chapter 4

Acute Gastrointestinal Emergencies

CHOLELITHIASIS AND CHOLECYSTITIS

Definition

Bile is an enzyme that is required for the breakdown and absorption of fats in the intestine. The biliary tract consists of the gallbladder, the hepatic bile canaliculi, the intrahepatic bile duct, the extrahepatic bile duct, and the common bile duct. Cholelithiasis is the formation of gallstones in any part of the biliary tract. Cholecystitis is an acute inflammation of the gallbladder with fever, nausea, vomiting, and often infection of the biliary tract. Cholecystitis is an acute surgical emergency. Cholangitis is usually an acute obstruction of the common bile duct by a gallstone.

Epidemiology

Approximately 20% of women and 8% of the men in the United States have gallstones. Common risk factors for formation of gall-stones are obesity, female gender, age greater than 40 years, multiparity, and oral contraceptives. Rapid weight loss and the drug clofibrate are also associated with gallstones. There is an increased familial tendency for the formation of gallstones and a high incidence in Pima Indians. Biliary colic is rare in children: however, if found in this age group, biliary colic is associated with sickle cell anemia or spherocytosis. Cholelithiasis is also common in the pregnant patient.

Cholecystitis occurs in 5 to 19% of patients with biliary tract disorders. Cholecystitis has the same risk factors as cholelithiasis. Gangrene and necrosis with perforation of the gallbladder are the main complications of cholecystitis.

Pathology

The gallbladder stores approximately 50 ml of bile at any one time. When the stomach receives food (especially fatty food), both vagal responses and secretion of cholecystokinin (pancreozymin) cause the gallbladder to contract. Gallstones can consist of two types: pigmented and cholesterol. Pigmented gallstones come in two types: brown and black. Black gallstones occur in the gallbladder and contain high concentrations of calcium bilirubinate. Black gallstones are found more often in the elderly and in those with sickle cell disease and hereditary spherocytosis. Brown gallstones are found in the gall-bladder, intrahepatic duct, and extrahepatic duct. Brown gallstones are more often associated with infection.

The purpose of the gallbladder is to concentrate and acidify the bile. When this process is increased or rapidly reproduced and when rising cholesterol levels are present, lecithin and bile acids act to solubilize cholesterol. While cholesterol levels rise and lecithin and bile acids decline, cholesterol comes out of solution and forms crystals. These crystals cannot be expressed by the gallbladder into the common bile duct during contractions, thus causing pain in the right upper quadrant of the abdomen.

In cholecystitis, the cystic duct is usually obstructed. Gallstones are found in 95% of the patients with cholecystitis. Duct obstruction can be from external causes such as tumor, parasites, fibrosis, or kinking of the duct. Infection and bacterial organisms can be isolated in 50 to 75% of patients with a diagnosis of cholecystitis, with *Escherichia coli* being the most frequent organism isolated.

Clinical Presentation/Examination

The most common presentation for a patient with cholelithiasis or cholecystitis is biliary colic, right upper quadrant pain after ingestion of fatty foods or dairy products, nausea, and vomiting. The pain often radiates to the right upper shoulder at the base of the scapula. The pain can be constant or intermittent. Symptoms can occur without ingestion of food. On physical examination there can be mild right upper quadrant or epigastric tenderness.

Patients with cholecystitis present much like those with cholelithiasis: They have right upper quadrant colicky pain, nausea, vomiting, and pain radiating to the base of the right scapula. Fever is often present, and the patient will be tachycardiac. Murphy's sign (tenderness on inspiration and palpation of the right upper quadrant) is usually present but is not specific for cholecystitis or cholelithiasis. Emphysematous cholecystitis occurs in 1% of patients with cholecystitis. Emphysematous cholecystitis is caused by gas-forming organisms (e.g., *Clostridium perfringens, Klebsiella*, and *E. coli*) in the gallbladder. The outcome is poor, and the patients present more acutely ill. Acalculous cholecystitis is more common in the elderly and has a predominance among males.

Diagnosis

A diagnosis is made by history, physical examination, and ultrasonography or by oral cholecystography with iopanoic acid. Nuclear scintigraphy is the best test for diagnosis of cholecystitis.

Laboratory Findings

A complete blood count (CBC), electrolytes, aspartate aminotransferase (AST), alanine aminotransferase (ALT), and liver function tests, including bilirubin, amylase, lipase, and urinalysis, should be performed on all patients suspected of having cholelithiasis or cholecystitis. All laboratory test results are usually normal in the case of cholelithiasis. With cholecystitis, there is usually leukocytosis with a shift to the left. Alkaline phosphatase, serum aminotransferase, and bilirubin levels are usually mildly elevated. Amylase is not usually elevated, and, if it is, pancreatitis should be considered in the differential diagnosis.

Radiography

An acute abdominal series should be performed to rule out other pathology of abdominal pain. Only 10% of all gallstones are radiopaque.

Treatment

Cholelithiasis consists of fluid and electrolyte replacement, control of vomiting with antiemetics, and nasogastric suctioning. Pain can usually be controlled with ketorolac tromethamine (Toradol), glycopyrrolate, or opiate analgesics. Morphine can cause the sphincter of Oddi to spasm, thus reducing the outflow of bile. It is suggested that morphine not be used in an acute setting until a definitive diagnosis is made. The definitive treatment is surgery. Lithotripsy has been used on a few selected patients.

Patients with cholecystitis are treated the same as patients with cholelithiasis in regard to fluid replacement, antiemetics, nasogastric suctioning, and pain management. Antibiotics are recommended for cholecystitis with a broad-spectrum antibiotic, a second- or third-generation cephalosporin. The patient is usually "cooled-off" prior to definitive surgery. If it is suspected that the gallbladder is necrotic or gangrenous, immediate surgery is recommended.

DIVERTICULOSIS AND DIVERTICULITIS

Definition

Diverticulosis is a false diverticulum (i.e., outpouching) of the mucosa and submucosa with the peritoneal covering intact, which has herniated through a defect in the circular muscular layer of the colon wall. It does not include all layers of the colon wall. Diverticulitis is an inflammatory process of the diverticulum of the colon.

Epidemiology

Diverticulosis rarely occurs in persons younger than 20 years of age. One third of the population will acquire diverticulosis by 45 years of age and two thirds by 85 years of age. Diverticulitis occurs in 10 to 25% of patients with diverticulosis. Diverticulitis is more commonly found in men, but it is on the increase in women.

Many patients will have recurrent attacks. In patients younger than 40 years of age with diverticulitis, the incidence of recurrent attacks is extremely high with 25% recurrence in 1 year, and 20% will require emergency surgery.

Pathology

The most common site of diverticular herniation is between the mesenteric and antimesenteric taenia, where the intramural blood vessels penetrate the muscularis muscle.

Laplace's law states that tension on a wall of a hollow cylinder is proportional to the radius of the cylinder multiplied by the pressure within the cylinder. Based on Laplace's law, the most common cause of diverticulosis is that diverticulosis is secondary to high intraluminal pressures in areas of weakness in the colon. The anatomy of the colon is important to this theorem. The sigmoid colon has the smallest lumen, thus this area is under the greatest pressure. The area of greatest diverticula is therefore present in the sigmoid colon.

Diverticulitis is caused by inflammation secondary to fecal material being inspissated into the neck of a diverticulum. This causes bacterial growth and an adjacent peridiverticulitis. Common organisms causing diverticulitis are aerobes (e.g., *Klebsiella, Enterobacter,* and *E. coli*) and anaerobes (e.g., *Clostridium, Peptostreptococcus,* and *Bacteroides fragilis*).

Clinical Presentation

The diagnosis of acute diverticulitis should always be considered in any patient older than 50 years of age with right or left lower abdominal pain. Patients often complain of a change in bowel habits that includes constipation or diarrhea. Patients with diverticulitis present most often with left lower abdominal pain with or without bloody stools. Patients with diverticulitis will present with a low-grade fever of 100.4° C. Patients often describe the pain as a steady or deep pain. The pain often mimics an acute appendicitis secondary to a redundant sigmoid colon laying on the right side of the abdomen over the appendix. Patients often complain of dysuria, pyuria, and frequency secondary to irritation of the bladder and ureter by an inflamed diverticulum.

On rare occasions a fistula can form from the colon to the bladder, and the patient will complain of pneumaturia or chronic urinary tract infections (UTIs). Small bowel obstructions, ileus, or free air from perforation can be the presenting complaint mimicking diverticulitis.

Examination

On physical examination the patient presents with a left lower abdominal tenderness with voluntary guarding and localized rebound tenderness. A mass can often be palpated in the left lower quadrant of the abdomen secondary to edema of the colon. All patients with abdominal pain should receive a rectal examination. Female patients should also receive a pelvic examination to rule out gynecologic pathology.

Diagnosis

In any patient who presents with abdominal pain, change in bowel habits, and bloody stool and is older than 40 years of age, ulcerative colitis, Crohn's disease, ischemic colitis, irritable bowel syndrome, or acute appendicitis should be considered in the differential diagnosis of diverticulitis.

Ulcerative colitis usually presents in patients younger than 30 years of age but peaks again in the sixth decade. These patients have frequent loose stools, rectal bleeding, and no abdominal tenderness. Ulcerative colitis starts in the lower colon and marches up the colon. It is cured by surgery.

Crohn's disease can occur from the tip of the tongue to the rectum. It can cause a transmural fistula or an abscess that can be difficult to differentiate from diverticulitis. Patients with Crohn's disease present with mucus in the stool, diarrhea, and rectal pain. They often have rectal skin tags and fissures or fistulas. These patients need a sigmoidoscopy with a tissue biopsy. Surgery is postponed as long as possible secondary to the ability of Crohn's disease to recur anywhere in the intestinal system.

Cancer of the colon causes a luminal narrowing of the colon or small bowel obstruction with a decreased size of stool. Patients can have diarrhea or constipation. The stools are often bloody, and the patient loses weight. A mass can usually be felt on rectal or abdominal examination and is usually nontender. Cancer patients often have anemia without an elevated white blood cell count.

Irritable bowel syndrome is a disease of exclusion. Patients with irritable bowel syndrome present with crampy or colicky pain that is caused by emotional upset or food, and the passage of flatus often brings relief of symptoms. The patient with an irritable bowel will alternate between bouts of constipation and diarrhea. The patient will be afebrile, and on abdominal examination a cord-like mass, the sigmoid colon, can often be felt in the left lower abdomen.

Laboratory Findings

All patients with suspected diverticulitis, or abdominal pathology, should have a CBC, electrolytes, BUN, creatinine, amylase, lipase, liver enzymes, and urinalysis performed. A pregnancy test should be performed on all females of child-bearing years.

An acute abdominal series should be performed on all patients to rule out ileus, and a check should be done for free air, small bowel obstruction, or foreign bodies that can all mimic diverticulitis. Abdominal computed tomography (CT) or ultrasound can be helpful in the diagnosis of diverticulitis and other abdominal pathology. A contrast or barium enema should not be performed in the acute phase of diverticulitis.

Treatment

Patients with diverticulitis should be treated with fluid replacement, bowel rest, and antibiotics. Most of the common organisms can be treated with ampicillin, cephalosporins, or metronidazole for 10 days. If the patient is allergic to penicillin, tetracycline can also be used.

If the patient has systemic signs of infection or sepsis, he or she should be admitted to the hospital and given intravenous (IV) fluids and IV antibiotics. Clindamycin, ampicillin, metronidazole, or an aminoglycoside is used for both aerobic and anaerobic coverage. Doses are:

1. Cefoxitin 2–3 g IV every 8 hours *or*
2. Gentamicin or tobramycin 1 to 1.66 mg/kg IV every 8 hours *plus* metronidazole or clindamycin 500 mg IV every 6 hours

Ten percent to 25% of patients treated for diverticulitis will have recurrent attacks. The current recommendation is that if the patient has two attacks or more, the patient should undergo elective resection of the involved part of the colon.

If hemorrhage from diverticulitis occurs, a transfusion is indicated. Colonoscopy or sigmoidoscopy is diagnostic 50% of the time for the bleeding site in patients with hemorrhage. Selective arterial catheterization can be diagnostic and therapeutic. When the bleeding source cannot be determined on colonoscopy or sigmoidoscopy, arterial catheterization can be performed, and infusion of vasopressin (0.2 units/min for 6 to 12 hours) can be given to slow or stop the bleeding from the diverticulum. Once the patient is in stable condition, surgery should be performed. Early consultation with a gastroenterologist or a surgeon is part of the management of bleeding diverticula.

ESOPHAGEAL TRAUMA

Definition

Esophageal trauma can be caused by swallowed foreign objects, perforation secondary to ingestion of caustic agents, sclerosing agents in an attempt to correct esophageal varices, lacerations of the mucosa or submucosa (Mallory-Weiss syndrome), or perforation of the full thickness of the thoracic and abdominal esophageal wall (Boerhaave's syndrome).

Epidemiology

Mallory-Weiss tears account for 5 to 9% of upper gastrointestinal (GI) bleeds. Mallory-Weiss tears are common in the alcoholic patient (75%). They are also common in a patient with a history of hiatal hernias (42%). Esophagitis and gastritis are common predisposing complaints. The bleeding is usually mild and resolves spontaneously in most cases.

Complete ruptures of the esophagus are caused by foreign bodies, iatrogenic procedures, blunt or penetrating trauma, caustic burns, chemical ingestion, pneumatic rupture, or postoperative breakdown of an anastomosis or violent vomiting or retching. Seventy percent of all esophageal perforations are iatrogenic. Boerhaave's syndrome is a spontaneous rupture of the esophagus.

Always consider myocardial infarction, pulmonary embolus, aortic aneurysm, spontaneous pneumomediastinum, perforated peptic ulcer, cholecystitis, mesenteric thrombosis, or pancreatitis in the differential diagnosis when considering Boerhaave's rupture or a Mallory-Weiss laceration.

Pathology

Mallory-Weiss lacerations are secondary to weakened mucosa, usually on the right posterolateral side of the esophagus. Mallory-Weiss lacerations are tears of the mucosa and submucosa. They occur secondary to violent vomiting or retching and increased intra-abdominal pressure secondary to blunt trauma, protracted coughing, and seizures. There are usually one or more tears in the esophagus in 70% of the cases.

Boerhaave's perforation is a complete perforation of the esophageal wall, causing the spillage of acidic gastric fluid in the mediastinum, thus causing mediastinitis. This also encourages bacteria to spread rapidly. It is usually secondary to violent vomiting or retching. The distal esophagus is often the site of rupture and usually involves a longitudinal tear in the left posterolateral part of the esophagus. Eighty percent of Boerhaave's perforations occur in middle-aged men who have a history of alcohol or large food intake in the last 24 hours. Eighty percent of ruptures occur in an esophagus in which there is no previous disease, and 25% of patients will have no history of vomiting. Fifty percent have a neurologic abnormality or are intoxicated at the time of rupture.

Clinical Presentation/Examination

The patient with a Mallory-Weiss tear presents with a history of multiple bouts of emesis and then sudden hematemesis. A history of retching is only present in half of the presentations.

A patient with Boerhaave's perforation will present with severe abdominal pain and chest pain that radiates to the neck. The patient will proceed rapidly to shock, septicemia, and death. On abdominal series of x-rays, air under the diaphragm and air-fluid levels in the pyopneumothorax and mediastinum are often noted. Subcutaneous emphysema is often noted. The patient often presents in cardiopulmonary collapse.

Often before subcutaneous emphysema is noted in the neck, the patient presents with an increased nasal quality in the voice. As the air increases in the mediastinum, a systolic crunching sound or Hamman's crunch is heard during a heart examination.

Diagnosis

Boerhaave's syndrome is diagnosed by history, clinical presentation, physical examination, and chest radiograph. On chest x-ray, the x-ray will classically show a pneumothorax, widened mediastinum, left-sided pleural effusion, and mediastinal air with or without subcutaneous emphysema. Lateral views of the cervical spine should also be obtained. These views will often show air or fluid in the retropharyngeal area if the rupture is a cervical rupture or perforation.

A patient presenting with a Mallory-Weiss laceration will present with a complaint or history of vomiting blood with or without chest pain, usually after alcohol intake or violent vomiting or retching.

Laboratory Findings

An examination of a CBC, electrolytes, cardiac enzymes, prothrombin time (PT), partial thromboplastin time (PTT), blood cultures, and type and cross of blood should be performed on all suspected patients with a Mallory-Weiss or Boerhaave lesion.

Treatment

Any patient who presents with the signs or symptoms of Mallory-Weiss or Boerhaave's rupture should have two large-gauge IVs placed with normal saline or lactated Ringer's solution, the aforementioned laboratory tests done, and chest, abdominal, and cervical spine x-rays performed. Also the aforementioned etiologies of chest pain must be ruled out. Antibiotics should be given immediately, and a surgical consultation should be obtained without delay. Surgical intervention is also required immediately.

GASTROINTESTINAL BLEEDING

Definition

GI bleeding can come from anywhere in the GI tract. Hematemesis is coffee-ground emesis that comes from an area proximal to the ligament of Treitz. Melena is from a source proximal to the right colon, and hematochezia is from a distal colorectal site. GI bleeding is defined as upper or lower GI bleeding. Upper GI bleeding is proximal to the ligament of Treitz (at the junction of the duodenum and jejunum). Lower GI bleeds are those distal to the ligament of Treitz.

Epidemiology

Mortality from GI bleeds is approximately 10%. The mortality rate has not changed in the past 4 decades for GI bleeds despite better diagnostic capabilities and treatment modalities. Upper GI bleeds occur in 50 to 150/100,000 persons per year. There are fewer lower GI bleeds that require hospitalization. Upper GI bleeds are most common in patients older than 50 years of age. Most acute hemorrhages occur in patients older than 60 years of age. Upper GI bleeds are more frequent in males than in females. Children have more lower GI bleeds than do adults. Eight percent of all GI bleeds stop spontaneously. Mortality rates approach 23% in those who require emergency surgery for a GI bleed.

Pathology

Numerous drugs, including nonsteroidal anti-inflammatory drugs (NSAIDs), salicylates, anticoagulants, and corticosteroids, have all been associated with GI bleeding. Peptic ulcer disease, esophageal varices, and erosive gastritis have all been associated with the ingestion of alcohol. Always obtain a history of ingestion of beets, which can stimulate hematochezia, or the ingestion of bismuth or iron, which can simulate melena.

A surgical history should always be obtained, especially from patients who have had an aortic graft. Consider an aortoenteric fistula if there is GI bleeding and a history of an aortic graft. A second GI bleed is not always from the same source as a prior GI bleed.

The most common upper GI bleed is caused by peptic ulcer disease (45%). The other 55% consist of gastric erosions, varices, Mallory-Weiss tears, esophagitis, and duodenitis. Lower GI bleeds are caused by diverticulosis, angiodysplasia, and polyps secondary to cancer, rectal disease, rectal fissures, and inflammatory bowel disease.

Clinical Presentation/Examination

Patients with suspected GI bleeds should have two large-gauge IVs placed and oxygen administered. The evaluation, diagnosis, resuscitation, and stabilization phases are usually performed simultaneously in the case of an acute GI bleed. The patient's vital signs should be monitored every 5 minutes until the patient's condition has stabilized.

The skin can be cool and clammy, and the patient will be hypotensive and tachycardic. Look for jaundice, palmar erythema, spider angiomata, or gynecomastia, which are all signs of chronic liver disease. Obtain a PT and PTT, especially if there is a history of liver disease. Petechiae and purpura are signs of underlying coagulopathy or signs of Gardner's syndrome, Peutz-Jeghers syndrome, or Rendu-Osler-Weber disease.

Examine the entire patient to include a complete eyes, ears, nose, and throat (EENT) examination. A posterior nasal bleed can simulate an upper GI bleed secondary to the swallowing of blood.

A rectal examination should be done to check the color of the stool and for the presence of blood. Bright red blood usually means a lower

GI bleed in the extreme distal portion of the colon; melena signifies a more proximal bleed.

The monitoring of vital signs are very important in a patient with an acute GI bleed. There will be no change in vital signs with the patient in the supine position until there is a 15% blood loss (10 ml/kg) or greater, but a patient with a 15 ml/kg blood loss will have postural changes of systolic pressure changes of equal to or greater than 20 mm Hg or a pulse equal to or greater than 20 beats/min.

A patient with a GI bleed will often be hypothermic. The patient will also often be hyperventilating on presentation. Remember that the foremost cause of anxiety in the emergency department (ED) is hypoxia. If the patient is very anxious, his or her oxygen-carrying capacity is compromised secondary to a lack of red blood cells. A capillary refill time greater than 2 seconds is a quick test of distal perfusion.

Diagnosis

Diagnosis of upper GI bleeding is made by placement of a nasogastric tube with gastric lavage or endoscopy. Barium swallows have limited value in the ED. Angiography can also be used, especially when vasopressors are being considered. Colonoscopy is used to diagnose lower GI bleeds.

Laboratory Findings

Every patient with a suspected GI bleed should have a CBC, PT, PTT, liver function tests to include amylase and lipase, electrolytes to include BUN and creatinine, urinalysis, and type and cross of 4 to 6 units of blood if the patient is hemodynamically unstable or is having increased bleeding. Remember that in cases of acute blood loss the hematocrit may be normal. An electrocardiogram (ECG) and x-rays of the chest and abdomen should be performed. An elevated PT is indicative of a vitamin K deficiency, warfarin therapy, liver disease, or consumptive coagulopathy. There is an 80% mortality rate for patients who present with a BUN level of greater than 100 mg/dl.

Treatment

All patients with suspected GI bleeds should have two large-gauge (14- or 16-g) IVs started. Crystalloid solutions should be utilized in resuscitation of the patient. Fluid should be given in 5- to 20-ml/kg boluses, and the patient's vital signs should be re-evaluated after each bolus of fluid until 50 ml/kg has been given. After 50 ml/kg has been given, blood products should be given. Patients with impending cardiopulmonary arrest from hemorrhagic shock should be given O negative blood immediately, but type and crossmatched blood is preferred. Whole blood is preferred but, if not available, the patient can be given packed red blood cells. Fresh frozen plasma (FFP) is needed to correct coagulopathies secondary to liver failure or warfarin therapy or when the total platelet count is less than 50,000/mm².

A nasogastric tube should be placed. Vital signs should be taken every 5 minutes, and the patient should be placed on oxygen and a Foley catheter placed to monitor urinary output. The patient should be placed on pulse oximetry and a cardiac monitor. Bright red blood expelled from the rectum is usually from a lower GI bleed; however, if a massive upper GI bleed is present, an upper GI source of bright red blood per rectum can give you a false sense of security. All GI bleeds should be treated as life threatening until the source of the bleed is defined.

Gastric lavage should be performed on every patient if awake. Remember that a negative lavage does not rule out an acute bleed. Pyloric spasm or edema might be present, thus preventing reflux of duodenal blood from an acute bleed. Iced solutions have no proven benefit over solutions at room temperature. Do not perform overvigorous suctioning after the lavage. A Foley catheter should be placed, and a goal of 30 ml/hr of urine output in an adult should be met.

Histamine H_2 antagonists should be used. Cimetidine (300 mg IV every 6 hours) or ranitidine (50 mg IV every 6 to 8 hours) should be used.

Patients who are unstable should be placed in the Trendelenburg position on their left side. Military anti-shock trousers (MAST) are controversial and are not usually recommended. Endoscopy is the most accurate diagnostic tool for detection of upper GI bleeds. It can identify a lesion in 78 to 95% of cases. If the bleed is a variceal bleed, sclerotherapy can be performed by a gastroenterologist. Angiography is still used, especially with lower GI bleeds and the use of vasopressors.

Colonoscopy is used when a lower GI bleed is suspected. Colonoscopy is usually performed 48 to 72 hours after presentation, after the bowel has been prepared. Colonoscopy is better than barium enema for evaluating lower GI bleeds.

Use of vasopressin (0.2 to 0.6 units/min IV) can be considered in management of massive GI bleeds. It is most commonly used for control of a variceal hemorrhage. IV nitroglycerin should be given when vasopressin is given to reduce the side effects of vasopressin.

In acute esophageal variceal bleeds, the Sengstaken-Blakemore or Linton tubes can be utilized to stop a variceal bleed. An endoscopy should be performed prior to their use. These tubes act by tamponading the variceal bleeding in a patient who is exsanguinating, and they are utilized when vasopressin has not slowed a variceal bleed.

Surgery is indicated in patients who are hemodynamically unstable, who have failed medical therapy, and who are actively bleeding.

All patients with unstable vital signs at time of admission, persistent bleeding, age greater than 75 years, large drop in hematocrit, or comorbid disease should be admitted to the hospital. Patients with true melena should also be admitted to the hospital. Melena is indicative of 20 ml of blood loss.

JAUNDICE AND HEPATITIS

Definition

Jaundice is a term used to describe the yellow color of the skin, sclera, and mucous membranes caused by the increased deposit of bilirubin. Hepatitis is a term used to describe inflammation of the liver. Hepatitis can be caused by a virus, bacteria, fungal, parasite, prescribed medication, immunologic disorder, or toxic exposure.

Epidemiology

Hepatitis A virus (HAV) is spread by the fecal-oral route or by contaminated food or water. Transmission via blood is theoretically possible with HAV. HAV is a ribonucleic acid (RNA) virus of the enteroviral picornaviruses group. HAV usually presents in epidemics. One half of persons living in cities in the United States are seropositive for HAV. Occult disease is more prevalent in the pediatric age group. Fecal shedding occurs before the onset of the prodrome, and there is no carrier state in HAV. There are about 30,000 cases of HAV in the United States annually, but this is probably a gross underestimate of the actual cases. Most cases are undiagnosed.

Hepatitis B virus (HBV) is a deoxyribonucleic acid (DNA) virus. There are eight subtypes of HBV that are defined by the surface antigens. HBV is transmitted by intimate contact and by parenteral exposure. Most transmission occurs between IV drug users, homosexual contact, and hemodialysis patients. Blood transfusion was the original mode of transmission, but with blood bank screening procedures this mode of transmission is rare today. There is usually no clear history of exposure.

Hepatitis non-A non-B (HNANB) is an RNA virus. There are two subtypes of transmission: (1) transfusion, and (2) fecal-oral. HNANB is now called hepatitis C. There is a 5 to 10% change of receiving the virus with a blood transfusion in the United States. Occupational exposure in health workers is also a concern. Fifty percent of those who are infected with hepatitis C go on to develop chronic hepatitis, and cirrhosis develops in 20% of those patients. HNANB accounts for 20 to 40% of parenterally transmitted forms of viral hepatitis and 80 to 90% of transfusion-related viral hepatitis.

Hepatitis delta virus (HDV) is an RNA virus. It can only infect patients who are actively producing hepatitis B surface antigen (HBsAg), thus a coinfection exists. Between 4% and 30% of patients who have HBV also have HDV. When coinfection is present, HBV is usually the dominant viral infection. HDV carries an increased risk of fulmination of disease. Chronic HDV results in chronic cirrhosis in 80% of patients in the chronic state. Fulminant liver failure is seen most often in IV drug users.

Toxic hepatitis can be caused by exposure to halothane, methyldopa, isoniazid, anabolic steroid, amrinone, acetaminophen, chlorpromazine, or alcohol.

Pathology

Bilirubin is the breakdown of hemoglobin. Hemoglobin is broken down secondary to an injury to the red blood cells and senescence of red blood cells. Bilirubin is carried on albumin. It is conjugated in the reticuloendothelial system mostly as diglucuronide and is excreted in the bile channels into the small intestine. A change in the destruction of red blood cells, an increase in the production of bilirubin, or a defect in the elimination pathway will produce jaundice and hyperbilirubinemia.

There are two subtypes of hyperbilirubinemia: conjugated and unconjugated. Conjugated hyperbilirubinemia is the result of the liver's inability to excrete bilirubin. This cholestasis is either intrahepatic or extrahepatic. Intrahepatic cholestasis is caused by hepatocellular damage, damage to the biliary endothelium, or decreased excretion of conjugated bilirubin. Obstructive or extrahepatic cholestasis is secondary to gallstones, mass lesions, congenital defect, or secondary inflammation due to another disease process (e.g., pancreatitis, pancreatic cancer).

Unconjugated hyperbilirubinemia is secondary to the increased bilirubin processing or load or a defect in the ability of the hepatocyte to take up conjugated bilirubin.

Viral hepatitis is the most common type of hepatitis: type A (infectious), type B (serum), type C (non-A non-B), and delta virus. Viral hepatitis causes liver inflammation and necrosis of the hepatic parenchymal cells.

Alcoholic hepatitis is caused by hepatocellular necrosis and by intrahepatic inflammation. Patients often present with dark urine, fever, and jaundice.

Clinical Presentation/Examination

A patient with viral hepatitis might present with a variety of symptoms, including nausea, vomiting, malaise, fatigue, and taste changes. Low-grade fever, pharyngitis, coryza, and headache are early symptoms and constitute the usual prodrome. The patient might complain of having the "flu." Dark urine and pruritus are common. Jaundice develops 1 to 2 weeks after the onset of the prodromal symptoms. If right upper quadrant pain is present, it is secondary to liver enlargement. Hepatomegaly or splenomegaly are often present.

HAV has a normal incubation period of 15 to 45 days before the onset of the prodrome. The symptoms are more abrupt in onset than are the other types of hepatitis. Jaundice, if it appears, is usually mild and there is no carrier state. Gamma M immunoglobulin (IgM) and anti-HAV appear in the acute phase of hepatitis then are replaced by gamma G immunoglobulin (IgG) and anti-HAV, which persists indefinitely and confers immunity against HAV.

HBV has an incubation period of 60 to 90 days, but serologic markers are present in 1 to 3 weeks after exposure. Ninety percent of neonates infected and 10% of adults infected become chronic carriers. Most cases are insidious in onset or present as a "serum sickness–like" onset with proteinuria, polyarthritis, and angioneurotic edema. The symptoms are more prolonged than those that occur with HAV. Ninety percent of the patients recover completely. Only 1% develop fulminant hepatitis with liver failure. Eighty percent of those who develop encephalopathy and coma do die. Hepatitis C has an incubation period of 20 to 90 days, whereas HDV is a coinfection with HBV.

On physical examination the patient often has liver tenderness even if the liver is not enlarged. In blacks, the sclera might appear more "muddy" than yellow, and the sublingual or subungual surfaces of the mouth should be checked for icterus. Icterus is usually not found until the bilirubin level is greater than 2.5 mg/dl. Stools can also be gray; however, this is uncommon. Spider angiomata are usually seen in those with chronic cirrhosis.

Diagnosis

HAV will have positive IgM and anti-HAV during the acute clinical phase. A positive IgG level and anti-HAV confers immunity.

HBV has three distinct HBV antigens. Hepatitis B surface antigen (HBsAg) is the outer protein coat of the viral particle. This will appear before a rise in transaminase elevation and clinical symptoms. It remains positive for 1 to 2 months after the icteric phase and up to 6 months after the antigenemic phase. Anti-HBs appears in the serum approximately 2 to 6 months after HBsAg disappears. A positive anti-HBs infers prior infection or vaccination against HBV. Chronic carriers do not develop anti-HBs but maintain HBsAg levels.

Hepatitis B core antigen (HBcAg) does not appear in the serum. Anti-HBc appears approximately 2 weeks after the appearance of HBsAg, and between the time of disappearance of HBsAg and the appearance of anti-HBs. Anti-HBc is a marker for recent infection. A high titer of IgM anti-HBc is a sign of severe infection. Low levels are found in chronic carriers. IgG anti-HBc with HBsAg connotes chronic hepatitis, but IgG with anti-HBs connotes remote HBV infection. Hepatitis B e antigen (HBeAg) is found in serum that has HBsAg. A high level of HBeAg implies a high state of viral replication and severe infection from HBV. It persists in chronic hepatitis.

HDV infection can be diagnosed by finding anti-HDV in the serum by radioimmunoassay.

Laboratory Findings

The following laboratory levels should be drawn: a CBC, electrolytes, liver function tests, AST (formerly serum glutamic-oxaloacetic transaminase [SGOT]), ALT (formerly serum glutamic-pyruvic transaminase [SGPT]), total bilirubin, gamma glutamyltransferase (GGT), PT, and PTT should be performed on all suspected patients with hepatitis. A liver panel of tests should be done including anti-HAV, anti-HAV IgM, HBsAg, HBeAg, HBsAb, HBcAb, HBcAb-IgM, HBeAb, anti-HDV, and anti-HCV. ALT is usually elevated more than AST. Bilirubin is usually between 5 and 10 mg/dl. An acute elevation of the PT is a clue to a complicated course.

Acetaminophen, alcohol, or aspirin levels should be drawn if the patient has possibly been exposed to these drugs. In alcoholic hepatitis, the AST will be a ratio to ALT of 1:5. The serum aminotransaminase level will range from two to ten times the normal level. Bilirubin and alkaline phosphatase levels are usually normal, but elevated levels imply severe liver damage. Alcoholics will also present with thrombocytopenia, anemia, and leukopenia and the PT will be prolonged. A PT level greater than 8 is a poor prognostic sign. A fever in an alcoholic patient mandates a search for infection (e.g., pneumonia, urinary tract infection, meningitis, sepsis, or peritonitis).

Alcohol cirrhosis or Laënnec's cirrhosis is end-stage irreversible alcoholic liver disease.

Treatment

The primary treatment of hepatitis is to treat the symptoms. Criteria for admission of a patient to the hospital include:

1. Encephalopathy
2. A PT prolonged greater than 3 sec
3. Severe dehydration
4. Hypoglycemia
5. Bilirubin greater than 20 mg/dl
6. Age older than 45 years
7. Immunosuppression
8. Uncertain diagnosis

Most patients present with poor fluid intake, dehydration, and diarrhea. These patients are treated with IV fluids and antiemetics. Medications that are metabolized in the liver should not be given, or, if required, the dose should be modified during the acute illness. Consumption of alcohol should be stopped.

There is a vaccine against HBV, and this vaccine should be given to those at high risk of exposure (e.g., homosexual men, IV drug users, health care workers, police, firemen, patients on chronic hemodialysis, and household and sexual contacts of HBV carriers). The vaccine is given in a series of three doses.

Immune globulin contains anti-HAV and low titer anti-HBs. Hepatitis B immune globlin (HBIG) is used to prevent infection of HAV if given within 14 days of exposure. HBIG consists of a two-dose regimen.

Infections such as pneumonia should be treated with antibiotics that are not metabolized in the liver.

PANCREATITIS

Definition

Pancreatitis is an acute or chronic inflammation of the pancreas. Acute pancreatitis is usually secondary to alcohol abuse or gallstones.

Epidemiology

Patients who are older than 50 years of age and present to a community hospital usually have "biliary pancreatitis," and those who present to an inner-city hospital usually have alcoholic pancreatitis. Pancreatitis affects 1.5 per 100,000 persons in the United States.

Patients with primary hyperlipidemias (Frederickson types I, IV, and V) have an increased susceptibility to pancreatitis. Drugs such as tetracyclines, azathioprine, cisplatin, furosemide, L-asparaginase, thiazides, and sulfonamides can induce pancreatitis. Trauma, pregnancy, postoperative complications, polyarteritis nodosa, uremia, diabetes mellitus, diabetic ketoacidosis, hereditary pancreatitis, hemochromatosis, penetrating peptic ulcers, tumors, scorpion bites, and postpancreatography have all been determined to cause acute pancreatitis. Hypercalcemia and infectious agents such as mumps, hepatitis B virus, ascariasis, coxsackie group B, systemic lupus erythematosus, scarlet fever, dysentery, *Salmonella typhimurium, Legionella*, and *Mycoplasma* can all cause acute pancreatitis.

Pathology

The pancreas produces exocrines of bicarbonate, elastase, carboxypeptidase, phospholipase, amylase, lipase, trypsin, and chymotrypsin. Endocrines include insulin, glucagon, and somatostatin. The true mechanism of the inflammatory process of pancreatitis is unknown. The major causes of pancreatitis in the United States are alcohol and biliary disease. Biliary pancreatitis is usually secondary to a gallstone distal to the common duct with secondary ductal hypertension and pancreatic enzyme activation.

Pancreatitis due to alcohol is thought to be caused by direct injury by the toxic metabolite acetaldehyde or by the change in the metabolism of lipids. A second theory is one in which large alcohol consumption causes an increased stimulation of pancreatic secretions, and thus ductal hypertension, which precipitates the sphincter of Oddi to spasm. It usually take 5 to 15 years of chronic alcohol ingestion to cause the first symptoms of pancreatitis.

Clinical Presentation/Examination

Clinical presentation is very broad. Epigastric abdominal pain with nausea and vomiting is the most common complaint. The pain can often be severe. The pain is usually constant and radiates to the midback and the thoracolumbar region. If the pain is colicky, it is probably not pancreatitis. Patients are often tachycardiac and tachypneic secondary to pain and vomiting. Guarding is more common than is rebound tenderness. Grey Turner's sign and Cullen's sign are signs of hemorrhage or hemorrhagic pancreatitis.

Pulmonary involvement is present in 18 to 30% of patients with pancreatitis. Pleural effusions and hypoxia are usually present without pulmonary infiltrates secondary to microatelectasis. Pleural fluid will be high in amylase content. Acute respiratory distress syndrome is common in severe pancreatitis. Disseminated intravascular coagulation has been seen in severe pancreatitis.

Diagnosis

A diagnosis is made by history and physical examination, elevation of amylase and lipase, and the amylase-creatinine ratio. The prognosis of pancreatitis can be determined by the Ranson criteria:

Prognosis of Pancreatitis	
Diagnosis at Admission	**Diagnosis 48 Hours Later**
Age older than 55 years	Change in hematocrit (falling) or decreased by >10%
Blood glucose >200 mg/dl	Calcium <8%
White blood cell count (WBC) >16,000/mm³	BUN >5 mg/dl
Serum LDH >350 IU/l	Arterial P_{O_2} <60 mm Hg
Serum SGOT >250 Sigma-Fanlal units/L	Base deficit >4 mEq/l Fluid sequestration >6 liters

See Ranson JHC: Etiologic and prognostic factors in human pancreatitis: A review. Am J Gastroenterol 77:663, 1982. ©Williams & Wilkins.

Laboratory Findings

The following laboratory levels should be drawn: a CBC, electrolytes, BUN, creatinine, liver function tests to include AST, ALT, GGT, total bilirubin, blood culture, amylase and lipase, and urinalysis. Amylase is elevated in most cases with a 95% sensitivity but is poorly specific. Amylase is a product of two genes on chromosome 1, AMY 1 and AMY 2. The pancreas is the only organ that makes AMY 2. The amylase-creatinine clearance ratio is helpful in the diagnosis of pancreatitis. The normal clearance ratio is 3%. A ratio greater than 5% is consistent with the diagnosis of pancreatitis. Other diseases can cause elevated ratios besides pancreatitis.

$$\frac{\text{Amylase clearance (\%)}}{\text{Creatinine clearance (\%)}} = \frac{\text{urine amylase}}{\text{serum amylase}} \times \frac{\text{serum creatinine}}{\text{urine creatinine}} \times 100$$

Hypocalcemia, hyperlipidemia, and hyperglycemia are common in acute pancreatitis. Hyperglycemia in a nondiabetic patient is a poor prognostic indicator.

Lipase is almost always elevated in acute pancreatitis. Lipase is more sensitive than amylase to pancreatitis but is not very specific to pancreatitis. In hemorrhagic pancreatitis, hemoglobin may be split by the action of pancreatic enzymes and if this occurs methemalbumin is formed.

Treatment

Fluid resuscitation is the mainstay of treatment of acute pancreatitis. The goal of fluid resuscitation is to keep the kidneys perfused. A falling hematocrit should suggest hemorrhagic pancreatitis. A nasogastric tube should be placed to reduce vomiting and gastric stimulation, and the patient should take nothing by mouth. Pain control is essential. Remember that morphine constricts the sphincter of Oddi and should not be used in acute pancreatitis. Antibiotics are not necessary unless a secondary infection is present. An infection from the biliary tract should be treated with ampicillin or a third-generation cephalosporin. Cimetidine (Tagamet) can be used to help control gastric upset and hasten recovery.

An x-ray of the abdomen should be taken to rule out other pathology. Rarely, a calcification is noted in the pancreas. Patients with pancreatitis will often have an ileus or air in the small bowel near the pancreas. The use of a computed tomography (CT) scan of the abdomen in suspected pancreatitis is diagnostic and prognostic.

If patients are not improving, a peritoneal lavage should be considered. Peritoneal lavage can dilute or remove the toxic substances released by the pancreatic necrosis. If the patient has not improved in 7 days, another cause should be considered, such as a pancreatic abscess, pseudocyst, or pancreatic ascites.

PEPTIC ULCER DISEASE

Definition

A peptic ulcer is a mucosal lesion beyond the muscularis mucosae of the stomach or the proximal duodenal areas. It must occur in acid-secreting epithelium.

Epidemiology

Ulcers occur more frequently in the spring and fall. Patients with chronic pancreatitis and emphysema have a higher occurrence of duodenal ulcers. Patients with cirrhosis or very heavy alcohol intake have an increased risk for gastric ulcers. Patients with hyperparathyroidism and Zollinger-Ellison syndrome also have a higher risk for peptic ulcers. In children, the ulcers are usually prepyloric or duodenal in location. Ulcers are increasing in the elderly, probably secondary to the increased use of steroids for emphysema, chronic obstructive pulmonary disease and NSAIDs for arthritis. Duodenal ulcers are more common than gastric ulcers. There is a high rate of recurrence of peptic ulcer disease within 1 year of presentation of the first episode.

Patients who have had surgery or who have suffered burns, shock, head trauma, or central nervous system tumors can present with "stress ulcers."

Pathology

Precipitating factors of peptic ulcer disease include use of NSAIDs, alcohol ingestion, coffee, cigarette smoking, and cola drinks. Most peptic ulcers occur along the lesser curvature of the stomach or in the proximal duodenum. They can also occur along surgical anastomoses, in the distal esophagus, and in Meckel's diverticulum.

In the normal digestive system, the mucosa is protected from acid secretions by mucosal resistance. When an imbalance in acid secretion occurs, there is a disruption of endogenous prostaglandins. An ulcer occurs secondary to the gastric mucosa's inability to resist hydrogen ions. The inability of the mucosa to prevent "back" diffusion causes the ulcer and bleeding.

Gastric ulcers usually occur secondary to prolonged gastric emptying with low or normal gastric acid secretion. On the other hand, duodenal ulcers are caused by hypersecretion of gastric acid without delay in gastric emptying. On pathologic examination of gastric mucosa from patients with peptic ulcer disease, there is a noted increase in the number of parietal cells and an increased sensitivity of the parietal cells to stimulation. This process causes an increased rate of gastric emptying and a faster loss of the buffering protection of the food in the stomach. Thus the mucosa in the stomach are exposed to a greater duration of unbuffered or unprotected gastric acid secretion secondary to the faster emptying rate.

Clinical Presentation

The most common presenting complaint of a patient with gastric ulcer disease is burning epigastric pain soon after ingestion of food. This pain often radiates straight through to the back through the pancreas. Gastric ulcer pain does not occur between meals.

Duodenal ulcer pain usually occurs between meals and often wakes the patient up from sleep. The pain is often worse when the stomach is empty. The patient often complains that the pain is periodic and recurs over several months or years before he or she seeks medical attention. The pain is almost always partially relieved by over-the-counter medications prior to presentation. The patient often presents with the complaint that he or she has tried several over-the-counter medications but none give complete relief.

Patients can present for the first time with a perforation of a peptic ulcer. They present with a sudden and acute episode of severe epigastric pain. The abdomen can be rigid and may mimic an acute appendicitis, secondary to the fluids that come from the perforation and run down the colonic gutter into the right lower quadrant, causing peritonitis. On upright or lateral decubitus x-ray examination, there will be free air under the diaphragm.

Examination

All patients should receive a complete physical examination that should include a rectal examination. Patients usually feel mildly tender in the epigastric region on physical examination. If pain occurs in the right upper quadrant of the abdomen and the pain is associated with fatty food, gallbladder disease should be considered. Pancreatitis can present with a burning epigastric pain that radiates through to the back as well. A history of alcohol, steroid, or NSAID use should always be obtained.

Diagnosis

A diagnosis is made by an upper GI test series, a barium swallow, or an endoscopic examination.

Laboratory Findings

A routine CBC is done to check the hematocrit and hemoglobin for longstanding bleeding, and electrolyte levels should be obtained. If a bleeding ulcer is considered, a type and crossmatch of blood is indicated. If pancreatitis or gallbladder disease is considered, liver function tests, amylase, and lipase should be drawn.

Treatment

Mild duodenal ulcers can be treated with antacids, 30 ml by mouth 1 to 2 hours after meals and at bedtime. H_2-blockers (histamine antagonists) inhibit gastric secretions. Cimetidine (Tagamet), 400 mg twice a day or at bedtime for several weeks, has been shown to cure ulcers in 68 to 95% of the time. Ranitidine (Zantac) and carafate can also be used to treat peptic ulcer disease.

H_2 agents should be used cautiously in patients who are taking theophylline, phenytoin, warfarin, diazepam, propranolol, or lidocaine IV secondary to the change in liver metabolism of these drugs in conjunction with H_2 agents.

If gastric hemorrhage (an acute GI bleed) is considered, two large-gauge IVs of normal saline or lactated Ringer's solution should be started. Type and crossmatched blood should be obtained and the aforementioned laboratory studies should be performed. Treatment should be for an acute GI bleed. Vital signs are taken every 5 minutes until fluid resuscitation is successful. Nasogastric suctioning should be started. Cimetidine, 300 mg IV every 6 hours, or ranitidine should be given. If the patient is unstable, a central venous pressure line should be started to monitor pressure and fluid response. The patient should be admitted to the intensive care unit, and a gastroenterologist consulted for an immediate endoscopic examination.

If the patient is stable, he or she can be placed on antacids or H_2 antagonists and referred for a barium swallow or endoscopic procedure. All patients with peptic ulcers must be referred for further follow-up.

BIBLIOGRAPHY

Gore RM, Levine MS, Laufer I (eds): Textbook of Gastrointestinal Radiology. Philadelphia, WB Saunders, 1994

Hamilton GC, Sanders AB, Strange GR, et al (eds): Emergency Medicine: An Approach to Clinical Problem-Solving. Philadelphia, WB Saunders, 1991

Kravis TC, Warner CG, Jacobs LM (eds): Emergency Medicine: A Comprehensive Review, 3rd ed. New York, Raven Press, 1993

May HL, Aghababian RV, Fleisher GR (eds): Emergency Medicine, 2nd ed. Boston, Little, Brown, 1992

Pearson RD, Guerrant RL, Isselbacher KJ, et al (eds): Harrison's Principles of Internal Medicine, 11th ed. New York, McGraw-Hill, 1987

Rosen P, Barkin RM (eds): Emergency Medicine: Concepts and Clinical Practice, 3rd ed. St Louis, Mosby-Year Book, 1992

Schiff L, Schiff ER (eds): Diseases of the Liver. Philadelphia, JB Lippincott, 1993

Schwartz GR, Cayten CG, Mangelsen MA, et al (eds): Principles and Practice of Emergency Medicine. Philadelphia, Lea & Febiger, 1992

Sleisenger MH, Fordtran JS (eds): Gastrointestinal Disease: Pathophysiology, Diagnosis, and Management, 4th ed. Philadelphia, WB Saunders, 1989

Tierney LM, McPhee SJ, Papadakis MA (eds): Current Medical Diagnosis and Treatment, 33rd ed. Norwalk, CT, Appleton & Lange, 1994

Tintinalli JE, Krone RL, Ruiz E (eds): Emergency Medicine: A Comprehensive Study Guide, 4th ed. New York, McGraw-Hill, 1996

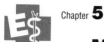

Chapter 5

Maxillofacial and Dental Emergencies

DENTAL EMERGENCIES

Definition

Patients can present to the emergency department (ED) with four general types of dental emergencies: (1) dentoalveolar trauma, (2) odontogenic pain, (3) hemorrhage, and (4) oral manifestations of systemic disease.

Pathology

There are 32 permanent teeth. There are four types of teeth: molars, premolars, canines, and incisors. From the midline of the front of the mouth posteriorly, there are: one central incisor, one lateral incisor, one canine, two premolars, and three permanent molars on each side (upper and lower). Additional teeth, called *supernumerary teeth*, can also be present.

The teeth are in, or affixed, to the mandible and the maxillary bones. The mandible is formed by two rami, which are divided into a horizontal portion and an ascending portion. The horizontal portion forms the mandible, and the ascending portion forms the coronoid process anteriorly and the condylar process posteriorly. The temporo-mandibular joint (TMJ) forms a diarthrosis between the mandibular fossa and the articular eminence of the temporal bone and the condyle of the mandible.

The muscles of the mouth, or muscles of mastication, are divided into the supramandibular group and the inframandibular group. The masseteric sling consists of the masseters, medial pterygoids, and temporalis muscles.

The tooth's anatomy is divided into the coronal portion, the part of the tooth seen in the mouth, and the root, which is the part that is embedded in the gingiva. The pulp of the tooth is the part of the tooth in which the neurovascular supply is formed. The coronal portion of the tooth, or the exposed part of the tooth, is the part of the tooth that is covered by the enamel. The unexposed root portion of the tooth is covered by cementum, which is softer than enamel. the coronal or crown of the tooth, from outside in, is made up of enamel, dentin, and pulp. The superior portion of the root is embedded in the gingiva, covered by the cementum, and held in place by the periodontal ligament to the alveolar bone. The apex of the tooth is where the dental nerve and vessels exit.

Clinical Presentation

Patients present to the ED most often with complaints of dental caries and periodontal disease. Dental caries is a multifactorial disease involving a susceptible host, cariogenic oral flora, and a substrate. Dental caries disease presents with toothache called *odontalgia*. The pain of odontalgia can be referred to the jaw, ear, eye, neck, or the opposite jaw.

Tooth eruptions are usually seen in infants and in children who are 5 to 8 years of age. There is controversy as to whether tooth eruption causes a low-grade fever in the infant. In adults, tooth eruption almost always involves the eruption of the third molar teeth. If food is impacted around the area of the third molar, subsequent inflammation can occur, causing *pericoronitis*.

Patients can also present with postextraction pain or *periosteitis*. If the patient presents with pain, foul odor, and foul taste in the mouth 2 to 3 days after a tooth extraction, the patient is suffering from a "dry socket" or *alveolar osteitis*. Alveolar osteitis is secondary to the loss of the blood clot and localized infection secondary to osteomyelitis.

A periodontal abscess is secondary to the entrapment of plaque and debris in a pocket between the tooth and the gingiva. The patient presents with swelling and pain of the gingiva or a *periodontal abscess*. If the periodontal abscess is left untreated, it can develop into acute necrotizing ulcerative gingivitis (ANUG), which is seen most commonly in young adults and adolescents. ANUG is caused by *Fusobacterium*, which invades the non-necrotic tissue. The patient will not only have signs of periodontal abscess, foul odor, and pain but will also present with fever, regional lymphadenopathy, and malaise. The gingiva will be edematous and fiery red. Ulcers will be present, and the tissue between the teeth will have a grayish pseudomembrane on the gingiva.

Patients will often present with complaints of oral lesions. These lesions can range from herpes zoster and stomatitis to viral or bacterial infections.

Patients can also present with nondental pain secondary to trigeminal neuralgia or tic douloureux, involving cranial nerve V. These patients will present with an acute, sharp, stabbing pain that starts suddenly and is separated by pain-free periods. It is diagnosed by history and by the patient pointing out the distribution of the pain in the fifth cranial nerve dermatome pattern. Trigger points or zones can often be found on examination. These trigger zones can reproduce the pain. Tic douloureux can be idiopathic or secondary to a cerebellopontine angle tumor, an acoustic neuroma, or a nasopharyngeal carcinoma or as a presenting complaint of multiple sclerosis.

Patients can also present with oral manifestations of systemic disease. Diabetes mellitus, acquired immunodeficiency syndrome, (AIDS), blood dyscrasias, granulomatous diseases, and collagen vascular disease can all present with oral manifestations. Patients with diabetes mellitus can present with gingival abscesses, dry mouth, gingival tenderness, pedunculated gingival proliferations, dry lips, increased tooth mobility, and gingival bleeding. Severe periodontal disease and chronic oral bleeding can also be present.

Patients with granulomatous disease can present with pyogenic granuloma, actinomycosis, or syphilitic ulcerations of the mouth. Pregnant females can present with a *pregnancy tumor* of the gingiva, which is a benign tumor that can recur if it is removed during pregnancy. If the tumor is still present 2 to 3 months after termination of pregnancy, it should be removed.

Patients with AIDS can present with numerous lesions of the oral mucosa secondary to countless causes. Many of these infections can be life threatening to the patient with AIDS and should never be taken lightly. The type of lesion should be determined and treated aggressively, and a referral should be made to a dentist who is experienced in treating dental problems in patients with AIDS. The patient should also be encouraged to follow up with a visit to an infectious disease specialist.

Acute leukemia can present with oral manifestations. The hyperplastic gingiva of acute granulocytic leukemia will present as bluish and edematous hyperplasia, which will almost completely cover the entire teeth. Chronic leukemia rarely involves the gingiva. Patients with leukemia can present with appetite loss, discomfort, gingival hemorrhage, and local infection.

Patients who take phenytoin for seizures or nifedipine for hypertension can present with phenytoin or nifedipine hyperplasia of the gingiva. This problem is found in younger patients and is not related to the dose or blood level. These patients present with severe hyperplasia and enlargement of the interdental papillae. The hyperplasia will encroach on the crown of the teeth. The gingiva will be pink, firm, and lobulated. The hyperplasia can be surgically removed, however, if either phenytoin or nifedipine therapy is continued, the hyperplasia can recur.

Examination

The patient should be given a complete physical examination. The sinuses should be percussed to rule out maxillary sinusitis. The ears should be examined to rule out acute otitis externa or media. Each tooth should be examined, and the gingiva should be palpated. The face should be examined for asymmetry secondary to an abscess or to facial cellulitis. The position of the eyeball should be examined to rule out a retrobulbar abscess causing referred pain.

Treatment

Dental caries odontalgia is treated acutely in the ED with analgesics, and/or the patient is referred to a dentist. If an abscess is present, the patient should be given penicillin or erythromycin, 250 to 500 mg four times a day (QID), and should be referred to a dentist. If a subperiosteal extension of the abscess or facial cellulitis with fluctuant swelling is present, an incision must be made and the site must be drained. The patient must be admitted to the hospital and given antibiotics intravenously (IV).

If the patient has recently undergone endodontic treatment with instrumentation, the patient can present with *pericementitis*, which is pain secondary to gas being sealed in the tooth during treatment. This patient should be referred back to the dentist or to an endodontist.

A patient with ANUG is treated with tetracycline 250 mg by mouth (po) QID or with penicillin 250 mg po QID, with warm saline rinses and application of topical local anesthetic agents to the gums (e.g., viscous lidocaine or 10% carbamide peroxide). These patients should be referred to the dentist or periodontist for 24-hour follow up.

A patient with postextraction pain is treated with copious irrigation of the socket with warm saline and then the socket is packed with medicated dental packing. If dental packing is not available, the socket should be packed with iodoform gauze that is slightly dampened with eugenol or Campho-Phenique. The patient should be referred back to his or her dentist within 12 to 24 hours.

Most lesions are herpangina or herpetic gingivostomatitis and are easily recognized. Lesions secondary to this type of infection are treated with viscous Xylocaine and oral acyclovir. It should always be determined if the patient is immunocompromised. The herpetic lesions are often secondarily infected. If secondary infections are present, treat with penicillin or erythromycin, 250 to 500 mg po QID. These patients should be referred to the dentist or primary care physician.

Tic douloureux may respond to treatment with carbamazepine, 100 mg twice a day (BID), and the dose should be increased gradually to a maximum dose of 1200 mg/day. Any patient with new-onset tic douloureux should be referred to a neurologist for a neurologic evaluation.

MAXILLOFACIAL FRACTURES

Definition

Maxillofacial fractures are usually secondary to blunt trauma. Good airway control is always a necessity in the management of any maxillofacial fracture. There are three basic principles of treatment to keep in mind when evaluating a patient with a maxillofacial fracture: (1) preservation of life by good airway control, (2) maintenance of function, specifically the masticatory apparatus, and (3) restoration of appearance.

Pathology

The face is divided into two areas. The arbitrary dividing line is the occlusal contact of the teeth. Above this line, fractures involve multiple frameworks of bone. They include the zygomatic arch, zygoma, nasal bones, orbital bones, and the maxilla. Fractures below this arbitrary line involve the mandible and its articulations and the TMJ. Types of fractures are classified as midfacial fractures, mandibular fractures, maxillary fractures, naso-orbital injuries, and TMJ injuries.

Clinical Presentation

Midfacial fractures include fractures and avulsions of the teeth and fractures of the zygomatic arch. A patient with a zygomatic arch injury or fracture will present with a depression or dimpling over the region of the zygomatic arch. There will be point tenderness at the fracture site. The patient may be unable to open his or her mouth secondary to impingement of the coronoid process of the mandible by the inward depressed fractured arch. It is rare to have an isolated fracture of the zygomatic arch, secondary to the amount of force that has to be directed over the arch, thus always look for a second fracture if a zygomatic arch fracture is present. Zygomatic arch fractures are best seen on a basal skull x-ray or submental-vertical view. These fractures are not life threatening, and treatment can be delayed. Cosmetic deformities can and should be corrected. If the fracture limits mandibular motion, it should be repaired immediately.

The zygomatic arch articulates with the maxilla, temporal bone, frontal bone, and the lateral wall of the maxillary sinus. Central portions of the orbital floor can fracture, affecting the function of the extraocular muscles. A patient may present with the following: facial flattening; circumorbital or subconjunctival ecchymosis; anesthesia of the cheek, upper lip, gum, or teeth; unilateral epistaxis; diplopia; and asymmetry of gaze or emphysema of the overlying tissue of the involved area of the face. If numbness of the cheek, teeth, gums, upper lip, and lateral ala nasi on the affected side is present, then the infraorbital nerve is injured at the zygomaticomaxillary fracture site.

Plain film x-rays can be taken along with a Water view. A computed tomography (CT) scan will often be necessary to define the magnitude and location of all fracture sites. Treatment is by surgery after the patient's airway has been stabilized and protected.

An *orbital floor fracture* is also a midfacial fracture. This fracture is present with a history of blunt trauma. Diplopia and lowering of the globe are the two most common physical findings. Diplopia is common with zygomaticomaxillary fractures, secondary to the zygomatic complex being depressed downward and medially. There will be a loss of extraocular motion of the affected muscles.

Visual acuity should be documented, and the eye should be examined for corneal abrasions or hyphemas. Diplopia may increase as swelling increases secondary to entrapment of the inferior rectus and oblique muscles, interruption of the muscle innervation, disruption of the muscular attachments, or orbital hemorrhage or edema. Serial examinations should therefore be performed. A good neurologic examination should be done on any patient who has a facial fracture. Surgical correction of the fracture is required. If ocular injury is present, an ophthalmologic consultation is necessary.

MANDIBULAR FRACTURES

Mandibular fractures present with 10 classic signs of fracture:

1. History of trauma
2. Malocclusion
3. Pain
4. Abnormal mobility or crepitus of the fractured segment
5. Interference with function and decreased range of motion
6. Deformity, either a facial deformity or a deformity of the dental arches
7. Deviation on opening
8. Swelling and ecchymosis
9. Mental nerve anesthesia
10. Radiologic confirmation

Examine the patient's ascending ramus and body of the mandible. Palpate the mandibular condyles, and check for a break in contour. Examine the dental arches for a step-off, loose teeth, bloody teeth, or malocclusion of the molars or frontal teeth. Remember that the mandible is a U-shaped arch. If one fracture exists, there is probably a second fracture on the other side of the arch. Examine the TMJ by placing your fingers into the patient's ear canals, and ask the patient to open and close his or her mouth. Note the patient's range of motion, disability, clicking, and pain, if any.

The most common area of fracture along the mandible is the alveolar area or the tooth-bearing segment of the mandible. The anterior and incisor areas are the most commonly fractured parts of the mandible. All avulsed or loose teeth should be preserved. If bleeding occurs, direct pressure should be applied with gauze sponges, and dental segments should be covered with a saline-soaked sponge if teeth are missing.

Fractures of the mandibular symphysis present with displacement of the lower incisor teeth and disruption of the arch's continuity. These teeth can be moved easily with bimanual palpation. Bilateral fractures in the mental region can result in a loss of anterior tongue support. Good airway support is a necessity in this type of fracture.

Condyle fractures will present with jaw deviation toward the side of the fracture on maximum opening of the mouth. If a bilateral subcondylar fracture is present, the patient will have an anterior bite with poor occlusion of the posterior molars and no incisor contact.

Edentulous fractures present with numerous teeth missing and lacerations of the gums. All dentures should be saved, because they can be used as splints for bony fragments and can also be used to maintain occlusal vertical dimensions. All open fractures should receive antibiotic therapy and tetanus prophylaxis.

MAXILLARY FRACTURES

Maxillary fractures can be divided into classes by the Le Fort system. Le Fort divided maxillary fractures into three types. Le Fort I is a horizontal maxillary fracture in which the jaw is free-floating. The fracture line is at the base of the nose, just above the level of the palate and below the attachment of the zygomatic process. It runs lateral to the maxillary sinuses and across the pterygomaxillary tissue to the lateral pterygoid. It would cover the area of a mustache in a male.

Le Fort I fractures are diagnosed by grasping the alveolar process and the anterior teeth between the thumb and the forefinger and by making a forward and backward movement. If movement occurs, then a Le Fort I fracture is present.

A Le Fort II fracture lies superior to the Le Fort I fracture line and is a pyramidal fracture. It is a vertical fracture through the facial aspects of the maxilla. It extends upward to the nasal and ethmoid bones. The Le Fort II fracture extends through the maxillary sinuses and the infraorbital rims bilaterally across the bridge of the nose.

If a patient has a Le Fort II fracture, the entire face will be swollen. Bilateral subconjunctival hemorrhage is often present, and the nose is often bleeding. Always examine the nasal discharge and ensure that the bloody discharge does not contain cerebrospinal fluid (CSF). If CSF is present, the patient also needs a neurosurgical evaluation. As little as possible movement of the facial bones is required to examine the patient for a facial fracture. If a Le Fort II fracture is present, the patient's entire face from the bridge of the nose down will move.

A Le Fort III fracture is one that extends through the frontozygomatic suture lines bilaterally. The fracture extends through the lateral orbital rim, through the base of the nose, and along the zygoma.

Surgical repair and stabilization are required for any Le Fort fracture by an oral surgeon. A CT scan is often needed to define the fracture lines and to rule out brain injury or bleeding, especially if CSF is noted.

Dislocation of the TMJ is a common presenting complaint. If the TMJ is dislocated, it can be manually manipulated back into place. The patient is often given diazepam, 10 mg IV, before reduction is attempted. The physician should then stand facing the patient and place his or her thumbs on the patient's third molars. The physician should grip his or her fingers around the patient's mandible and exert downward pressure until the condyles return into the fossa. After reduction is complete, the patient should not open his or her mouth wide and should eat a soft diet for 1 week. The patient should receive analgesics and muscle relaxants for effective pain control. If the patient has a chronic dislocation, a Barton bandage should be applied for 1 week. In a severe case, internal wiring may be needed.

OPHTHALMOLOGIC EMERGENCIES

Definition

Any eye problems that include acute sudden onset of eye pain, sudden vision loss with or without pain, chemical eye injury, or any blunt or penetrating eye trauma need an immediate evaluation. Common nonemergent eye problems seen in the ED are conjunctivitis, foreign bodies, corneal ulcers, blepharitis, hordeolum, and chalazion. True ophthalmologic emergencies include herpes simplex keratitis, central retinal artery or vein occlusion, amaurosis fugax, retinal detachment, and acute angle-closure glaucoma. Trauma emergencies can involve any part of the eye, including the lid, cornea, globe, and fractures of the orbit.

Pathology

The eye is protected by the eyelids. The eyelids terminate at the medial and lateral canthi. The upper eyelid is supported by the dense fibrous band of the tarsal plate. A fascial plane called the orbital septum separates the eyelids from the orbit.

The muscles of the eye include the orbicularis oculi muscle, which is arranged circumferentially around the eye. Its function is to close the eyelids, and this muscle is innervated by cranial nerve VI. The levator palpebrae muscle closes the eyelids and is innervated by cranial nerve III. Cranial nerve V is responsible for the sensory function of the eyelids. Cranial nerve V, the trigeminal nerve, has two branches—the infraorbital and supraorbital nerves. The infraorbital nerve, which is located in the infraorbital ridge, enters the orbit through its foramina and runs along the floor of the bony orbit. If a blow-out fracture occurs, this nerve can be damaged. The ophthalmic artery supplies the eyelids with blood.

The lacrimal glands secrete tears. The lacrimal glands are located on the lateral side of the eye, underneath the upper lid at the superior temporal border of the orbit. The tears roll over the cornea and sclera to the medial lacrimal puncta into the lacrimal sac via the upper and lower canaliculi. The tears then drain into the nose via the nasolacrimal duct and drain in the area of the inferior turbinate.

There are two types of conjunctiva: the palpebral conjunctiva and the bulbar conjunctiva. The palpebral conjunctiva lines the eyelids. The bulbar conjunctiva covers the anterior surface of the eyeball and serves to protect the eyeball.

The cornea is an avascular clear tissue that serves to protect the eye and has a refractive power of a 40+ diopter lens. The cornea is extremely sensitive to pain. It is made up of five layers: epithelium,

Bowman's membrane, stroma, Descemet's membrane, and endothelium.

The eye has two chambers—an anterior chamber and a posterior chamber. The anterior chamber is located between the posterior side of the cornea and the anterior side of the iris. The posterior chamber is located between the posterior side of the iris and the anterior side of the lens. Aqueous humor fills both chambers and can pass through the pupil of the eye. The lens is a clear, biconvexed, oval-shaped object that can alter its shape and refraction. The ciliary body is a circular band that forms the anterior part of the pigmented choroid to the root of the iris. The ciliary muscle changes the shape of the lens, and the ciliary process manufactures aqueous humor.

The space posterior to the lens is filled with vitreous humor, a gelatinous substance that helps to maintain the shape of the eyeball. The retina is located in the most posterior area of the eyeball. The retina receives light that has passed through the cornea, aqueous and vitreous humor, and lens.

The following cranial nerves and muscles can be checked by testing the six cardinal positions of gaze:

Cranial nerve VI—lateral gaze, the lateral rectus muscle

Cranial nerve III—medial gaze, the medial rectus muscle

Cranial nerve III—medial and inferior gaze, the inferior rectus muscle

Cranial nerve III—superior and medial gaze, the superior rectus muscle

Cranial nerve IV—lateral and inferior gaze, the superior oblique muscle

Cranial nerve III—lateral and superior gaze, the inferior oblique

Examination

Every patient who presents with even a trivial eye complaint should have his or her visual acuity documented using the Snellen chart. If the Snellen chart is not available, ask the patient to read newsprint and document the patient's ability to read print of different sizes. If the patient cannot read or visual acuity is such that he or she cannot read newsprint, ask the patient to count fingers or document the patient's ability to see hand motion. If the patient usually wears glasses, check the patient's visual acuity with and without glasses. If the patient does not have his or her eyeglasses available, a pinhole occluder can be used to approximate lens correction.

A slit lamp examination is preferred for all eye examinations. Use a slit lamp to examine the cornea, limbus, sclera, anterior chamber, iris, lens, lids, and conjunctiva. A fluorescein examination should be performed on all patients to rule out foreign bodies, lesions, or abrasions of the cornea. The patient's direct and consensual pupillary response to light should be tested and documented. The patient's extraocular movements should be tested in all six positions of gaze.

A funduscopic examination should be performed to examine and visualize the retina, optic disk, blood vessels, and vitreous. The optic disk is less than one third of the diameter of the disk and should be clear and crisp. If you are having trouble examining the disk, you can use a mydriatic such as 2.5% phenylephrine (Neo-Synephrine) or Paradrine to dilate the pupil. Always examine the pupillary function prior to instillation of the mydriatic of your choice.

When examining the vessels of the eyes, the veins should be larger than the arteries by 3:2. Retinal detachment, open-angle glaucoma, optic neuritis, and branch retinal arterial occlusion can all cause visual field loss. To examine a patient for visual field defects, ask the patient to sit approximately 1 meter from you. Ask the patient to occlude one eye. Tell the patient to look at your nose or pupil, then with one or two fingers, bring your fingers from the lateral, medial, inferior, and superior visual field areas. Note when the patient sees your fingers.

If glaucoma is suspected, the patient's intraocular pressure should be measured with a Schitz tonometer, Tono-pen or Goldmann applanation tonometer, or air-puff tonometer on a slit lamp.

Always examine the limbus, where the cornea and sclera come together, because this is the most common site of globe rupture. Always evert the superior eyelid to examine for lesions or foreign bodies and to inspect the cul-de-sac of the upper lid. Eversion can be performed with a cotton-tipped applicator.

Mydriatics dilate the pupil for a better examination of the optic disk and retina. Mydriatics are contraindicated in any patient with a history of glaucoma or increased intraocular pressure.

Topical anesthetics block neurotransmission along the sensory nerve fibers of the cornea.

Cycloplegics produce mydriasis by blocking the muscarinic receptors and produce paralysis and cycloplegia of lens accommodation by paralyzing the ciliary muscles. Cycloplegics are used to relieve photophobia secondary to ciliary spasms, corneal abrasion, ocular trauma, or iridocyclitis. Cyclopentolate and homatropine methylbromide are the two most commonly used cycloplegics. Scopolamine can also be used, but this agent has an onset of 40 to 60 minutes and lasts up to 6 hours. Atropine is also a cycloplegic but has an onset of 10 to 15 minutes and lasts up to 36 to 48 hours. Mydriasis from atropine can last from 3 to 7 days.

DISEASES OF THE EYE

Conjunctivitis can be caused either by bacteria or by viral etiologies. Bacterial conjunctivitis presents with a painful granular foreign body sensation and a mucopurulent discharge. Visual acuity is usually not affected, and pupillary function is not affected.

If *staphylococcal allergic conjunctivitis* is present, a small white ulcer will be present at the limbus. This white exudate is secondary to an allergy to the staphylococcal toxin. The treatment for bacterial conjunctivitis is a 10% solution of sulfacetamide drops. Place two drops in each eye four times a day for 7 to 10 days. Tobramycin or erythromycin ointment or drops can also be used. If staphylococcal allergic conjunctivitis is present, a dilute corticosteroid can be used for 5 to 7 days to decrease inflammation. The eye should not be patched if bacterial conjunctivitis is considered as a diagnosis.

Viral conjunctivitis presents with red, itching, irritated eyes. The discharge is clear instead of purulent as in bacterial conjunctivitis. Viral conjunctivitis is treated as bacterial conjunctivitis secondary to the risk of co-bacterial infection and the inability to differentiate between viral and bacterial conjunctivitis in many cases. Neomycin ointment should not be used, because it can cause a hypersensitivity dermatitis in 15% of patients.

Allergic conjunctivitis is secondary to environmental contacts. Vernal conjunctivitis is diagnosed by the presence of cobblestone papillae under the upper lid and intense itching and tearing and is usually seen in the spring and fall when plants are pollinating. Chemosis, swelling of the bulbar conjunctiva, can occur when small gnats fly into the eye and become lodged in the conjunctiva. The conjunctiva will be extremely red and swollen. Allergic conjunctivitis is usually uniocular. A chemical conjunctival allergic reaction can occur secondary to the use of atropine or neomycin.

All cases of allergic conjunctivitis are treated with topical antihistamines, vasoconstrictors, and dilute corticosteroids. Oral antihistamines and cool compresses are often helpful.

Herpes zoster conjunctivitis is a devastating uniocular viral infection that usually involves cranial nerve V. Its cause is presumed to be secondary to an infection of the nerve root by the herpes virus. Always examine the tip of the nose for shingles, a herpes lesion. The tip of the nose is innervated by the same nasociliary nerve as the cornea. Keratitis and anterior uveitis are often involved. If keratitis is present and is not properly treated, loss of vision can occur. Usually large doses of topical and systemic steroids are required for treatment. Any patient who presents with a dendritic lesion of herpes keratitis should be referred immediately to an ophthalmologist.

Keratoconjunctivitis occurs in epidemics secondary to the adenovirus type 8. Upon examination, the patient will have a tender ipsilateral perauricular lymph node on the same side as the infected eye. Keratitis appears, which is seen as scattered subepithelial infiltrates, approximately 1 week after the onset of symptoms. There is no specific treatment for the infection, but topical antibiotics are usually given to prevent a secondary bacterial infection.

Chemical conjunctivitis can be secondary to either an alkali or an acid substance. Alkali chemicals causes a liquefaction of the cornea and conjunctiva. The corrosive action, if unobstructed, continues to dissolve soft tissue until this process is stopped. Acid chemicals cause a coagulation necrosis of the cornea. The invasion is limited by the coagulum that is formed in the acute burning process.

Both type of burns are treated with immediate copious irrigation for 30 to 60 minutes at the site of the burn, and the irrigation should continue upon the patient's arrival at the ED. Both burns should be referred to an ophthalmologist. Neutralization of the acid or alkali chemicals should not be attempted.

Foreign bodies of the conjunctiva or cornea are common presentations in the ED. Conjunctival foreign bodies can often be seen by the unaided eye. Any patient who presents to the ED with pain, redness, and excessive tearing in one eye should be suspected of having a foreign body in the eye. The upper eyelid should always be everted to examine the superior cul-de-sac for foreign bodies. The inferior cul-de-sac should also be examined for foreign bodies. Proparacaine hydrochloride should be placed into the eye for pain control, and then a cotton-tipped applicator can be used to remove any foreign body in the conjunctiva. A mild antibiotic ointment can be applied to the eye twice a day from 2 to 3 days after removal of the foreign body. If the abrasions are very large, patching may be required for 24 hours.

Corneal foreign bodies present with pain, photophobia, redness, and tearing. Proparacaine can be applied to the eye to control the pain and make the examination easier for the patient. After the foreign body has been identified, it can be removed with a sterile hypodermic needle, cornea spud, or bur with the use of a slit lamp. Oral and topical antibiotics should be given for 5 to 7 days along with an updated tetanus immunization and good pain control medication. The eye should be patched after application of antibiotic ointment. The pressure patch should be left in place for 24 hours, and the eye should be checked again in 24 hours.

If the foreign body was a metal object, there is an increased risk of a rust ring forming. If present, the rust ring should be removed with a bur. If it is very difficult to remove the foreign body in the cornea, place an antibiotic ointment in the eye and double-patch the eye for 24 hours. This will cause the corneal epithelium to soften in 24 hours, and then the foreign body can often be removed easily. Corneal ulcers can occur secondary to corneal foreign bodies and infections. They present with severe pain and redness. On examination of the anterior chamber, white inflammatory exudate, or hypopyon, is often seen. Do not treat the eye until cultures have been collected and an ophthalmologist has been consulted. If iritis is present secondary to ciliary spasm, cyclopentolate 1% can be applied to the affected eye to relieve the ciliary spasm.

Subconjunctival hemorrhage is secondary to the rupture of small vessels in or beneath the bulbar conjunctiva. The eye will be very red and free of pain. Subconjunctival hemorrhage can be secondary to vomiting, coughing, Valsalva maneuver, or trauma. The hemorrhage resolves spontaneously in 10 to 14 days.

Blepharitis is a chronic inflammation of the lid margins secondary to a chronic staphylococcal infection of the skin and oil glands adjacent to the lash follicles. Treatment with sulfacetamide drops and scrubbing of the eyelashes and lid margin with a no tears–type baby shampoo will help to resolve the blepharitis in a few days.

Corneal flash burns or *ultraviolet keratitis* is secondary to the direct absorption of ultraviolet light by the corneal epithelium. Snow blindness, which is a reflection of light off of snow, and welder's blindness are two common causes of ultraviolet keratitis. On examination, a diffuse punctate keratitis is seen with fluorescein staining and cobalt blue illumination. There will be multiple areas of pinpoint staining that are indicative of ruptured corneal epithelial cells. Use topical anesthetics for examination purposes, and then topical anesthetics should not be used secondary to inhibited healing and decreased protective reflexes of the cornea. The eyes should be pressure-patched for 24 to 36 hours and good oral pain medication should be given.

Hordeolum (also commonly called a stye) is an acute inflammation of the meibomian gland of the eyelid. Treat the hordeolum with warm compresses and topical antibiotics. If it does not resolve, a referral to an ophthalmologist is required for incision and drainage of the gland.

Chalazion is a chronic granulomatous inflammation of the meibomian gland. If present, the patient will require a referral to an ophthalmologist for surgical removal of the chalazion.

Glaucoma occurs in two types: acute angle-closure glaucoma and open-angle glaucoma. Open-angle glaucoma is a chronic condition of elevated intraocular pressure. If this condition is not treated, damage to the optic disk can occur. On examination of the optic disk, the optic cup-disk ratio is increased and the patient may complain of scotomas, secondary to a physiologic blind spot caused by the glaucoma.

Acute angle-closure glaucoma is a congenital narrowing of the anterior chamber angle, secondary to the anterior iris leaf and the posterior surface of the cornea closing acutely, preventing the exit of aqueous humor. The patient presents with acute unilateral dull, aching ocular pain and blurred vision. The patient often presents with nausea and vomiting. Halos are often present. On examination, the eye appears very red with decreased visual acuity. The pupil is mid-dilated or fixed to light, and the cornea is often hazy.

The goal of therapy for acute angle-closure glaucoma is to increase aqueous humor outflow and to decrease the production of aqueous humor. Acetazolamide (Diamox) is given as a 500-mg bolus IV to decrease the formation of aqueous humor and thus decrease intraocular pressure. Topical timolol 0.25% to 0.5% (Timoptic), one drop to the affected eye with a second drop in 10 minutes, can also be used to decrease the formation of aqueous humor and intraocular pressure. If the patient has underlying pulmonary disease such as asthma or chronic obstructive pulmonary disease (COPD), betaxolol (Betoptic) can be used instead of timolol. Timolol is a nonselective β-adrenergic receptor blocker.

Glycerol in a 50% oral solution can be given in a dose of 1 ml/kg. Glycerol decreases intraocular volume and deepens the anterior chamber, thus reducing intraocular pressure. Mannitol 1 to 2 g/kg can be given IV instead of glycerol, if the patient cannot tolerate the sweet taste of glycerol.

Pilocarpine 2% can be given to cause miosis. It should be given every 15 minutes for the first hour and then one drop every 30 to 60 minutes. Miosis will increase outflow of aqueous humor into the anterior chamber and through the trabecular meshwork, after intraocular pressure starts to decrease. An ophthalmologist should be consulted by any patient with acute angle-closure glaucoma.

Central retinal artery or *vein occlusion* can be a cause of acute vision loss. Central artery occlusion is usually secondary to atherosclerosis secondary to thromboemboli, thrombosis, or vasospasm. The onset of vision loss is acute and painless. Upon examination of the fundi, the retina will be pale and a small pink dot will be present in the vicinity of the fovea. The retinal arteries will not be visible. Acute vigorous digital massage of the globe and the anterior chamber are required to reduce intraocular pressure enough to allow the atheromas to move peripherally. An ophthalmologist should be consulted immediately for paracentesis to be performed.

Central retinal vein occlusion is secondary to a rigid atheromatous artery next to the vein, exerts direct pressure on the vein and thus decreases or occludes the blood flow of the vein. This is usually a slow process that presents as a painless decrease of vision in one eye. On funduscopic examination, a chaotically blood-streaked retina with prominent dilated and congested veins will be present. An ophthalmologic consultation is required.

Retrobulbar neuritis is an acute loss of central vision in one eye, with the peripheral vision being preserved in the affected eye. This is usually a painless event and is diagnostic for multiple sclerosis in 25% of the cases of retrobulbar neuritis.

Retinal detachment is an acute painless loss of vision. The patient presents with a complaint of a curtain coming down over the visual field. The patient often gives a history of flashing lights or drifting dust or spiders across the visual field. Retinal detachments are secondary to the seepage of the posterior vitreous body through a retinal tear, causing a separation of the retina from the posterior eyeball. On examination of the fundus, the undulated gray detachment can be seen. If the detachment is inferior, the treatment consists of keeping the patient calm with the head elevated. If the detachment is superior, the patient should lie flat. An immediate ophthalmologic consultation is indicated.

Hysterical blindness is a common finding in young females. It is secondary to an acute psychiatric trauma. On examination the fundus and pupil appear to be normal. Direct and consensual pupillary examination will be normal. An optokinetic drum or strip will elicit opticokinetic nystagmus, thus confirming intact visual pathways. The patient will need a psychiatric referral.

OCULAR TRAUMA

Ocular trauma is a common complaint in the ED. Trauma of the orbit, lid, cornea, conjunctiva, lens, or penetrating trauma can occur.

Penetrating trauma can cause laceration to the eyelids. Lacerations of the lids can involve the lid margins, canalicular system, levator or canthal tendons, and lacerations through the orbital septum. All lacerations of the lid margin should be referred to an ophthalmologist for repair.

Conjunctival lacerations, if small and uncomplicated, will heal on their own. A prophylactic antibiotic ointment should be given. If the conjunctival laceration is larger than 1 cm, an ophthalmologist should be consulted for repair.

Corneoscleral lacerations and *puncture wounds* should be treated by an ophthalmologist. If a penetrating object is in the cornea, the object should be left alone until the ophthalmologist arrives. Removal of the object can precipitate leakage of vitreous humor. A classic sign of corneal perforation is a teardrop-shaped pupil. If it is questionable that there is a penetrating object in the eye, perform the Seidel test. This test is performed by instilling fluorescein dye into the eye and by examining the site of possible penetration under cobalt blue light. If the dye appears as a flowing stream of green fluid, secondary to flowing vitreous humor, surrounded by a pool of orange solution, then a corneal perforation is present. An ophthalmologist should be consulted.

Orbital or *intraocular foreign bodies* can have associated intracranial injuries. If an intraocular foreign body is suspected of being metallic, a lateral radiogram can be taken in an attempt to locate the object. A CT scan can also be used for suspected metallic objects. Magnetic resonance imaging (MRI) can be used in nonmetallic objects. B-mode ultrasonography can also be used, if available.

If the object is metal and is left in the globe, siderosis can occur. Siderosis is caused by the slow oxidization of a metallic object, which causes the binding of metallic substances to proteins and thus can cause blindness or degenerative changes in the eye. Chalcosis can also occur secondary to copper-containing foreign bodies that are left in the globe. Chalcosis is sterile pyogenic endophthalmitis. An ophthalmologist should be consulted with regard to any penetrating foreign bodies to ensure that chalcosis or siderosis does not occur.

Endophthalmitis can occur secondary to a deep infection of the vitreous and aqueous humor, secondary to bacterial contamination from ocular penetrating trauma. This infection is usually secondary to gram-positive *Staphylococcus*, *Streptococcus*, and *Bacillus*. Endophthalmitis should be treated by an ophthalmologist with topical and intraocular antibiotics. It is often found in immunocompromised patients and in IV drug abusers.

Corneal abrasions present with a foreign body sensation of the eye with photophobia, redness, and pain. An examination is performed with fluorescein dye and a cobalt light. If a corneal abrasion is present, there will be fluorescein uptake in the abrasion. A short-acting cycloplegic and antibiotic ointment can be placed in the eye to relieve ciliary spasm and prevent infection. A double-pressure patch should be applied to the eye for 24 hours. Most corneal abrasions heal in 24 to 36 hours with a good pressure patch. The eye should be checked in 24 hours for continued healing and to ensure that there is no ulcer formation. Post-traumatic corneal ulcers can occur secondary to corneal abrasions. If present, an ophthalmologist should be consulted and cultures should be taken.

Hyphemas are usually secondary to trauma. If the patient has been struck in the eye, a traumatic hyphema may be present. A hyphema is a small amount of blood in the anterior chamber. The blood is secondary to a rupture of the vessels of the ciliary body or iris. Hyphemas are graded on a scale of I to II based on the involvement of the anterior chamber. Patients present with photophobia, pain, and blurred vision. Hyphemas can cause an increase in intraocular pressure. Nausea and vomiting may be present. Always consider intracranial trauma in the presence of a hyphema secondary to the force required to cause a hyphema. Acute treatment for a hyphema is to keep the patient calm and elevate the head of the bed by 30 to 45 degrees. A Fox eye shield should be place to protect the eye.

The definitive treatment of a hyphema is directed at decreasing the intraocular pressure with IV mannitol, topical timolol, and acetazolamide. Antifibrinolytics and transexamic acid are used by some authors. Patients who have sickle cell disease or sickle cell thalassemia are at increased risk for hyphemas. The sickled cells can block the trabecular meshwork and occlude the outflow of aqueous humor. Acetazolamide is not used in a patient with sickle disease, secondary to the lowering of the pH in the anterior chamber. Methazolamide should be used for these patients. Sickling is increased in the hypoxic, acidic anterior chamber. Any patient who presents with a hyphema should have an ophthalmologic consultation.

Iritis is an acute inflammation of the iris and ciliary bodies of the eye. The patient presents with a complaint of a deep, aching, eye pain, and photophobia. On examination with a slit lamp, a perilimbal injection, known as a ciliary flush, may be present. "Cells and flare" may be present on slit lamp examination also. This condition is secondary to the leakage of white blood cells and protein from the inflamed ciliary body. Intraocular pressure is usually decreased in iritis. Treatment of iritis includes a long-acting cycloplegic such as homatropine for 7 to 10 days to relieve the ciliary spasm and control the pain.

Sympathetic ophthalmia is a rare granulomatous inflammation secondary to ocular trauma. It occurs weeks or months after penetrating trauma. It is believed to be an autoimmune response to the normal immunologic sequestered uveal tissues of the injured eye. It presents as pain, photophobia, and blurred vision in the uninjured eye. Treatment is enucleation of the blind eye.

Lens subluxation or *dislocation* is usually secondary to trauma. On examination, the edge of the lens is often visible and may be prolapsed into the anterior chamber. If complete anterior dislocation is present, an acute pupillary glaucoma may be present. The patient will present with monocular diplopia or distortion with subluxation and marked gross blurring of vision. Lens subluxation is common in a patient with Marfan's syndrome, coloboma of the lens, homocystinuria, and tertiary syphilis. An ophthalmologic consultation is required.

OTOLARYNGOLOGIC EMERGENCIES

Definition

Ear pain and decreased hearing are common primary complaints secondary to ear pathology in a patient presenting to the ED. Otitis media, otitis externa, or foreign bodies in the ear are common presentations in both adults and children. Other otolaryngologic problems are sinusitis, tonsillitis, pharyngitis, peritonsillar abscess or retropharyngeal abscess, epistaxis, and trauma.

Ears

The middle ear is made up of the tympanic membrane, the incus, the malleus, and stapes bones, the round and oval windows, and the mucous membrane of the middle ear. The eustachian tube drains the middle ear into the nasopharynx.

Pain from the ear can be caused by infection of the external canal, middle ear, TMJ, maxilla, or any of the sounding structures of the ear. Otalgia, ear pain, can also be caused by herpes zoster, Bell's palsy, cervical arthritis, occipital neuralgia, and teeth pain.

OTITIS MEDIA

Otitis media can be caused by a viral or bacterial infection. The common bacterial causes of otitis media are *Streptococcus pneumoniae, Haemophilus influenzae*, group A *Streptococcus*, and *Branhamella catarrhalis*. Common viral causes of otitis media are: respiratory syncytial virus, parainfluenza virus, adenovirus, influenza, and enterovirus. *Mycoplasma pneumoniae* is associated with bullous myringitis.

Patients with an acute otitis media present with fever, pain in the ear, hearing loss, and discharge from the ear (if the tympanic membrane has ruptured). On examination the tympanic membrane will be red and bulging and will have decreased mobility with insufflation. Acute otitis media can be treated with amoxicillin (Augmentin), erythromycin, sulfisoxazole, trimethoprim-sulfamethoxazole, penicillin V, or cephalosporins. Topical heat and analgesic ear drops can be used if the pain is severe. A myringotomy is indicated if severe pain, high fever, marked toxicity or facial nerve paralysis, meningitis, or brain abscess is present.

OTITIS EXTERNA

Otitis externa is an acute infection of the ear canal. The external canal is usually protected by a coat of waxy cerumen and an acid pH. If an abrasion in the ear canal occurs or water persists in the ear canal, both conditions destroy the natural barrier, and an acute overgrowth of normal flora can occur. *Pseudomonas* is the most common cause of an acute otitis externa. The patient presents with edema of the tissue of the bony ear canal, the pinna, and the auricular region. Herpes zoster can also present as acute otitis media. Herpes zoster in the ear canal can present as the Ramsay Hunt syndrome. This syndrome is secondary to a herpes zoster virus infection of the geniculate ganglion, which presents as ear pain, decreased hearing, facial palsy, and adjacent cranial nerve involvement.

Otitis externa is treated with gentle curettage of the debris in the canal, with irrigation or suction and antibiotic drops in the canal for 7 to 10 days. Gentamicin ophthalmalogic drops are often used to treat otitis externa. If the canal is swollen and closed, a wick should be gently inserted, using alligator forceps. Malignant external otitis should be suspected in undiagnosed diabetic patients or in the immunocompromised patient.

FURUNCLE

A furuncle is a localized abscess of the ear canal. A furuncle in the ear canal can be very painful. It usually ruptures and drains on its own without further treatment. It presents with pain, redness, and edema of the canal. If a patient with a furuncle presents to the ED and the furuncle has not ruptured, a trial of penicillin-VK 250 mg QID and hot compresses can be tried for a few days. If the furuncle does not resolve in a few days or if it becomes larger, then the furuncle should be drained via an incision. Oral antibiotic should be continued and topical antibiotic ear drops should be started.

BULLOUS MYRINGITIS

Bullous myringitis presents with a persistent painful ear and mild hearing loss. It can be secondary to a viral or mycoplasmal origin. On examination the tympanic membrane will have blisters that can contain either clear or hemorrhagic fluid. Treatment consists of heat, analgesics, and erythromycin or tetracycline oral antibiotics.

ACUTE HEARING LOSS

Acute hearing loss can be divided into two types: conduction and sensory loss. Acute conduction hearing loss can be secondary to an obstruction by cerumen, otitis externa edema, perforated tympanic membrane, otosclerosis, acute serous otitis, or tympanosclerosis.

Acute unilateral sensory hearing loss can be secondary to viral neuritis, chronic or acute noise exposure, or an acoustic neuroma. Acute bilateral hearing loss can be secondary to antibiotics, such as the antimalarials, aminoglycosides, and vancomycin. Nonsteroidal anti-inflammatory drugs can also cause an acute unilateral or bilateral hearing loss. Antineoplastic agents such as cisplatin and nitrogen mustard, which are used to treat cancer, can also cause an acute bilateral hearing loss. Loop diuretics such as furosemide and ethacrinic acid can cause acute hearing loss, and acute exposure to noise can also cause acute bilateral hearing loss.

The two tests that can be done in the ED to differentiate between a conductive hearing loss and a sensory hearing loss are the Rinne and Weber tests. The Rinne test is performed by placing a vibrating 512-Hz tuning fork against the mastoid process and by allowing the amplitude to decrease naturally. When the patient no longer feels the vibration of the tuning fork, the tuning fork is placed next to the patient's ear, where it should normally still be heard. If a conductive hearing loss is present, then the patient is unable to hear the tuning fork when it is brought to the ear.

The Weber test is performed by placing a vibrating tuning fork against the midline of the forehead. In a normal Weber test, the sound will be midline and will be equal in both ears. If a conductive hearing loss is present, the sound will lateralize to the side with the conductive loss because the vibrations are detected more readily by the ear that is not being distracted by environmental noise.

A unilateral sensory hearing loss will cause a normal Rinne test and a Weber test to lateralize the unaffected ear. Bilateral sensory hearing loss is usually accompanied by tinnitus secondary to medications or loud noise. Excessive ingestion of aspirin is a common cause of tinnitus.

Treatment is directed at the underlying cause. If the ears are packed with cerumen, this wax should be removed. If hearing loss or tinnitus is secondary to medications, the medications should be discontinued. If loss is secondary to otitis media, the condition should be treated. If otitis media or a sensory or conductive hearing loss lasts longer than 3 weeks, with treatment, then the patient should be referred to an otologist.

EPISTAXIS

Epistaxis, or an acute nosebleed, is usually secondary to trauma. Epistaxis can be caused by atherosclerosis, hypertension, coagulopathy, tumors, foreign bodies, changes in atmospheric pressure, or exposure to caustic materials in the air.

Anterior epistaxis is usually secondary to an acute bleed from Kiesselbach's plexus, which lies anteriorly on the septum. Kiesselbach's plexus is supplied by branches of the anterior ethmoidal and nasopalatine arteries. Anterior bleeds can also occur at the site of the lateral walls of the turbinates, which are supplied by the sphenopalatine artery.

Anterior bleeding can be caused by trauma, nose picking, or viral, allergic or vasomotor etiologies. Excessive blowing of the nose or bacterial rhinitis can also cause anterior bleeding. During the winter when the humidity of the air is very low, the dry air will dry out the nasal mucosa, producing hypertrophied mucosa, rhinitis sicca, which causes increased nose bleeding. Patients who use cocaine for recreational purposes by sniffing cocaine into the nares can cause vasoconstriction of the arteries and even small infarctions of the nasal vascular system. Chronic use of cocaine can cause septal perforation and thus epistaxis.

Posterior epistaxis is secondary to bleeding from a branch of the sphenopalatine artery. Posterior bleeds are more common in the elderly and are more profuse than are anterior bleeds. There is no specific cause for posterior bleeds.

Treatment of anterior bleeds consists of pinching the nose for 10 minutes, application of ice, and application of vasoconstrictors such as cocaine 2 to 5%–soaked cotton balls, into the bleeding nares or a solution of epinephrine (1:1000) and oxymetazoline 0.05% or phenylephrine 1% solution mixed in equal parts and applied to the septal area. The anterior nares can also be packed with petroleum jelly ribbon gauze. After the bleeding is stopped, the patient should be taught how to keep the nasal mucosa moist with petroleum jelly, bacitracin ointment, or any other moisturizing ointment.

In the case of posterior bleeding, a posterior pack should be applied. There are numerous ways to pack the posterior nose. A 4 × 4-in. gauze can be rolled up in a log form as a pack. A No. 16 French Foley catheter can be introduced into the nares and pushed forward until it is seen in the posterior pharynx. The catheter is then grabbed by a hemostat and brought out of the mouth. A string is tied at one end of the catheter, and the 4 × 4-in. gauze is tied to the other end. The Foley catheter is then pulled back through the nose along with the string until the packing is lodged in the posterior nasopharynx. A second piece of string should be tied to the 4 × 4-in. gauze and should hang out of the mouth and be taped to the face to preclude the loss of the gauze pack. The gauze should be placed firmly into the nasopharynx. The gauze should have been soaked with cocaine 2 to 5% or the aforementioned epinephrine and phenylephrine solution. Any patient who has a posterior pack should be admitted to the hospital for pain control, sedation, antibiotic therapy, and an ear, nose, throat (ENT) consultation.

SEPTAL HEMATOMAS

Septal hematomas are usually secondary to blunt trauma to the nose. Bleeding occurs between the cartilage and the perichondrium covering. If the hematoma is not drained, necrosis of the cartilaginous septum can occur. The hematoma should be drained by aspiration;

the nose should be packed to stop rebleeding; and oral antibiotics should be given.

CAULIFLOWER EAR

A cauliflower ear involves the same principle as a septal hematoma. This also needs to be drained, or a deformity of the ear can occur.

BLOCKED SALIVARY GLAND

Occasionally, one of the salivary glands will become blocked at the Stensen (parotid gland) or Wharton (submandibular gland) duct. This will present as a painful swelling of the parotid or submandibular areas, often at mealtime. It can also occur in diabetic or dehydrated patients. If a stone is blocking a duct, sialolithiasis can occur. This will present with little pain, but swelling of the parotid submandibular gland. Often if the patient sucks on tart lozenges, salivation can be stimulated and the stone can be released. If the ducts are chronically blocked, a referral to an otolaryngologist should be made for dilation of the ducts or incision and drainage of the stone.

In rare cases, an acute involvement of the submandibular gland may cause Ludwig's angina and may threaten to obstruct the patient's airway. If Ludwig's angina is present, an incision should be made and the gland should be drained immediately. Good airway control is necessitated.

Postadenotonsillectomy bleeding can occur acutely, in the first 24 hours, or can be delayed for 5 to 7 days. If a patient presents with bleeding secondary to surgery, good airway control is a necessity, and an otolaryngologic consultation should be made immediately.

SINUSITIS

Definition

Acute sinusitis can be caused by viral or bacterial etiologies. Paranasal sinusitis is usually of viral etiology secondary to an acute upper respiratory tract infection.

Pathology

When swelling occurs in the paranasal sinus, swollen nasal mucous membranes obstruct the ostium of the sinus. This ostium obstruction impedes sinus drainage. When drainage cannot occur, oxygen in the sinus is reabsorbed, and a relative negative pressure causes an acute vacuum in the sinus and pain. If this vacuum is not relieved, a transudate of serum from the vessels of the mucous membrane drains into the sinus. This can be seen on x-rays as air-fluid levels. If bacteria are present, then an acute suppurative sinusitis can occur. Most sinus infections are secondary to gram-positive cocci. Chronic sinusitis is usually secondary to gram-negative or anaerobic organisms.

Clinical Presentation

Acute maxillary sinusitis will cause pain in the maxillary areas of the face or can cause an acute toothache type of pain, secondary to the maxillary sinuses sitting on top of the upper molars. Frontal sinusitis will cause a frontal headache, and ethmoid sinusitis will cause pain in the retro-orbital area between the eyes. An acute sphenoid sinusitis will cause referred pain to the frontal or occipital areas of the head.

Examination

The patient should be given a complete examination. The ears, nose, throat, and neck should especially be noted. Green or yellow purulent rhinorrhea is often present. Upon examining the nose the mucous membranes will be swollen and red, and there will be tenderness on percussion of the infected sinus. If the patient presents with fever or chills, a secondary infection should be suspected.

Diagnosis

Sinusitis is a clinical diagnosis that can be confirmed by radiographs, CT, or MRI. An upright Water view or lateral or submental vertex views are often helpful in the diagnosis of mucosal thickening of sinusitis.

Treatment

The treatment for an acute sinusitis is 3 weeks of therapy with antibiotics, analgesics, and a topical vasoconstrictor. Penicillin, erythromycin, ampicillin, amoxicillin, cephalosporins, or sulfamethoxazole (Septra) are all excellent choices for treatment of acute sinusitis.

In complicated or chronic sinusitis, drainage can be useful. Ethmoid sinusitis can cause a secondary orbital cellulitis or abscess, especially in children. Swelling of the orbit or eyelid, proptosis, and displacement of the globe laterally or interiorly are all signs of abscess formation. Any patient with a suspected orbital abscess should be admitted to the hospital, and an ENT consultation is necessary.

Frontal sinusitis can cause osteomyelitis of the posterior table of the frontal bone. If this takes place, meningitis, epidural abscess, brain abscess, or subdural empyema may occur. Pott's puffy tumor, or forehead abscess, is secondary to the destruction of the anterior table of the forehead. All patients with true frontal sinusitis should be admitted to the hospital.

TRAUMATIC DENTAL EMERGENCIES

TOOTH FRACTURES

Fractures to the teeth are usually classified by the Ellis system, which divides fractures of the anterior teeth into three classifications. *Ellis type I* is a fracture that involves just the enamel portion of the tooth. It is usually more cosmetic than painful. Pain is usually secondary to a sharp piece of tooth rubbing the soft tissue of the gingiva. Treatment involves a referral to a dentist for smoothing of the rough edges and cosmetic restoration.

Ellis type II fracture involves the enamel and dentin of the tooth where the dentin is exposed. The patient presents with sensitivity to heat, cold, or air. On examination, a pinkish color of the dentin can be noted. Children younger than 12 years of age will have less dentin than adults. The open dentin is susceptible to contamination of the pulp by microorganisms. In the ED, the fractured tooth should be covered with calcium hydroxide to protect the dentin. If calcium hydroxide is not available, the exposed dentin should be covered with dry gauze or tinfoil for protection. The patient will require a referral to a dentist within 24 hours. The patient should be treated with analgesics and should be advised that the tooth may develop pulpal necrosis or resorption secondary to disruption of the tooth's neurovascular supply.

Patients with an *Ellis class III* fracture of a tooth have involvement of the enamel, dentin, and pulp. These patients may present with or without severe pain depending on the trauma to the neurovascular pulp. On examination the dentin will be exposed with blood seeping from the pulp. The patient should be referred immediately to a dentist or endodontist. No over-the-counter topical dental analgesic preparations should be applied to the exposed tooth secondary to the irritation of the soft tissue or the likelihood of the formation of a sterile abscess in the fractured tooth. The patient's pain should be treated with oral analgesics, and the tooth should be covered with tinfoil to decrease the irritation of the pulp. All fractured parts of the tooth should be saved for the dentist.

AVULSED OR SUBLUXATED TEETH

Any motion of a permanent tooth upon examination should be considered a subluxation of that tooth, especially if there is a ring of blood around the gingival crevice. Treatment of minimal subluxation involves a soft diet for several days and a follow up. If the tooth is very mobile, the tooth will require stabilization by a dentist for 10 days to 2 weeks. These patients should be referred to a dentist or endodontist.

A completely avulsed tooth is a true dental emergency. A completely avulsed permanent tooth, of less than 2 to 3 hours, should be replaced into the socket from which it came. If several teeth are avulsed, an x-ray can be taken to help guide the replacement of the avulsed teeth. It is important to remember that a percentage point is lost for each minute that the tooth is out of the socket in regard to successful replantation. If the patient presents to the ED with the avulsed tooth, the tooth should be quickly rinsed with running tap water and should be reinserted into the socket by only holding the crown, not the root. If the patient or you cannot replace the tooth into the socket, it should be placed in milk or wrapped in moist gauze. If there is no danger of the patient swallowing or aspirating the tooth, ask the patient to hold the tooth in his or her own mouth so that it can be bathed in the patient's own saliva. Never allow an intoxicated patient or a patient with an altered mental status to hold the tooth in his or her mouth. Milk is the preferred solution to preserve the tooth because of its osmolarity and ion concentration of Ca^{2+} and Mg^{2+}. The goal is to preserve the periodontal ligament fibers on the root of the avulsed tooth. There are numerous commercial transport mediums, including Hank's solution and Tooth Preserving Systems to preserve and transport an avulsed tooth to a dentist. If the avulsed tooth is a primary tooth, 6 months to 5 years of age, the tooth is not replaced into the socket. There is increased risk of ankylosis and fusion of the tooth to the bone itself, resulting in a facial deformity. Any patient with an avulsed tooth should be referred immediately to a dentist for stabilization of the tooth to avoid ankylosis. The patient should be placed on oral penicillin, 250 to 500 mg po QID.

LACERATIONS

Lacerations of the oral mucosa, tongue, and palate are very common secondary to falls, motor vehicle accidents, or assaults. Small mucosa, gingiva, hard palate, and tongue lacerations usually require no suturing. Lacerations greater than 1.5 cm should be sutured secondary to the increased risk of infection and fibrotic healing. All foreign debris should be removed by irrigation or with hemostats. Nonviable tissue should be removed. The wounds should be closed with a 3–0, 4–0, or 5–0 chromic suture. Silk can also be used but must be removed in 7 to 10 days; furthermore, silk has an increased risk of secondary infection. If there is extensive loss of tissue, a dirty wound, or crushed tissue, the patient should be given penicillin or erythromycin, 250 to 500 mg po QID for 7 to 10 days.

All lip lacerations should be closed with meticulous care, especially if they involve the vermilion border, secondary to a long-lasting cosmetic deformity. Deep lip lacerations should be closed from the inside out, and reabsorbable suture material should be used for deep lacerations to ensure that premature separation of the wound does not occur secondary to the tension placed on the wound by the lip musculature. The vermilion border should be approximated with the greatest care. A surgical ink pen can be used to place a dot at the edge of the vermilion border to help approximate placement of the sutures.

Through-and-through lacerations should be irrigated copiously and should be closed from the inside out, thus ensuring that all foreign debris has been removed. The patient should be placed on penicillin or erythromycin 250 to 500 mg po QID for 7 to 10 days. The wound should be checked in 24 to 48 hours to ensure that there is no infection. All lacerations require current tetanus prophylaxis.

BIBLIOGRAPHY

Braunwald E, Isselbacher KJ, Petersdorf RG, et al (eds): Harrison's Principles of Internal Medicine, 11th ed. New York, McGraw-Hill, 1987

Hamilton GC, Sanders AB, Strange GR, et al (eds): Emergency Medicine: An Approach to Clinical Problem-Solving. Philadelphia, WB Saunders, 1991

Kravis TC, Warner CG, Jacobs LM (eds): Emergency Medicine: A Comprehensive Review, 3rd ed. New York, Raven Press, 1993

May HL, Aghababian RV, Fleisher GR (eds): Emergency Medicine, 2nd ed. Boston, Little, Brown, 1992

Rosen P, Barkin RM (eds): Emergency Medicine: Concepts and Clinical Practice, 3rd ed. St. Louis, Mosby-Year Book, 1992

Schwartz GR, Cayten CG, Mangelsen MA, et al (eds): Principles and Practice of Emergency Medicine. Philadelphia, Lea & Febiger, 1992

Tierney LM, McPhee SJ, Papadakis MA (eds): Current Medical Diagnosis and Treatment, 33rd ed. Norwalk, CT, Appleton & Lange, 1994

Tintinalli JE, Krone RL, Ruiz E (eds): Emergency Medicine: A Comprehensive Study Guide, 4th ed. New York, McGraw-Hill, 1996

Chapter **6**

Environmental Emergencies

CHEMICAL BURNS

Definition

Chemical burns are secondary to exposure to single compounds, or to mixtures. Burns are usually secondary to exposure either to alkalis or to acids. Acids cause coagulation necrosis and protein precipitation. Alkalis produce liquefaction necrosis, which causes a deeper penetrating wound. Acids cause eschars and limit penetration of the agent.

Acids such as sulfuric, sulfosalicylic, picric, tungstic, formic, trichloroacetic, acetic, cresylic, chromic, and hydrofluoric are major causes of industrial burns. Alkalis can also cause severe burns and include hydroxide salts of sodium, potassium, ammonium, barium, lithium, and calcium derivatives. White phosphorus is also commonly used in ammunitions, pesticides, and rodenticides and can cause severe burns.

There are six types of chemicals classified by the manner in which they damage proteins:

1. Vesicants produce blisters.
2. Reducing agents cause the binding of free electrons in tissue protein.
3. Corrosives cause protein denaturation, causing eschars and indolent ulcers.
4. Oxidizing agents cause damage when the agent comes in contact with the skin, and often a toxic moiety is released.
5. Desiccants cause cellular dehydration and thermal injuries by an exothermic reaction.
6. Protoplasmic poisons cause protein denaturation by salt formation or by metabolic competition or inhibition.

Epidemiology

Chemical burns can occur in the home, in school, on the farm, in laboratories, or at the workplace. More than 30,000 products sold in the United States can cause chemical burns. Some of the more common chemical burns are secondary to hair dye and hair treatment products. Approximately 40% of all occupational injuries involve the skin, secondary to chemical exposure, and 25% are chemical burns.

The face, eyes, and extremities are the most commonly burned parts of the body. Usually less than 5% of the total body surface is burned by chemicals. Chemical burns have lower mortality and morbidity rates than do thermal burns.

Pathology

The skin's three layers: the epidermis, dermis, and adipose/connective tissue layers serve as a barrier against foreign agents. Reactions are based on the morphologic reaction of the skin to a toxic agent and consist of simple erythemal reactions, blistering, and full-thickness burns. Erythema, or first-degree burns, cause capillary and arterial dilatation. Patients present with pruritus, burning, and pain. Partial-thickness or second-degree burns present as first-degree burns; furthermore, there is an outpouring of fluid into the extracellular spaces that causes edema, vesicles, or bullae. Full-thickness burns cause total tissue destruction.

Absorption of an agent is determined by the area of the body that is exposed, the integrity of the skin, the nature of the chemical agent, and the presence of garments. There is a higher absorption rate for agents that are highly lipid soluble and have a high pH.

Diagnosis

A diagnosis is made by determining the following:

1. The manner of contact with the agent
2. The concentration of the agent involved
3. The quantity of the agent involved
4. The duration of contact with the agent
5. The mechanism of action—acid or alkali
6. The extent of penetration by the agent

Treatment

Any burn whether acid or alkali should be irrigated immediately with copious amounts of water. This irrigation should continue for a minimum of 30 minutes. If the patient is still wearing garments with the chemical on them, remove the garments immediately. If the chemical is dry, brush off as much as you can before applying irrigation. Exceptions to these rules are sodium metals or related compounds, which should be covered with mineral oil or excised as soon as possible. Water can cause a severe exothermic reaction. Water on phenol (carbolic acid) can enhance penetration, thus treat phenol as follows. The mainstay of treatment is to decontaminate, débride, or neutralize any chemicals on the skin.

Phenol (carbolic acid) is a corrosive organic acid that causes chemical burns. It is commercially available in concentrations of 1 to 90%. Phenol is used in medicine and in industry, and it denatures proteins. Patients with exposure to phenol present with white-to-brown–colored coagulum that is almost painless. Hexylresorcinol is a phenol derivative that is chemically related to creosol, creosote, and cresylic acid. Phenol burns cause coagulation necrosis and can become trapped under the eschar.

Copious irrigation is the main treatment. Polyethylene glycol 300 (PEG 300) and industrial methylated spirits (IMS) in a 2:1 mixture have been effective in reducing the extent of cutaneous corrosion; however, this mixture does not reduce systemic toxicity. Isopropyl alcohol can also be used to decontaminate phenol instead of water or the mixture of PEG and IMS.

Acetic acid is found in hair wave neutralizer solutions and can cause burns to the scalp with prolonged contact. Acetic acid can cause partial-thickness burns that can become infected with bacterial flora. Treatment consists of copious irrigation with water and oral antibiotic therapy.

Formic acid is used in airplane–glue making, tanning works, and cellulose formate works. If formic acid comes into contact with the skin, coagulation necrosis occurs and the skin should be irrigated immediately with copious amounts of water, which is the mainstay of treatment. If large areas of necrotic skin are present, they should be débrided or application of healing skin grafts should be considered.

Nitric acid is used in the casting of steel and iron, engraving, electroplating, and fertilizer manufacturing. Injury is secondary to oxidation and can leave the skin yellow. Copious irrigation is the mainstay of treatment.

Chromic acid injury is secondary to the oxidizing action of the hexavalent compounds. Chromate ions will penetrate the skin and cause ulcerating lesions. A patient may present with lacrimation, ulceration of the nasal septum, conjunctivitis, and systemic chromium toxicity. Fatalities have been reported with a 10% body surface exposure. Copious irrigation with water and observation for systemic toxicity are the mainstays of treatment.

Sulfuric and *hydrochloric acids* turn the skin dark brown or black and are found in toilet bowl cleaners, drain cleansers, ammunitions, and fertilizer manufacturing. Automotive batteries often contain as much as 25% sulfuric acid. Copious irrigation and débridement of damaged tissue are the mainstay of treatment.

Hydofluoric acid is a protoplasmic poison that causes progressive tissue loss, including bone destruction. Hydrofluoric acid penetrates the skin, dissociates, and causes the release of fluoride ions. Fluoride ions cause the immobilization of intracellular magnesium and calcium and can poison the cellular enzyme reactions. Fluoride ions also cause the spontaneous depolarization of nerve tissue and pain secondary to the increased permeability of potassium.

Hydrofluoric acid is used in fire-proofing material, high-octane fuels, frosting and etching glass, microelectronics, microinstruments, and the semiconductor industry. This acid is used to remove rust, clean stones, and make dyes.

A patient who has been exposed to hydrofluoric acid presents with both systemic and localized reactions. Hypomagnesemia, hypocalcemia, and hyperkalemia are hallmarks of hydrofluoric acid poisoning. Solutions of less than 20% might take 12 to 24 hours before symptoms occur. The stronger the solution, the faster symptoms will occur. On examination the skin often appears blue-gray.

Treatment of hydrofluoric acid poisoning consists of two phases.

The first phase is the immediate treatment of the contaminated area with copious irrigation with water for 15 to 30 minutes. The second phase is the detoxification stage, which can be achieved by giving the patient calcium gluconate by subcutaneous or intradermal injection, topical application, or intra-arterial infusion. Calcium gluconate can be applied to the area after it is mixed with Surgilube or dimethyl sulfoxide (DMSO). This gel mixture will cause binding of hydrofluoric acid to the gel. The drawback to this therapy is that calcium is not very permeable in the skin.

Subcutaneous or intradermal injection of a 10% calcium gluconate solution through a 30-gauge needle into the affected area of skin is the best treatment. The maximum dose of 0.5 ml/cm^2 of skin is recommended for treatment. After the administration of calcium, pain is almost immediately abated. Extinction of pain is a good guide to the correct amount of calcium therapy.

Intra-arterial infusion of calcium gluconate can be used to prevent tissue necrosis and to stop pain in large burns caused by hydrofluoric acid. This treatment must be performed with an intra-arterial catheter in the appropriate vascular supply of the burned extremity and with a three-way stopcock that is attached to an arterial pressure monitoring device. Ten milliliters of a 10% calcium gluconate solution in 40 ml of 5% dextrose should be infused over 2 to 4 hours. Infusion of calcium deep into the tissues only increases the change of tissue damage and ensures intra-arterial infusion of calcium. Calcium should not be injected intra-arterially.

Alkalis cause liquefaction necrosis and can cause toxic systemic absorption. Proteins and lipids form soluble protein complexes and soaps, which permit further passage of hydroxyl ions into deep tissues. Skin exposure to lime and lye is treated with copious irrigation. Any ocular burn should be irrigated copiously for a minimum of 30 minutes after the pH has been determined. Acids quickly precipitate, and penetration is limited secondary to the localized buffering and barriers of the eye. Alklali burns can be disastrous to the eye. The higher the pH, the more damage can occur. Alkali can penetrate the cornea, anterior chamber, and retina. Alkalis can disrupt the cellular membrane lipid metabolism. A follow-up visit to an eye specialist is required for treatment of acid or alkali burns to the eye.

FROSTBITE

Definition

Frostbite is a localized freezing that usually occurs in the distal extremities, fingers, hands, toes, and feet. If the face is exposed, facial tissue including the nose can freeze. Nonfreezing injuries include trench foot and chilblains (pernio).

Epidemiology

Peripheral cold injuries are unique to humans. Most animals that live in cold climates have adapted mechanisms for cold weather (i.e., fur or fat). Most cold injuries are accidental secondary to routine exposure without consideration of risk factors. The military has had a long experience with cold weather injuries, and cold injuries have caused wars to be won or lost.

Pathology

Frostbite occurs when actual freezing of the macrovascular and microvascular takes place. Rapid freezing can occur when the skin comes into contact with volatile hydrocarbons (e.g., gasoline) at low temperatures. As the skin cools, capillary circulation slows until it stops completely and cold-induced vasospasm occurs. Arterioles constrict to protect any heat that is still present, until capillary shunting occurs with arteriole-to-venule blood flow. This entire process is known as the "hunting response." This response is the body's attempt to retain as much heat as possible and to keep enough blood circulating to perfuse the tissues.

As the cool blood returns from the extremities to the central circulation, the core temperature drops and more body temperature is lost. As the core temperature continues to drop, shunting stops and the extremity then freezes. Actual ice crystals form in the intracellular and extracellular tissues of the extremity. Freezing causes an intracellular dehydration, increased intracellular osmolality, and denaturation of intracellular proteins. Blood viscosity increases as blood temperature decreases, causing occlusion of venules, platelet aggregation, and arteriolar vascular damage within 1 to 2 hours after the onset of freezing. When frozen tissue is thawed, a protein-rich fluid leaks from the injured vasculature and leaks into the interstitial space, which leads to more venous stasis and occlusion.

Clinical Presentation

Patients initially present with "frostnip." These patients complain of numbness, blanched skin, and the cessation of cold and discomfort. The onset of pain and cold is the first sign of frostbite.

If the extremity is rewarmed at this stage, no tissue death occurs; however, pain and hypersensitivity can be present for several days or weeks. If partial tissue destruction occurs, significant pain will be present along with a throbbing sensation, which will be present for 48 to 72 hours and can persist for weeks or months.

Chilblains or pernio constitute a mild form of dry-cold exposure that is repetitive. "Cold sores" are often present on the face and palms of the hands and feet. If the patient has Raynaud's phenomenon, pain can be intense with exposure to cold. Patients have pruritus, edema, erythema, plaques, ulcerations, and blue nodules.

Trench foot or immersion foot is caused by prolonged exposure to cold temperatures at temperatures that are just above freezing. The patient presents with cold, edematous, and cyanotic feet and often complains of numbness and leg cramps. Bullae can develop with ulceration and liquefaction. After rewarming, the skin remains very painful to touch, dry, and erythematous.

A patient with true frostbite presents with large, clear blisters in 24 to 48 hours after freezing. Frostbite is divided into superficial injury and deep frostbite injury. In superficial frostbite, the skin remains pliable, and the tissue is soft beneath the surface. In deep frostbite, the tissues feel woody or stony upon palpation.

It often takes several weeks before lines of demarcation between blackened dead tissue and healthy viable tissue are formed.

Examination

Serial examinations over several weeks are required to determine the full extent of the frostbitten tissue.

Diagnosis

A diagnosis is made by a history of long-term exposure to cold weather and by physical examination and presenting symptoms. Surgical amputation should be delayed as long as possible secondary to the weeks or months it will take for declaration of demarcation lines of cold injury between good tissue and dead tissue.

Laboratory Findings

A complete blood count (CBC), prothrombin time (PT), partial thromboplastin time (PTT), blood urea nitrogen (BUN), electrolytes, creatinine, calcium, magnesium, phosphorus, and cardiac and liver enzymes should be drawn on all patients with frostbite or hypothermia. Specific laboratory tests are not available for diagnosis of frostbite. Technetium pertechnetate scanning has shown a correlation between persistent tissue perfusion and tissue defects.

Treatment

Rewarming should begin as soon as possible in the field. Rewarming by skin to skin contact, without rubbing, should be the initial treatment. Rewarming should not take place in the field if there is a possibility of refreezing before definitive therapy, because refreezing causes more damage to the tissue.

Remember that if frostbite is present, hypothermia can also be present. Ensure placement of a large-gauge intravenous (IV) line of normal saline or lactated Ringer's solution at room temperature. Place the patient on a cardiac monitor, and take the patient's temperature rectally to rule out core hypothermia. An electrocardiogram (ECG) should be performed to rule out cardiac arrhythmias secondary to hypothermia. If the patient is hypothermic, do not handle the patient roughly, because this can precipitate cardiac arrhythmias. Most patients with frostbite are at least partially hypothermic. Remember to rewarm the patient's entire body.

Rapid rewarming is the mainstay of treatment. Rewarming should begin as soon as possible with warm gently circulating water at 40 to 43° C. Rewarming should continue until the extremity is pliable and erythema is present. This process usually takes 15 to 30 minutes. The entire extremity must be thawed.

As reperfusion of the frost bitten body part occurs, extreme pain will occur. If parenteral analgesia is required, give morphine, meperidine, or butorphanol tartrate (Stadol).

After the extremity is thawed, keep it elevated to reduce edema. Evaluate the extremity for signs and symptoms of compartment syndrome. If this condition is suspected, obtain compartment pressures. If the compartment pressures are elevated, consult a surgeon or orthopedic specialist regarding an escharotomy or a fasciotomy. Blisters should be débrided, or sterile aspirations should be done. If hemorrhagic blisters are present, do not débride the blisters; perform sterile aspiration instead. The patient should receive whirlpool treatments twice daily with warm antibiotic solutions for débridment. Do not place a pressure dressing on the patient's extremities, because this may decrease blood flow. If a secondary infection is present, parenteral penicillin is the drug of choice. Always perform a Gram stain and a culture of the damaged or infected skin before starting the patient on parenteral antibiotics. Again surgical treatment—amputation—should be a last resort, and should not be performed acutely secondary to the weeks or months before the extent of true damage is known.

The pain from chronic chilblains can be treated with nifedipine, 20 to 60 mg/day.

DYSBARIC DIVING INJURIES

Definition

Diving injuries are caused by the change of pressure from ascent to descent and vice versa in freshwater or saltwater bodies. Barotrauma is the name given to pressure injuries that occur during a diver's descent and ascent. Decompression sickness is a multisystem disorder caused by the release of liberated inert gases from solution when ambient pressures decrease too rapidly. The result is that gas bubbles form in the blood and body tissues.

Epidemiology

In the United States, more than 3 million persons dive professionally, commercially, and recreationally. Numerous accidents occur secondary to inexperienced divers and equipment malfunction.

Pathology

Pressure is a force on an object or unit area that is measured in units. Air at sea level is 14.7 lb/in^2 (psi). Water pressure is measured in atmosphere absolute (ATA). At sea level the ATA is 1. At 33 ft of sea water (fsw) the ATA is 2 ATA, and at 165 ft the ATA is 6. Fresh water is less dense than sea water (34 ft of fresh water [FFW] = 1 ATA).

The physiology of gaseous changes under pressure are described by Henry's law, Dalton's law, and Boyle's law. Henry's law states that the amount of gas dissolved in a given volume of fluid is proportional to the pressure of the gas with which it is in equilibrium.

Dalton's law states that the pressure exerted by each gas in a mixture of gases is the same as would be exerted if that gas alone occupied the same volume, or, alternatively, the total pressure of mixture of gases is equal to the sum of the partial pressures of the component gas. Boyle's law states that the volume of a gas is inversely proportional to its pressure at a constant temperature.

What this all means is that as a diver descends, the gases in the body are "squeezed" in enclosed spaces and ambient pressures increase with underwater descent. The body will attempt to maintain equilibrium, but if there is an obstruction to the portals of gas exchange, equalization cannot occur. If equalization does not take place, then there is a pressure imbalance, distortion of the affected tissue, vascular engorgement, hemorrhage, and mucosal edema. This is termed *barotrauma.* Barotrauma of descent or "squeeze" can affect the ears and sinuses as gases are retracted. Organs and tissue also contract with descent.

Barotrauma of ascent is caused by expansion of gases. If the air-filled spaces during descent cannot equalize secondary to obstruction, then as the diver ascends the expanding gases will distend the surrounding tissues and cause the reverse effect of squeeze. Organs and tissue bulge and expand.

Barotrauma can cause reverse squeeze and can injure the middle ear. Alternobaric vertigo can result from the asymmetric middle ear pressure during the diver's ascent. This condition is usually transient and resolves in a few hours.

Pulmonary barotrauma is caused by overpressurization syndrome or "burst lung" injury. Diving equipment is designed to deliver the same amount of pressure as the surrounding environment. Compressed gas expands during the diver's ascent. The diver must ascend slowly enough to allow expanding gases to escape from the lungs. If the gas does not escape, it will dissect into surrounding tissues or rupture the lungs. The seriousness of the injury depends on the amount of gas that has escaped and on the location of the injury.

Dysbaric air embolisms are the result of gas bubbles entering the systemic circulation through a ruptured pulmonary vein. These bubbles leave the lungs via veins, go through the heart, and lodge in small arteries of the distal circulation. When the diver surfaces, the high intrapulmonic pressure from lung overexpansion is relieved.

This allows bubble-laden blood to return to the heart. The brain is the most commonly affected organ, followed by the heart.

Nitrogen narcosis is a result of breathing gases at a higher-than-normal atmospheric pressure. Nitrogen is a lipid-soluble gas and is an anesthetic at elevated partial pressures. This anesthetic effect occurs at 70 to 100 fsw. Decreased work impairment occurs at 200 fsw, and unconsciousness occurs at 300 fsw.

Decompression sickness is a multisystem disorder secondary to the liberation of inert gases from a solution and the secondary formation of gas bubbles in the blood and body tissues when ambient pressures are decreased. There is increased tissue absorption of inert gas, usually nitrogen.

The physiology of decompression sickness is as the diver descends, the ambient pressure increases and a positive gradient of nitrogen from the alveoli into the tissues develops. As the diver's depth stabilizes, so does the gradient, which equalizes to zero. The rate at which the diver reaches a new inert gas equilibrium will be an exponential function of the diffusion and perfusion of the different tissues. Equilibrium is achieved based on the gradient of inert gas from the alveoli to the tissues, the ratio of blood-to-tissue inert gas solubility, and the blood flow to the tissues. When the ambient pressure is decreased too rapidly for the diffusion of inert gas from the tissues to occur, decompression sickness occurs.

Decompression sickness is caused by the mechanical vascular occlusion of bubbles that usually impair venous return. Bubbles also cause an inflammatory reaction secondary to an immune system response. The bubble is viewed by the immune system as a foreign body. This immune response triggers the Hageman factor, which activates the intrinsic clotting mechanism and kinin complement system. This action causes platelet activation, cellular clumping, increased vascular permeability, lipid embolization, microvascular slugging, and interstitial edema. These processes cause decreased tissue perfusion and tissue ischemia.

Clinical Presentation/Examination

Patients with barotrauma caused by descent injuries present with three types of aural barotrauma: (1) external ear squeeze or barotitis externa, (2) middle ear squeeze or barotitis media, and (3) inner ear barotrauma. Barotitis externa is caused by the occlusion of the ear canal by cerumen, exostoses, foreign bodies, or earplugs. Water cannot go into the external canal and, therefore, the air that is trapped in the external canal (behind the tympanic membrane) will push on the tympanic membrane and cause the tympanic membrane to outwardly bulge, rupture, or hemorrhage.

On examination, the canal or tympanic membrane presents with petechiae or blood-filled cutaneous blebs along the canal or a ruptured tympanic membrane.

Barotitis media results from a failure to equalize the middle ear to its new environmental pressures, secondary to a dysfunction or an occlusion of the eustachian tube. The purpose of the eustachian tube is to equalize the pressure from the outside environment and the middle ear when the pressure between the pharynx and the middle ear is greater than 20 mm Hg. Pain occurs when pressures reach 1100 to 1500 mm Hg. At these pressures the tympanic membrane begins to bulge inward, and edema with mucosal engorgement and hemorrhage occur. If this process continues, the tympanic membrane will rupture.

On examination the tympanic membrane will have hemorrhagic changes. There can be blood around the nose and mouth, and a conductive hearing loss will be present, which usually resolves without treatment.

Inner ear barotrauma presents with the classic trio of vertigo, tinnitus, and deafness. These symptoms can be permanent and disabling to the cochleovestibular system. They are usually secondary to a rapid change in pressures between the middle ear and the inner ear. Divers suffering from inner ear barotrauma can also present with nausea, vomiting, nystagmus, disorientation, diaphoresis, and ataxia. The onset of symptoms can be acute or delayed.

The patient can present with four types of injuries of the inner ear due to barotrauma:

1. Hemorrhage within the inner ear at the basal turn of the cochlea
2. Rupture of Reissner's membrane, which causes a mixing of endolymph and perilymph
3. Fistulation of the round and oval window
4. A mixed injury of the membranous labyrinth

Any one of these injuries can cause severe sensorineural hearing loss.

On physical examination the results will depend on the associated barotrauma to the tympanic membrane. It can be hemorrhagic or normal. There will be a mild or severe sensorineural hearing loss.

Barotrauma of ascent presents with three different types of symptoms. Barodontalgia or "tooth squeeze" occurs when pulp decay, periodontal infections, or a recent extraction of a tooth has taken place and there is an empty socket. It is caused by disequilibrium of an air-filled space in or around the tooth. It is almost always self-limiting and requires no treatment.

Aerogastria or "gas in the gut" is a painful type of barotrauma that usually occurs in the inexperienced diver. If a diver drinks carbonated beverages or eats a heavy meal before a dive, this can precipitate aerogastria. The patient presents with a colicky abdominal pain, abdominal fullness, belching, and flatulence. It rarely causes long-term harm. Flatulence during ascent usually resolves the problem, but syncope, shock-like states, and actual rupture of the bowel have been reported.

A patient with lung barotrauma presents with gradually increasing hoarseness, substernal chest pain, and neck fullness either immediately upon surfacing, or symptoms may be delayed for hours. As symptoms and the time before treatment increase, dysphagia, dyspnea, or syncope can occur. With pulmonary overpressurization syndrome (POPS), subcutaneous emphysema or mediastinal emphysema can be the presenting complaint.

Divers with dysbaric air embolism (DAE) have an abrupt onset of pain and air panic after a rapid ascent. A rapid ascent is not always part of the history prior to an acute DAE. Neurologic presentations include acute stroke, menoplegia or multiplegia, convulsions, aphasia confusion, vertigo, dizziness, blindness, deafness, focal paralysis, and sensory disturbances. Asymmetric multiplegias are very common.

On physical examination, the patient can be awake or unconscious. On retinal examination, visualization of bubbles in the retinal arteries has been noted. This is called Libermeister's sign, described as a sharply circumscribed area of glossy pallor. This is a very rare finding.

The physical presentation of decompression sickness or "the bends" involves musculoskeletal, joint, and spinal cord pain. The bends are described as type I (with mild symptoms) or type II (with more severe symptoms, including neurologic symptoms). The patient presents with subcutaneous emphysema, pruritus, and scarlatiniform, erysipeloid, or mottled rash. The hallmark of the bends is joint pain. The pain is often described as a dull ache or a deep, throbbing, or sharp pain. Movement is extremely painful, and there may be some numbness or dysesthesia around the painful joint. The elbows and shoulders are the most commonly affected joints. Often if a blood pressure cuff is inflated around the involved joint, the patient will receive some relief of symptoms. Neurologic symptoms include lower-extremity paresthesias, paraplegia, paraparesis, and bladder dysfunction. Urinary retention is a a hallmark of spinal cord decompression sickness.

Diagnosis

A diagnosis is made by determining the type of diving equipment used, the number of dives, the depth of the dives, surface interval times between repetitive dives for all dives in the past 48 to 72 hours, and the onset of symptoms. Always ask whether the dive was done in fresh water or in sea water. The water temperature and predisposing factors like alcohol, cigarette use, obesity, prior history of pulmonary embolism, dehydration, and vigorous exercise prior to injury should always be obtained. The onset of clinical symptoms and presentation in relationship to the last dive are all important factors in determining the likelihood of dysbaric injury.

Laboratory Findings

A CBC, electrolytes, BUN, creatinine, calcium, magnesium, phosphorus, liver and cardiac enzymes, urinalysis, and arterial blood gas should be performed on all persons with diving injuries.

Treatment

Any patient with an acute case of DAE should be placed on 100% supplemental oxygen via facemask at 6 to 8 l/min. Oxygen increases offgasing of nitrogen bubbles and improves oxygenation to tissue that has been damaged already. Remember that patients who have been injured during a dive may often also suffer from hypothermia, thus a rectal temperature should be taken to determine the patient's core temperature. Do not place the patient in the Trendelenburg or Durant position secondary to the patient's ability to aggravate cerebral edema. Advanced life support should be administered according to protocol. A high dose of steroids is recommended by some authors secondary to the ability of steroids to reduce cerebral edema. There are no good anecdotal studies that prove this to be true. The patient must be transferred immediately to a hyperbaric chamber for decompression.

Treatment for acute barotitis externa involves keeping the canal dry and precludes swimming or diving until the canal has healed. Antibiotics and analgesics are prescribed as needed.

Treatment for acute barotitis media involves long-acting spray decongestants, antihistamines, and abstinence from diving until the tympanic membrane heals. If the tympanic membrane is ruptured in the water, antibiotics should be used. Oral analgesics can be given for pain. Ear drops should not be used when a ruptured eardrum is present. Treatment of inner ear barotrauma often involves bed rest, elevation of the patient's head, avoidance of strenuous activities, and symptomatic treatment of dizziness.

Uncomplicated lung barotrauma and uncomplicated POPS are treated with rest, supplemental oxygen, and observation. If a pneumothorax is present, immediate treatment is required with needle aspiration or tube thoracostomy. If symptoms are severe, recompression is required. If a diver suddenly loses consciousness after surfacing, this is a sign of a DAE that requires aggressive hyperbaric treatment. Patients who suffer from any type of severe decompression sickness require immediate hyperbaric treatment. Remember that hemoconcentration and dehydration are both common in serious decompression sickness, and fluid replacement is essential for treatment.

HIGH-ALTITUDE ILLNESS

Definition

Persons who live or travel to a high-altitude area can suffer frostbite, hypothermia, trauma, dehydration, lighting injuries, ultraviolet keratitis, and high-altitude sickness. The oxygen content at sea level is 21%. The barometric pressure is decreased as altitude increases, thus the oxygen content of air decreases. At very high altitudes (>18,000 ft) the percentage of oxygen in the air decreases by 90%. High altitude is considered 1500 to 3500 m (4900 to 11,500 ft) above sea level.

Patients with high-altitude illness can present with acute mountain sickness (AMS), high-altitude cerebral edema (HACE), high-altitude pulmonary edema (HAPE), re-entry pulmonary edema (RPE), high-altitude retinopathy (HAR), high-altitude pharyngitis, bronchitis, and chronic mountain polycythemia (CMP).

Epidemiology

High-altitude hypoxia is secondary to long periods of strenuous exercise at high altitudes and rapid or abrupt descents without acclimatization. Underlying disease like chronic obstructive pulmonary disease (COPD), heart disease, poor physical conditions, sickle cell disease, and pregnancy can all affect cell metabolism at high altitudes.

Pathology

The main problem with a rapid ascent to high altitudes without acclimatization is that the mitochondria struggle to respond to the acute decrease in oxygen levels and cell metabolism is interrupted. The alveolar PO_2 is inadequate for cellular respiration. The hypoxic ventilatory response (HVR) is affected by the carotid body. The decrease in oxygen level causes the respiratory center in the medulla to increase ventilation. This causes hyperventilation and respiratory alkalosis, which acts as a brake for the respiratory system. Extreme hypoxemia can develop during sleep. The respiratory rate and pH will return to normal after 4 to 7 days of acclimatization. During this acclimatization period, the ventilation rate continues to increase until the chemoreceptors are reset to lower PCO_2 levels. Acclimatization is determined by the arterial PCO_2 levels. If the person's ascent continues to another height, this process is repeated.

Within 2 hours of ascent, erythropoietin is increased in the plasma, thus causing an increase in red blood cell mass in the plasma. The oxyhemoglobin dissociation curve is shifted minimally, secondary to the increase in 2,3 diphosphoglyceric acid, which is proportional to the severity of hypoxia, and the curve shifts back to the right. The presence of alkalosis secondary to hyperventilation shifts the curve back to the left.

An acute ascent to high altitudes causes the baroreceptors to suppress the antidiuretic hormone (ADH) and aldosterone, which induces diuresis. Bicarbonate diuresis and respiratory alkalosis decrease plasma volume and cause hyperosmolality. The osmoreceptor center of the brain effectively handles this hyperosmolar state without much problem.

As ascent progresses, stroke volume decreases initially and the heart rate increases. Blood pressure is mildly elevated. The pulmonary circulation constricts when exposed to hypoxia, and pulmonary pressures increase. If the pressures are extremely high, pulmonary edema occurs.

Sleep stages III and IV are reduced at high altitudes, and stage I is increased. There is only a small decrease in rapid eye movement (REM) time, but the person spends more time in a state of arousal and awake at high altitudes. Cheyne-Stokes breathing can occur at high altitudes (> 9000 ft) with apneic pauses that last from 6 to 12 seconds, thus causing the person to awaken frequently.

AMS is due to hypobaric hypoxia. Two theories have been proposed as to why hypobaric hypoxia occurs in AMS. One theory is that the edema is caused by a cytotoxic reaction due to the failure of the sodium-potassium pump, which causes intracellular accumulation of sodium and water and thus a toxic reaction to hypernatremia and water. The secondary theory is that the edema is vasogenic secondary to a leaky blood-brain barrier.

HAPE is caused by noncardiogenic edema. Cardiac output is low, and pulmonary vascular resistance and pulmonary artery pressures are markedly elevated. Left ventricular function is normal, and end-diastolic pressure, wedge pressure, and left atrial pressure are normal to low. Increased pulmonary hypertension plays an important role in HAPE, but the exact mechanism is still unknown. It is believed that the exaggerated pulmonary pressures are secondary to the pressor response to hypoxia of high altitude. The combination of pulmonary venous constriction, fibrin and platelet thrombi, and uneven arterial vasoconstriction of the lungs has also been suggested to cause or increase the likelihood of pulmonary edema.

CMP is also called Monge's disease. CMP is greater in males than in females and is seen in persons who live for a long time in high-altitude areas of the world or in lowlanders who relocate to high altitudes. CMP is caused by a chronic elevation of hemoglobin, which is higher than the expected hemoglobin for that altitude (usually 20 to 22 g/dl). It is often seen in patients with chronic COPD or in those who suffer from sleep apnea.

HAR is believed to be caused by a lack of oxygen (i.e., hypoxia) to the eye. On examination, retinal hemorrhages, dilatation of retinal veins, retinal edema, tortuous veins, disk hyperemia, and cotton wool exudates can be seen and are found commonly in mountain climbers who sleep at heights above 5000 m. These hemorrhages require no treatment and resolve usually in 10 to 14 days.

RPE occurs secondary to a sojourn when the patient who lives at a high altitude, leaves the normal high altitude and goes to a lower elevation, and then returns to the normal high-altitude home. RPE is believed to be caused by acute pulmonary vasoconstriction and pulmonary hypertension, secondary to re-exposure of the lung's pulmonary muscularization at lower levels of oxygen.

Persons exposed to altitudes greater than 2500 m can develop a dry hacking cough, secondary to the dry, cold air. Bronchospasms can also occur secondary to the dry, cold air, which can exacerbate symptoms of asthma and COPD. The entire oral mucosa of the nose and pharynx can become dry and cracked secondary to hyperventilation and dehydration. Antibiotics are usually not helpful secondary to the lack of pathogens. Candies or throat lozenges or breathing of steam can help to keep the mucosa moist.

Clinical Presentation/Examination

AMS presents as an acute hypoxic syndrome of gradual onset and occurs above 6600 ft. Children are slightly more susceptible than are adults. Susceptibility is reduced by repeated exposure to high altitudes.

A patient with AMS presents with lightheadedness and slight breathlessness after exercise, 1 to 6 hours after arrival. The patient often complains of a bifrontal headache that is made worse by bending over or the Valsalva maneuver. The patient often complains of feeling "hungover." He or she is often very irritable and anorexic and has symptoms of nausea and vomiting. As symptoms progress, dyspnea increases and oliguria is present. Severe lassitude can occur, and AMS can develop into HACE within 24 hours if treatment is delayed. The patient's blood pressure and pulse rate will be increased. On funduscopic examination, tortuous and dilated veins and retinal hemorrhage are common findings. On lung examination, rales secondary to pulmonary edema can be present. If mental status changes occur, cerebral edema may be present. Fluid retention is the hallmark of AMS, and, unlike when acclimatization is taking place, diuresis is usually present.

HACE occurs in the presence of AMS or HAPE. A patient with HACE presents with altered mental status, stupor, ataxia, and a progression to coma and death. Nausea, vomiting, and headache are not always present. The patient presents with focal neurologic symptoms, such as third and sixth cranial nerve palsies, secondary to intracranial compression.

HAPE has the greatest mortality of all the high-altitude illnesses. Children are at greater risk than are adults, and women are less susceptible than are men. Cold, excessive salt ingestion, heavy exertion, rapid ascent, and use of sleeping medications all predispose the patient to an increased risk of HAPE.

A patient with HAPE presents with dyspnea on exertion, decreased exercise performance, increased recovery time from exercise, and localized rales, usually in the right midlung. As the patient gets sicker, he or she develops tachycardia, increased dyspnea, dyspnea at rest, increased weakness, cyanosis, productive cough, and increased rales. HAPE is usually exacerbated at night and a fever higher than 38.5° C is often present. A prominent P2 and a right ventricular heave are often noted on auscultation. An ECG will often show a right axis deviation and a right ventricular strain pattern of pulmonary hypertension. Patients then become unconscious and progress to coma and die.

Patients with CMP present with difficulty sleeping, drowsiness, headache, muddled thinking, impaired peripheral circulation, and chronic chest congestion.

Laboratory Findings

A CBC, PT, PTT, electrolytes, BUN, creatinine, calcium, magnesium, phosphorus, liver and cardiac function tests, and a urinalysis should be performed on all patients with suspected high-altitude sickness. An arterial blood gas is the mainstay of diagnostic testing for altitude sickness.

Treatment

Any patient suspected of suffering from altitude sickness should be placed on oxygen via facemask or nasal cannula, have at least one large-gauge IV placed, and the aforementioned laboratory tests drawn. The patient should also have an ECG, arterial blood gas, and a chest radiograph performed.

The treatment of AMS is to prevent progression of the illness, improve acclimatization, and abort the illness. There are three principles of treatment of AMS: (1) no higher ascent in the presence of symptoms should be attempted, (2) descend if symptoms do not abate or become worse, and (3) descend and treat immediately if changes in consciousness, ataxia, or pulmonary edema occur.

Generally AMS is a mild self-limiting illness that improves on its own within 12 to 36 hours with acclimatization and rest. Often a change in just 500 to 1000 ft will be all that is needed to treat and resolve symptoms of AMS. Oxygen should be given to all symptomatic patients with AMS. Oxygen will relieve the headache and dizziness.

If symptoms are severe, acetazolamide 250 mg twice a day (BID) can speed up the resolution of symptoms. Acetazolamide acts by inhibiting the enzyme carbonic anhydrase and slows the hydration of carbon dioxide to hydrogen and bicarbonate ions. The drug mimics the process of ventilatory acclimatization and causes a higher arterial Po_2 level. The drug also maintains a higher cerebral blood flow and acts as a diuretic for fluid retention. Acetazolamide should be used for any patient who has a history of altitude illness, abrupt ascent to higher than 10,000 ft, or treatment for AMS or annoying periodic breathing during sleep.

Dexamethasone 4 mg by mouth (PO), intramuscularly (IM), or IV can be used to treat AMS. It reduces vasogenic edema, lowers intracranial pressure, and acts as an antiemetic and mood elevator. Diuretics can be used to treat edema. Prochlorperazine, 5 to 10 mg, can be given to the patient for nausea and vomiting. Any patient with a change in mental status, pulmonary edema, or ataxia should be admitted to the hospital and should then be transferred to a hospital at a lower altitude.

The goal of treatment of HACE is complete immediate reversal of the pulmonary and cerebral edema. HACE is treated much like AMS, with oxygen, descent to a lower altitude, steroids, hyperbaric chamber therapy, and acetazolamide. If the patient is in a coma, place a Foley catheter, intubate, and hyperventilate the patient to decrease the acute intracranial pressure. Remember that the P_{CO_2} is already low and the pH is high. Aggressive hyperventilation can produce cerebral ischemia; therefore, do not be too aggressive with hyperventilation of the patient.

Give loop diuretics, such as furosemide 40 to 80 mg or bumetanide 1 to 2 mg IV or mannitol 1 to 2 g/kg for cerebral edema. The patient should be evacuated to a lower altitude as soon as possible. Even after aggressive treatment, the patient can remain in a coma for several weeks after he or she has been evacuated to a lower altitude.

The main treatment of HAPE consists of early recognition of symptoms. Chest x-rays will show progressive interstitial or localized alveolar infiltrates. Oxygen therapy and removal of the patient to a lower altitude are critical for the severe symptoms of HAPE. Bed rest in a warm environment is often enough to improve the patient who has mild symptoms. Loop diuretics (furosemide 40 to 80 mg *or* bumetanide 1 to 2 mg) and morphine 2 to 10 mg IV can both be used in the treatment of pulmonary edema. Nifedipine 10 to 30 mg has been used to reduce pulmonary artery pressure by 30 to 50% and to increase arterial oxygen saturation. All patients with HAPE should be hospitalized until pulmonary edema has resolved.

CMP is treated with relocation of the patient to a lower altitude, home oxygen use, or phlebotomy. Acetazolamide 250 mg BID has been used with some success in the treatment of CMP. Therapy with medroxyprogesterone acetate 20 to 50 mg/day has also been used.

HEAT INJURIES

Definition

Patients present with three types of heat injures: (1) heat cramps, (2) heat exhaustion, and (3) heat stroke. They are all the result of the body's inability to respond to environmental heat conditions with an inadequate correction of extracellular fluid and electrolyte deficiencies. These three types of heat injuries overlie each other and often form a continuum.

Epidemiology

Heat injuries have been recorded throughout time. Many military battles have been won or lost because of heat injuries. Heat injuries are usually secondary to heat exposure without proper acclimatization. Heat injuries often affect those at the extremes of age—the very old and the very young—and those whose occupations require them to work in a hot environment.

Pathology

Heat is generated through metabolism. Biochemical reactions generate energy and produce byproducts of water and carbon dioxide, sulfates, phosphates, urea, and other chemicals. The chemically generated heat byproducts are measured as the basal metabolic rate. This rate is defined as 50 to 60 kcal/hr/m^2 of body surface area or 100 kcal/hr for a 70-kg man. These biochemical reactions produce about 1.1° C (2° F) of hourly body temperature. Body temperature can rise due to strenuous exertion, hyperthyroidism, sympathomimetic drug ingestion, and environmental heat. *Conduction* is the transfer of heat from a warm object to a cooler object. *Conversion* is heat lost from air and the circulation of water vapor molecules around the body. *Radiation* is the transfer of electromagnetic waves, and *evaporation* is the conversion of a liquid to a gaseous form. All of the aforementioned processes affect the body's ability to lose and conserve heat.

Thermoregulation is controlled by heat sensors in the skin and by central organs of the body. The main center of temperature regulation is in the anterior hypothalamus. When the body senses an increase in core temperature, the main response is sweating and cutaneous vasodilation. Cutaneous vasodilation increases heat loss from the skin by convection and radiation by increasing the amount of sweat lost by evaporation. In extremely hot weather, up to 1 to 4 l/hr of sweat can be lost. Each liter of sweat contains approximately 580 kcal of heat. Humidity affects the amount of heat lost by sweating. As the humidity approaches 100%, less and less heat is lost. At 100% humidity, no heat loss will occur. Winds greater than 0.5 to 5 m/sec do not increase heat loss.

Excessive or increased heat affects all organs of the body. The main effects of a climate change on the body are the alterations of sodium and water balance through acclimatization, which is mediated by aldosterone over several days or weeks. If the person is not acclimated to the heat, an acute contraction of extracellular fluid volume occurs; renal plasma flow decreases; and secretion of aldosterone increases. This action is the body's attempt to retain sodium and water and to expand extracellular fluid volume. Less sodium is found in sweat and urine, but potassium continues to be secreted in both the urine and sweat.

Drugs that interfere with heat metabolism are the phenothiazines and the cyclic antidepressants secondary to their anticholinergic properties, which interfere with sweating.

Clinical Presentation

A patient with heat cramp presents with painful spasm of the skeletal muscles and the abdominal muscles. Heat cramps usually occur after strenuous physical activity. The patient often hyperventilates and produces large amounts of sweat that has a high sodium content. The patient often knows that he or she is getting hot and drinks large amounts of tap water, which is low in sodium; thus, only free water is ingested and, with the continued high loss of sodium via sweating, hyponatremia occurs. An onset of heat cramps occurs secondary to this free water intake and hypernatremic sweating. There is usually a large accumulation of lactate secondary to hyperventilation, causing respiratory alkalosis. Respiratory alkalosis causes an acute hypokalemia, which causes muscle cramps, paresthesias, and tetany. The core temperature is usually normal in a patient with heat cramps.

Heat exhaustion is secondary to true volume depletion and electrolyte loss due to sweating. Hypovolemia often leads to hypoperfusion. The patient presents with nausea, vomiting, lightheadedness, headache, tachycardia, and hyperventilation. The patient's body temperature is usually normal or slightly elevated.

Heat stroke is a true life-threatening emergency. Heat stroke is defined as a core temperature higher than 40° C (106° F) with neurologic symptoms. Temperatures higher than 42° C (107.6° F) are associated with a poor prognosis. True heat stroke can cause severe end-organ damage in minutes if it is not treated. The patient presents with sudden loss of consciousness, irritability, bizarre behavior, hallucinations, combativeness, or coma. The patient can present with virtually any neurologic abnormality from pupillary abnormalities to an acute cerebrovascular accident.

Often it is said that a patient in true heat stroke does not sweat, but in early heat stroke the patient will sweat in attempt to cool the body through thermoregulation. A patient with true heat stroke often presents with hot dry skin. Remember that the most common cause of decreased sweating involves anticholinergic drugs. Always ask if the patient is taking any anticholinergic medications. Heat stroke is not always induced by exercise. Persons at the extremes of age—the very elderly and the very young—are susceptible to heat injury.

Remember that fluid and electrolyte abnormalities and dehydration are usually not present in the heat stroke victim. Vigorous administration of IV fluids can cause pulmonary edema, especially in the elderly, in the patient with COPD, and in the patient with congestive heart failure.

Examination

The patient should be given a complete examination. The patient's skin needs to be examined for sweating, temperature, and color. A complete baseline neurologic examination should be performed, followed by serial neurologic examinations.

Diagnosis

A diagnosis of heat cramps, heat exhaustion, or heat stroke is made by clinical presentation, laboratory studies, serum sodium and potassium levels, core rectal temperature, and neurologic status of the patient at the time of presentation.

Laboratory Findings

A CBC, PT, PTT, electrolytes, BUN, creatinine, liver function tests to include CPK and CPK-MB and MM fractions, urinalysis, and a urine or serum myoglobin should be performed on all patients. If heat stroke or rhabdomyolysis is suspected, fibrin degradation products should be drawn. On urinalysis, hematuria, casts, proteinuria, mild myoglobinuria, and white blood cells can be found in the urine of any heat-injured victim. These symptoms are usually secondary to decreased renal blood flow. Sodium and potassium are both lost in sweat. Dehydration can cause both hyponatremia or hypernatremia and hypokalemia or hyperkalemia. There can be decreased or increased liver function test results with a heat injury, and a prolonged prothrombin time can be noted. The white blood cell count is often elevated. Respiratory alkalosis is often present on arterial blood gas analysis.

With heat cramps, hyponatremia, hypokalemia, hypomagnesemia, and respiratory alkalosis can be present.

With heat exhaustion, victims who have not taken in PO fluids will usually present with hypernatremia. If salt-containing fluids have been taken, the sodium and potassium levels will usually be normal.

In rhabdomyolysis, the CPK and serum myoglobin will be elevated, along with myoglobinuria on urinalysis. Hyperkalemia is often present in severe exertional rhabdomyolysis. Hyperkalemia can cause cardiac dysrhythmias and death.

Treatment

Any patient with a suspected heat injury should have two large-gauge IVs placed. The patient should be placed on a cardiac monitor and on pulse oximetry. The patient should be given 2 liters of oxygen via nasal cannula and should have the abovementioned laboratory tests drawn. An arterial blood gas should be analyzed if acidosis or alkalosis is suspected. If hyperkalemia or hypokalemia is suspected, or if heat stroke is present, an ECG should be done. Serial blood pressure, pulse, and rectal temperatures should be taken until a diagnosis is made or the patient's core temperature is back to normal.

Heat cramps respond to hypotonic salt solutions (0.9% normal saline). If severe hyponatremia is present, 3% hypertonic saline solution may be required for treatment.

The treatment of hypovolemia due to heat exhaustion is with rapid administration of IV fluids, 1 or 2 liters of 0.9% normal saline, rest, and PO fluids. Heat exhaustion due to salt depletion is treated based on the BUN, serum sodium level, potassium level, hematocrit changes, and the patient's total body water deficit. The total body water deficit should be calculated and then replaced slowly over 48 hours. A correction that is too rapid can cause hypernatremia and seizures.

Heat stroke is treated by rapid cooling of the patient to at least 39° C

(102.2° F). The goal temperature for cooling should not be exceeded. Immersion in a tub of ice water, cooling blankets, and air cooling with fans can be utilized. Protection of the patient's airway is of greatest importance. If the patient is hypotensive, a Swan-Ganz catheter should be placed to monitor central venous pressure (CVP). A Foley catheter should be placed to monitor urine output. The patient should be placed on 5 to 10 liters of oxygen by facemask, and Dextrostix should be performed.

If the patient is suffering from severe shivering or seizures, treat the patient with diazepam or chlorpromazine therapy. All heat stroke victims should be admitted to the intensive care unit. Patients who have had heat cramps and heat exhaustion can usually be discharged to home unless they have underlying cardiac or pulmonary disease.

HYPOTHERMIA

Definition

The history of cold injuries goes as far back as Hippocrates, Aristotle, and Galen. Napoleon's army suffered devastating losses from the cold in Russia, and Hannibal lost half of his army crossing the Pyrenees Alps. Hypothermia is defined as a core temperature of less than 35° C (95° F). Hypothermia almost always occurs accidentally when a person is exposed to outdoor temperatures.

Epidemiology

Approximately 1500 fatalities are caused by cold weather in the United States each year. The mortality rate can reach 50% when a patient has significant underlying disease. Age, basic health status, nutritional status, current medications, intoxicants, and time of exposure are factors that contribute to hypothermia.

Pathology

Body temperature falls from loss of heat by conduction. Conduction is the transfer of heat from a warm object to a cold object. Conduction is 30 times greater in water than in air, thus body heat is lost at a greater rate when the person is immersed in water. Convection is the transfer of heat by actual movement of heated material from one object to another. Winds increase the loss of heat by convection. Evaporation and radiation also cause the loss of heat from the body.

The hypothalamus regulates heat in the body. Heat is conserved by peripheral vasoconstriction and behavioral responses to cold. Shivering is a mechanism by which heat is generated by the body. Heat can also be produced by an increased metabolic rate by stimulation of the adrenal and thyroid glands.

Hypothermia is usually divided into immersion and nonimmersion accidental exposure. Metabolic heat loss can be caused by hypopituitarism, hypothyroidism, and hypoadrenalism. Severe hypoglycemia can also lead to hypothermia. A patient presenting with disease of the central nervous system (CNS), stroke, acute head trauma, Wernicke's disease, or brain tumor can also present with hypothermia.

Alcoholics who live on the street and who are chronically intoxicated are often victims of hypothermia. Ethanol is a vasodilator, anesthetic, and CNS depressant. Often alcoholics do not realize that it is extremely cold, and they are anesthetized secondary to intoxication and consequently suffer from hypothermia.

Use of barbiturates, insulin, and phenothiazines can precipitate hypothermia. Burns or sepsis can also cause hypothermia. Burns can cause hypothermia through the loss of direct body heat through the burn site. In the septic patient, the hypothalamic temperature set point is altered secondary to direct damage to the hypothalamus.

Hypothyroidism or myxedema coma can often present much like hypothermia. Therapy with thyroxine in large doses is needed to treat myxedema coma.

Clinical Presentation

The patient's presentation correlates with the patient's core temperature. Mild hypothermia is defined as a core body temperature of between 32° C (90° F) and 35° C (95° F). The patient is awake, and his or her body attempts to adjust to the cold environment and the acute decrease in core temperature by creating an excitation (responsive) stage of shivering and behavioral stimulation to dress warmer. The result is that the heart rate increases, blood pressure rises, and cardiac output increases.

As the core temperature drops to below 32° C, the metabolism slows and there is a decrease in both CO_2 and oxygen production. Shivering stops somewhere between 30° C (86° F) and 32° C (90° F). In this phase, the heart rate, blood pressure, and cardiac output decrease.

As hypothermia increases and core temperature decreases the cardiac effects of hypothermia increase. The patient's ECG will appear abnormal. Life-threatening arrhythmias can ensue. The classic Osborn "J" wave can be present. A J wave is a positive deflection at the end of the QRS complex. It is not pathognomonic of hypothermia but is characteristic of hypothermia. Sinus bradycardia and atrial fibrillation occur with a slow ventricular response. Ventricular fibrillation occurs as the core temperature drops until finally asystole occurs. A cold heart is extremely irritable, and rough handling of the patient can precipitate deadly ventricular cardiac arrhythmias.

Pulmonary effects of hypothermia include tachypnea and decreased respiratory rate and tidal volume. Cold also decreases the gag reflex and cough reflexes and causes bronchorrhea, thus increasing the risk of aspiration pneumonia. The oxyhemoglobin dissociation curve shifts to the left, thus indicating that less oxygen is being released in the tissues. If an arterial blood gas is drawn, corrections must be made on a nomogram to determine the actual oxygen saturation level of the blood.

As the patient's body temperature decreases, neurologic symptoms of depressed consciousness will ensue. The patient will become confused, then lethargic, and then comatose.

Cold will actually cause a cold diuresis, which can lead to a significant volume loss. Intravascular volume is also shifted to extravascular spaces to attempt to conserve heat. Thus blood viscosity increases, hemoconcentration occurs, and intravascular thrombosis and embolic events can also occur. Cold also suppresses the enzymatic function of the liver and the pancreas. A decreased hepatic metabolism causes a decrease in drug metabolism and detoxification of toxic substances. Pancreatitis has been noted in hypothermia.

Examination

The patient should be given a thorough examination. Particular attention should be paid to the neck. The patient should be checked for the presence of a thyroidectomy scar, because this can be a clue to myxedema coma.

Diagnosis

The diagnosis is made after taking the patient's history of cold exposure, rectal temperature, and clinical presentation.

Laboratory Findings

A CBC, PT, PTT, electrolytes, BUN, creatinine, cardiac and liver enzymes, thyroid function tests, and urinalysis should be performed. If sepsis is suspected, blood and urine cultures should be taken.

Treatment

A patient with suspected hypothermia should have two large-gauge IV lines started and should be given warm normal saline or lactated Ringer's solution. The patient should be placed on a cardiac monitor and given warmed 100% oxygen via facemask. The aforementioned laboratory tests should be performed. A Foley catheter should be placed gently to monitor the patient's urine output.

The first rule in treating the hypothermic patient is that the patient is not dead until he or she is warm and dead, especially in the case of hypothermia caused by cold weather. The second rule is that one should never handle a hypothermic patient roughly, because this can precipitate deadly cardiac arrhythmias. CPR should be performed on all patients after a 1-minute evaluation for pulse and blood pressure.

If the patient has no pulse or blood pressure after 1 minute, CPR and rewarming should be started.

Do not treat cardiac arrhythmias in severe hypothermia, because these arrhythmias usually resolve with warming. Antiarrhythmic drugs in hypothermia are unpredictable, and the hypothermic heart is resistant to atropine, pacing, and countershock. If the patient is in ventricular fibrillation, give one or two electrical defibrillations and then continue rewarming and CPR. As the myocardium rewarms, the patient's cardiac rhythm usually converts to a sinus rhythm on its own.

Remember that a large number of hypothermic patients are alcoholics who live on the streets. They are usually deficient in thiamine. Give 100 mg of thiamine after 100 ml of 50% dextrose IV. Always give naloxone 1 to 4 mg to any unconscious patient to antagonize any opiates that are present.

The patient can be rewarmed by active or passive core rewarming methods. Passive rewarming is performed by removing the patient from the cold environment and by letting the patient rewarm on his or her own with blankets and in a warm environment. Active external rewarming is performed by application of exogenous heat to the patient. Be careful with rapid active external rewarming. This method can cause peripheral vasodilation and venous pooling, which can cause a rewarming shock secondary to acute hypotension and hypovolemia from peripheral dilation. A rewarming acidosis can occur secondary to the rapid release of lactic acid from the tissues. This condition is corrected with 100% oxygen therapy.

Active core rewarming is achieved by giving the patient warmed oxygen by facemask or intubation; heated IV fluids; gastric lavage with warm water, warm bladder lavage, warm peritoneal lavage, or warm pleural lavage. If peritoneal lavage is performed, the dialysis solution should be between 40° C (104° F) and 45° C (113° F). In the case of severe hypothermia if available, heated hemodialysis and cardiopulmonary bypass can be performed.

Death from hypothermia can be defined as a failure to revive the patient after the patient's body temperature has reached 30° C (86° F) to 32° C (90° F). Any patient suffering from hypothermia should be admitted to the hospital for at least 24 hours for monitoring of potential cardiac arrhythmias. Remember that no patient is dead until he or she is warm and dead!

INSECT BITES

Definition

Hymenoptera is the order to which the families of bees, wasps, yellow jackets, ants, and hornets belong. Insects have modified ovipositors that protrude from the abdomen and act like a hypodermic needle when administering venom.

Epidemiology

Reactions to hymenoptera are very common in the United States. Fortunately, very few deaths actually occur from envenomization.

Pathology

Hymenoptera produce venom in one or two tubular glands, which collect the venom in a venom reservoir. The venom reservoir connects to the stinger. The venom consists of several different kinds of substances depending on the species of hymenoptera. Venom is made up of proteins, peptides, carbohydrates, lipids, and amino acids. Phospholipase A and hyaluronidase are the two most common enzymes in the venom. The toxicity of the venom is a result of the low-molecular-weight substances acetylcholine, bradykinin, histamine, serotonin, and dopamine.

All stings and their reactions are IgE-mediated. When a person is stung by a hymenoptera, there is an immediate increase in IgE antibodies, which are released and attach to and stimulate mast cells and basophils. The patient is now sensitized to the antibodies. On subsequent stings, an antigen-antibody interaction activates histamine, which causes the release of the slow-reacting substance of anaphylaxis (SRS-A), an acidic sulfate ester. Re-envenomation also causes the eosinophil chemotactic factor of anaphylaxis (ECF-A) to be released. The histamine SRS-A and the ECF-A cause the reaction to the envenomation.

An acute histamine release will cause urticaria, angioedema, vasodilation, a decrease in the blood pressure, an increase or decrease in the respiratory rate, vomiting, and tenesmus. Histamine and SRS-A release are believed to cause the bronchial smooth muscle constriction related to the sting. Release of histamine also causes platelet aggregation and degranulation.

Each species has its own brand of venom. The venom of the fire ant is very alkaloid and can cause necrosis. The venom is not a protein and exhibits antibiotic activity, which cause pustules to form. Honeybee venom contains histamine; wasp venom contains serotonin and histamine; hornet venom contains acetycholine, histamine, and serotonin.

Clinical Presentation/Examination

Patients who are stung by bees or wasps present to the emergency department (ED) with five different reactions. *Local reactions* consist of edema at the sting site. There is no systemic reaction. Localized edema of the mouth or throat area, secondary to a sting, can compromise the airway. Stings to the area around the eye can cause capsular cataracts, lens abscess, glaucoma, perforation of the globe, atrophy of the iris, and refractive changes.

A *toxic reaction* occurs when there is a history of 10 stings or more at one time. The patient presents with nausea, vomiting, syncope, lightheadedness, diarrhea, edema without urticaria, involuntary muscle spasms, headache, and convulsions. The difference between a systemic or anaphylactic reaction and a toxic reaction is the absence of urticaria and bronchospasm. Diarrhea is also more intense in a toxic reaction than in an anaphylactic reaction.

Systemic or anaphylactic reactions are caused by a generalized systemic reaction to hymenoptera venom. It can occur from a single sting or from multiple stings. Symptoms can range from a mild reaction to death within minutes. It is often stated that the shorter the interval between the sting and the systemic reaction, the more severe the reaction will be.

A patient with a mild systemic reaction presents with facial flushing, generalized urticaria, itching eyes, and a dry cough. As the systemic reaction progresses, the patient develops dyspnea, wheezing, cyanosis, nausea, vomiting, diarrhea, fever, chills, abdominal cramps, laryngeal stridor, loss of bowel and bladder control, loss of consciousness, bloody and frothy sputum, and finally shock. The onset of symptoms from shock to death can last from 2 to 3 minutes to 30 minutes.

A patient with a *delayed reaction* presents with a serum-sickness–like syndrome—fever, generalized malaise, headache, urticaria, lymphadenopathy, and polyarthritis 10 to 14 days after the sting.

Unusual reactions involve cardiovascular, neurologic, or urologic symptoms of encephalopathy, vasculitis, neuritis, or nephrosis from days or weeks after the sting.

Diagnosis

A diagnosis of hymenoptera sting with a local, toxic, systemic, anaphylactic, or delayed reaction is based on a history of envenomation, the patient's clinical presentation, and physical examination.

Laboratory Findings

A laboratory examination in the ED for hymenoptera stings is nonspecific. A baseline CBC, PT, PTT, electrolytes, BUN, creatinine, and urinalysis should be performed.

Treatment

Any patient who presents to the ED with a suspected anaphylactic reaction to envenomation should have two large-gauge IV lines of 0.9% normal saline placed and should be given 100% oxygen via facemask. The patient should also be placed on the cardiac monitor. An arterial blood gas should be drawn, and the aforementioned laboratory tests performed. The patient should receive epinephrine hydrochloride 1:1000, 0.3 to 0.5 ml SQ for adults and 0.01 ml SQ for a child. Diphenhydramine hydrochloride 25 to 50 mg IM, IV, or PO should be given. Cimetidine (Tagamet) 300 mg IV should be given along with methylpredinsolone sodium succinate (Solu-Medrol) 125 mg IV. If severe bronchospasm occurs, give albuterol nebulizer treatments. If a very severe reaction is taking place, give aminophylline 500 mg IV for an adult and 5 mg/kg for a child.

A patient with laryngeal edema should be intubated. If the patient is hypotensive, give dopamine 200 mg in 250 ml of 0.9% normal saline, starting at 5 µg/kg/min and titrating to the desired pressure. Crystalloid infusions and CVP monitoring should be performed.

In localized reactions or toxic reactions, an adult patient can be treated with prednisone, 60 mg PO for 5 days, and oral antihistamines. A child should be treated with the appropriate dose of antihistamine and prednisone.

Any patient with involvement of three or more body systems should be admitted to the hospital for 24-hour observation. Any patient with an anaphylactic reaction should be admitted to the hospital and should be referred to an allergist for testing and immunotherapy. The patient should be given an EpiPen or an Ana-Kit at time of discharge from the hospital. This kit contains epinephrine 1:1000, 0.5 ml, and antihistamine tablets until immunotherapy is completed. The patient should be advised to wear a Medic-Alert tag at all times.

LIGHTNING INJURIES

Definition

Lightning injuries can always be severe. The mechanism of injury caused by lightning injuries differs from that of high-voltage electrocution. Lightning injuries are caused by direct strikes, side flash or splash, thermal burns, ground or stride voltage, contact voltage, or blunt injury secondary to being thrown by the strike blast.

Epidemiology

Approximately 100 to 200 persons are killed by lightning in the United States annually. This accident can occur in occupational settings, camping, fishing trips, or in one's own back yard.

Pathology

Injury is caused by the voltage, current, and duration of the lightning strike. Electricity produces alternating current, and death usually occurs secondary to ventricular fibrillation. Lightning causes direct current injuries and acts as massive countershock, which causes acute respiratory arrest and asystole. The voltage of lighting averages from 10 to 30 million volts, but it can range from a few million volts to 2 billion volts. The effect of lightning lasts for a very short time in comparison with injury due to generated electrical power. A person is often only exposed to lightning for 1 to 10 msec.

Lightning has an explosive effect. As it passes through the atmosphere, it heats the air channel through which it passes to a temperature higher than 8000° C. This rapid expansion of the air channel causes a shock wave, which is the thunder clap heard with lightning, and thus an explosion. The air cools to 1500 to 2000° C rapidly after the explosion. Unlike generated electrical current, lightning passes over the body, secondary to the short duration of exposure. Lightning does not have time to break down tissue, enter the body, and cause deep thermal burns. This is called the "flashover" phenomenon. If the victim is in the water, the current will remain longer and can cause first- or second-degree burns to the skin. Usually no entry or exit wound is found in lightning injuries, unlike generated electrical injuries.

Clinical Presentation

The patient who is struck directly by lightning usually presents in asystole and is unconscious. A victim of contact voltage is touching or holding an object when it is struck by lightning. Side flash or splash occurs when the victim is struck by the off-splash of the lightning being reflected off of a building or tree, and the victim is "splashed" by the reflection of the lightning. Step or stride voltage or ground voltage injuries occur when one body part, which is closer than another body part and which is also touching the ground, is struck by current. This creates a potential difference between the body parts; thus, conduction of the electricity passes from one body part to the other. If the victim is wearing potentially thermal objects, these objects can ignite or become superheated and cause thermal burns to the body. The victim can be thrown secondary to the voltage and suffer blunt trauma when landing, secondary to the explosive properties of lightning.

Examination

A patient who is acutely struck by lightning is usually in cardiopulmonary shock. The patient should be given a complete examination and should be treated as a trauma patient. Head injury, extremity fractures, rib fractures, pulmonary contusion, pelvis fracture, and cervical spine fractures should all be considered during an examination of a patient with injuries caused by lightning. The patient must be examined thoroughly for entrance and exit wounds, burns, and lacerations.

Diagnosis

A diagnosis is made after consideration of the history of a lightning strike, the setting in which the strike occurred, the clinical presentation, and the physical examination of the patient.

Laboratory Findings

A CBC, PT, PTT, electrolytes, BUN, creatinine, cardiac enzymes, liver function tests, and urinalysis should all be performed. The CPK should be fractionated to include the MM and MB fractions. The urine should be examined for myoglobin. A check of serial cardiac enzymes with the MM and MB fractions of the CPK should also be performed for 24 hours to rule out cardiac injury or rhabdomyolysis.

Treatment

Any patient who is struck by lightning should be placed on a cardiac monitor and have at least two large-gauge IV lines of normal saline placed. The patient should also be placed on oxygen; have x-rays done of the cervical spine, chest, and pelvis; and have an ECG performed. Treatment is mainly supportive care. A patient with cardiac arrhythmias should be treated per protocol. Treatment of fractures is based on the results of the x-rays. If the patient loses or lost consciousness, a CT scan of the head should be done to rule out an intracranial bleed.

Severe burns are treated in the standard fashion with surgical consultation. If compartment syndrome occurs, the patient should have a fasciotomy and an escharotomy. Neurologic injuries can present as paralysis of the extremity, seizures, or psychiatric disorders. A patient can have permanent neuritis, neuralgia, paresis, hemoplegia, and difficulty with mental functioning. The patient often has a mild form of post-traumatic stress disorder.

Fifty percent of persons injured by lightning will have ruptured tympanic membranes. A consultation with an ENT physician should be ensured. Cataracts can occur in a patient up to 2 years after he or she has been struck by lightning. Furthermore, retinal separation or perforation, optic nerve damage, iritis, or uveitis can also occur.

All persons struck by lightning, whether symptomatic or asymptomatic, should be admitted to the intensive care unit secondary to the delayed possibility of congestive heart failure or acute cardiac arrhythmias.

MARINE FAUNA ENVENOMATIONS

Definition

Several types of animals that live in the ocean can inflict harm on humans. The types of injuries can be divided into those caused by shock, stinging, trauma, and ingestion of poison. These injuries can cause hemorrhage, lacerations, infections, envenomations, or infection from foreign bodies.

Epidemiology

Hundreds of thousands of marine injuries occur in the United States each year. Fortunately, few injuries prove fatal. Severe bites from sharks and barracudas have a high mortality and morbidity rate. Approximately 50 to 100 shark attacks occur annually worldwide. The biting force of some sharks can reach 18 tons per square inch. Fifteen to 25% of all shark bites prove fatal. The major cause of death is drowning and hemorrhage.

There are more than 4000 species of sponges that can inflict pain from horny elastic skeletons. Over 9000 species of coelenterates exist, and more than 100 species are dangerous to humans. Coelenterates are divided to three groups: *hydrozoans,* Portuguese man-of-war; *scyphozoans,* jellyfish; and *anthozoans,* anemones. Coelenterates possess venom-charged stinging cells called nematocysts. The stinging nematocysts are located on single organelles on the surfaces of the tentacles, and they are triggered by contact with the victim.

The Atlantic Portuguese man-of-war *(Physalia physalis)* is a floating sail that inhabits the surface of the ocean. It has multiple nematocyst-bearing tentacles that can measure up to 30 m in length. These tentacles can break off, and they are often found on the beach. They have the ability to discharge venom for months after breaking off.

Jellyfish *(Chironex fleckeri)* are scyphozoan animals that have some of the most potent venoms in existence. There is a 15 to 20% mortality rate from box jellyfish stings.

Pathology

Specialized glands of marine fauna produce *crinotoxins.* These toxins are usually gastric secretions or slimes and are administered without the aid of traumatogenic devices. Bacterial toxins are products of decomposition that are eaten and are called *oral toxins.* Venoms that are produced in specialized glands and delivered by special traumatogenic devices are called *parenteral toxins.*

Most marine bacteria are halophilic, motile, and heterotropic and are gram-negative rod forms. Protozoa, yeasts, croalgae, and viruses are present in sea water, marine life, and marine sediments.

Bites from sharks and barracudas cause massive tissue loss and destruction. They can also cause fractures and infections.

Sponges have spicules made up of silicon dioxide and calcium carbonate, which can cause a severe dermatitis or "sponge diver's disease." Sponges also produce crinotoxins, which are direct dermal irrititants in the form of okadaic acid, halitoxin, and subcritine.

Clinical Presentation/Examination

Cuts caused by coral present with erythema, stinging pain, and pruritus. Erythema occurs within minutes after the person is cut. If the cut is not treated, cellulitis and ulceration with sloughing of tissue occur. These wounds heal very slowly (usually in 3 to 6 weeks).

Wound necrosis, reactive bursitis, local ulceration, and deep cellulitis with lymphangitis can develop.

A person who comes in contact with a sponge presents with a pruritic dermatitis in the first few hours. After a few hours, itching and a burning sensation ensues and can progress to localized joint edema, soft tissue edema, joint stiffness, and vesiculation.

The skin may become purpuric and mottled. Mild symptoms usually resolve in 3 to 7 days without treatment. If the patient's skin comes in contact with a large sponge, this envenomation can cause systemic symptoms of malaise, dizziness, nausea, fever, and muscle cramps, and the area of contact can become bullous and purulent over several hours. An anaphylactoid reaction or a systemic erythema multiforme reaction can develop 7 to 14 days after exposure to a large sponge.

Calcium carbonate can cause an irritant dermatitis. Surface desquamation can occur 10 days to 2 months after contact.

Contact with a coelenterate produces an itching, burning, and urticarial reaction. Mild contact causes a mild erythematous reaction. Severe envenomation can cause a delayed, hemorrhagic, or zoster form of reaction in 4 to 12 hours after contact.

The fire coral (*Millepora* species) can cause severe, intense, painful burning and itching within seconds after contact. Within 30 minutes, warmth, redness, and pruritus ensue. The lesions usually resolve in 3 to 7 days, but hyperpigmentation can remain for 4 to 8 weeks.

Jellyfish stings can present with hypotension, muscle spasms, respiratory and muscle paralysis, and death. A patient presents with immediate intense pain. The victim collapses within minutes. Wheals and vesicles and a dark reddish-brown or purple whip-like flare pattern with stripes occur within 8 to 10 minutes of envenomation. Blisters can occur within 6 hours, and superficial necrosis can occur in 12 to 18 hours. On occasion, a "frosted" pathognomonic, transverse cross-hatched pattern presents at the sting site.

Diagnosis

A diagnosis of envenomation caused by marine fauna is made by a history of exposure and clinical presentation.

Laboratory Findings

There are no specific laboratory tests for marine fauna envenomations. If cellulitis or sepsis is suspected, a CBC, blood cultures, and electrolytes tests should be performed.

Treatment

All marine injuries are subject to infections with gram-negative rods. Even minor cuts caused by coral should be treated with antibiotics. Treat the patient with trimethoprim-sulfamethoxazole or ciprofloxacin. Cultures should be taken from all wounds. If rapidly progressive cellulitis or myositis develops, treat the patient for *Vibrio parahemo-lyticus* or *V. vulnificus.* If a wound has the classic erysipeloid reaction, treat the patient for *Erysipelothrix rhusiopathiae.* Cephalexin, penicillin, or erythromycin can be used to treat most of these infections. The *Vibrio* species can be treated with third-generation cephalosporins. If IV antibiotics are required, give tobramycin, mezlocillin, azlocillin, tetracycline, gentamicin, chloramphenicol, piperacillin, trimethoprim-sulfamethoxazole, or ciprofloxacin.

Bites are subject to infection, crush injury, and lacerations. *Clostridia* is a major infective organism in bites. All bite injuries should receive tetanus 0.5 ml IM and tetanus immune globulin 250 to 500 mg IM. All bites should be x-rayed to check for foreign bodies, teeth, coral fragments, or fractures secondary to crush injuries. An orthopedic or general surgery consultation is needed if fractures or a large tissue loss is present.

Cuts caused by coral are treated with antibiotic therapy. If stinging is severe, rinse the cut site with diluted acetic acid (vinegar) or isopropyl alcohol 20%. Always x-ray the wound to check if a fragment of coral was left behind. All wounds should be examined thoroughly for foreign bodies. If the wound is deep, do not close the wound with sutures; rather, close the wound with adhesive tape and débride the wound again in 3 to 4 days. The wound should be dressed with a sterile wet-to-dry dressing and should be cleaned twice daily with normal saline or dilute povidone-iodine solution 1 to 5%. Bacitracin or polymyxin B-bacitracin-neomycin ointment can be used if the patient is allergic to povidone or iodine.

All injuries caused by sponges should be x-rayed, especially if the interphalangeal or metacarpophalangeal joints are involved. Broken pieces of sponge are often retained by the skin, and frequently they are not radiolucent. The skin should be dried, very gently and any spicules should be removed carefully. Adhesive tape can be used to remove the spicules, and facial peel can be used for large areas. There is no treatment for the irritant dermatitis or desquamation of skin caused by contact with calcium carbonate particles in the sponge.

Pain can be treated with acetic acid (vinegar) 5% or isopropyl alcohol 40 to 70%. The site should be soaked for 10 to 30 minutes up to four times a day. Do not apply topical steroids, because they will worsen the primary reaction if applied before acetic acid. If erythema multiforme occurs, then give the patient systemic corticosteroids—prednisone 60 to 100 mg PO for 2 to 3 weeks. After acetic acid has been applied and decontamination is complete, then topical steroids can be applied to reduce itching. If severe pruritus is present, antihistamines can be given.

Treatment of large or severe jellyfish stings includes supportive care, airway ventilation assistance, and hemodynamic support. All victims who are stung by coelenterates should be observed for at least 8 hours. All stings should be rinsed immediately with sea water and *not* with fresh water. Do not rub the wound. Remove tentacles with forceps and a well-gloved hand to prevent self-envenomation. Apply ice packs to the sting site.

Apply acetic acid (vinegar) 5% or isopropyl alcohol 40 to 70% to the sting site for at least 30 minutes to decontaminate the area. The remaining nematocysts can be removed by applying shaving cream or a paste of baking soda, flour, or talc and then shaving the area with a razor. Tetanus should be given, and antibiotic therapy should be started. Local anesthetic or mild steroid lotions can be applied to stop itching along with oral antihistamines. If left untreated, symptoms resolve in 1 to 2 weeks.

NEAR-DROWNING

Definition

Drowning is divided into several different syndromes. Near-drowning is the temporary suffocation by submersion of a person in a body of water. Drowning is defined as death after suffocation by submersion.

Epidemiology

Drowning is the third leading cause of death in the United States, and approximately 4500 people drown each year. The total number of near-drownings that take place each year in the United States is unknown. Children younger than 4 years of age and teenagers have the highest mortality rate for freshwater drownings. Elderly often drown in the bathtub. Drugs and alcohol contribute greatly to the morbidity and mortality rates connected with water injuries. Alcohol in particular contributes to diving injuries and to cervical spine injuries. Drownings can also be attributed to people having seizure disorders and poor swimming skills.

Pathology

Drowning is caused by respiratory failure and neurologic injury secondary to hypoxia. The swimmer panics and attempts to hold his or her breath, which results in hyperventilation. Vomiting and aspiration then occur. The term "dry drowning" is used to describe a drowning in which there is no aspiration secondary to laryngospasm and glottal closure. This occurs in 10 to 15% of all drownings.

A great deal has been said about which is better—freshwater or saltwater drownings. Drowning is still drowning! Surfactant is washed out of the alveoli by both fresh water and salt water. Fresh water also changes the surface tension of surfactant. When surfactant is lost, ventilation-perfusion mismatch ensues, then atelectasis and alveolar capillary membrane breakdown occur. This leads to noncardiogenic pulmonary edema and cerebral hypoxia. Metabolic acidosis occurs secondary to hypoxemia and decreased perfusion.

Clinical Presentation

Near-drowning victims can be found in the water or on shore. Patients with diving injuries or spinal cord injuries can present with priapism, paradoxical respirations, flaccidity, bradycardia, and hypotension. Most diving injuries involving the spinal cord are lower cervical spine injuries involving the ventral spine.

Near-drowning victims present with tachycardia, dyspnea, and accessory muscle use with inspiration. On physical examination, the patient can present with rales, rhonchi, wheezing, or a normal lung examination.

Examination

The patient should be given a thorough physical examination. If a patient is unconscious, assume that the patient has a spinal cord injury until proven otherwise. Divers can have other fractures besides neck fractures. Any victim of a near-drowning (and thus has hypoxia), needs a complete neurologic examination.

Diagnosis

A diagnosis is made by history, clinical presentation, and physical examination.

Laboratory Findings

A CBC, PT, PTT, electrolytes, BUN, creatinine, urinalysis, and an arterial blood gas should be performed on all near-drowning victims. If an acute myocardial infarct is suggested, cardiac enzymes should be drawn. In near-drowning victims, there are usually no significant electrolyte abnormalities. There are usually no BUN or creatinine abnormalities. Hemoglobinuria can occur after hemolysis. A rapid glucose stick should always be done to rule out hypoglycemia. If hypoglycemia is present, treat the patient with 50% D5W.

Treatment

All drowning victims should be removed from the water, and care should be taken to protect the spinal cord secondary to the likelihood of a diving injury. Airway maintenance and assisted ventilation are essential if a spinal cord injury is suspected or if the patient is unconscious. Cardiopulmonary resuscitation should be started if the patient is pulseless and breathless.

All victims of near-drowning should receive 100% oxygen via facemask to keep the Po_2 to at least 60 mm Hg in adults and 80 mm Hg in children. If these levels of Po_2 cannot be maintained with oxygen via facemask, then the patient should be intubated and positive end-expiratory pressure (PEEP) or continuous positive airway pressure (CPAP) should be used. If cerebral edema is present, the patient should be hyperventilated to a Pco_2 of 30 mm Hg.

At least one large-gauge IV line of 0.9% normal saline should be started. The patient should be placed on a cardiac monitor and have a chest x-ray performed. The patient should also be placed on pulse oximetry and have the aforementioned laboratory studies drawn, including an arterial blood gas. An ECG should also be performed, and arrhythmias should be treated per protocol.

Always take a rectal temperature on a near-drowning victim to rule out hypothermia. If hypothermia is present, treat the patient as per protocol. Remember that no one is dead until he or she is warm and dead! A near-drowning victim who is hypothermic should be warmed to at least 86 to 90° F before he or she is pronounced dead. Patients have survived prolonged submersions in cold water. Cold water often has a protective effect on the brain and heart by slowing metabolism and through preferential shunting of blood to the brain.

If bronchospasm is present, treat the patient with nebulized albuterol. Treat electrolyte abnormalities when necessary. Place a Foley catheter to monitor the patient's urine output, and place a nasogastric tube to prevent vomiting and aspiration.

Increased intracranial pressure (ICP) is more common in children than in adults (ICP>20 mm Hg) and must be watched carefully. Often ICP monitoring is used to check on the ICP in children.

All patients who are victims of near-drowning should be admitted to the hospital for at least 24 hours of monitoring. Any victim of a near-drowning, even if he or she is asymptomatic upon arrival of the emergency medical service, should be transported to the hospital for evaluation.

REPTILE AND SNAKEBITE INJURIES

Definition

Snakes are poikilothermic, and they hibernate or undergo denning in cool temperatures. There are basically two types of poisonous snakes: pit vipers (Crotalidae) and coral snakes (Elapidae).

There are three types of poisonous pit vipers. The *Crotalus* includes 20 different kinds of rattlesnakes. The massasauga and pygmy rattlesnakes belong to the *Sistrurus* genus of rattlesnakes. The *Agkistrodon* genus of pit viper includes the water moccasin *(A. piscivorus)* and the copperhead *(A. contortrix).* The water moccasin or "cottonmouth" has a very white buccal mucosa and is amphibious. It is smaller than a rattlesnake. The copperhead is so called because of its copper-like color when it becomes an adult. The number and size of the rattles does not tell the age of the rattlesnake, but the more rattles the snake has, the older it is.

There are two species of the Elapidae family of coral snakes in the United States. They are related to the cobras and kraits of the Old World. Coral snakes are small and shy and have a distinctive pattern of red and black bands on wider interspaces of yellow rings. The eastern coral snake *(Micrurus fulvius)* has a black snout. The Arizona or Sonoran coral snake *(Micruroides euryxanthus)* has a black head, and the yellow rings may be narrower. The mnemonic rhyme "Red on yellow, kill a fellow—coral snake. Red on black, venom lack— harmless snake," can be used to remember the difference between a poisonous coral snake and a nonpoisonous coral snake.

Snakes are nonaggressive by nature and prefer to retreat rather than attack. They attack when cornered, except when they are emerging from hibernation or just before they hibernate. After hibernation, snakes are dehydrated and have lost body fat. Unexpected variations in climate or temperature confuse snakes and make them more aggressive. Their venom is the most potent at this time. Snakes can inject varying amounts of venom at the time of biting.

Harmless snakes usually have round pupils, a single nostril, and a round head. On the ventral side of a harmless snake, the scales of the anal plate (distal part of the snake) are whitish and loose. A pit viper has vertical pupils and a "pit" or second nostril proximal to the main nostril, and the head is more triangular or arrowhead shaped. The scales of pit vipers on the ventral side of the snake form single rows from the anal plate to a point approximately a third of the distance away from the tail of the snake.

The pit is a thermoreceptor organ that allows the snake to track and approach warm-blooded animals. Pit vipers have anteriorly positioned hollow, retractable fangs on the maxillary area of the head. The venom is made and kept until it is needed in an anlage of the parotid glands. When the glands are squeezed by the palatine muscles, venom is pushed through the hollow fangs and injected into the victim.

Epidemiology

There are approximately 8000 snakebites in the United States each year. Approximately 50 persons die of snakebites each year in the United States. The most snakebites occur in North Carolina, followed by Arkansas, Texas, Georgia, West Virginia, Mississippi, and Louisiana. Most snakebites occur in July and August. Bites usually occur between the hours of 6:00 AM and 9:00 PM. Hikers, fishermen, hunters, farmers, and cowboys are the usual persons bitten by snakes. Snakes are also used in religious ceremonies, and snake handlers are commonly exposed to snakes in certain areas of Appalachia.

Pathology

There are numerous variables with regard to how much poison a snake injects. The larger the snake, the more available venom is present for envenomation. If a snake is angry, disturbed, or alert, that snake is more dangerous. The angle of the bite will determine the depth and the duration of the bite.

There are two basic types of venom: neurotoxic and hemopatholytic. The venom of the snake consists of several different biochemical compounds. Snake venom can contain anticoagulants and agglutinins that can affect red blood cells. Cytolysins, proteolysins, and antibactericidin can affect cellular blood components and the endothelium of blood vessels. Neurotoxins A and B, which affect the cardiorespiratory centers of the brain and CNS, are found in the venom of the coral snake. Cardiotoxins affect the heart. Hyaluronidase facilitates the spread of venom, and cholinesterase and anticholinesterase will affect the myoneural junctions of the victim. Proteolytic enzymes and phospholipases are also present.

The type of victim also affects the reaction to a venomous snakebite. Children, infants, patients with hypertension, diabetes, the elderly, or debilitated are at greater risk from snakebites. A woman who is menstruating may bleed excessively after being bitten by a pit viper. A woman with endometriosis may also bleed excessively and have severe pain from a pit viper bite. A pregnant woman who is bitten by a pit viper is also at greater risk of having a spontaneous abortion.

The location of the bite is also important. The more proximal the bite is to the heart, head, or trunk, the more dangerous the bite. Bites on the patient's upper extremities are more dangerous than those on the lower extremities.

Clinical Presentation

A patient may present in two different ways depending on the kind of venom injected. Neurotoxic venom, from neurotoxins A and B, cause CNS manifestations of convulsions, dysphagia, and psychotic behavior. Neurotoxin B affects the myoneural junctions and causes weakness of muscles, locomotor disturbances, paresthesias, paralysis, and fasciculation. Coral snakes are the main harborers of neurotoxins.

Hemopathic snakebites present with extravasation of blood; swelling; edema; ecchymoses; and bleeding from the lungs, kidneys, rectum, peritoneum, and vagina. Hemopathic venom causes changes in red blood cells, causing decreased transportation ability of oxygen by the red blood cells and consequently tissue anoxia and necrosis. Disseminated intravascular coagulation, thrombocytopenia, hypofibrinogenemia, and fibrinolysis can occur. Hemopathic venom is seen primarily in pit vipers.

Examination

Examine the area around the bite for redness and edema. Fang marks greater than 15 mm of separation are indicative of a very large snake. Fang marks less than 8 mm are indicative of a smaller snake.

Diagnosis

A diagnosis is made by a history of a snakebite, the location of the bite, the area of the United States in which the bite took place, the physical examination, and the clinical presentation.

Laboratory Findings

A CBC, PT, PTT, electrolytes, BUN, creatinine, magnesium, calcium, phosphorus, liver function, cardiac tests, and type and crossmatch of blood should be performed on any patient who has a snakebite.

Treatment

Any patient with a suspected snakebite should have at least one large-gauge IV line of 0.9% normal saline placed, and the patient should be placed on a cardiac monitor. The patient should receive 2 liters of oxygen via nasal cannula, and the aforementioned laboratory tests should be performed. The patient should be placed supine to decrease metabolism and absorption of venom. The bitten extremity should be immobilized and placed in a dependent position. Antivenin is available for both pit vipers and coral snakes.

The treatment for a pit viper bite is supportive and, if severe bleeding is present, blood transfusions should be given. If seizures are present, give calcium gluconate 10 ml of a 10% solution. Serial circumferential measurements should be taken of the patient's limbs to rule out compartment syndrome. Pressures greater than 30 mm Hg will require a fasciotomy. All snakebite victims should be given IV antibiotics, either cephalosporins or tetracyclines.

A polyvalent antivenin against pit viper bites of North and South America is available. It is made from horse serum, thus skin testing should be performed to check for an allergic reaction before administration of the serum. The serum is good for treatment of bites of the eastern diamondback rattlesnake, western diamondback rattlesnake, tropical rattlesnake, water moccasin, fer-de-lance, and the bushmaster. The biggest mistake made in treating snakebites is not giving enough antivenin. Pit viper bites should be treated aggressively, especially in the very young and the very old or in those with underlying disease, secondary to the increased risk of tissue necrosis and sloughing of tissue.

Coral snakebite victims are treated with coral snake antivenin. Wyeth Laboratories makes a specific antivenin that should be given to a person bitten by an eastern coral snake. Neostigmine, 2.5 mg every 30 to 60 minutes, has shown to be beneficial for coral snakebites. The patient must have good respiratory care after being bitten by a coral snake.

Treat the patient's pain with narcotics, but do not give meperidine to the patient if a Gila monster bite is suspected. Meperidine has a synergistic effect with the venom of a Gila monster. Local injections of lidocaine or procaine can be given to relieve localized pain; however, do not use epinephrine secondary to its vasoconstrictive properties, which can potentiate tissue ischemia. Do not given the patient steroids unless a serum sickness–like syndrome is present. All patients with snakebites should receive a tetanus immunization booster. If compartment syndrome is present, a surgical consultation is necessitated. All patients with snakebites should be admitted to the hospital for serial limb measures, CBCs, PTs, PTTs, and airway management.

SPIDER AND SCORPION BITES

Definition

Spiders and scorpions belong to the Arachnida class. There are approximately 20,000 different species of venomous spiders and 500 species of scorpions. Only 50 species of arachnids pose a threat to the population of the United States.

Venomous species that live in the United States include the black widow spider and the brown recluse spider. Scorpions are arachnids who resemble crustaceans, and their potential for harm is different for each scorpion's venom.

Epidemiology

Scorpions are found throughout the world. In the United States, scorpions are found mostly in the southwestern states. Only the *Centruroides sculpturatus,* found mostly in Arizona, is dangerous. The black widow *(Latrodectus mactans)* spider is found throughout the United States. The *L. hesperus* is found in Arizona and the western states. The brown recluse *(Loxosceles reclusa)* spider is found primarily in the central part of the United States.

The black widow spider is a glossy black, with occasional red stripes, and has bright red markings on the abdomen. It is shaped like an hourglass. The female is twice as big as the male. It is about ½ inch in length from the head to the abdomen, with feet that are approximately 1½ inches long.

The black widow spider likes to live in outhouses, stables, woodpiles, and under rocks. This spider is not aggressive, except when she is guarding eggs. The first appendage of the spider is called the chelicera. There are two accessory glands at the end of the chelicera where the spider's fangs are found. The spider is able to control the amount of venom that it injects into its victim. The venom consists of both protein and nonprotein compounds. The venom paralyzes the prey and helps to digest the victim. In humans, it acts as a neurotoxin. The toxin causes depletion of acetylcholine at the presynaptic nerve terminal.

The brown recluse spider is about 1 inch in length, including legs, and is tan to dark brown. Its classic distinguishing mark is a violin-shaped darker area found on the cephalothorax. It also has only three pairs of eyes instead of the usual four sets. This spider is found under rocks, in woodpiles, attics, and closets, and it is not aggressive in nature.

The venom consists of one enzyme, sphingomyelinase D. This enzyme causes a direct lytic action on the red blood cells. It is not a neurotoxin. The local effects of the venom are thought to be primarily from the hemolytic enzymes levarterenol-like substances that cause severe vasoconstriction. The systemic effects of envenomation are thought to be caused be an allergic reaction.

Scorpions are arachnids and are some of the oldest living animals. The scorpion has a tail-like structure that is actually the last six segments of its abdomen. This structure has two venom glands and a stinger.

Scorpions live under rocks, logs, trees, and stony crevices. The *C. sculpturatus* scorpion lives on or near trees. This scorpion is a nocturnal predatory animal.

The scorpion's venom varies from one species to another, and it can produce both local and systemic reactions. The venom can cause hemolysis, hemorrhage, and destruction of local tissue. The *C. sculpturatus* scorpion attacks with a neurotoxin venom, which activates repetitive firing of the axons by activation of the sodium channels.

Clinical Presentation

A person who is bitten by a *black widow spider* will complain of a pinprick. In a few minutes, edema and redness will ensue. Two fang marks will be noted. In approximately 15 to 60 minutes, the pinprick will turn into a dull crampy pain in the area of the bite, which will spread to the entire body. The pain goes from the chest, to the upper extremities, and then to the abdomen. The classic symptom of a black widow spider bite is that the patient presents with a board-like abdomen and severe cramping pain.

Often, without a history of a spider bite, the patient will present as if he or she has acute appendicitis, pancreatitis, or a peptic ulcer. Headache, vomiting, weakness, ptosis, dyspnea, conjunctivitis, anxiety, difficulty speaking, and crampy pain in all muscle groups will be present.

The patient will often be hypertensive and cerebrospinal fluid pressure will sometimes be elevated. ECG changes can mimic digitalis toxicity. All symptoms usually resolve in 2 to 3 days.

When the victim is bitten acutely by a *brown recluse spider,* the patient will complain of a burning pain at the bite site. The venom apparatus is similar to that of the black widow spider. During the next 2 to 3 hours, a white area of vasoconstriction begins around the site of the bite, and pain increases. An erythematous ring then forms, and a central bleb is noted. The ring looks much like a bull's eye. During the next 24 to 72 hours, the bleb darkens and the tissue at the site of the bite starts to become necrotic. This necrosis then spreads from the center of the lesion to surrounding tissue. The necrosis now involves the skin and subcutaneous fat.

At about this time, systemic symptoms occur. The patient will complain of chills, fever, rash, petechiae, nausea, vomiting, weakness, and malaise. In severe envenomation, the patient can present with thrombocytopenia, hemolysis, jaundice, renal failure, pulmonary edema, and shock. Fatalities can occur in children.

Scorpion bites present with immediate pain and stinging at the sting site. Immediate localized redness and edema occur. Nausea, vomiting, sweating, blurred vision, excessive salivation, itching of the nose and throat, anxiety, restlessness, hyperthermia, muscle spasms, blurred vision, hypertension, hemiplegia, syncope, pseudoseizures, cardiac arrhythmia, and respiratory failure can occur within 30 minutes of envenomation. The *C. sculpturatus* scorpion bite can cause sensitivity to touch, numbness, and weakness.

Laboratory Findings

A CBC, PT, PTT, electrolytes, BUN, creatinine, and urinalysis should be performed. No laboratory tests are specific for hymenoptera bites.

Treatment

The initial treatment for *black widow spider* bite consists of applying ice packs to the bite site, supportive care, and monitoring the patient for symptoms of hypertension. A tetanus immunization should be given to all victims of spider bites. If pain symptoms are severe, calcium gluconate 10 ml of a 10% solution should be given over 20 minutes. Calcium gluconate has been shown to alleviate the symptoms of a black widow spider bite. If the patient is asymptomatic in 2 hours after the bite, he or she can be discharged to home. If hypertension occurs, the patient should be treated with sodium nitroprusside and admitted to the hospital. If severe muscle spasms are present give methocarbamol or diazepam IV. If the patient is younger than 16 years of age, or older than 65 years of age, he or she should be given the *Latrodectus* antivenin. This antivenin is a derivative of a horse serum, thus an anaphylactic reaction may occur. Skin testing should be performed prior to administration of the antivenin. The antivenin is made by Merck Sharp & Dohme. The dose consists of one vial of antivenin administered over 15 minutes and diluted in 50 ml of normal saline.

Treatment for a bite from a *brown recluse spider* involves early use of systemic steroids within 24 hours of the bite. Methylprednisolone 100 mg IV and oral prednisone for 5 days is the treatment of choice. Dapsone 50 to 200 mg/day has also been used. There is an antivenin, but it is not available in the United States. Any patient who is bitten by a brown recluse spider should be admitted to the hospital for treatment, daily blood count, and monitoring of urine output. If acute renal failure occurs, dialysis should be performed. A surgical consultation should be obtained for possible surgical débridement of the wound, but there is controversy as to whether surgical débridement improves wound healing.

The treatment for a *scorpion* bite is to apply ice to the bite site and treat the patient symptomatically. *C. sculpturatus* scorpion antivenin is available from the Antivenom Production Laboratory of Arizona

State University. Antivenin should be given in the case of severe envenomations. All children and elderly persons should be admitted to the hospital for observation. Pain is treated with narcotics and barbiturates.

BIBLIOGRAPHY

Auerbach PS: Clinical therapy of marine envenomation and poisoning. In Tu At (ed): Handbook of Natural Toxins. Vol. 3: Marine Toxins and Venoms. New York, Dekker, 1988

Auerbach PS, Halstead BW: Hazardous aquatic life. In Auerbach PS, Geehr ED (eds): Management of Wilderness and Environmental Emergencies, 2nd ed. St Louis, CV Mosby, 1989

Braunwald E, Isselbacher KJ, Petersdorf RG, et al (eds): Harrison's Principles of Internal Medicine, 11th ed. New York, McGraw-Hill, 1987

May HL, Aghababian RV, Fleisher GR (eds): Emergency Medicine, 2nd ed. Boston, Little Brown, 1992

Rosen P, Barkin RM (eds): Emergency Medicine: Concepts and Clinical Practice, 3rd ed. St Louis, Mosby-Year Book, 1992

Schwartz GR, Cayten CG, Mangelsen MA, et al (eds): Principles and Practice of Emergency Medicine. Philadelphia, Lea & Febiger, 1992

Steinman AM: Cardiopulmonary resuscitation and hypothermia. Circulation 74 (Suppl 4):29, 1986

Tierney LM, McPhee SJ, Papadakis MA (eds): Current Medical Diagnosis and Treatment, 33rd ed. E. Norwalk, CT, Appleton & Lange, 1994

Tintinalli JE, Krone RL, Ruiz E (eds): Emergency Medicine: A Comprehensive Study Guide, 3rd ed. New York, McGraw-Hill, 1992

Zell SC, Kurtz KJ: Severe exposure to hypothermia: A resuscitation protocol. Ann Emerg Med 14:339, 1985

Chapter 7

Infectious Disease Emergencies

HIV INFECTIONS AND THE PATIENT WITH AIDS

Definition

Human immunodeficiency virus (HIV) type 1 (HIV-1) is the virus that causes acquired immmunodeficiency syndrome (AIDS).

Epidemiology

The first case of AIDS was reported in 1981. Two rare diseases, Kaposi's sarcoma and *Pneumocystis carinii* pneumonia (PCP), were found commonly in the ill homosexual male population in California. The Centers for Disease Control and Prevention (CDC) first defined the criteria for AIDS in 1982 as "a case of a disease at least moderately predictive of a defect in cell-mediated immunity occurring in a person with no known cause for diminished resistance to that disease." In 1985, serologic testing was available for the general population. In 1987, the CDC published a revised edition of HIV/AIDS criteria. Currently, at time of writing, the CDC is in the process of revising the 1987 criteria for AIDS.

More than 174,000 persons have been reported to have AIDS in the United States, and there have been more than 266,098 cases of AIDS worldwide since 1990. It is estimated that there are 1.2 million cases of HIV-positive persons in the United States and more than 4 million persons worldwide with AIDS. Both of these figures are probably grossly underestimated. Rates of infection are greater in the inner cities. Concentrations in the United States remain high in the cities of Miami, New York, and San Francisco. Eighty percent of the HIV infection in the United States is in adult males. The average ages of those infected are between 20 and 49 years of age. Black males account for 27% of the HIV-positive population, and 15% of the HIV-positive population are Hispanic. Infection among the female and pediatric populations is increasing, whereas infection in the white male homosexual population is decreasing. The mean time from exposure to the HIV virus to the development of AIDS is 8.23 years in adults and 1.97 years in children younger than 5 years of age. The average survival time following the diagnosis of full-blown AIDS is 9 months.

Risk factors for acquiring HIV are homosexuality, bisexuality, intravenous (IV) drug use, heterosexual exposure, maternal-neonatal transmission by an HIV-positive mother, shared use of IV needles, sexual contact with prostitutes, and a blood transfusion prior to 1985. Heterosexual transmission is increasing.

Pathology

HIV is a cytopathic retrovirus that selectively attacks the primary T4-helper cells and kills the infected cells. The viral gene is carried as a single-stranded ribonucleic acid (RNA) with the viral particle. The RNA template is reverse-transcribed into deoxyribonucleic acid (DNA), which then becomes permanently integrated into the host's DNA. This infection thus causes a qualitative T4-lymphocytic function defect, lymphopenia, autoimmune phenomena, and circulation immune complexes. The cellular immunity defect causes devastating opportunistic infections and neoplasms.

Transmission of the virus is usually by or through contact with body fluid, such as blood, semen, vaginal secretions, or transportation in utero. HIV has been isolated from breast milk, tears, cerebrospinal fluid (CSF), alveolar fluid, synovial fluid, and amniotic fluid. There has been no reported transmission from casual contact.

Clinical Presentation

A patient can present asymptomatically with AIDS-related complex or with full-blown AIDS to the emergency department (ED).

A patient who is infected with HIV will present with fever, weight loss, fatigue, malaise, arthralgia, and lymphadenopathy within a few weeks of exposure to HIV. These initial symptoms resolve in a few days or weeks but can recur at any time and for any duration.

Patients with known HIV or AIDS complexes often present to the ED with complaints of fever, headache, cough, anemia, anorexia, malaise, colitis, abdominal pain, or diarrhea. Fever-related AIDS-associated diseases include *Mycobacterium avium-intracellulare* (MAI), cytomegalovirus (CMV), Hodgkin's lymphoma, and Hodgkin's disease. CMV causes retinitis.

A patient with AIDS often presents with a dermal complaint of xerosis, pruritus, or skin infections (e.g., from *Staphylococcus aureus* as folliculitis, bullae, or ecthyma). Herpes simplex, herpes zoster, syphilis, and scabies are also common dermal complaints. Kaposi's sarcoma is a common cancer in a patient with AIDS. Molluscum contagiosum is also very common. Fungal skin infections are also very common, including *Candida* and *Trichophyton* organisms. In the female patient, there is an increase in the human papillomavirus. Seborrheic dermatitis with scaling plaques, hyperkeratosis, is also very common in the patient with AIDS.

By the time of death from AIDS, 75 to 90% for patients will have neurologic complications. In 10 to 20% of patients with AIDS, neurologic problems will be the presenting complaint. These patients present to the ED with headache, seizures, meningitis, altered mental status, and neuropathy. The CSF of these patients should be evaluated (including the opening pressure). The most common causes of altered mental status and neurologic changes in the patient with AIDS are AIDS dementia, herpes simplex, *M. tuberculosis, Toxoplasma gondii,* and *Cryptococcus neoformans.*

The patient often presents with a mental disorder or psychiatric complaint such as depression, psychosis, dementia, or delirium. This patient will need to have a computed tomography (CT) scan of the head and a lumbar puncture to evaluate the CSF.

Organisms that can cause diarrhea in the patient with AIDS include *Salmonella, Shigella, Giardia, Campylobacter jejuni, Cryptosporidium,* and *Isospora* species. Kaposi's sarcoma, MAI, HSV-1, HSV-2, and CMV also cause diarrhea in the patient with AIDS. A patient will present with abdominal pain, cramping, bloody diarrhea, and vomiting. The fluid and electrolyte balance status of these patients must be evaluated and addressed. Always examine the mouth of the patient with AIDS. Eighty percent of all patients with AIDS will have oral candidiasis of the buccal mucosa and tongue. Treatment with clotrimazole troches five times a day can help to control these infections. Remember that *Shigella* can cause seizures in the very young, and *Salmonella* can cause bacteremia in the patient with AIDS.

Patients often present to the ED with pulmonary complaints. Any patient with HIV or AIDS who presents to the ED with pulmonary complaints will need sputum cultures with a Gram stain, acid-fast stain, blood culture, and chest x-ray. If leukocytes are present in the sputum, this suggests a bacterial infection. The most common bacterial infection in the patient with AIDS is PCP (80%) followed by mycoplasmal tuberculosis (MTB), CMV, *C. neoformans, Histoplasma capsulatum,* and new neoplasms. A patient with PCP presents with a nonproductive cough and shortness of breath. Any patient with AIDS who has shortness of breath will need pulse oximetry and an arterial blood gas drawn as part of the evaluation.

A patient with AIDS can present with ophthalmologic complaints of redness of the eyes, photophobia, eye pain, or changes in visual acuity. All eye complaints must be taken very seriously secondary to the possibility of CMV retinitis (which occurs in 10 to 15% of all patients with AIDS). The lesion will be a fluffy white retinal lesion that is often perivascular in nature. Herpes lesions of the cornea and Kaposi's sarcoma can also be present.

Radiographs

If a diffuse infiltrate is present on the chest x-ray and the patient presents with no cough, CMV, PCP, or Kaposi's sarcoma is suggested.

Cryptococcosis, mycobacterial pneumonia, *M. tuberculosis,* histoplasmosis, or neoplasm can be present with hilar adenopathy and a diffuse pulmonary infiltrate.

Fungal lesions, bacterial infections, PCP, and *M. tuberculosis* will present as cavitary lesions. Nodular lesions will be present with fungal lesions, toxoplasmosis, *M. tuberculosis, M. avium,* and Kaposi's sarcoma. Coccidioidomycosis, histoplasmosis, lymphoid interstitial pneumonitis, CMV, *P. carinii, M. tuberculosis,* and *M. avium* can present as diffuse interstitial infiltrates. *P. carinii, M. pneumon-*

iae, M. tuberculosis, M. avium, and bacterial pneumonia can present with focal consolidations.

Examination

Any patient who is known to be HIV positive or who presents with a common complaint of AIDS should have a complete physical examination, including a rectal examination for blood, and special attention should be paid to the oral mucosal for *Candida* and to the skin for lesions. A complete history should always be taken and should include the patient's sexual habits and preference, IV drug use, blood transfusions, and knowledge of how the patient acquired HIV and his or her sexual partners. A history of weight loss, skin changes, diarrhea, headaches, or recurrent infections should also be obtained. The immunization status of the patient with AIDS should be obtained as part of the history. Any patient with AIDS who has a severe headache or mental status change should preferably have a contrast-enhanced CT scan to show ring-enhanced lesions of toxoplasmosis. Often a magnetic resonance imaging (MRI) scan is needed to make a final diagnosis. A biopsy of the brain is often needed for a definitive diagnosis.

Diagnosis

A diagnosis is made by a positive result on an enzyme-linked immunosorbent assay (ELISA) and the Western blot test. The CD4 cell count is utilized to follow the course of the disease. The CD4 cell surface marker helper induces immunologic reactions. CD4 cells respond to the class II major histocompatibility complex antigens and release cytokines, which activate and augment the immunologic response. CD4-positive lymphocytes are the primary targets of HIV infection, and the CD4 receptor is the primary binding site of HIV-1. As the HIV/AIDS illness progresses, the CD4 count drops. A CD4 count below 100 is considered to be full-blown AIDS.

The patient with HIV is staged according to his or her current symptoms, CD4 cell count, and related diseases. There are several types of staging, which include the five-stage Walter Reed staging system. There is also a system with three stages that is commonly used. At an early stage, the CD4 count is greater than 500 cells/mm³. At the middle stage, the CD4 count is 200 to 500 cells/mm³. At the late stage, the CD4 count is less than 200 cells/mm³.

Laboratory Findings

CBC, electrolytes, blood cultures (including aerobic, anaerobic, and fungal organisms), and a urinalysis should be obtained. Liver function tests (LFTs), BUN, creatinine, HIV or CD4 count, serologic testing for syphilis, and blood antigen for cryptococcal and *Toxoplasma* and *Coccidioides* serologies should also be drawn.

If meningitis is suspected, the CSF should be examined for *Tox-*

oplasma and *Cryptococcus* antigens, along with a red and white blood cell count, glucose, protein, Gram's stain, India ink stain, bacterial, fungal, and viral cultures, and coccidioidomycosis titer.

In 50% of all patients with AIDS, there will be liver involvement with elevation of alkaline phosphatase, and often jaundice is present.

Stool cultures should be obtained from any patient who presents with diarrhea.

Treatment

Specific complaints and disease should be addressed. The CD4 count and underlying illness will determine if the patient should be admitted to the hospital. The patient's fluid balance and electrolyte status should always be addressed along with a complaint of headache or fever. Always ask if the patient is eating, drinking, or vomiting up food and liquid. If a patient with AIDS is not admitted to the hospital, he or she should be referred to an infectious disease physician within 72 hours of the ED visit for a follow-up examination.

Cutaneous Complaints

Varicella zoster is treated with IV acyclovir 30 mg/kg/day and varicella immune globulin immunization.

Herpes simplex is treated with acyclovir, 200 mg five times a day for 10 days. If herpes simplex is overwhelming, the patient should be admitted to the hospital and treated with IV acyclovir 25 to 30 mg/kg/day.

Candida and *Trichophyton* are treated with miconazole, clotrimazole, or ketoconazole.

Ophthalmologic Complaints

CMV is treated with ganciclovir, 7.4 to 15 mg/kg/day.

Pulmonary Complaints

P. carinii is treated with trimethoprim-sulfamethoxazole (TMP-SMX)—TMP 15 to 20 mg/kg/day and 75 to 100 mg/kg/day of SMX orally (PO) for 3 weeks; however, if the patient is seriously ill, he or she should be admitted to the hospital and given pentamidine, 4 mg/kg/day IV or intramuscularly (IM) for 3 weeks.

Tuberculosis is treated with a three-, four-, or six-drug combination regimen.

1. Isoniazid, 5 to 10 mg/kg/day PO, *plus*
2. Rifampin, 9 mg/kg/day *plus*
3. Pyrazinamide, 25 mg/kg/day PO, *or*
4. Streptomycin, 0.75 to 1 mg/kg/day IM

Gastrointestinal Complaints

Salmonellosis is treated with TMP-SMX, TMP 10 mg/kg/day and SMX 50 mg/kg/day PO, or ampicillin 12 g/day IV. Candidiasis is treated with clotrimazole, 30 to 50 mg/day, or ketoconazole, 200 to 400 mg/day. Cryptosporidiosis has no effective therapy. Diarrhea can be treated with psyllium (Metamucil), attapulgite (Kaopectate), and in extreme cases with atropine sulfate (Lomotil).

Central Nervous System Complaints

Treatment of toxoplasmosis is with pyrimethamine, 25 to 50 mg/day PO or streptomycin, 0.75 to 1 mg/kg/day IM plus sulfadiazine, 100 mg/kg/day for 3 to 6 months. Cryptococcosis is treated with amphotericin B, 0.4 to 0.6 mg/kg/day.

MALARIA

Definition

Malaria is an infectious protozoal disease caused by the bite of the female *Anopheles* mosquito, which is infected by one of four genera of *Plasmodium.*

Epidemiology

More than 200 million persons worldwide acquire malaria annually, and 1.5 million persons die each year of the disease. The anopheline mosquito is found mostly in the tropical and subtropical regions of the world below 8200 feet. Malaria is found in the Caribbean, sub-Sahara Africa, Central and South America, Southeast Asia, the Middle East, the Indian subcontinent, and Oceania.

The incidence of malaria is increasing in the nontropical regions of the world, secondary to international travel to the tropical regions of the world by nontropical living persons. The CDC reported 3436 cases of malaria in the United States from 1980 to 1988.

Pathology

Malaria is caused by four different species of the genus *Plasmodium: P. vivax, P. ovale, P. malariae,* and *P. falciparum.* After direct injection of the organism into the bloodstream by the female anopheline mosquito, the organism is carried to the host's liver, where asexual reproduction of the parasite takes place in the hepatic parenchymal cells. This stage is called the *pre-erythrocytic* or *exoerythrocytic stage.* When the parenchymal liver cells are completely filled with the daughter merozoites, the parenchymal cells rupture and thousands of daughter merozoites are released back into the bloodstream. These newly released cells invade other erythrocytes, spreading the infection and causing the recurrent paroxysms of malaria—chills and fever followed by diaphoresis. This stage is called the *erythrocytic stage.* If the host is infected with *P. vivax* or *P. ovale* malaria, a portion of the intrahepatic sporozoites can remain dormant in the liver for months, thus causing a "relapsing" form of malaria. Malaria at an early stage can often be confused with influenza, viral syndrome, or hepatitis. During the erythrocytic stage, the merozoites mature and never reinvade the liver. Erythrocyte target cells develop, and new merozoites invade uninfected red blood cells. This lysogeny occurs every 2 to 3 days, and the classic symptoms—fever, chills, and diaphoresis—will recur in a regular pattern. After several cycles, the merozoites develop into sexual, gametocytic forms. The host is then able to pass on the disease to other feeding anopheline mosquitoes as infective sporozoites.

Clinical Presentation

The incubation period ranges from 8 days to several weeks prior to symptoms of infection. Patients with acute malaria present with a prodrome of headache, low-grade fever, chills, myalgia, chest pain, cough, abdominal pain, diarrhea, and arthralgias. The illness will progress to very high-grade fevers, nausea, orthostatic dizziness, tachycardia, and weakness. These high-grade fevers will last for several hours and then abate, leaving the patient with exhaustion and diaphoresis. The chills, fever, and diaphoresis will become cyclic and correspond to the asexual erythrocytic cycles. Noncardiac pulmonary edema, renal failure, and cerebral malaria can occur in infected persons secondary to hemolysis, especially with *P. falciparum. P. falciparum* can also cause glomerulonephritis, nephrotic syndrome, polyclonal antibody stimulation, and thrombocytopenia secondary to an obstruction of capillary blood flow from hemolysis. If the malaria is left untreated, hypersplenism can occur and result in pancytopenia.

P. falciparum presents 8 to 25 days (a mean of 12 days) after the bite. The asexual erythrocytic cycle is 48 hours, and there is no relapse. On red blood cell examination, the morphologic characteristics include a high degree of parasitemia. The trophozoites are ring forms and have a thread-like cytoplasm with double chromic dots. *P. falciparum* prefers reticulocytes. Mature trophozoites and schizonts are rarely seen. The gametocytes are shaped like a banana.

P. malariae has an incubation period of 15 to 30 days and an asexual erythrocytic cycle of 72 hours with no relapse. The organism prefers older red blood cells. On microscopic examination, the degree of parasitemia is low, the trophozoites are compacted in the cytoplasm, and mature trophozoites and schizonts are seen. The gametocytes are round.

P. ovale has an incubation of 9 to 17 days with a mean of 15 days' incubation time. The asexual erythrocytic cycle lasts for 48 hours, and then the patient has a relapse of illness. The organism prefers reticulocytes, and the degree of parasitemia is low. The trophozoites are compacted into the cytoplasm. Schizonts and mature trophozoites are observed on a smear. The gametocytes are round.

P. vivax has an incubation period of 8 to 27 days, with a mean of 14 days. The asexual erythrocytic cycle is 48 hours. There is a relapse, and the organism prefers reticulocytes. The degree of parasitemia is low, and the trophozoites are ameboid in the cytoplasm. The gametocytes are round, and mature trophozoites and schizonts are seen on examination.

Examination

The patient can present with splenomegaly, high fever, tender abdomen, tachycardia, and tachypnea. The liver may or may not be enlarged on examination of the abdomen. Atypical presentations of malaria include a maculopapular skin rash and lymphadenopathy.

Diagnosis

A diagnosis is made by visualizing the parasites on Giemsa-stained thick and thin blood smears. If the infection is in its very early stages, especially with *P. falciparum,* the parasite may not be detectable. It is best to obtain a blood sample when the patient's fever is on the rise and when the patient feels chilled. At this point, the blood contains the schizonts. If no parasites are visualized, the smear should be repeated in 3 days. The degree of parasitemia correlates with the prognosis.

Laboratory Findings

A complete CBC, electrolytes, BUN, creatinine, calcium, magnesium, LFTs, and phosphorus should be drawn. An erythrocyte sedimentation rate should be performed along with stool cultures. Normochromic normocytic anemia is often present. The leukocyte count is often mildly depressed, and thrombocytopenia is often present. LFT, BUN, and creatinine levels are often mildly elevated. An examination of the electrolyte levels will often show hypoglycemia and hyponatremia. If a Venereal Disease Research Laboratory (VDRL) test is taken, it will often give a false-positive result.

Treatment

If no parasites are noted on a Giemsa stain, therapy should not be withheld in highly suspicious cases. Any patient with *P. falciparum* or a 1 to 2% parasitemia should be treated in the hospital.

The treatment of the patient is based on the severity of illness and on whether the patient is infected by chloroquine-resistant *P. falciparum.* Most patients with non–*P. falciparum* malaria can be treated as outpatients. Any patient with severe underlying chronic illness, a pregnant patient, an infant, or a patient with severe hemolysis should also be hospitalized for treatment.

A patient with *P. vivax, P. malariae,* or *P. ovale* can be treated with outpatient therapy with chloroquine. Chloroquine is given in a loading dose of a 1-g load (600-mg base), then 500 mg (300-mg base) in 6 hours, then 500 mg/day (300-mg base) for 2 days up to a total dose of 2.5 g. Children are given a 10-mg/kg base to a maximum loading dose of 600 mg, then 5 mg/kg base in 6 hours, followed by 5 mg/kg base per day for 2 days.

Primaquine phosphate in a 26.3-mg loading dose (15-mg base) per day for 14 days can be given *upon completion* of chloroquine therapy. Children receive 0.3 mg/kg base for 13 days *upon completion* of chloroquine therapy.

In uncomplicated *P. falciparum,* chloroquine-resistant infections, give quinine sulfate 650 mg PO three times a day (TID) for 5 to 7 days. A child under 12 years of age should receive 8.3 mg/kg PO TID for 5 to 7 days.

Pyrimethamine/sulfadoxine (Fansidar) can also be given–3 tablets (75 mg/1500 mg) PO for one dose—children older than 2 months of age:

>50 kg	give 3 tablets
30–50 kg	give 2 tablets
15–29 kg	give 2 tablets
10–14 kg	give ½ tablet
4–9 kg	give ¼ tablet

Doxycycline 100 mg PO BID for 10 days can also be given. Do not give this drug to children younger than 8 years of age. Mefloquine, 1250 mg PO can be given in one dose for adults. In children, mefloquine is given in 1 tablet/10kg for one dose.

In complicated *P. falciparum* chloroquine-resistant infections, give quinidine gluconate IV as a 24 mg/kg loading dose (15-mg base) over 4 hours, then 7.5 mg base/kg over 4 hours every 8 hours until the patient's condition stabilizes and the patient is able to take PO therapy. When the patient can take PO therapy give quinine sulfate, sulfadoxine (Fansidar), doxycycline, and mefloquine as above. In children, give quinidine gluconate IV as a 6.2 mg base/kg loading dose over 2 hours, then a continuous infusion at a rate of 0.0125 mg base/kg/min until PO therapy can be started.

Doxycycline, 100 mg IV every 12 hours can also be given until PO therapy can be started. Do not give IV or PO doxycycline to children younger than 8 years of age. Parenteral quinine sulfate is the drug of choice for the severely ill patient with *P. falciparum.* This drug is only available from the CDC. Quinine and quinidine can induce severe hypoglycemia and are potent myocardial depressants. If IV quinidine gluconate is used, cardiac monitoring is a necessity. Primaquine should not be used in patients with glucose-6-phosphate dehydrogenase (G6PD) deficiency, secondary to its ability to produce massive hemolysis of erythrocytes.

Any patient with dehydration secondary to vomiting, who is unable to keep oral medications down, and who is hemodynamically unstable should be admitted to the hospital. In severe parasitemia, exchange transfusions have proved to be lifesaving. Any person who is traveling to an area where malaria is endemic should take the appropriate chemoprophylactic drugs before traveling to that region. The CDC malaria hot-line is (404) 332–4555.

TETANUS

Definition

Tetanus is secondary to a wound infection contaminated by *Clostridium tetani*. *C. tetani* is a gram-positive, anaerobic, spore-forming, rod-shaped motile organism.

Epidemiology

C. tetani is found in the soil, feces of animals and humans, and dust. The tetanus spores can live in the soil for months or years. The organisms are very hardy and are heat resistant. Due to the required immunization program in the United States, the death rate from tetanus is very low (approximately 21% for the 50 to 100 reported cases a year). Approximately 300,000 to 500,000 cases of tetanus are reported worldwide each year with an overall mortality rate of 45%. Most of these cases are in the underdeveloped world. Patients older than 50 years of age, who are inadequately immunized, are the majority of victims of tetanus.

Tetanus is more common in wet and damp areas of the world and rarely occurs in cold areas. Reported cases of tetanus also occur after abdominal surgery and in IV drug abusers. There is a 25 to 50% mortality rate for generalized tetanus. Death results from respiratory failure, pulmonary embolus, pneumonia, and dysrhythmias. Long-term complications are few for those who survive.

Pathology

Tetanus is a toxin-mediated disease that causes generalized muscular rigidity and violent muscular contractions. These contractions and muscular rigidity can cause spasms of the respiratory system that can lead to hypoxia and eventually to death. Most cases are secondary to a break in the skin from puncture wounds, lacerations, or abrasions. Three conditions must be present for tetanus to occur: (1) an environment that promotes the germination of the tetanus spores, (2) actual growth of the organism and toxin production, and (3) the lack of the host organism's immunologic protection from the organism. There is an increased risk of infection if a foreign body is present. If other bacteria are present or the local tissue has been damaged or devitalized, this increases the risk of tetanus growth and toxin release. When these conditions are present, the oxidation-reduction potential of the local tissues is reduced and the spores that are present revert to the vegetative form of bacterial production, causing the bacilli to produce toxins and thus clinical illness. The tetanus organism produces three exotoxins: (1) tetanospasmin, (2) tetanolysin, and (3) nonconvulsive neurotoxin. Nonconvulsive neurotoxin and tetanolysin do not produce clinical disease. Tetanospasmin causes the clinical symptoms of tetanus. The tetanospasmin exotoxin is spread by the blood from the original site of infection to the brain, spinal cord, sympathetic nervous system, and skeletal muscles. Tetanospasmin is then taken up by inhibitory neurotransmitters and causes disinhibition of individual motor groups and thus uncontrollable muscle spasm and rigidity.

Tetanus can be categorized into four forms or types: (1) generalized, (2) local, (3) cephalic, and (4) neonatal. Generalized tetanus is usually caused by minor trauma and is the most common form of tetanus.

Local tetanus occurs only in the local area of injury. Local tetanus usually resolves in weeks or months without residual effects. Local tetanus can progress to the generalized form of tetanus.

Neonatal tetanus occurs in Third-World or underdeveloped countries and has a very high mortality rate. Neonatal tetanus is secondary to cuts or abrasions or contamination during the cutting of the umbilical cord of the newborn. The illness occurs during the first week of life.

Cephalic tetanus can be caused by local injury to the head or by otitis media. Only 1 to 3% of all tetanus is cephalic tetanus. One third of patients with cephalic tetanus recover completely; two thirds develop general tetanus.

Clinical Presentation/Examination

The incubation period for tetanus varies from 24 hours to over 1 month, usually from 3 to 14 days. Patients with generalized tetanus present with stiffness and pain in the jaw and trunk muscles. Trismus is a common presenting complaint. Lockjaw is the common term used for masseter muscle rigidity in an infected patient. As the organism continues to spread, the patient develops a risus sardonicus (or sardonic) smile. These patients will present with opisthotonos, drooling, hydrophobia, weakness, myalgias, irritability, muscle cramps, dysphagia, clenching of fists, flexing of arms, and extension of lower extremities. In severe cases, even light touch, light, or noise can cause muscle spasm. These patients are alert and awake unless tetanus has affected the laryngeal muscles. During the second week of the disease process, patients become hypersympathetic. These patients develop profuse sweating, tachycardia, labile hypertension, increased excretion of urinary catecholamines, and hyperpyrexia. The illness progresses over the first three days to maximum symptomatology, and the symptoms persists for 5 to 7 days. If the patient survives, the symptoms will resolve completely in about 4 weeks. Local tetanus presents with persistent rigidity of muscle, which is in close proximity to the site of injury.

Patients with cephalic tetanus usually present with trismus and dysfunction of cranial nerves III, IV, IX, X, XII, and especially VII. The nerve dysfunctions are ipsilateral to the site of infection. There is also a high mortality rate for those with cephalic tetanus.

Infants with neonatal tetanus present with symptoms of poor sucking or swallowing and generalized muscle spasms that develop rapidly with very high mortality rates.

The primary complication of all persons infected with tetanus is respiratory failure secondary to asphyxia from hypertonic respiratory muscles. The patient also has problems with clearing secretions, which can lead to bronchiolitis, pneumonia, or atelectasis. The increased hyperactivity of the nervous system can lead to cardiac complications, such as cardiac arrest secondary to dysrhythmias, hypertension, tachycardia, myocarditis, and pulmonary edema. Muscle contractions can be so severe that they can cause subluxations and fractures of long bones and joints. Rhabdomyolysis can also occur and cause myoglobinuria and acute renal failure. Dehydration and renal vein thrombosis are common. Patients can also be hyperthermic secondary to muscle contractions.

The differential diagnosis of tetanus includes rabies, strychnine poisoning, hypocalcemic tetany, dystonic reactions secondary to phenothiazines, peritonitis, temporomandibular joint disease, and meningeal irritation secondary to subarachnoid hemorrhage and bacterial meningitis. Black widow spider bites, status epilepticus, peritonsillar abscess, and dislocation of the mandible can all mimic tetanus.

Diagnosis

The diagnosis of tetanus is a clinical diagnosis based on physical examination, history, and presenting complaints.

Laboratory Findings

A CBC, electrolytes, calcium, magnesium, and phosphorus should all be evaluated. There are no diagnostic tests to rule in or out tetanus. Cultures for *C. tetani* are only positive in one third of infected persons. Hypocalcemia can also mimic tetanus, thus a calcium level should always be drawn. A CT scan should be performed if there are any focal neurologic changes. A lumbar puncture should be performed if meningitis is suspected. Electromyography can be used to diagnose cephalic or localized tetanus.

Treatment

The best treatment for tetanus is prevention. Current CDC recommendations for routine diphtheria, tetanus, and pertussis immunization for children are for immunization at 6 weeks of age for the first dose; with a second dose 4 to 8 weeks after the first dose; a third dose 4 to 8 weeks after the second dose; and a fourth dose 6 to 12 months after the third dose, followed by a booster at 4 to 6 years of age. Adults should have a booster every 10 years, or if the wound is other than clean or minor in nature. The patient should have a tetanus booster if older than 7 years of age. Tetanus comes as a single antigen (T) diphtheria toxoid and tetanus (DT) for children younger than 7 years of age and as a diphtheria toxin for patients older than 7 years of age.

Acute treatment consists of four basic principles of management: (1) aggressive supportive care, (2) administration of the antitoxin, (3) elimination of toxin production, and (4) active immunization. Any patient who is suspected of having an acute tetanus infection should be treated very carefully. Quick or rough handling can cause the patient to have a muscle spasm. Cardiac and respiratory monitoring should be ensured in the ED. Aggressive airway management should be standard treatment with aggressive ventilatory support. Muscle spasms should be treated with IV benzodiazepines. If the patient has to be paralyzed to maintain airway support, succinylcholine, pancuronium, or atracurium can be used. Dantrolene is a direct muscle-relaxing agent that does not act on the central nervous system. This drug has been recommended as an adjunct muscle relaxant agent in tetanus.

Meticulous fluid and electrolyte management should be maintained. If the patient shows sympathetic overactivity, labetalol or propranolol can be used to control this sympathetic overactivity. Magnesium sulfate is recommended to treat autonomic dysfunction in severe tetanus. Hypertensive episodes can be treated with sodium nitroprusside. Bradydysrhythmias could be treated with temporary pacing instead of atropine or sympathetic drugs. Continuous spinal anesthesia has been reported to be beneficial in patients who have severe tetanus associated with autonomic instability.

Human tetanus immune globulin (TIG) should be used to neutralize circulating tetanospasmin and toxins that have not already affixed to the nervous system. TIG should be administered early, especially before surgical débridement or antibiotic administration. Surgical débridement and antibiotics will both release more toxins into the bloodstream and thus increase circulating toxins in the bloodstream and muscle spasm. TIG is administered in a dose of 3000 to 10,000 units IM. Blood levels are achieved in 48 to 72 hours and last up to 25 days. Only one dose is needed.

After TIG is administered, give penicillin 10 to 24 million units/day IV in divided doses for adults. In children, give 100,000 units/kg/day in divided doses for 10 to 14 days. Metronidazole, 500 mg PO every 6 hours, has also been recommended as a treatment. Tetracycline and erythromycin have both also been used in patients who are allergic to penicillin.

TICK-BORNE ILLNESSES

Definition

There are three families of ticks, two of which cause disease in humans and animals. These two families of ticks are the Ixodidae (hard ticks) and the Argasidae (soft ticks). Ticks are hematophagous parasites of the phylum Arthropoda, class Arachnida and Acarina order. Ticks can transmit Rocky Mountain spotted fever (RMSF), Lyme disease, tularemia, tick paralysis, relapsing fever, and babesiosis.

Epidemiology

Ticks are found worldwide in wilderness areas and are second only to mosquitoes in the transmission of disease to humans.

Pathology

Ticks require several blood meals during their life cycle. Their mouth parts are barbed and are very capable of burrowing and embedding themselves into animals and humans. All ticks start as eggs and go through three stages of growth: larva, nymph, and adult. The life of a tick lasts from 1 to 3 years. Ticks usually take a blood meal between each of these cycles and can be infective at any stage. The duration of feeding time depends on the type of tick.

LYME DISEASE

Symptoms of Lyme disease were first described in Old Lyme, Connecticut in 1975. The disease was first described in 1977 after the discovery of a new species of tick called *Ixodes dammini*. Lyme disease presented as several cases of juvenile rheumatoid arthritis (JRA). In 1981, the *I. dammini* tick was discovered on Long Island, New York, and was found to contain a spirochete that could be grown in an artificial medium. This spirochete was named *Borrelia burgdorferi*. The *B. burgdorferi* spirochete was found to cause Lyme disease. The spirochete can be found in the CSF, blood, and skin lesions of infected persons.

Lyme disease is now found throughout the United States and is worldwide. There were more than 7000 cases of Lyme disease reported to the CDC in 1989 and 7997 cases in 1990. This disease occurs most often in young adults and children. It has three areas of concentration: the coastal Northeast (Massachusetts to Maryland), the Midwest (Minnesota and Wisconsin), and the West (California, Oregon, Utah, and Nevada). In the Midwest, the *I. dammini* tick is the principal vector, and in the Midwest the *I. pacificus* tick is the principal vector.

Lyme disease, if left untreated, can present in one of three stages. *Stage I* is the most common presenting stage. The patient presents with erythema chronicum migrans (ECM). ECM is an erythematous, annular lesion with central clearing, which expands from the site of the tick bite. ECM occurs from 3 to 32 days after the tick bite, with a median of 7 days. Eighty-five percent of patients who are bitten have accompanying fatigue and generalized malaise. Sixty-four percent of patients present with headache; 59% with fever and chills; and 48%

with stiff neck and arthralgias. ECM usually fades completely in 4 weeks.

Stage II begins approximately 4 weeks after the onset of ECM and can last for several months. Stage II patients can present with ophthalmitis, radiculoneuropathy, and first-, second-, or third-degree cardiac atrioventricular (AV) blocks. Ten percent of patients who progress to stage II and who are not treated will develop unilateral or bilateral facial nerve palsy, chronic headaches, or meningoencephalitis.

Stage III is seen in 60% of patients who are not treated. Stage III consists of arthritis, which can present or persist for several weeks or years after the onset of skin lesions. Stage III presents with brief exacerbations of recurrent episodes of migratory oligoarthritis with periods of remission, where remissions last longer than do the exacerbations. The knees, shoulders, elbows, temporomandibular joint, ankle, wrists, hip, and small joints of hands and feet (in this order) are the most common presenting arthritic joint complaints.

Diagnosis

The diagnosis of Lyme disease is very difficult to make. The primary diagnosis is made by a history and physical examination. Only one third of patients present with a history of a tick bite. The disease should be considered in any patient who lives in an endemic area and who presents with a rash or nonspecific symptoms of a viral illness, meningitis, new heart block, arthritis, multiple neurologic abnormalities, or joint pain.

Laboratory tests do not usually prove very helpful. The erythrocyte sedimentation rate is mildly elevated, and there can be mild anemia with a normal white blood cell count and an absolute lymphocyte decrease. Proteinuria, microhematuria, and an increased serum glutamic ixaloacetic transaminase (LDH) level may all be present. Blood, CSF, and synovial fluid cultures are not helpful in the diagnosis. Serologic testing of gamma G immunoglobulin (IgG) and gamma M immunoglobulin (IgM) with indirect fluorescent antibody and ELISA are sometimes helpful.

A patient with suspected tick bites should be completely undressed, and the patient's skin should be inspected for ticks. If a tick is found, it should be removed.

Treatment

Treatment of stage I Lyme disease is accomplished with doxycycline 100 mg PO BID or tetracycline 250 mg PO four times a day (QID) for 10 to 21 days. Tetracycline should not be given to pregnant women or children younger than 8 years of age. In children younger than 8 years of age, amoxicillin 250 to 500 mg PO TID can be used. IV penicillin in pregnant women at 5 million units QID for 10 to 14 days has been recommended or penicillin 250 to 500 mg PO or erythromycin 250 mg PO QID can be used.

Patients who have stage II Lyme disease with neurologic disease can be treated with oral medication as described earlier or, if neurologic disease is severe, ceftriaxone (Rocephin) 2 to 4 g/day IV can be given for 14 days. Children can receive 50 to 80 mg/kg/day for 14 days. Penicillin can also be used in an increased dose of 20 to 24 million units/day for 10 to 14 days.

If the patient has a first-degree AV block, the patient can be treated with PO medication as described earlier. In severe cardiac disease, second- or third-degree block, the patient should be admitted to the hospital and have either IV penicillin or IV ceftriaxone. Aspirin 4 g/day PO has shown some effect in persistent high-degree AV block in Lyme disease.

In stage II arthritis, penicillin 20 million units IV for 2 to 3 weeks should be given. Ceftriaxone 2 g/day for 2 weeks is usually more effective than is penicillin. The results of the antibiotics might be delayed for several weeks or months. Thirty-day oral regimens of doxycycline 100 mg PO BID or amoxicillin 500 mg PO TID with probenecid 500 mg PO TID have also been successful in treating Lyme disease.

A special concern in the case of the pregnant patient is the effect of Lyme disease on the fetus. The *B. burgdorferi* spirochete can pass transplacentally and cause harm to the fetus. Gestational Lyme's borreliosis can cause hydrocephalus, prematurity, cardiovascular anomalies, fetal death, neonatal respiratory distress, cortical blindness, hyperbilirubinemia, intrauterine growth retardation, sudden infant death syndrome, syndactyly, rash, and maternal toxemia of pregnancy. Pregnant patients with Lyme disease should be treated aggressively and followed closely.

ROCKY MOUNTAIN SPOTTED FEVER

RMSF is an acute febrile systemic illness caused by the organism *Rickettsia rickettsii.* RMSF is transmitted by Ixodid ticks. The wood tick, *Dermacentor andersoni,* in the western United States and the American dog tick, *D. variabilis,* in the southeastern United States are the two ticks that transmit RMSF in the United States. RMSF is the second most commonly acquired tick-borne disease in the United States.

There are between 500 and 1000 reported cases of RMSF in the United States each year, and approximately 40 deaths occur annually. The peak incidence for RMSF is in late spring to early fall.

RMSF can present with a very wide clinical spectrum. Only two thirds of patients have an identifiable tick bite. Only 3% of patients present with the classic triad of fever, rash, and a history of tick exposure in the first 3 days of illness. The ticks invade the small blood vessels of the body and cause vascular damage and vasculitis secondary to an immunologic response. The patient usually presents with a generalized vasculitis, causing a petechial rash and thrombocytopenia. The immunologic response can cause rash, fever, disseminated intravascular coagulation (DIC), third spacing of fluid, myocardial necrosis, encephalitis, pulmonary interstitial disorders, and adult respiratory distress syndrome.

The incubation period is from 2 to 14 days after the bite. The shorter the incubation period, usually the more severe is the illness. The patient usually presents with a very high fever 40° C (104° F), followed by the rash. The rash presents initially as an erythematous, macular, blanching rash that progresses to a very deep red papular rash, which becomes petechial in nature. The rash usually begins on the flexor surfaces of the wrists and ankles and spreads to the rest of the body in a centripetal and centrifugal pattern. Seventy-five to 85% of patients present with headache, 66% with nausea and vomiting, 20 to 25% with meningoencephalitic involvement, 33% with a cough, and 85% with myalgias.

Diagnosis

It is very difficult to diagnose RMSF, and there are no good laboratory tests to diagnose RMSF. The white blood cell count may be slightly elevated, and other laboratory tests will be organ specific for invasion. Immunofluorescent antibody staining can be performed on skin tissue obtained from an area of rash. This result is 100% specific and 70% sensitive. Serologic tests are only helpful in the first few days of illness. The complement fixation, Weil-Felix reaction, is the most diagnostic check for RMSF. A titer greater than 1:64 or a fourfold rise in paired sera is diagnostic of RMSF.

Treatment

Treatment of suspected RMSF should not be withheld pending results of complement fixation. Tetracycline is the drug of choice for adults and children older than 8 years of age. Tetracycline is given as 10 to 20 mg/kg IV BID up to 500 mg per dose or 25 to 50 mg/kg PO QID. In children younger than 8 years of age, chloramphenicol 50 mg/kg/day IV or PO is given.

TICK PARALYSIS

Tick paralysis was first reported in the United States in 1912. Tick paralysis occurs when the female *Dermacentor* tick, which is infected, bites a human. In Australia, the *I. holocyclus* tick is the primary carrier. Most cases occur in the spring and summer and involve children. Tick paralysis is uncommon in the United States. If the tick is not removed, the paralysis can be fatal. The onset of symptoms occur 4 to 7 days after attachment of the tick. Tick paralysis is thought to be caused by a toxin secreted by the tick during one of its blood meals.

Diagnosis

The patient presents with restlessness and irritability, then an ascending flaccid paralysis occurs with acute ataxia or a combination of these symptoms can occur simultaneously. Deep tendon reflexes are lost at an early stage. The paralysis progresses to bulbar paralysis, respiratory paralysis, and death. Ataxia and cerebellar findings can be present in the absence of muscular weakness. Isolated facial paralysis has also been reported in patients with a tick embedded in the ear.

Treatment

Any patient with possible exposure to ticks with flaccid paralysis or acute ataxia should be undressed completely, and the patient's entire skin surface should be inspected, including the scalp and hair for ticks. Removal of the tick is curative. Supportive care that includes mechanical ventilation is sometimes necessary. Symptoms usually resolve, and the patient recovers completely in 48 hours. Guillain-Barré syndrome, Eaton-Lambert syndrome, poliomyelitis, botulism, myasthenia gravis, and polyneuropathy should always be considered in any patient with an ascending flaccid paralysis or acute ataxia.

BABESIOSIS

Babesiosis is a malaria-like illness caused by a parasite of the genus *Babesia. Babesia* is an intrathyrocytic protozoan parasite. There are more than 70 species of *Babesia.* Babesiosis is a rare disease in the United States. It was first described in the United States in 1957, and only 200 cases have been reported since 1957. It is transmitted by the *I. dammini* tick, the same tick that transmits Lyme disease. *B. microti* is the most common species that causes disease in the United States. Most causes are reported in the New England states of Massachusetts and Rhode Island. *B. microti* is found on mice and deer in the United States. It was first described in 1888 by Babes as the cause of febrile hemoglobinuria in cattle. It is proposed that babesiosis was the cause of the fifth plague in the Book of Exodus in the Bible.

The nymph stage of the tick's life cycle is the only stage in which transmission can occur. The incubation period is from 1 to 4 weeks. A patient presents with flu-like symptoms of fever, chills, headache, anorexia, and fatigue. Lesser symptoms of myalgia, photophobia, depression, diaphoresis, arthralgias, dark urine, emotional liability, and hyperesthesias can occur. Patients with severe disease can present with acute respiratory distress syndrome, renal insufficiency, hemolytic anemia, hemoglobinuria, and disseminated intravascular coagulation. These symptoms occur more often in splenectomized patients.

Diagnosis

A diagnosis is made by examination of blood smears with Giemsa-stained thick and thin smears. Intraerythrocytic pyriform, ring, or tetrad forms may be seen. The budding forms will look like a Maltese cross. Indirect fluorescent antibody testing for *B. microti* is available through the CDC. A titer of 1:1024 is suggestive of babesiosis. Other laboratory tests are nonspecific. The bilirubin and serum lactate dehydrogenase levels can be elevated. Hemolytic anemia can also be present.

Treatment

A patient who still has his or her spleen usually recovers without sequelae. In a patient who has been splenectomized, the combination of quinine (650 mg PO QID) and clindamycin (600 mg IV QID for 10 days) is recommended.

RELAPSING FEVER

Relapsing fever is caused by a spirochete of the *Borrelia* species from a bite of the ticks of the genus *Ornithodoros.* The Argasidae ticks like to live in burrows and caves and feed on various rodents (endemic). *Borrelia* causes an acute febrile illness characterized by cyclic periods of fever and spirochetemia that last for several days. There is also an epidemic form that can be transmitted by body lice (*B. recurrentis*) in an epidemic form. This form has not been reported in the United States. Ticks in all stages of the tick life cycle can transmit *Borrelia.*

The epidemic form of relapsing fever, or louse-borne form, is transmitted by person-to-person contact. It is not transmitted by louse bites, rather it is transmitted when the louse is crushed against the infested patient. The spirochetes are liberated, and they penetrate through a bite site, abrasion, or intact skin. The relapsing phenomenon is due to the spirochete undergoing antigenic variation in the body of the infected host. Epidemic relapsing fever is still found in the Sudan and Ethiopia and in parts of Asia, South America, and Europe.

The endemic, tick-borne form of relapsing fever is found in the United States. The Argasidae tick is found on mice, rats, chipmunks, squirrels, and rabbits. The *Borrelia* spirochete can be transmitted transovarily from one generation to the next. Infection can take place in as little as 15 to 30 minutes during the tick feedings. Saliva is transmitted through a bite site or intact skin. The incubation period takes from 4 to 18 days. Patients present with abrupt onset of fever, headache, chills, arthralgias, myalgias, nausea, and vomiting. Pruritic eschar is noted occasionally at the site of the tick bite.

On physical examination, splenomegaly, jaundice, and hepatomegaly are often noted. Nuchal rigidity, delirium, peripheral neuropathy, and pupillary abnormalities are noted. A petechial or macular rash is often noted on the trunk. The initial fever usually lasts for 3 days, and a relapse occurs in approximately 7 days. The relapsing cycles usually recur on an average of thee times, in which the successive relapses are less severe.

Diagnosis

To diagnose relapsing fever, *Borrelia,* the borreliae have to be demonstrated in the peripheral blood during a febrile episode. A blood specimen should be obtained as the patient's temperature rises. The spirochete can be visualized on a Wright or Giemsa stain. The spirochete is approximately 5 to 20 μm in length and lies in the plasma spaces between the red blood cells or may overlie the red blood cells.

Treatment

Treatment is with tetracycline in adults and children older than 8 years of age. Give the patient tetracycline, 500 mg PO QID for 10 days. Erythromycin, 500 mg PO QID, can also be used for children younger than 8 years of age and in adults who are allergic to tetracycline. Ceftriaxone (Rocefin), chloramphenicol, streptomycin, and penicillin have all been used successfully to treat relapsing fever.

A complication in the treatment of relapsing fever is the occurrence of a Jarisch-Herxheimer reaction secondary to the administration of antibiotics. Fever, severe rigors, and a drop in the patient's leukocyte count and platelet count occur with severe hypotension. Any patient who is treated for relapsing fever should be admitted to the hospital, and one or two IV lines should be started in anticipation of a Jarisch-Herxheimer reaction.

TULAREMIA

Tularemia is caused by a zoonotic bacterium called *Francisella tularensis*. *F. tularensis* is a small gram-negative pleomorphic nonmotile rod that is transmitted to humans by insects or infected animals. Two types of *F. tularensis* are found in the United States. Jellison type A is found in North America and is associated with rabbits and ticks. Jellison type B is found in Europe and Asia. This type is associated with rodents and causes a more minor illness. The ticks *Dermacentor variabilis* and *Amblyomma americanum* are the primary tick vectors in the United States. Transmission can occur in any stage and is transovarial.

Peak occurrence is during the summer in May to August and again in December and January. Tularemia is found worldwide from a latitude of 30 to 71 degrees north. Rabbits and mice are believed to be the main vectors of the bacteria, but the bacteria have been found in more than 100 animals. Transmission can occur with ingestion of infected fomites, water, or soil or with inhalation of dust or water that has been infected. Person-to-person transmission is rare.

Patients with tularemia present in six different classes or groups: (1) oropharyngeal, (2) glandular, (3) ulceroglandular, (4) typhoid, (5) pneumonic, and (6) oculoglandular. The ulceroglandular type is the most common, and the pneumonic and typhoid types are ranked second and third. Lymphadenopathy is the most common presenting sign and is present in 65 to 95% of patients. Children will present with cervical adenopathy (82%), inguinal adenopathy (54%), and fever (87%). Ulcerations are more common in adults than in children. The ulcer occurs on an extremity at the site of the bite. There is regional lymphadenopathy and fever. The regional adenopathy reflects the primary entry site. The typhoid type presents with fever, chills, abdominal pain, diarrhea, debility, weight loss, and anorexia. Patients who acquire tularemia from rabbits usually have axillary or epitrochlear nodal adenopathy. Nodes can sometimes become suppurative and drain.

Glandular tularemia is the second most common form of tularemia and presents with cervical lymphadenopathy but with no skin ulcers. A person with pulmonary tularemia presents as a patient with pneumonia, chills, fever, nonproductive cough, and substernal burning with malaise, dyspnea, and prostration. Pulmonary tularemia can occur from either direct inhalation of the aerosolized organisms or bacterial spread from the original site of infection.

Diagnosis

A diagnosis is made by having a high index of suspicion. Acute specific agglutination titers greater than 1:160 or a fourfold increase is confirmatory. A skin test for tularemia is available, and the result is positive during the first few weeks of infection. This skin test can be obtained from the CDC. Aspiration of an affected lymph node is not recommended due to the possibility of the spread of the *F. tularensis* organism. If aspiration is performed, special precautions should be taken when handling the specimen.

Treatment

Streptomycin, 30 to 40 mg/kg/day IM BID for 3 days then 20 mg/kg/day IM BID for 4 to 7 days, is the treatment of choice. Tetracycline, 50 to 60 mg/kg PO QID for 14 days, is an alternative choice.

ACUTE GASTROENTERITIS

Definition

Diarrhea is usually self-limiting and is the passage of rapidly successive and excessive fluid stool. *Enteritis* is synonymous for diarrhea. When nausea and vomiting also occur with diarrhea, this is called *gastroenteritis.* When the diarrhea contains mucus, pus, or blood, this is called *dysentery.*

Etiology

Viruses cause 50 to 70% of all diarrhea; bacterial agents cause 15 to 20%; and parasites cause 10 to 15%. The remaining 5 to 15% of diarrhea has no known cause. The usual modes of transmission are fecal-oral transmission; zoonotic transmission from wild or domestic animals; or person-to-person transmission.

Epidemiology

Diarrhea occurs worldwide in 3 to 5 billion persons annually.

Pathology

The average colon only passes 100 ml of fluid per day, which is from 8 to 9 liters of secretions from ingested fluids per day. The sodium-osmotic gradient protects large amounts of water from being excreted from the small intestine and colon. Diarrhea can be produced by three mechanisms: (1) increased intestinal motility from stress, chemical ingestion, cholinergic drugs, antacids, bile salts, and caffeine; (2) decreased absorptive bowel capacity; and (3) increased fluid volume.

When organisms invade bowel mucosa, they disrupt the integrity of the mucosa. They can cause an inflammatory disease process, causing exudate with poor absorption. This inflammatory exudate can cause blood, pus, or mucus to be discharged in stool. Viral organisms do not alter bowel mucosa.

Five factors that affect or protect the host against diarrhea are: (1) gastrointestinal (GI) mucus, (2) secretory immunoglobulins and phagocytic cells, (3) gastric acidity, (4) the normal flora of the intestine, and (5) the motility of the intestine.

Questions to Ask During History Taking

1. Did the diarrhea start abruptly? An abrupt onset of diarrhea is usually caused by an exogenous agent, exotoxins, or toxins. Chronic or recurrent diarrhea usually involves an underlying intestinal disease.
2. Does the diarrhea start during the day or night? Functional diarrhea occurs only during the daytime, and the patient is symptom free at night. Diarrhea that occurs at night (i.e., nocturnal diarrhea) is usually a sign of organic disease (e.g., hyperthyroidism, inflammatory bowel disease, or diabetic visceral neuropathy).
3. What do the stools look like? Bloody stool with pus or mucus indicates an infection or inflammatory process of the colon. Copious watery stools are a sign of small bowel etiology for diarrhea. Pale, foul-smelling stools are usually caused by a malabsorption syndrome.
4. Have there been any changes in diet? Milk will cause diarrhea in patients who are lactose intolerant. Food allergies can cause diarrhea. Foods that contain mannitol or sorbitol can cause osmotic diarrhea (e.g., dietetic candies and foods).
5. Is anyone else affected by diarrhea? If more than one person in a family is affected by diarrhea, food poisoning should be suspected. A history of ingesting foods such as rewarmed rice, eggs, or seafood can confirm the diagnosis.
6. Has the patient been outside the United States? The person may have traveler's diarrhea.

7. Is the patient taking any antibiotics? Antibiotics can frequently trigger diarrhea.
8. If elderly, is the patient a chronic laxative abuser or user?
9. Does the patient consume large amounts of alcohol?
10. Is there a new psychosocial stress in the patient's life?
11. Is the patient a homosexual male?
12. Is the patient a food handler?
13. Does the patient work in a day care center?
14. Is the patient an athlete? Diarrhea can occur in long-distance runners secondary to intestinal ischemia.
15. Has the patient lost weight over a specific period of time? Weight loss over a period of time indicates a malabsorption etiology.
16. Has the patient's appetite changed? Weakness and depressed appetite are signs of parasitic infection, cancer, or inflammatory bowel disease.
17. Is the patient immunocompromised? Is the patient HIV positive, or does the patient have an acquired immunodeficiency syndrome (AIDS)-related complex?

Diagnosis/Physical Examination

First look at the patient's vital signs. Does he or she have a fever? A fever suggests an infective etiology or an inflammatory process and does not usually occur in the enterotoxin-induced diarrheas. Is the patient tachycardiac? An elevated pulse in lieu of decreased blood pressure is a sign of dehydration. Take the patient's orthostatic vital signs. Fever, tachycardia, and chills in a toxic-looking patient could be signs of sepsis or bacteremia. Does the patient have nausea or vomiting? A sudden onset of nausea and vomiting is an indication of toxin-induced gastroenteritis.

Look at the patient's skin turgor. Decreased skin turgor and dry mucous membranes are signs of dehydration. Does the patient have mental status changes? Mental status changes can be caused by hypotension or acidosis.

Hyporeflexia is a sign of hypokalemia caused by a loss of potassium in stool. Is the patient's abdomen tender? A tender abdomen is a sign of *Yersinia* or *Campylobacter*. Bacterial enteritis can look like acute appendicitis in these patients. A patient with viral or toxin-induced diarrhea does not usually have a very tender abdomen.

A rectal examination should be performed on all patients with diarrhea to obtain information on whether the result of a hemoculture of the stool is positive. Is there is a perianal fissure or fistula causing the bleeding. Is there a foreign body in the rectum?

A definite sign of toxigenic diarrhea is an acute onset of diarrhea in 2 to 12 hours of exposure. The patient usually does not appear toxic but has a mild, generalized abdominal tenderness and some cramping pain that is usually intermittent. No systemic symptoms are present. The onset of the diarrhea is sudden and lasts for 10 to

24 hours. The patient does not usually have a fever. There is no mucus, blood, or fecal leukocytes in the stool.

Infectious diarrhea is marked by a fever that starts gradually over 1 to 3 days, with abdominal tenderness and tenesmus. Systemic symptoms are often present with vomiting, chills, malaise, nausea, and headache. The patient looks "sick" or "toxic." The patient will have abdominal tenderness, which often mimics acute appendicitis. There is usually blood, mucus, or fecal leukocytes in the stool.

Laboratory Findings

In toxic-looking patients, especially children and the elderly, obtain a complete blood count (CBC), looking for eosinophilia in parasitic infections, electrolytes, blood urea nitrogen (BUN), and creatinine. Perform a fecal leukocyte examination. Take blood cultures, and culture the patient's stool for parasites.

Treatment

Most infectious diarrhea can be cured with ciprofloxacin, ampicillin, or trimethoprim-sulfamethoxazole (TMP-SMX). Ciprofloxacin has not been approved for use in children or pregnant women.

Intravenous (IV) fluid treatment of dehydration includes:

> *Adult:* To 1 liter of D5W/.45 normal saline (NS) add 10 to 20 mEq of KCl and 50 mEq NaHCO (1 amp)
> *Child:* To 1 liter of D5W/.25NS add 10 to 20 mEq of KCl and 50 mEq NaHCO
> *Oral rehydration:* World Health Organization (WHO): To 1 liter of water add:
> > 20 g of glucose
> > 3.5 g of sodium chloride
> > 2.5 g of sodium bicarbonate
> > 1.5 g of potassium chloride

Do not use antimotility drugs. Bismuth subsalicylate (Pepto-Bismol) may be used.

Prevention

All or most diarrhea can be prevented by sanitary hand-washing, terminal cleaning, adequate sewage disposal, early recognition of the organism, and proper early treatment.

	A	B	C	D	E	F	G	H
1	Organism	Pathogenesis of Mucosal Damage	Character of Stool	Incubation Period	Duration of Symptoms	Fecal Leukocytes	Epidemiology	Treatment
2	Adenovirus	Invasion without destruction	Watery diarrhea	3–10 days	5–12 days	None	Usually in children infancy to 7 years old, winter, person-to-person	Fluid and electrolyte support
3	Aeromonas hydrophila	Invasive destruction	Watery, bloody diarrhea	—	2–10 weeks	Yes	Brackish drinking water, AIDS patients, immunocompromised patients, children	Ciprofloxacin 500 mg PO BID × 7 days or TMP-SMX 160 mg/800 mg PO × 7 days
4	Bacillus cereus	Preformed toxins	Only 25% of exposed persons will have diarrhea	2–3 hours	Less than 10 hours	None	Warmed-up fried rice, vegetables, and meats	Antiemetics, IV fluids, no antibiotics
5	Blastocystis hominis	Alteration without invasion	Watery stools	3–10 days	Days to weeks untreated	None	Immunocompromised patients, AIDS patients, a protozoan	Metronidazole 250–750 mg PO TID × 10 days or iodoquinol 650 mg PO TID × 20 days

Table continued on following page

	A	B	C	D	E	F	G	H
	Organism	Pathogenesis of Mucosal Damage	Character of Stool	Incubation Period	Duration of Symptoms	Fecal Leukocytes	Epidemiology	Treatment
6	*Campylobacter* sp.	Invasive destruction	Bloody stools	2–5 days	5–14 days	Yes	Contaminated food and water, birds, animals; may mimic appendicitis	Ciprofloxacin 500 mg BID × 7 days, erythromycin 500 mg PO QID × 7 days
7	Ciguatera fish poison	Preformed toxins, neurotoxin	Watery diarrhea	2–6 hours	1–8 weeks	None	Contaminated fish around Florida and Hawaii, barracuda	IV fluid, supportive of anticholinesterase activity, H₁ blockers for pruritus
8	*Clostridium difficile*	Cytopathic toxins	Watery, sometimes bloody	While on antibiotics	Resolves with antibiotic treatment	Yes	Antibiotic treatment, especially clindamycin	Metronidazole 250 mg PO QID × 10 to 14 days, vancomycin 125 mg PO QID × 10–14 days

#	Organism	Mechanism	Stool	Incubation	Duration		Source	Treatment
9	*Clostridium perfringens*	Does not invade mucosa	Watery stool, enteritis necroticans will have blood in stool	6–12 hours	Less than 24 hours	None, enteritis-yes	Rewarmed meats and poultry	Self-limiting, antitoxin to beta-toxins in enteritis necroticans
10	Crohn's disease	Inflammatory destruction	Watery, bloody stools, with mucus	Intermittent	Years	Yes	Not an infection, a disease that causes bloody diarrhea	Sulfasalazine, corticosteroids, metronidazole
11	*Cryptosporidium*	Alteration without invasion	Watery diarrhea	Days to weeks	Chronic	None	AIDS patients	Spiramycin 1 g PO TID × 14 days?, indomethacin 50 mg PO TID
12	Cytomegalovirus	Invasive destruction	Watery diarrhea	Days to weeks	Recurrence in 8–9 weeks after treatment	None	AIDS patients, immunocompromised patients	Ganciclovir 5 mg/kg q12hr IV for 14 days
13	*Entamoeba histolytica*	Invasive destruction	Blood or mucus in stool	Days to weeks	Months to years	Yes	Passers of cysts in poor hygiene areas	Iodoquinol, tetracycline dehydroemitine, chloroquine phosphate

Table continued on following page

	A	B	C	D	E	F	G	H
	Organism	**Pathogenesis of Mucosal Damage**	**Character of Stool**	**Incubation Period**	**Duration of Symptoms**	**Fecal Leukocytes**	**Epidemiology**	**Treatment**
14	Enterohemorrhagic *Escherichia coli* 0157:H7	Cytopathic toxins	Bloody stool, hemorrhagic colitis, thrombotic thrombocytopenic purpura	3–8 days	5–10 days	Yes	Raw beef, ground beef, milk, meats, person-to-person	Ciprofloxacin 500 mg PO BID × 7 days or TMP-SMX 160 mg/ 800mg PO × 7 days
15	*Enteromonas hominis*	Alteration without invasion	Chronic watery diarrhea	Days to weeks	Chronic if not treated	None	Fecal-oral route, male homosexuals	Metronidazole 250–750 mg PO × 10 days
16	Enterotoxigenic *Escherichia coli*	Colonization produces toxins	Watery without blood, abrupt onset	24–72 hours	48–72 hours	None	Traveler's diarrhea, unpeeled fruits or vegetables, contaminated ice	TMP-SMX 160 mg/800 mg PO BID × 7 days
17	*Giardia lamblia*	Alteration without invasion	Watery stools	1–3 weeks	Chronic if not treated	None	Male homosexuals, water-borne, day care centers, backpackers, travelers	Metronidazole 250 mg PO TID × 5 days, furazolidone 100 mg PO QID × 7–10 days

18	*Isospora belli*	Alteration without invasion	Watery stools	Days to weeks	Chronic	None	AIDS patients, immunocompromised patients	TMP-SMX 160 mg/800 mg PO QID × 10days then BID × 3 weeks
19	*Mycobacterium avium-intracellulare*	Invasive destruction	Profound diarrhea	Days to weeks	Chronic	Yes	AIDS patients, immunocompromised patients	Multiple drug therapy
20	Noncholera vibrios	Colonization produces toxins	Copious watery diarrhea	24–48 hours	7 days	None	Shellfish	Rehydration and tetracyclines
21	Norwalk virus	Invasion without destruction	Watery diarrhea	20–36 hours	4–7 days	None	Children, day care centers, family contact	Rehydration IV or PO
22	*Plesiomonas hominis*	Alteration without invasion	Watery diarrhea	1–2 days	5–40 days	Yes	Shellfish, AIDS patients, immunocompromised patients	Ciprofloxacin 500 mg PO BID × 7 days or TMP-SMX 160 mg/800 mg PO × 7 days
23	*Plesiomonas shigelloides*	Invasive destruction	Bloody stools	1–2 days	5–40 days	Yes	Shellfish, immunocompromised patients, AIDS patients	Ciprofloxacin 500 mg PO BID × 7 days or TMP-SMX 160 mg/800 mg PO × 7 days

Table continued on following page

	A	B	C	D	E	F	G	H
	Organism	Pathogenesis of Mucosal Damage	Character of Stool	Incubation Period	Duration of Symptoms	Fecal Leukocytes	Epidemiology	Treatment
24	Rotavirus	Invasion without destruction	Watery stools	20–36 hours	4–7 days	None	Day care centers, children	PO, IV rehydration
25	*Salmonella* sp.	Invasive destruction	Watery stools	8–24 hours	2–5 days	Yes	Poultry, eggs, egg products, pets, turtles, milk	Ciprofloxacin 500 mg PO BID × 7 days or TMP-SMX 160 mg/800 mg PO × 7 days
26	Scombroid fish poison	Preformed toxins	Mild diarrhea	20–30 minutes	6 hours	None	Dark meat fish, tuna, mackerel, blue fish, mahimahi	Diphenhydramine 50 mg IM, cimetidine 300 mg IV
27	*Shigella* sp.	Invasive destruction	Watery stools, dysentery	24–48 hours	4–7 days	Yes	Fecal-oral, person-to-person	Ciprofloxacin 500 mg PO BID × 7 days or TMP-SMX 160 mg/800 mg PO × 7 days

No.	Organism	Mechanism	Stool				Source	Treatment
28	*Staphylococcus aureus*	Preformed toxins	Little or very mild diarrhea, toxin absent	1–6 hours	<10 hours	None	Protein-rich foods, mayonnaise, eggs, potato salad, pastries, ham	IV fluids, antibiotics can make the diarrhea worse
29	*Strongyloides stercoralis*	Invasive destruction	Watery, bloody stool, larvae found in stool	Days to weeks	Chronic	Yes	AIDS patients, immunocompromised patients	Thiabendazole 50 mg/kg/day BID × 2 days (max of 3 g/day)
30	Ulcerative colitis	Inflammatory destruction	Mucus and blood containing stool	Days to weeks	Chronic	Yes	Family?	Surgery
31	*Vibrio cholerae*	Colonization produces toxins	Massive watery diarrhea	12–48 hours	2–7 days	None	Shellfish and epidemics	IV therapy with sodium and potassium
32	*Vibrio parahemolyticus*	Causes patchy mucosal damage	Watery stools	6–48 hours	Under 24 hours	Yes	Gram-negative bacillus, fresh or frozen seafood	Tetracycline 500 mg PO QID × 7 days or doxycycline 100 mg PO × 7 days
33	*Yersinia enterocolitica*	Invasive destruction	Long duration of excretion of organism, up to 6 weeks	12–48 hours	5–14 days	Yes	May mimic appendicitis, terminal ileitis syndrome, polyarthritis	Ciprofloxacin 500 mg PO BID × 7 days or TMP-SMX 160 mg/800 mg PO × 7 days

BIBLIOGRAPHY

Benenson AB (ed): Control of Communicable Diseases in Man, 14th ed. Springfield, VA, American Public Health Association, 1985

Braunwald E, Isselbacher KJ, Petersdorf RG, et al (eds): Harrison's Principles of Internal Medicine, 11th ed. New York, McGraw-Hill, 1987

Hamilton GC, Sanders AB, Strange GR, et al (eds): Emergency Medicine: An Approach to Clinical Problem-Solving. Philadelphia, WB Saunders, 1991

Hoephrich PD, Jordan MC, Ronald AR (eds): Infectious Diseases, 5th ed. Philadelphia, JB Lippincott, 1994

Keisch GT, Formal SB, Bennish ML: Shigellosis. In Warren KS, Mahmoud AAF (eds): Tropical and Geographical Medicine, 2nd ed. New York, McGraw-Hill, 1990

Kravis TC, Warner CG, Jacobs LM (eds): Emergency Medicine: A Comprehensive Review, 3rd ed. New York, Raven Press, 1993

May HL, Aghababian RV, Fleisher GR (eds): Emergency Medicine, 2nd ed. Boston, Little, Brown, 1992

Pearson RD, Guerrant RL, Isselbacher KJ, et al (eds): Harrison's Principles of Internal Medicine, 11th ed. New York, McGraw-Hill, 1987

Rosen P, Barkin RM (eds): Emergency Medicine: Concepts and Clinical Practice, 3rd ed. St Louis, Mosby-Year Book, 1992

Schwartz GR, Cayton CG, Manglesen MA, et al (eds): Principles and Practice of Emergency Medicine, 3rd ed. Philadelphia, Lea & Febiger, 1992

Sleisenger MH, Fordtran JS (eds): Gastrointestinal Disease: Pathophysiology Diagnosis, Management, 4th ed. Philadelphia, WB Saunders, 1989

Tierney LM, McPhee SJ, Papadakis MA (eds): Current Medical Diagnosis and Treatment, 33rd ed. Norwalk, CT, Appleton & Lange, 1994

Tintinalli JE, Krone RL, Ruiz E (eds): Emergency Medicine: A Comprehensive Study Guide, 4th ed. New York, McGraw-Hill, 1996

Chapter 8

Medical Emergencies

ACID-BASE PROBLEMS

Definition

The acidity of any solution is based on the hydrogen ion activity of that particular solution. The level of activity of hydrogen ions is directly proportional within a solution to the concentration of the hydrogen ions in that solution multiplied by an activity coefficient. Thus, the acidity of a solution is equal to the ratio of activity of the acid to its corresponding base multiplied by its dissociation constant.

The pH is the concentration of hydrogen ions expressed as a negative logarithm. A neutral solution exists when the number of hydrogen ions equals the number of hydroxyl (OH^-) ions in water at $25°$ C ($77°$ F) or the number of ions is 10^{-7} mol/l. A solution with a pH of 1.0 will be very acidic and have a hydrogen ion concentration of 1×1.0^{-1}. A solution with a pH of 14.0 will have a hydrogen concentration of 1×14^{-14} and will be extremely alkaline. The pH is computed by the Henderson-Hasselbach equation as a negative log.

$$pH + pK + \log \frac{\text{proton acceptor (base)}}{\text{proton donor (acid)}}$$

In humans and animals, the pH must remain fairly constant. This is achieved by cellular consumption of nonvolatile acids, physicochemical buffering, and the transfer of acid or alkali between the cytosol and the organelles.

Carbon dioxide (or CO_2, which is a volatile acid) is produced as a byproduct of the body's metabolism of proteins, fats, and carbohydrates and is excreted mainly by the lungs. CO_2 is transported from the tissues to the lungs by plasma bicarbonate and hemoglobin. CO_2 is present as carbonic acid in the arterial blood at a P_{CO_2} of 40 mm Hg, on the average.

Nonvolatile acid is excreted by the kidneys in three ways: (1) ammonia, which is produced in the distal tubule cells from glutamine and other precursors, is excreted by the kidneys (the majority of acid excretion), (2) the direct excretion of hydrogen (a very small amount of acid is excreted in this manner), and (3) the excretion of acid with urine buffers by the HaH_2PO_4 system.

Numerous factors affect the excretion of acid by the kidneys. Sodium and bicarbonate are absorbed in the proximal tubules and are independent of aldosterone. Thus, if a patient is dehydrated or volume depleted, an increased amount of sodium and bicarbonate will be absorbed by the proximal tubule. If the patient is volume overloaded, then less sodium and bicarbonate are absorbed. If there is an increase in aldosterone or a decreased metabolism of aldosterone by the liver or a sodium deficiency, then there is an increase in the absorption of sodium and bicarbonate in the proximal tubules. H_2CO_3 is dissociated into H^+ and HCO_3^-, where H^+ and K^+ are excreted in the urine in exchange for Na^+. HCO_3^- is formed in cells. Na^+ is absorbed from the opposite side of the tubule lumen back into the bloodstream and becomes $NaHCO_3$.

Renal tubular acidosis can be classified as either distal or proximal. In distal tubular acidosis the distal tubule is damaged and is unable to create transepithelial pH gradients, which causes impairment of the filtering of bicarbonate and thus an acidification of the urine by the distal nephron. Proximal tubular acidosis is caused by an increased pH secondary to failure of the proximal nephron to reabsorb the normal load of bicarbonate; however, this increased load is usually handled by the distal tubule if it is not damaged also.

Buffers neutralize acids or bases and allow a steady state of the pH in the body. Without buffers, there would be wide swings in the pH of the body. Buffers are usually metabolic or respiratory in nature. The main buffers in the blood are hemoglobin in the cell and bicarbonate and protein in the plasma. The average buffer base or buffering capacity in an adult is approximately 1000 mEq. Intracellular buffers are phosphate and protein. Anemia, decreased muscle mass, and low protein levels all affect the body's ability to buffer hydrogen ions. Patients with anemia, low protein, or decreased muscle mass are at a higher risk of severe acidosis.

The *base excess* or *base deficit* is the measure of the deviation of buffer base from its normal value. Base deficit (negative base excess) represents the amount of bicarbonate (in mEq/l) that is required to restore the total buffer base of extracellular fluid (ECF) to its normal value. At a pH of 7.35 to 7.45, if bicarbonate is 24 mEq, the base deficit will be 0. At a pH of 7.10 to 7.19 and a bicarbonate level of 24 mEq, the base deficit will be 6. At a pH of 7.45 to 7.49 and a bicarbonate level of 24 mEq, the base deficit will be -1. P_{CO_2}, pH, and bicarbonate affect base excess or deficit in the following ways:

If P_{CO_2} is increased by 10 mm Hg, the pH will decrease by about 0.10.

If P_{CO_2} is increased by 10 mm Hg, the pH will rise by 0.13.

If HCO_3 rises by 5 mEq/l, then the pH will rise by about 0.08.

If HCO_3 falls by 5 mEq/l, then the pH will fall by about 0.10.

The normal level of CO_2 of the blood is 24 to 31 mEq/l. CO_2 in the blood contains bicarbonate, carbonic acid, and carbamino compounds. Arterial CO_2 is usually 1.5 to 2 mEq/l higher than the arterial bicarbonate level on electrolyte analysis. Venous P_{CO_2} is usually 6 torr higher than an arterial sample. Venous bicarbonate is 1.1 mEq/l higher than arterial bicarbonate.

Potassium also has an inverse relationship with the pH. An increase or decrease in the pH of 0.10 causes an inverse increase or decrease in the potassium level of 0.5 mEq/l in the serum potassium.

Chloride and bicarbonate concentrations also have an inverse relationship. If there is a high bicarbonate level, then the chloride levels will be low (e.g., in metabolic alkalosis). Those patients with low plasma bicarbonate and normal to elevated chloride levels will be in metabolic acidosis. The exception to this rule is when there is a high anion gap metabolic acidosis. When there is a unmeasured amount of anions such as lactate, this can cause low levels of bicarbonate and chloride.

The anion gap is based on the sodium, chloride, and bicarbonate concentrations in the serum. Potassium is usually ignored because of its small, changing values. The anion gap is based on the electroneutrality of the electrolytes. Thus:

$$Na + UC = Cl + HCO_3 + UA$$

Where UC = unmeasured cations; UA = unmeasured anions; Na = sodium; Cl = chloride; HCO_3 = bicarbonate.)

$$Anion\ gap = Na^- (Cl + HCO_3)$$

An increase in the anion gap is usually secondary to an increase in organic acids, ethylene glycol, methanol, hyperglycemic hyperosmolar states, or lactic acidosis. Salicylate, paraldehyde, toluene, formaldehyde, and sulfur can all cause a high anion gap acidosis. A decrease in the anion gap (<7) is rare. It is usually secondary to hypoalbuminemia, syndrome of inappropriate diuretic hormone (SIADH), or hypoosmolar states. Whenever the anion gap changes more or less than the bicarbonate, a coexisting or mixed acid base disorder may be present.

METABOLIC ACIDOSIS

Metabolic acidosis is divided into normal anion gap metabolic acidosis and the increased anion gap metabolic acidosis. In normal anion gap metabolic acidosis, there is a loss of bicarbonate or an addition of chloride. In increased anion gap metabolic acidosis, there is an increased production of organic acids. Methanol, ethanol, ethylene glycol, and salicylates are major causes. Ketoacidosis may be caused by starvation, alcohol, or diabetes. The most common cause of increased anion gap acidosis in the injured or ill patient is lactic acidosis. Thiamine deficiency is an important cause of lactic acidosis in the alcoholic patient. Patients with lactic acidosis are further divided into patients who have poor tissue oxygenation (type A) and those with normal tissue oxygenation (type B).

Pyruvic acid is a three-carbon acid that is transformed into fat or amino acids. It can be transported into the mitochondria where it is used in the Krebs[3] cycle. After oxidization, it becomes acetyl-coenzyme A (CoA). Pyruvic acid is the immediate precursor of lactic acid. The kidney and the liver contain enzymes that can catalyze the conversion of pyruvate back into glucose—the process of gluconeogenesis. If pyruvic acid becomes lactic acid, the only way it can be metabolized is via the reaction of lactate dehydrogenase (LDH), which regenerates pyruvate and converts nicotine adenine dinucleotide (NAD) to its reduced form (NADH).

Normal anion gap metabolic acidosis is caused by the loss of bicarbonate from severe diarrhea, adrenal insufficiency, pancreatic fistulas, ammonium chloride, carbonic anhydrase inhibitors, arginine hydrochloride, or amino acid hydrochoride.

The diagnosis of metabolic acidosis is based on the low pH and low bicarbonate levels. The anion gap can determine which type of metabolic acidosis is present.

The mnemonics MUKSLEEP and MUDPILES can be used to remember the causes of anion gap acidosis:

M—methanol	M—methanol
U—uremia	U—uremia
K—ketoacidosis	D—DKA
S—salicylates	P—paraldehyde
L—lactate	I—iron or isoniazid
E—ethanol	L—lactate
E—ethylene glycol	E—ethylene
P—paraldehyde	S—salicylate

And you can use CAT for:

C—CO_2, CN
A—anticholic/ketacidosis, alcoholic lactic acidosis, alcohol, and aspirin
T—toluene (See the toxicology section for specific treatment.)

The mainstay of treatment of metabolic acidosis is improved tissue perfusion and ventilation, correction of the underlying cause, and administration of sodium bicarbonate as needed. If the serum pH is less than 7.10, then bicarbonate therapy should be considered. The dose of sodium bicarbonate is 1 mEq/kg. Each 0.1 rise in pH will decrease the oxygen availability of tissues by about 10% secondary to the shift of the oxyhemoglobin dissociation curve to the left. It is dangerous to give bicarbonate to patients in diabetic ketoacidosis (DKA), which can cause severe central nervous system (CNS) changes. In the hypoxic patient or the patient with a right-to-left heart shunt, rapid administration of bicarbonate can lower the PO_2 to dangerous levels.

METABOLIC ALKALOSIS

Metabolic alkalosis is usually caused by an excessive loss of hydrogen and chloride through excessive loss of gastric secretions or excessive diuresis with the loss of chloride, hydrogen, and potassium. Vomiting and diarrhea are the most common causes of gastric loss. Duodenal ulcers can also cause an increased loss of gastric acid. Pyloric stenosis and excessive suctioning by way of a nasogastric tube can also produce excessive loss of gastric acid. Diuresis with excessive loss of potassium can lead to hypokalemia. Diarrhea or excessive colostomy or ileostomy drainage can cause hypokalemia and acid loss.

Other causes of metabolic acidosis include mineralocorticoid use, which results in renal absorption of sodium and bicarbonate at the expense or loss of hydrogen, chloride, and potassium. Blood transfusions can also produce alkalosis with the infusion of citrate, thus increasing the levels of bicarbonate and producing alkalosis. Lactated Ringer's solution, if given in very large amounts, can cause a patient to become alkalotic. Patients who ingest large amounts of antacids can also become alkalotic.

Alkalosis can cause the release of endogenous catecholamines and can accentuate adrenergic vasodilator effects. It reduces the amount of plasma potassium by 0.5 mEq/l for every 0.10 rise in the pH. Magnesium and calcium also fall in metabolic alkalosis. Oxygen availability falls by 10% for every 0.1 rise in the pH.

The diagnosis of metabolic alkalosis is made by a pH above 7.45 and a bicarbonate level above 26 mEq/l. Hypochloremia and hypokalemia are usually present. Patients present with shallow respirations. Treatment is divided into the two types of metabolic alkalosis: (1) chloride-responsive alkalosis, often caused by vomiting, which is generally very responsive to fluid and chloride, and (2) chloride-resistant alkalosis, which is nonhypovolemic. Metabolic alkalosis is caused by increased excretion of H^+ and K^+ while Na^+ is reabsorbed, secondary to increased amounts of large quantities of Na^+ and Cl^- being filtered through the kidneys. Treatment for chloride-resistant alkalosis is: if the pH is greater than 7.55 or the patient has tetany, give one half of the chloride deficit as sodium chloride, one fourth as potassium chloride, and one fourth as some type of hypochloride (NH_4Cl, arginine hydrochloride, or 0.1 N hydrochloric acid). Large amounts of potassium may be required in these patients to correct the alkalosis.

RESPIRATORY ACIDOSIS

Respiratory acidosis is secondary to an inadequate minute ventilation or increased dead space in the respiratory system. Respiratory acidosis can also be caused by increased carbohydrate metabolism if pulmonary function is marginal. Causes of inadequate minute ventilation include head trauma, excess sedation, or chest trauma. Severe chronic obstructive pulmonary disease (COPD) causes increased dead space in the lungs and thus a decreased minute volume. In severely obese patients, chronic hypoventilation secondary to obesity can cause the *pickwickian syndrome,* named after the character in Charles Dickens' *Pickwick Papers.*

A P_{CO_2} above 45 mm Hg is usually caused by one of the aforementioned causes. A rise in the P_{CO_2} stimulates the respiratory center in the brain and thus increases the minute ventilation and respiratory rate. In patients with COPD, who often have terminal disease, the P_{CO_2} will rise to 60 to 70 mm Hg. At these levels, respiratory acidosis can occur and can depress the respiratory center of the brain. In these patients, stimulation for breaths is driven by chronic hypoxia as regulated by the chemoreceptors in the aortic and carotid bodies. Oxygen decreases the person's stimulus to breathe and thus can cause respiratory arrest.

A diagnosis is made on the basis of a P_{CO_2} greater than 45 mm Hg and a pH less than 7.39. If the arterial pH is less than 7.30, then metabolic acidosis is often present. On an electrolyte panel, look at the CO_2. If the CO_2 level is high, then respiratory acidosis is usually chronic. If the potassium and chloride levels are high or normal, then the person has acute respiratory acidosis. Metabolic acidosis is usually associated with hypochloremia and hypokalemia.

The goal of treatment of respiratory acidosis is to improve alveolar ventilation and increase minute ventilation. If minute ventilation is doubled, P_{CO_2} will be reduced by 50%. Do not correct chronic respiratory acidosis too quickly, because this can cause a sudden development of metabolic and respiratory alkalosis, which can lead to sudden cardiac arrhythmias or seizures, secondary to hypocalcemia. Patients with chronic respiratory acidosis should not have their arterial P_{CO_2} lowered by more than 5 mEq/hr.

RESPIRATORY ALKALOSIS

Respiratory alkalosis is caused by trauma, sepsis, shock, hyperventilation, hypoxia, or metabolic acidosis. Any stressful situation can cause hyperventilation and thus respiratory alkalosis. Respiratory alkalosis exists when the P_{CO_2} is less than 25 to 35 mm Hg. As respiratory alkalosis increases, it perpetuates more hyperventilation and thus an increase in respiratory alkalosis.

For each 1-mm Hg decrease in P_{CO_2} there is a decrease in cerebral blood flow of about 2 to 4%, thus causing cerebral vasoconstriction, which can cause cerebral metabolic acidosis. Cerebral metabolic acidosis will stimulate the breathing center of the brain. Ventilation will therefore increase, causing a progressive respiratory alkalosis. The oxyhemoglobin dissociation curve is shifted to the left. For every increase of 0.10 in pH, the P_{O_2} decreases by about 10%.

A diagnosis is made by a pH greater than 7.40 and a Pa_{CO_2} less than 35 mm Hg. Treatment is directed at solving the underlying cause. Hysterical hyperventilation, hypoxia, pulmonary embolism, and sepsis are major causes of respiratory alkalosis. Instruct the hysterical patient to rebreathe expired air that has an increased P_{CO_2}. Remember that the primary cause of agitation in the emergency department (ED) is hypoxia. Critically ill patients can present with hyperventilation; however, do not assume that all hyperventilation is secondary to hysterical hyperventilation. A hyperventilating patient should be sedated very carefully because any decrease in respiration in a patient with a pulmonary embolism can cause acute respiratory arrest.

ADRENAL CRISIS AND ADRENAL INSUFFICIENCY

Definition

Adrenal insufficiency is an acute or chronic decreased or absent level of circulating hormones—aldosterone and cortisol—which are produced by the adrenal cortex. It can be caused by structural or functional lesions of the adrenal or anterior pituitary glands. Adrenal crisis is a continuum of adrenal insufficiency, in which there is adrenal insufficiency that is life-threatening.

Primary, chronic adrenal insufficiency, or Addison's disease, is caused by a primary failure of the adrenal glands. Failure can also be secondary to failure of the hypothalamus, pituitary gland, or hypopituitarism, or it can have an iatrogenic cause secondary to chronic use of steroids or acute withdrawal of steroids.

Pathology

The adrenal gland consists of two parts: the adrenal cortex and the medulla. The adrenal cortex produces glucocorticoids, androgenic steroids, and mineralocorticoids. The medulla secretes the catecholamines epinephrine and norepinephrine and is under neural control.

Cortisol is the major glucocorticoid that is secreted by the cortex. It is released in direct response to stimulation of the cortex by adrenocorticotropic hormone (ACTH). ACTH is secreted by the anterior pituitary gland. ACTH is secreted after the anterior pituitary gland is stimulated by corticotropin-releasing factor (CRF) by the hypothalamus. This entire process has a diurnal rhythm with higher secretion in the morning and less in the evening. The plasma cortisol level acts to suppress the release of ACTH as a negative feedback inhibition. When any stress occurs (either physical or emotional), CRF is released, thus causing the release of ACTH and an increase in the release of cortisol. The CRF that is released is resistant to suppression through the negative feedback inhibition.

Cortisol maintains blood glucose levels by limiting glucose uptake at extrahepatic sites and by providing the precursors for gluconeogenesis of fat and protein breakdown. Cortisol also has a minor sodium-retaining effect on the kidneys and plays a large part in maintaining intracellular and extracellular water distribution.

Cortisol also enhances the pressor effects of catecholamines on the heart muscles and arterioles. In extremely large amounts, cortisol can inhibit allergic and inflammatory reactions. Cortisol is inhibited by negative feedback by the suppression of the secretion of ACTH from the anterior pituitary gland. It also suppresses the release of melanocyte-stimulating hormone (MSH).

Aldosterone is the primary mineralocorticoid. Aldosterone is regulated via a negative feedback system by the renin-angiotensin system and the plasma potassium concentration. ACTH also has some aldosterone-stimulating effects. Aldosterone primarily affects the distal tubules of the kidneys. Aldosterone increases sodium reabsorption and potassium excretion at the distal tubules of the kidneys. There is also some androgen hormone production by the adrenal glands, and this excretion is regulated by ACTH; however, this source of androgenic production is minimal compared with the production by the gonads.

Addison's disease is caused by primary adrenal insufficiency secondary to the destruction or disease of the adrenal cortex. Ninety percent of the adrenal cortex must be diseased or destroyed before symptoms appear. Idiopathic atrophy is the leading cause of primary adrenal insufficiency—75% is autoimmune and 25% is idiopathic.

Hashimoto's disease, diabetes mellitus, primary ovarian failure, pernicious anemia, chronic active hepatitis, chronic mucocutaneous candidiasis, vitiligo, and alopecia have all been associated with Addison's disease. Fungal infections that are disseminated and adrenal tuberculosis are frequent causes of Addison's disease. Addison's disease has been reported in patients with acquired immunodeficiency syndrome (AIDS). Sarcoidosis, amyloidosis, neoplastic disease, congenital adrenal hyperplasia, and hemorrhage or infarction of the adrenal glands have been reported.

Bilateral adrenal hemorrhage (adrenal apoplexy) is usually secondary to a stress-related event. Anticoagulant therapy is a major cause of adrenal apoplexy. The hemorrhage usually occurs between the third and the 18th day of new anticoagulant therapy. These patients present with a sudden onset of flank pain, costovertebral ankle pain, hypotension, or epigastric pain. Surgery, burns, pregnancy, trauma, convulsions, and adrenal vein thrombosis can all precipitate adrenal hemorrhage.

In the infant or newborn child, hemorrhage can be precipitated by septicemia usually secondary to *Pneumococcus, Meningococcus, Staphylococcus, Haemophilus,* and gram-negative organisms. Adrenal hemorrhage is often present in Waterhouse-Friderichsen syndrome, which is described as an overwhelming septicemia secondary to meningococcemia. Petechial rash, fever, chills, headache, and purpura are often present. There is usually bilateral hemorrhage with this syndrome, and death occurs if it is not treated promptly.

Metastatic breast or prostate cancer or Cushing's syndrome can also cause primary adrenal failure. Cushing's syndrome is treated with the chemotherapeutic agent mitotane, which can by itself precipitate adrenal failure. Drugs such as rifampin, methadone, and ketoconazole can cause adrenal insufficiency.

Clinical Presentation/Examination

The clinical presentation of primary or chronic adrenal insufficiency is one of gradual onset. Symptoms are associated with the decreased amounts of aldosterone and cortisol in the plasma and the lack of feedback suppression of MSH and ACTH. By knowing what each of these hormones do, you can predict the symptoms.

Low cortisol presents with hypoglycemia, anorexia, nausea, vomiting, lethargy, and poor response to even minor stressors. The patient is usually fluid overloaded secondary to the inability to regulate fluids and often presents with water intoxication.

Low aldosterone impairs the ability to conserve sodium and excrete potassium. Patients with low aldosterone present with the symptoms of dehydration, hypotension, low sodium, postural syncope, and decreased cardiac output and size.

Deficient cortisol levels cause the lack of suppression of MSH and ACTH. These patients present with increased pigmentation. The brown pigmentation is usually distributed over the exposed parts of the body: the face, neck, arms, hands, nipples, elbows, and knees. The mucous membranes can also be darken. Nevi and hair can become darker. Mucocutaneous candidiasis, vitiligo, and alopecia can occur. Women with Addison's disease have decreased growth of axillary and pubic hair secondary to adrenal androgen deficiency. Men with Addison's disease will not lose hair secondary to adequate testicular androgens. Longitudinal pigmented bands can be seen in the nails.

On cardiac examination, the heart sounds are very soft and almost inaudible. Gastrointestinal (GI) symptoms of nausea, vomiting, weight loss, and diarrhea with abdominal pain are common complaints.

A patient may present as being confused but will often state that his or her sense of taste, hearing, and olfaction are increased. Paralysis due to hyperkalemia can also be present. If these symptoms are present, the patient rapidly proceeds to a ascending muscular weakness, which leads to flaccid quadriplegia.

Secondary adrenal insufficiency is caused by the destruction or diseased pituitary gland or hypothalamus, causing the inability of the pituitary gland to secrete ACTH. Prolonged steroid use is the most common cause of secondary adrenal insufficiency. Rapid withdrawal of steroids in the chronic user can cause collapse and death, secondary to adrenal atrophy. Atrophy is caused by the exogenous administration of glucocorticoids, which cause a hypothalamic-pituitary-adrenal (HPA) suppression and thus adrenal atrophy. Adrenal atrophy can occur in patients who have had as little as 20 to 30 mg/day of prednisone for 1 week.

Sarcoidosis, histiocytosis X, hemochromatosis, Sheehan's syndrome, pituitary hemorrhage, pituitary tumor, internal carotid artery aneurysm, head trauma, meningitis, cavernous sinus thrombosis, pituitary gland irradiation, iatrogenic HPA, and acute discontinuation of steroids can all cause secondary adrenal failure.

Patients with secondary adrenal failure present with symptoms of ACTH impairment. Their presentation is due to the lack of adrenal androgens and cortisol. Hyperpigmentation does not occur in secondary adrenal insufficiency. Both men and women present with androgen deficiency signs secondary to insufficient gonadotropic hormone release from the pituitary gland.

Diagnosis

A diagnosis of primary adrenal insufficiency is made by demonstrating a low baseline plasma cortisol level and failure to increase the cortisol level with exogenous administration of ACTH. The patient's failure to respond to ACTH proves that the adrenal cortex is damaged or diseased and has no capacity to respond to exogenous ACTH.

Secondary adrenal insufficiency is diagnosed by demonstrating low plasma cortisol and urinary metabolite levels that increase in a stepwise fashion with repetitive ACTH stimulation over several days.

A rapid test can be utilized to determine if the adrenal glands are functional. A serum cortisol level is determined. The patient is then given 25 units of corticotropin (synthetic ACTH) intramuscularly (IM), intravenously (IV), or subcutaneously (SC). A second serum cortisol level is then drawn in 30 to 60 minutes. This test is based on the fact that a single injection of ACTH will cause a response by the adrenal glands within 1 hour, and in the normal adrenal glands the baseline cortisol level will double within 1 hour. Patients with primary insufficiency will show no increase in plasma cortisol level, and patients with secondary insufficiency will show no or a slight increase in plasma cortisol. A normal response to this test is a peak cortisol level equal to or greater than 20 µg/dl. A more prolonged test is required for a definitive diagnosis.

Laboratory Findings

A complete blood count (CBC), electrolytes, blood urea nitrogen (BUN), creatinine, glucose, cortisol level, aldosterone level, 24-hour urine, and urinalysis should be performed on all patients with suspected adrenal insufficiency.

In primary adrenal insufficiency hypoglycemia, mild hyperkalemia, hyponatremia, (<120 mEq/l) and azotemia are often found. The BUN is usually mildly elevated.

In secondary insufficiency the aldosterone level is largely unaffected secondary to the renin-angiotensin system and the stability of the plasma potassium. There is no hyponatremia, hypokalemia, and azomia in secondary insufficiency. However, hypoglycemia is often present in patients with hypopituitarism.

Treatment

Any patient with suspected adrenal insufficiency should have an electrocardiogram (ECG) performed. In primary adrenal insufficiency, the T wave is flat or inverted. The QT interval is prolonged. The PR and/or QRS interval is also prolonged, and the ST segment is depressed.

A chest x-ray should also be performed. It usually shows a small, narrow cardiac silhouette secondary to decreased vascular volume. A flat plate of the abdomen should also be performed. In adrenal tuberculosis, adrenal calcifications are often present. Hemorrhage or infections can also show adrenal calcifications. If azotemia is present, it is reversed with rehydration.

The mainstay of treatment for primary adrenal insufficiency is replacement of aldosterone and cortisol. Androgen therapy is often required in the female patient. Glucocorticoid replacement can be achieved by giving 5 mg of prednisone in the morning and 25 mg in the evening or 25 mg of cortisol acetate in the morning and 12.5 mg in the evening. This therapy mimics the normal diurnal variation of cortisol secretion.

Mineralocorticoid replacement is accomplished by giving the patient fludrocortisone acetate (Florinef), 0.05 to 0.2 mg/day by mouth (PO). A patient with Addison's disease also needs adequate salt intake.

In the female patient with primary adrenal insufficiency, androgen therapy is often required. When there is a decreased androgen hormone level, there is decreased pubic and axillary hair growth. If this condition is present, give fluoxymesterone (Halotestin) 2 to 5 mg/day PO.

Patients with secondary adrenal insufficiency usually do not require mineralocorticoid therapy. If hypotension is present, and the patient cannot maintain a diet generous in sodium, give fludrocortisone acetate 0.05 to 0.1 mg/day.

In the presence of hypopituitarism, androgen insufficiency can present in both males and females. If present in females, give fluoxymesterone, 2 to 5 mg/day. If larger doses are required in the female, long-acting testosterone (Depo-Testosterone) can be given.

Patients who present in true adrenal crisis are treated on clinical presentation as if they have a life-threatening emergency. Adrenal crisis is secondary to an acute cortisol insufficiency. There is usually an aldosterone insufficiency present also. Adrenal crisis occurs when the physiologic demand for cortisol and aldosterone exceeds the capacity of the adrenal glands to produce them. There is usually a precipitating event, which is often a sudden withdrawal of steroids.

These patients present with anorexia, nausea, vomiting, and abdominal pain. They are usually very weak and confused and appear acutely ill. Postural hypotension is present, and circulatory collapse is imminent. The heart sounds will be distant and soft, and the pulse will be feeble.

These patients need rapid infusions of 5% dextrose and isotonic saline. This type of IV fluid corrects the dehydration, hypotension, hypoglycemia, and hyponatremia. The dehydration is usually about 20% of the total body water (TBW).

These patients need steroids in the form of hydrocortisone sodium succinate (Solu-Cortef), which should be given as an IV bolus. Hydrocortisone, 100 mg, should be added to the first bag of IV solution and given over the first hour. After this bolus, 100 mg of hydrocortisone should be given every 6 hours for the first 24 hours. This helps to correct hyponatremia, hyperkalemia, hypotension, and hypoglycemia.

As the patient's dose of glucocorticoids is reduced to 100 mg in a 24-hour period, mineralocorticoid therapy can be started with desoxycorticosterone acetate (Percorten), 2.5 to 5 mg IM once or twice daily. If hypotension is not relieved, then additional corticosteroids should be given. Vasopressors can be used if hypotension is life threatening.

The patient can be treated and tested at the same time. The patient is given normal saline and, instead of hydrocortisone, the patient is given 4 mg of dexamethasone and 25 units of corticotropin as an infusion over the first hour. Cortisol levels are obtained before and after the infusion. Corticotropin is then infused at a rate of 3 units/hr for the next 8 hours. Cortisol levels are then drawn at the sixth and eighth hours. A 24-hour urine collection is made to determine the level of 17-hydroxycorticosteroid.

If the patient has primary adrenal insufficiency, all cortisol levels will be less than 15 μg/dl and the urinary 17-hydroxycorticosteroid (OHCS) will also be low. This means that the adrenal glands are unable to respond to ACTH stimulation. If there is an adequate response (i.e., a normal cortisol level), then the diagnosis of adrenal insufficiency is excluded. If a partial response is present, then the diagnosis is secondary adrenal insufficiency; however, further testing is needed for a definitive diagnosis.

The primary cause of death in acute adrenal crisis is circulatory collapse and hyperkalemia-induced arrhythmias. Patients with flaccid quadriplegia, secondary to hyperkalemia, are treated with glucose, insulin, and bicarbonate.

All patients with renal insufficiency should be admitted to the hospital for a diagnostic work-up.

ALCOHOLIC KETOACIDOSIS

Definition

Alcoholic ketoacidosis occurs in both the alcoholic and nonalcoholic patient. It is secondary to alcohol abuse and can be seen in first-time alcohol users in which food intake is minimal.

Epidemiology

The incidence of alcoholic ketoacidosis is unknown but is related to the incidence of alcoholism in a particular population.

Pathology

Alcoholic ketoacidosis is related to the increased mobilization of free fatty acids from adipose tissue and the liver's increased ability to convert free fatty acids into the substrates acetoacetate and beta-hydroxybutyrate. In the liver's metabolism of alcohol, the rate of nicotinamide adenine dinucleotide (NAD) reduction exceeds the rate of mitochondrial NADH oxidation. The decreased rate of production of NAD causes a decrease in the amount of NAD that is available. This situation persists for days even after the patient discontinues use of alcohol consumption. NAD metabolism is a step-dependent part of the oxidation of fatty acids in the mitochondria of the hepatocytes of the liver. When there is limited NAD, the hepatocytes form ketone bodies.

In alcoholic ketoacidosis, the insulin levels are low and the cortisol, glucagon, growth hormone, and epinephrine levels are increased. Unlike in diabetic ketoacidosis, the serum glucose is low. These increased hormonal levels, combined with hypoglycemia, promote lipolysis, which increases the levels of free fatty acids available for conversion to ketones. These patients often present with vomiting, starvation, or chronic malnutrition, which also contributes to ketoacidosis.

Clinical Presentation

The typical patient with alcoholic ketoacidosis is a heavy drinker who is binge-drinking and has a decreased food intake over several days. The patient often stops both alcohol and food intake with the onset of nausea, vomiting, and abdominal pain.

The patient appears very ill and shows signs of dehydration, tachycardia, tachypnea, and generalized abdominal pain. The patient can present in an alert or a comatose state with hypothermia, normal temperature, or hyperthermia. The patient often co-presents with pancreatitis, hepatitis, or gastritis. The initial presentation can be delirium tremens, sepsis, meningitis, pneumonia, or pyelonephritis.

Examination

The patient should be given a complete examination, including a neurologic and rectal examination. If the patient is comatose, special attention should be paid to an examination of the head to rule out head trauma. Often the alcoholic patient becomes hypoglycemic, faints, and strikes his or her head. Do not blame altered mental status on alcoholic ketoacidosis or alcohol intoxication alone.

Diagnosis

A diagnosis is made by a history of binge alcohol intake, decreased food intake, abdominal pain on examination, and the presence of metabolic acidosis. A low or mildly elevated glucose level and a positive result on a nitroprusside test also help to establish the diagnosis of alcoholic ketoacidosis.

Soffer and Hamburger's criteria for alcoholic ketoacidosis include: a serum glucose level below 300 mg/dl; a recent history of alcohol intake or a relative or absolute decline in alcohol consumption in the past 24 to 72 hours with a history of vomiting; the presence of metabolic acidosis; and no other causes attributed to metabolic acidosis, including diabetic ketoacidosis, lactic acidosis, renal failure, or toxic drug ingestion.

Laboratory Findings

A CBC, electrolytes, creatinine, BUN, glucose, liver function tests (LFTs), amylase, lipase, magnesium, calcium, phosphate, alcohol level, serum osmolality, complete urinalysis, and an arterial blood gas (ABG) should be performed on all patients with suspected alcoholic ketoacidosis.

There will be a large anion-gap metabolic acidosis present secondary to the high level of ketones in the blood. The pH will be higher in a patient with alcoholic ketoacidosis than in a patient with diabetic ketoacidosis. The serum potassium and chloride levels are usually lower in the patient with alcoholic ketoacidosis than in the patient with diabetic ketoacidosis. This lower chloride level is attributed to the increased vomiting seen in the alcoholic patient.

Metabolic acidosis is secondary to the increased ketones acetoacetate and beta-hydroxybutyrate, which are intermediates in the oxidation of fatty acids. Because of the lack of NAD in the alcoholic patient, beta-hydroxybutyrate accumulates more rapidly than does acetoacetate.

The nitroprusside test is a quick test for ketones. It can be utilized to test for ketones in both the blood and the urine. It is a better test for acetoacetate and does not react to beta-hydroxybutyrate at any level.

Glucosuria is often mild or absent in the urine. Hypoglycemia is usually secondary to starvation and malnutrition. A blood alcohol test should be performed; however, the patient may have stopped alcohol consumption hours or days before presentation.

Treatment

Any patient with suspected alcoholic ketoacidosis should have two large-gauge IV lines of normal saline 0.9% established and should be placed on 2 liters of oxygen via nasal cannula. The patient should also be placed on a cardiac monitor; and the aforementioned laboratory studies should be drawn. The mainstay of treatment for alcoholic ketoacidosis is the administration of a saline solution and glucose. Every patient should also receive thiamine, 50 to 100 mg IV, before the administration of glucose to prevent Wernicke's disease. It usually takes 12 to 18 hours to reverse ketoacidosis. It is recommended that the IV solutions be alternated between saline solutions and glucose-containing solutions. The patient should also receive multivitamins PO or IV.

Insulin and sodium bicarbonate are not part of the treatment of alcoholic ketoacidosis unless the pH falls below 6.9. Any patient with alcoholic ketoacidosis should be admitted to the intensive care unit (ICU). The patient should have good nutritional support and should be encouraged to stop drinking alcohol.

DIABETIC KETOACIDOSIS

Definition

Diabetic ketoacidosis (DKA) occurs in the diabetic population, and the patient presents with hyperglycemia and ketonemia. DKA is usually secondary to the presence of an excess of stress hormones in the absence of insulin.

Epidemiology

There is often no precipitating cause of diabetes or DKA. However, trauma, myocardial infarction, infections, stroke, pregnancy, pancreatitis, stressful events, omission of daily insulin injections, and hyperthyroidism can all precipitate DKA. The greater the presenting serum osmolarity, blood glucose level, and BUN, the greater the mortality. There is also an increased mortality rate for patients who present with a serum bicarbonate level of less than 10 mEq/l. The two main precipitating factors for DKA in the diabetic are myocardial infarction and infection.

Pathology

Insulin is responsible for the metabolism and storage of fats, carbohydrates, and proteins. Stress hormones that are associated with DKA are glucagon, cortisol, catecholamines, and growth hormone. Diabetic ketoacidosis is secondary to a relative insufficiency of insulin and an excess of stress hormones, which causes hyperglycemia and ketonemia.

Insulin is released by the beta cells of the pancreas, stimulated by the ingestion of glucose. Insulin causes the liver to take up ingested glucose and convert glucose to glycogen. Insulin inhibits glycogen breakdown (glycogenolysis), and it also suppresses gluconeogenesis.

Insulin causes lipid metabolism by increasing lipogenesis in the liver and adipose cells. This process also prevents lipolysis. Insulin promotes the storage of fat and the production of triglycerides from free fatty acids. Insulin also inhibits the breakdown of triglycerides into free fatty acids and glycerol. This whole process causes the breakdown and storage of glucose into glycogen.

In muscle tissue, insulin stimulates the uptake of amino acids into muscle cells and mediates the incorporation of amino acids into muscle protein. Insulin also prevents the release of amino acids from muscle protein and from hepatic protein sources. Diabetes mellitus is caused by the lack of an insulin-secretory mechanism for the beta cells of the pancreas. A total lack of insulin production is usually found only in adult onset diabetes, and there is usually a primary failure of the initial rapid-release phase of insulin secretion, causing a decrease in stored fuels. This has been proved by the inadequate response to a glucose load, which causes an abnormal finding on the glucose tolerance test. As the insulin beta cell secretory mechanism failure worsens, the fuel storage process is also impaired. The process is mobilized during fasting, thus hyperglycemia occurs. As blood glucose levels increase secondary to glycogenolysis, the reserves of insulin are utilized and the blood glucose level may return to normal. In the presence of relative or absolute insulin depletion, catabolism, hyperglycemia, and ketonemia occur, thus causing DKA. As this process is taking place during insulin insufficiency, the transportation of glucose into the cells is inhibited.

The normal cellular response to the lack of glucose or cellular starvation is to increase the circulation of catecholamines, glucagon, cortisol, and growth hormone. These hormones are the counter-regulatory hormones in regard to insulin utilization. An increase in the circulation of these hormones causes an anti-insulin effect on cells. The excessive counter-regulatory hormones in the presence of relative insulin deficiency causes DKA. All of these counter-regulatory hormones are catabolic and cause the reverse effect produced by the insulin that is present until there is total insulin depletion. These hormones cause further carbohydrate metabolism by increasing the processes of gluconeogenesis and glycogenolysis. Catecholamines and glucagon are stimulated by lipolysis, which causes an increase in the circulation of free fatty acids for the conversion of ketones. There is increased protein (usually muscle) breakdown, which provides more amino acids for gluconeogenesis. The relative insulin insufficiency and excess of counter-regulatory hormones cause hyperglycemia and ketonemia, with hyperglycemia occurring before ketonemia. Hyperglycemia is secondary to enhanced gluconeogenesis and glycogenolysis and the relative lack of insulin.

Ketonemia is secondary to the breakdown of large amounts triglycerides into fatty acids into the circulation. The liver takes up these fatty acids and converts them into ketone bodies. Without the presence of insulin, the utilization of the peripheral ketones is decreased and ketones accumulate in the ratio of 3:1 (beta-hydroxybutyrate to acetoacetate).

Clinical Presentation

Patients with DKA often present with symptoms secondary to the osmotic diuresis associated with hyperglycemia. Nausea, vomiting, weight loss, and abdominal pain are the most common presenting complaints. Patients can present with paralytic ileus, pain from gastric dilatation, and abdominal tenderness. Hyperglycemia causes an increased osmotic load secondary to the inability of the cell to freely exchange water in the presence of hyperglycemia. Intracellular water is lost, thus osmotic diuresis causes total body fluid depletion. A patient with DKA will therefore present with tachycardia, hypotension, and dehydration. Patients who have DKA secondary to the osmotic diuresis lose potassium, calcium, magnesium, sodium, chloride, and phosphorus. This loss of electrolytes can also be increased if the patient is vomiting. Remember that for every 180 mg/dl increase in serum glucose, the serum sodium level is decreased by 5 mEq/l.

Circulating ketone bodies, when the hydrogen ions dissociate, cause a fall in serum bicarbonate, and thus acidosis develops. The ketone bodies oxidize to acetone, and this causes the fruity odor on the patient's breath that is associated with DKA. These patients also present with hyperventilation secondary to the acidosis.

Patients can be either awake with altered mental status or in a coma. There is no correlation between the conscious state of the patient and the degree or severity of ketonemia, electrolyte imbalance, acidosis, or hyperglycemia. A patient can also present with pancreatitis or hemorrhagic pancreatitis secondary to ketoacidosis.

Examination

The vital signs of a patient in DKA should be watched closely. The acidosis can cause a severe peripheral vasodilatation and vascular collapse. On examination of the liver, the patient may present with hepatomegaly secondary to an accumulation of fat within the liver, but this usually resolves when ketogenesis is reversed. The entire patient needs to be examined, with particular attention to signs of infection. A rectal examination, a complete neurologic examination, and a fundoscopic examination also need to be performed. A history of any recent illness must be obtained. Common sites of infections in the diabetic are the lungs and the urinary tract system.

Diagnosis

A diagnosis is made by the finding of a serum glucose level greater than 300 mg/dl, a bicarbonate level of less than 15 mEq/l, a pH less than 7.3, and a serum acetone level greater than 2:1 dilution. The differential diagnosis of DKA is alcoholic ketoacidosis, lactic acidosis, nonketotic hyperosmolar coma, or hypoglycemia.

Laboratory Findings

A CBC, potassium, sodium, chloride, BUN, creatinine, glucose, amylase, lipase, calcium, magnesium, acetone, phosphorus, LFTs, serum osmolarity levels, serum ketones, a complete urinalysis with culture, a blood culture if the patient looks septic, or extremes of age are present along with an ABG should be performed on all patients.

There is an exchange of H^+ and K^+ across the intracellular membranes that causes the increased serum potassium levels seen in DKA.

Serum osmolarity has a direct correlation between the conscious level of the patient and the osmolarity level. Mental confusion or coma is often present at levels above 340 mOsm/kg. A serum lactate level should be drawn to determine if lactic acid is contributing to the metabolic acidosis.

On examination of the urine, there will be glycosuria and ketonuria. On arterial blood gas, the pH will be decreased with a low serum bicarbonate, and decreased P_{CO_2} will be present secondary to the metabolic acidosis with respiratory compensation. Serum sodium is usually low secondary to total body fluid loss.

Potassium is initially normal or high; however, as the hyperglycemia is corrected, the serum potassium shifts intracellularly and becomes extremely low. Serum chloride is low secondary to vomiting. There is an increased anion gap secondary to ketonemia.

A rapid bedside glucose stick with reagent strips can rapidly identify hyperglycemia. A drop of blood can be placed on a nitroprusside-impregnated tablet to evaluate for ketones. Nitroprusside reacts with acetoacetate but not with beta-hydroxybutyrate, thus this test can sometimes be a misleading.

Treatment

Any patient who presents with the symptoms of DKA should have two large-gauge IV lines placed with normal saline 0.9% and should be given 2 liters of oxygen via nasal cannula. The patient should be placed on a cardiac monitor and have the aforementioned laboratory examinations performed. A rapid bedside glucose level should be obtained. An ECG should be performed to identify an acute myocardial infarction and to monitor the presence of hyperkalemia. A chest x-ray should be performed to rule out infection in the diabetic patient as a precipitating cause of DKA.

If it is determined that the patient is hyperglycemic and is in DKA, and there is no history of congestive heart failure, the main treatment for DKA is fluids. The average water deficit is 5 to 10 liters with a sodium deficit of 450 to 500 mEq. The first liter should be administered rapidly over 30 minutes to 1 hour, and the patient's vital signs should be checked. If the patient is hypotensive, 3 to 5 liters might be required in the first hour. The normalization of body fluid restores perfusion and increases renal blood flow, which precipitates ketone excretion. As the serum sodium level reaches 155 mEq/l, the IV solutions should be replaced with a hypotonic solution or ½ normal saline 0.45%.

If the pH is less than 7.0, bicarbonate should be considered. Respiratory depression and CNS depression can occur at a pH of less than 6.8. Give 44 to 100 mEq of bicarbonate if the pH is less than 6.9.

The initial serum potassium level is normal or high, but the intracellular potassium is extremely low. There is usually a potassium deficit of 5 to 10 mEq/kg in the patient with DKA. If the initial serum potassium level is low, this indicates a massive intracellular potassium loss. Massive potassium replacement is required during the next 24 hours. As IV fluids are given, the serum potassium falls. As insulin is given, potassium will return to the cells. If DKA therapy with fluids and insulin is administrated too rapidly, precipitous hypokalemia can occur and can cause fatal respiratory paralysis, cardiac arrhythmias, or paralytic ileus. Potassium should be given in small doses of 20 mEq/l of fluid. If oliguria or renal failure is present, then potassium should be given much slower. There should be continuous cardiac monitoring when the potassium is given. Usually 100 to 200 mEq are required in the first 12 to 24 hours of treatment.

A low dose of insulin is the best technique for treating DKA. A continuous insulin infusion of 5 to 10 units/hr of insulin should be administered. A continuous insulin infusion of 1 unit/hr raises the plasma insulin concentration by 20 μg/ml. At insulin blood concentrations of 20 to 200 uU/ml, gluconeogenesis and lipogenesis are inhibited and peripheral tissue potassium uptake is stimulated. A priming IV bolus is not required. Low-dose insulin therapy provides a greater stabilization of the extracellular potassium concentration. When the serum glucose level reaches 250 mg/dl, glucose should be added to the IV solution (D5W ½NS).

The mainstay of treatment for DKA is a slow, steady lowering of the serum glucose level to allow a slow, steady correction of electrolytes and glucose levels. Insulin can also be administered SC or IM, when good nursing care is not available. Twenty units of glucose can be given in an IM bolus, then 5 to 10 units/hr IM.

As the glucose level normalizes on an IV insulin infusion and the ketones clear, the IV insulin should not be abruptly discontinued. There should be an overlap between the start of SC insulin and the discontinuation of the insulin infusion.

There is controversy about the replacement of phosphate in the patient with DKA. Hypophosphatemia has been associated with neuromuscular paralysis, leading to myocardial dysfunction and respiratory failure. Phosphate is part of the conversion of energy from adenosine triphosphate (ATP) and the delivery of oxygen at the tissue level through 2,3-diphosphoglyceric acid (2,3-DPG). Phosphate must also be present for many cofactors, enzymes, and biochemical intermediates to metabolize. DKA causes a shift of phosphate from an extracellular to intracellular position when insulin is administered. Insulin also accelerates glucose storage. Dangerous hypophosphatemia is defined as a serum phosphate level of less than 1 mg/dl.

Phosphate replacement can be given in either PO or IV form. Five milliliters of potassium phosphate (KH_2PO_4 plus K_2HPO_4) containing 4 mEq/ml and phosphorus 96 mg/ml, can be added to 1 liter of IV fluids and given to the patient. Administration of phosphate can cause hypocalcemia, hypomagnesemia, hyperphosphatemia, metastatic soft tissue calcification, hypernatremia, and dehydration secondary to osmotic diuresis.

Any patient who is diagnosed with DKA should be admitted to the ICU.

DISSEMINATED INTRAVASCULAR COAGULATION

Definition

Disseminated intravascular coagulation (DIC) can be caused by obstetric complications, trauma, malignancy, infections, and shock. DIC is a result of out-of-control coagulation and the fibrinolytic cascade within the systemic circulation.

Pathology

DIC is caused by the consumption of platelets and coagulation factors, particularly fibrinogen and factors V, VIII, and XIII. This increased consumption occurs because thrombin is formed in excessive amounts. Thrombin overwhelms the inhibitor system, which accelerates the coagulation process and directly activates fibrinogen. The increased fibrin is deposited in small vessels and in multiple organs. The fibrinolytic system lyses fibrin and impairs thrombin formation. This fibrin lysis causes fibrin-degraded products to be released. Platelet function is then affected and inhibits fibrin polymerization.

This cascade causes an increase in bleeding diathesis secondary to decreased platelet function and clotting factors. Small blood vessels are then obstructed by fibrin degradation products, which then cause tissue ischemia. The red blood cells are injured, and anemia occurs as a result of fibrin deposition.

Clinical Presentation

Patients with DIC present with purpura, signs of end-organ injuries, and an increased bleeding tendency.

Patients with obstetric history present with a history of amniotic fluid embolism, hydatidiform mole, abruptio placentae, toxemia of pregnancy, or retained products of conception. Any malignancy of the pancreas, prostate, breast, or lung, or acute promyelocytic leukemia can present with DIC. Heat stroke, aortic aneurysm, snakebite, hemorrhagic pancreatitis, giant hemangioma, or transfusion reactions can cause DIC. Gram-negative sepsis, gram-positive sepsis, Rocky Mountain spotted fever, scrub typhus, *Plasmodium falciparum* malaria, histoplasmosis, rubella, varicella, arboviruses, and influenza A can also cause DIC. Severe liver disease and primary fibrinolysis are also rare causes of DIC.

Examination

The patient should be given a complete examination, including a fundoscopic and rectal examination.

Diagnosis

A diagnosis is made by clinical presentation, history of infection, obstetric complication, trauma, malignancy, presence of shock, and snakebite. On blood examination, the following findings can be helpful in diagnosing DIC:

1. The fibrinogen level will be low.
2. The prothrombin time (PT) will be prolonged.
3. The partial thromboplastin time (PTT) will be prolonged.
4. The thrombin time will be prolonged.
5. The platelet count will be less than $100,00/mm^3$.
6. Fibrin degradation products (fibrin split products) will be zero to large, depending on fibrinolysis.
7. Serum creatinine or urinalysis may be abnormal.
8. A peripheral smear will show schistocytes and red blood cell fragments.

Laboratory Findings

CBC, PT, PTT, fibrinogen, fibrin split products, electrolytes, aspartate amino transferase (AST), alanine aminotransferase (ALT), gamma glutamyltransferase, total protein, bilirubin, BUN, creatinine, fibrin monomers, euglobulin lyses time and factor V and VIII assays should be obtained for any case of suspected DIC. A urinalysis and urine cultures should be performed if sepsis is suspected. Blood cultures should also be performed if sepsis is suspected.

Treatment

The mainstay of therapy in treating acute DIC is treatment of the underlying condition that caused DIC and reversal of the triggering mechanism. Many episodes of DIC are self-limiting. When treatment of DIC is necessary, the therapy is directed at one of the two major pathologic components of DIC. If the patient is hemorrhaging, the patient should receive platelets, coagulation factors found in cryoprecipitate (factors I, V, VIII), and blood. The goal of replacement therapy is to elevate the platelet counts and fibrinogen level. The PT and PTT lag behind therapeutic changes.

If DIC is predominantly caused by fibrin deposition and thrombosis, then heparin therapy should be considered in selected patients. Patients who present with gram-negative sepsis in pregnancy, retained products of conception of fetal death, giant hemangioma, or acute promyelocytic leukemia are at increased risk of fibrin deposition and thus respond better to heparin therapy. There is little benefit from the use heparin in patients with an underlying diagnosis of abruptio placentae, liver disease, meningococcemia, or trauma. Start with a 5000- to 10,000-unit bolus of heparin, then 1000 to 1500 units/hr.

All patients with suspected DIC should be admitted to the ICU for careful monitoring of fluid status.

FLUID AND ELECTROLYTE EMERGENCIES

SODIUM

The normal sodium concentration of the adult body is about 40 mEq/kg. Sodium is 98% in the ECF. The normal serum sodium is 140 mEq/l.

Hyponatremia

Hyponatremia is usually caused by too much TBW or dilutional hyponatremia. Patients with chronic malnutrition, sepsis, congestive heart failure, renal failure, or trauma are at greater risk of water retention and thus hyponatremia. Hyponatremia can also be caused by diarrhea, vomiting, and excessive sweating. Children will often present to the ED with hyponatremia secondary to their mothers' attempt to rehydrate them with tap water (free water), water that does not contain sodium, and thus severe hyponatremia occurs. Adrenal insufficiency, diuretics, salt-losing nephritis, renal disease of the medulla, acute vasomotor nephropathy, renal transplantation, or relief of a urinary obstruction can all cause hyponatremia.

Factitious hyponatremia can be caused by hyperlipidemia, hyperproteinemia, or hyperglycemia. Glucose causes water to be drawn out of the cells and into the intracellular fluid (ICF), thus creating a factitious hyponatremia. For each 100-mg/dl increase in glucose, sodium will fall about 1.6 to 1.8 mEq/l.

The four main causes of hyponatremia can be classified as:

1. Hyponatremia with decreased ECF
   a. Extrarenal losses, urinary Na <20 mEq/l
   b. Renal losses, urinary N >20 mEq/l
2. Hyponatremia with normal ECF, urinary Na >20 mEq/l
3. Hyponatremia with increased ECF
4. Pseudohyponatremia

Hyponatremia can be further divided. *Hypovolemic hyponatremia* involves the loss of both sodium and water, with more replacement of free water than with sodium. The most common cause of hypovolemic hyponatremia is diarrhea and vomiting. Excessive sweating, cystic fibrosis, and adrenal insufficiency are also causes. Mineralocorticoid deficiency, diuretics, and primary kidney disorders can all cause hypovolemic hyponatremia.

Euvolemic hyponatremia is found in patients who have hyponatremia with normal or slightly increased ECF, without edema, with a near-normal total body sodium content. These patients usually present with CNS systems. A common cause of euvolemic hyponatremia is SIADH. In children, there is hypotonicity and hyponatremia (plasma osmolality <280 mOsm/kg H_2O); inappropriately concentrated urine (urine osmolality >100 mOsm/kg H_2O); high urine sodium concentration; no hypervolemia or hypovolemia; and normal cardiac, renal, adrenal, hepatic, and thyroid functions. Hyponatremia is corrected by severe water restriction. Serum osmolality will also be greater than 300 mOsm/l, and the urine osmolality will be less than 600 to 1200 mOsm/l. If serum osmolality is less than 270 to 280 mOsm/l, then urine osmolality should be 50 mOsm/l or less. A "reset osmostat" is common in the chronically ill or malnourished patient. Hyponatremia in this case is usually asymptomatic and is managed by treating the underlying disease.

Hypervolemic hyponatremia presents in patients who have an increase in TBW. It is found in patients with congestive heart failure, nephrotic syndrome, cirrhosis of the liver, and acute or chronic renal insufficiency. The patient presents with peripheral edema or pulmonary edema. In the patient with cirrhosis of the liver, edema is caused by a decrease in the effective arterial blood volume secondary to a decreased peripheral resistance with arteriovenous shunting and splanchnic venous pooling. In heart failure, edema is caused secondary to low cardiac output. In patients with nephrotic syndrome, edema is caused by low capillary oncotic pressure, which causes a loss of fluid from the intravascular spaces to the interstitial spaces.

Hyponatremia at levels below 120 mEq/l will cause CNS changes. Mortality rates for serum sodium concentrations less than 120 mEq/l are at 50%. When hyponatremia is present, the brain moves interstitial fluid into the cerebrospinal fluid (CSF), and there is a loss of cellular potassium and organic osmolytes. As the brain loses sodium into the CSF along with potassium and chloride losses, over several hours, the brain loses its protective mechanisms. The brain slowly loses other intracellular osmolytes and amino acids. Thus, the brain can become dehydrated, which can lead to *osmotic demyelination syndrome* or *central pontine myelinolysis* when hyponatremia is corrected too rapidly.

A diagnosis is made by a serum sodium level of less than 120 to 125 mEq/l or a urine sodium less than 10 to 20 mEq/l. In the presence of adequate renal perfusion, this suggests that the ECF or body content of sodium is low.

Hyponatremia in the stable asymptomatic patient, secondary to hemodilution, is treated by fluid restriction; however, complications can arise if water is restricted too severely. The total sodium deficit can be calculated by using TBW multiplied by 60% of the patient's body weight, multiplied by the normal sodium (140), minus the current sodium level:

Sodium deficit =
(weight in kilograms $\times$ 60%) (140 − serum sodium) = mEq deficit

The equation is used for a normovolemic patient. Most patients who are hyponatremic are hypervolemic, thus the 60% weight has to be adjusted. Twenty percent body weight is used in the hypervolemic patient.

Sodium deficit =
$$\text{(weight in kilograms} \times 20\%) (140 - \text{serum sodium}) = \text{mEq deficit}$$

The underlying cause of the hyponatremia must also be treated. If hyponatremia is less than 120 mEq/l and CNS symptoms are present, then give 3% saline solution at 25 to 100 ml/hr. The serum and urine sodium levels should be watched very carefully for changes, and careful attention to the possibility of fluid overload. Furosemide should be given with the 3% saline solution to prevent fluid overload. In pseudohyponatremia, as in hyperglycemia, the serum sodium will correct itself as the hyperglycemia is corrected.

In the patient with chronic hyponatremia, the sodium level should not be corrected any faster than 0.5 mEq/l/hr or 12 mEq/l/day. Severe neurologic complications can occur if the sodium is corrected too fast.

Hypernatremia

Hypernatremia is usually caused by a TBW deficit secondary to excessive loss or reduced intake. Sweating, diarrhea, vomiting, and hyperpyrexia are the most common causes of hypernatremia. Mannitol, glycerol, or an increased intake of salt can also cause hypernatremia.

The causes of hypernatremia can be classified into types of water loss; (1) reduced intake of water, (2) increased water loss and gain of sodium, (3) increased intake, or (4) renal salt retention. Hyponatremia can also be classified by its relationship to blood volume, hypovolemia, euvolemia, and hypervolemia.

In patients with hypernatremia and hypovolemia, the cause is from either a nonrenal cause or a renal cause. The major nonrenal causes are GI loss, respiratory loss, or sweating. If renal-associated failure is present, the causes are from adrenal failure, diuretics, renal disease, osmoreceptor failure, and relief of urinary obstruction.

In patients with euvolemia and hypernatremia, hypernatremia is caused by impaired thirst secondary to coma, nonrenal losses from the respiratory system, skin, and GI system. Renal causes involve use of osmotic diuretics, renal disease, reset osmostat, GI loss, or relief of urinary obstruction.

In patients with hypovolemia and hypernatremia, the cause is usually secondary to excessive use of mineralocorticoids, Cushing's syndrome, congenital adrenal hyperplasia, hyperaldosteronism, or exogenous corticosteroids. Hypernatremia with hypervolemia can also be caused by giving hypertonic saline.

Diabetes insipidus (DI) can also present with hypernatremia. DI is caused by the failure of secretion of ADH, a central cause, or a nonresponse to ADH at the kidneys, or nephrogenic cause. Seventy percent of DI is secondary to neoplasms; 30% of DI is idiopathic (10% trauma and 20% secondary to pituitary surgery).

Aneurysms, tuberculosis, sarcoidosis, eosinophilic granuloma, and Sheehan's syndrome are other causes of DI. Medications such as amphotericin B, aminoglycosides, lithium, and cisplatin can also cause DI (secondary). DI can also be primary, secondary to a familial predisposition. If DI is secondary to trauma, it 'presents in three phases. In the first phase, an initial polyuria secondary to insufficient ADH secretion by the hypothalamic cells will be present, then a transient phase in which the previously formed hormone from the posterior pituitary is released, and thus polyuria resolves for a few days. In the third phase, after all of the released (stored) ADH has been used, polyuria returns. The damaged cells in the hypothalamus can regenerate, but it can take weeks to months before DI resolves.

Nephrogenic and central DI can be differentiated by giving 5 units SC aqueous vasopressin and noting the response. If there is a response to the vasopressin, urine osmolarity greater than 800 mOsm/l, then DI is secondary to a central etiology. Also note the response to water deprivation after vasopressin is given. In patients with central DI, there will be no response to water deprivation but a response to vasopressin. In nephrogenic DI, there will be no response to water deprivation, dehydration, or vasopressin.

Patients become acutely symptomatic at serum sodium levels greater than 158 mEq/l. Infants with hypernatremia will present with a high-pitched cry and will alternate between wailing and lethargy. Adults will become very irritable. At serum osmolality between 350 and 375 mOsm/l, irritability and restlessness occur and between 375 and 400 mOsm/l tremulousness and ataxia occur. With a serum osmolality greater than 400 mOsm/l, asynchronous jerks and tonic spasm are observed. At levels greater than 430 mOsm/l, death is the outcome.

Thrombosis, multiple small hemorrhages, or massive brain hemorrhage can occur secondary to hypernatremia. In children and infants with a serum sodium level between 160 and 165 mEq, 16% will develop chronic neurologic deficits. Mortality rates for hypernatremia are as high as 10%.

Treatment of hypernatremia is achieved by replacing fluid in the dehydrated patient with plasma-expanding fluids, such as normal saline or Ringer's lactate. After tissue perfusion is normalized, the IV solution should be changed to 0.45% saline, until urine output is 0.5 ml/hr. Serum sodium concentration should not be reduced greater than 10 to 15 mEq/day. The formula for the amount of water needed to correct hypernatremia is:

$$\text{Water deficit (in liters)} = \text{TBW} \left(1 - \frac{\text{Na2}}{\text{Na1}}\right)$$

Where Na1 is the current serum sodium and Na2 is the desired serum sodium. TBW is 60%.

$$\text{Water deficit} + (60\% \times \text{weight in kg}) \left(1 - \frac{145}{\text{current Na}}\right)$$

Each liter of H_2O deficit will result in a rise of the serum sodium of 3 to 5 mEq/l or 8 to 15 mOsm/l. Each liter of sodium should contain 80 to 100 mEq of sodium. If cardiac failure is present, rehydration should be performed even more slowly with a central venous pressure (CVP) or pulmonary artery wedge pressure (PAWP) being monitored to monitor fluid overload.

Children have a predilection to develop hyperglycemia when they are hypernatremic. Glucose should be given to children as a 2.5% solution until glucose levels normalize. After urine output is established, then add 20 to 40 mEq/l of potassium chloride to each liter of fluid. If severe sodium (180 to 200 mEq/l) is present, consider peritoneal dialysis using 7.5% high-glucose, low-sodium dialysate. Rapid correction of serum sodium should take place to about 155 mEq/l and then slowly correct to 145 mEq/l. Hypercalcemia is often present with hypernatremia, but the use of insulin to lower the serum calcium is not recommended secondary to its ability to increase the idiogenic osmole content of the brain. If DI is of central nature, the treatment is vasopressin or 1-deamino-(8-D-arginine)-vasopressin (DDAVP).

POTASSIUM

Potassium is primarily an intracellular cation. In the cells, the K^+ concentration is approximately 110 to 150 mEq/l. In the plasma or serum, the potassium concentration is 3.5 to 5 mEq/l. Total body potassium is about 50 to 55 mEq/l or 3500 mEq in the normal 70-kg man. Seventy-five percent of all potassium is in the muscle. The normal daily potassium intake is around 50 to 150 mEq/day.

Hypokalemia

Hypokalemia is usually secondary to intracellular shifts or increased losses by urinary excretion. Intracellular shifts are usually secondary to increased serum bicarbonate levels. Remember that for every rise in pH of 0.10, the serum potassium will fall by 0.5 mEq/l, secondary to increased serum bicarbonate levels.

In excessive vomiting, hypokalemia is secondary to metabolic alkalosis created by the loss of gastric fluid. In diabetic ketoacidosis, potassium follows glucose into the cells and thus hypokalemia occurs.

Other causes of hypokalemia include malignant hypertension, Bartter's syndrome, hyperaldosteronism secondary to diuretic use, renal artery stenosis, renal tubular acidosis, magnesium deficiency, hypercalcemia, myelocytic and monocytic leukemias, and GI loss secondary to fistulas, diarrhea, and vomiting. Hyperaldosteronism causes the kidneys to excrete potassium and chloride and retain sodium and bicarbonate. This is primarily driven by aldosterone. Hyperaldosteronism presents with hypertension, hypokalemia, and metabolic alkalosis. Chronic ingestion of licorice can also cause hypokalemia.

In children presenting with metabolic alkalosis, juxtaglomerular hyperplasia, hyperreninemia, hyperaldosteronism, kaliuresis, hypokalemia with sodium, and bicarbonate retention without hypertension or edema, always consider Bartter's syndrome. A patient with Liddle's syndrome presents with a familial type of pseudoaldosteronism, but with a normal aldosterone level.

In a seriously ill patient who is on an epinephrine infusion drip, epinephrine can cause the serum potassium to fall by 0.5 mEq/l. In a patient who is on chronic theophylline therapy, theophylline can potentiate the increase influx of potassium into the cells and thus worsen hypokalemia.

Patients with hypokalemia present with symptoms related to their serum potassium levels. At levels below 2 to 2.5 mEq/l, muscle weakness occurs and there is an increased incidence of intestinal ileus. At levels of 1.5 to 2 mEq/l, respiratory paralysis can be noted. Remember that the patient who is taking digitalis has an increased risk of digitalis toxicity and arrhythmias in the presence of hypokalemia.

A diagnosis is made after checking the serum potassium value. At a potassium level of less than 3 mEq/l, ECG changes can be noted. The QRS complex and T waves flatten; the ST segment is depressed; and prominent P or U waves can be present and also prolonged QT and PR intervals.

Treatment consists of infusing 10 to 15 mEq/l of KCl per hour in 50 to 100 ml of 5% dextrose or normal saline over for 3 to 4 hours. When giving KCl, the patient should be on a cardiac monitor, and no more than 40 mEq of potassium should ever be put into a single liter of IV fluid. It will take 40 to 50 mEq of potassium to raise the serum potassium by 1 mEq. Remember that as the serum potassium deficit increases, the total body potassium deficit increases at a greater percentage. To determine the correct total body potassium deficit, look at the corrected pH level for the serum potassium level (a rise in the pH of 0.10 will lower the potassium by 0.5 mEq/l) and correlate these two values to determine the correct potassium loss.

Hyperkalemia

Hyperkalemia is caused by many different etiologies: factitious, abnormal potassium distribution, primary renal tubular potassium secretory defect, metabolic acidemia, increased intake into the plasma, oliguric renal failure, and impaired renin-aldosterone axis. Pseudohyperkalemia secondary to hemolysis, leukocytosis, and thrombocytosis are very common. If the blood specimen is not analyzed within 30 minutes of being drawn, this can cause a factitious increase in the serum potassium. Also excessive opening and closing of a clenched fist can elevate the potassium level while a tourniquet is on the arm.

Hyperglycemia with DKA is a common cause of hyperkalemia, but this is not true hyperkalemia. Acute chronic renal failure with oliguria is the most common cause of dangerous hyperkalemia. Succinyl-choline and the breakdown of muscle mass in sepsis can also raise the potassium level.

At serum potassium levels greater than 6 mEq/l, cardiac conductivity and contractility are affected. At levels between 6.5 and 7 mEq/l, intracardiac blocks can be produced. First atrioventricular (AV) node blocks occur, then ventricular blocks occur, and finally the heart stops in diastole. In severe hyperkalemia, respiratory failure can occur secondary to respiratory muscle weakness.

Always correlate serum potassium levels with the arterial pH levels. Suspect hyperkalemia in any patient with excessive tissue breakdown, oliguric renal failure, or severe hemolysis. Acidosis is almost always present with hyperkalemia.

On an ECG, as the potassium level reaches 5.6 to 6 mEq/l, the T waves will become tall and peaked in the precordial leads. At levels of 6 to 6.5 mEq/l, the impulse conduction decreases and the PR and QT intervals are prolonged. At levels of 6.5 to 7.0 mEq/l, the P wave diminishes and the ST segment becomes depressed. At levels above 7 mEq/l, AV conduction is delayed and idioventricular rhythms occur. At levels above 7.5 to 8 mEq/l, the P wave completely disappears, the QRS complex widens, the S and T waves merge, and the ventricular rhythm becomes irregular. At levels greater than 10 to 12 mEq/l, the classic sine wave is seen. Patients die of ventricular fibrillation or diastolic arrest caused by the blocking of the distal Purkinje fibers.

Treatment is directed at correcting the serum potassium level. At levels of 5 to 5.5 mEq/l, diuresis is helpful. At levels of 5.5 to 6 mEq/l, diuresis and ion-exchange resin such as sodium polystyrene sulfonate (Kayexalate) should be used. Each gram of sodium resin will eliminate 1 mEq of potassium. The dose is 15 to 25 g of Kayexalate with 50 ml of a 20% sorbitol solution every 4 to 6 hours orally. It can also be given rectally as a 20-g dose with 20% sorbitol every 4 hours. Be careful in giving Kayexalate to patients who have impaired cardiac function. The sodium in Kayexalate can cause acute water retention and thus heart failure. If serum potassium is greater than 6.5 mEq/l, insulin and glucose should be given. Glucose pulls potassium, magnesium, and phosphorus into the cells. Give 50 ml of 50% IV glucose and then 5 to 10 units of regular insulin. In 1 liter of 20% glucose, place 40 to 80 units of insulin that should be given over the next 2 to 4 hours. Potassium and glucose levels should be monitored every hour.

Sodium bicarbonate causes alkalosis and can reduce serum potassium levels. An ampule of 50 ml of a 7.5% solution can be given as an IV drip over 10 to 20 minutes. Hypertonic sodium chloride 3% solution can also be given to antagonize potassium, forcing potassium into the cells. Calcium gluconate or calcium chloride can be given if the serum potassium is greater than 7 to 7.5 mEq/l. Ten milliliters of a 10% calcium gluconate can be given very slowly over 10 to 20 minutes. Be very careful when giving calcium to patients who are also on digitalis therapy. Hypercalcemia can potentiate the toxic effects of digitalis on the heart muscle. If calcium is given to a patient who is on digitalis, place 10 ml of a 10% calcium gluconate in 100 ml of D5W and infuse slowly over 20 to 30 minutes while the patient is on a cardiac monitor. If the patient is in a life-threatening tachyarrhythmia, all of the aforementioned measures should be performed at the same time.

Calcium gluconate 10% solution	10 to 20 ml IV
Sodium bicarbonate	50 to 100 mEq IV
Insulin	20 units of regular insulin over 1 hour with glucose
Glucose	50 g of glucose IV over 1 hour
Diuretics	
Furosemide	40 mg IV
Ethacrynic acid	50 mg IV
Cation-exchange resin Kayexalate	15 to 50 g PO or rectally with sorbitol

Peritoneal dialysis or hemodialysis for patients in oliguric renal failure

CALCIUM

Calcium is 99% stored in the bones as mineral abate. Calcium homeostasis is under the direct control of the parathyroid gland, parathyroid hormone (PTH), calcitonin, and vitamin D metabolites (namely, calcitrol). The parathyroid gland secretes PTH when ionized calcium or magnesium levels are low. Calcium levels are increased by the stimulation of osteoclasts by PTH to increase bone resorption. Calcitonin on the other hand decreases the release of calcium from bone by inhibiting the activity of the osteoclasts, thus lowering the serum calcium levels. Vitamin D is absorbed directly from the GI tract or can be produced nonenzymatically by ultraviolet light.

Calcium is essential for muscle depolarization, release of neurotransmitters in the CNS and peripheral nervous system, and in the clotting cascade for activation or conversion of factors IX, VII, VIII, prothrombin, and fibrinogen. It is also necessary for platelet aggregation and granule release. It acts as a membrane stabilizer and is needed for neutrophil chemotaxis and lymphocyte activation.

Calcium is found in three forms in the blood: protein-bound, complexed, and ionized. Total plasma calcium ranges from 8.5 to 10.5 mg/dl.

Hypocalcemia

Hypocalcemia is usually caused by sepsis or shock, pancreatitis, hypomagnesemia, alkalosis, hypoparathyroidism, fat embolism syndrome, osteoblastic metastasis, impaired production of vitamin D secondary to renal failure, hepatic failure, malabsorption, and anticonvulsant therapy. Decreased albumin levels can also cause hypocalcemia.

Hypoparathyroidism is usually secondary to postparathyroidectomy secondary to thyroidectomy surgery. Hungry bone syndrome can be seen after postparathyroidectomy. Hypocalcemia is secondary to a rapid remineralization of the skeleton after the tumor has been removed. This rapid remineralization can cause hypocalcemia and hypophosphatemia, which can cause tetany. These patients require large amounts of calcium and vitamin D replacement.

Hypocalcemia is seen in renal failure secondary to hyperphosphatemia, but there is usually no decrease in vitamin D in hypocalcemia secondary to renal failure. Acute trauma, hyperpyrexia, and rhabdomyolysis can all cause an acute hyperphosphatemia, which can lead to an acute hypocalcemia. Excessive use of phosphate can also lead to hyperphosphatemia in patients given phosphate enemas or cathartics.

Hypocalcemia and hypomagnesemia are often seen together in renal failure, diuretic use, alcoholism, and epilepsy. Hypomagnesemia lowers the secretion of PTH, which lowers the calcium levels. Addison's disease, Hashimoto's disease, pernicious anemia, moniliasis, and exostoses can cause idiopathic hypoparathyroidism. Pseudoparathyroidism is a familial disease noted by decreased end-organ responsiveness to PTH, which causes hyperphosphatemia, hypocalcemia, parathyroid hyperplasia, and excessive serum PTH concentrations. This is an x-linked dominant trait with a female:male ratio of 2:1. Patients will have short, round faces, brachycephaly, pudgy fingers and toes, and growth failure of the fourth and fifth metacarpals. They have seizures and are often mentally retarded. Their skin is coarse and dry with brittle hair.

Rickets or vitamin D deficiency is rare in the United States. Breastfeeding without sun exposure can lead to infantile rickets. Breast milk is low in vitamin D.

A diagnosis of hypocalcemia is made by a history of thyroid surgery or a lack of vitamin D intake. After thyroid or parathyroid surgery, if the patient has hypocalcemia he or she will present with parathesias around the mouth and in the fingertips. The deep tendon reflexes will also be weak, and the patient is usually irritable. The patient can also present acutely, or many years later, with seizures.

Trousseau's sign is a positive carpal spasm when a blood pressure cuff is applied to the upper arm and a pressure is maintained for 3 minutes above the systolic pressure. The fingers will extend at the interphalangeal joints, and the fingers at the metacarpophalangeal joint will be flexed. The wrist will be flexed, and the forearm will be pronated.

Chvostek's sign is a twitch at the corner of the mouth when the examiner taps over the facial nerve anterior to the ear. This sign can be present in up to 30% of the normal population, thus it is not as reliable a test as Trousseau's sign.

Remember that each rise in the arterial pH will lower ionized calcium by 3 to 8%. If the patient is alkalotic, the patient may have a normal serum total calcium but may have ionic hypocalcemia. On an ECG, when the serum calcium is below 6 mg/dl, the QT intervals can be prolonged, with the T wave of normal length, and the ST segment prolonged.

On x-rays, if rickets is present, you will find craniotabes on an x-ray of the frontal skull, with widened rib cage (Harrison's groove), bowed legs, and often fractures in many healing stages. There can be cupping and splaying of the metaphyseal ends of long bones and widening of the metaphyses and epiphysis. Also there is thinning of cortical bone, which becomes demineralized over time.

Treatment is based on replacement of calcium and treating the underlying cause of hypocalcemia. Oral calcium can be given in the form of calcium ascorbate, calcium lactate, calcium glubionate, calcium carbonate, and calcium gluconate. Milk is a poor source of calcium secondary to its large phosphate content. If calcium levels are dangerously low after thyroid or parathyroid surgery, calcium can be given parenterally. Ten milliliters of 10% $CaCl_2$ or calcium gluconate can be given over 10 to 20 minutes while the patient is on a cardiac monitor. Calcium should be given very slowly. A continuous drip of 1 g of $CaCl_2$ can be given over 6 to 12 hours if necessary.

Patients who are receiving massive blood transfusions also require calcium. If blood is being given faster than 1 unit every 5 minutes, 10 ml of 10% calcium chloride should be given every 4 to 6 hours if the patient is in shock or heart failure.

Rickets is treated with daily doses of vitamin D at 5000 to 10,000 international units (IU) until electrolyte and bone changes have been corrected.

Hypercalcemia

Hypercalcemia is defined as an ionized calcium level above 2.7 mEq/l or a total calcium level above 10.5 mEq/l. The mnemonic "Pam P. Schmidt" can be used to remember the causes of hypercalcemia:

P—parahormone
A—Addison's disease
M—multiple myeloma
P—Paget's disease
S—sarcoidosis
C—cancer
H—hyperthyroidism
M—milk alkali syndrome
I—immobilization
D—excess vitamin D
T—thiazides

These pathologies can be generalized into categories: malignancy, endocrinopathy, drug, granuloma, immobilization, and miscellaneous (e.g., Paget's disease, postrenal transplantation, recovery from acute renal failure, and phosphate depletion syndrome). In malignant causes of hypercalcemia, women with breast cancer often have hypercalcemia as do men with lung cancer. The rule of hypercalcemia is that the higher the calcium level over 14 mg/dl, the more likely it is secondary to a malignancy.

The second most common cause of hypercalcemia is primary hyperparathyroidism. This is usually secondary to a parathyroid adenoma (80%) and parathyroid hyperplasia (20%). Hyperparathyroidism is seldom caused by parathyroid carcinoma.

Several *endocrine adenomas* from the pituitary gland, adrenal gland, and pancreas can cause hypercalcemia. Examples are Werner's syndrome, multiple endocrine neoplasia type I, and Sipple's syndrome, which consists of pheochromocytoma and medullary cell carcinoma of the thyroid gland. These can all cause hypercalcemia.

Any patient who is immobilized secondary to trauma or illness can develop hypercalcemia secondary to the body's suppression of the parathyroid-vitamin D axis. This causes calcium to leave the bones, thus producing a transient hypercalcemia. There can be a tremendous urinary excretion of calcium in these patients (300 mg/day). Patients with Paget's disease who are on bed rest for chronic pain can also develop hypercalcemia.

Patients who are on thiazide diuretics often present with hypercalcemia secondary to the increased renal tubular reabsorption of calcium and decreased plasma volume. Many of the other types of diuretics cause increased calcium excretion and thus hypocalcemia.

When a patient is hypercalcemic, the heart's conduction rate is slowed and the refractory period of the heart is decreased. This increases the person's sensitivity to digitalis medications. This patient also has decreased gastric motility and increased gastric secretion in response to increased gastrin levels.

The kidneys are affected by hypercalcemia. The kidney loses its concentrating ability, which causes a reversible tubular defect. This tubular defect causes polyuria, dehydration, and polydipsia. If hypercalcemia happens on a long-term basis, microscopic calcium deposits can occur in the kidneys and can progress to renal insufficiency. A patient can present with nephrolithiasis and nephrocalcinosis secondary to hypercalcemia in the presence of dehydration.

A patient with a calcium level above 14 to 15 mg/dl will present with lethargy, muscle weakness, confusion, and sometimes coma. Calcium levels below 12 mg/dl are usually asymptomatic. These patients present with polyuria, polydipsia, and dehydration. A patient with a calcium level higher than 15 mg/dl presents with stupor, somnolence, and coma.

In patients with hypercalcemia on an ECG, the ST segment can be depressed, with a widened T wave and a shortened ST segment and QT intervals. As the calcium level increases, bradyarrhythmias, bundle branch blocks, progressing to second-degree blocks, and then complete heart blocks, can be seen. At levels greater than 20 mg/dl, cardiac arrest occurs.

The mnemonic *stones, bones, psychic moans,* and *abdominal groans* can be used to remember the signs and symptoms of hypercalcemia:

Stones—renal calculi

Bones—osteolysis

Psychic moans—psychiatric disorders

Abdominal groans—peptic ulcer disease and pancreatitis

Patients who require treatment are those who present with an inability to maintain a fluid intake, a calcium level higher than 12 mg/dl and/or abnormal renal functions. All of these patients are usually dehydrated and have reduced TBW secondary to the ability of calcium in high levels to interfere with the excretion of ADH. The main treatment, therefore, is to give the patient large amounts of saline (5 to 10 l) IV. If the patient also has severe cardiac or renal disease, hemodialysis or peritoneal dialysis is required. Diuretics should be used to maintain urine output, but thiazide diuretics should not be used. Furosemide (Lasix), 1 to 3 mg/kg, can be used. Hypokalemia and hypomagnesemia are treated as needed.

Drug therapy with mithramycin or calcitonin (Calcimar) has been advocated, especially in patients with metastatic bone disease. Mithramycin is cytotoxic and suppresses bone reabsorption and calcium release from bone. Fifteen to 25 µg/kg in a 5% dextrose solution IV, 3 hours a day for 3 days, can lower calcium levels within 48 hours, but maintains suppression for up to 7 days.

Calcitonin inhibits osteoclasts and is much less toxic than is mithramycin. This drug is given as 0.5 to 4 MRC units/kg IM every 12 hours, with a maximum dose of 8 MRC units/kg every 6 hours. The action of calcitonin can be prolonged when given with corticosteroids.

Patients with multiple myeloma, leukemia, sarcoidosis, vitamins A or D, intoxication, or breast cancer can benefit from glucocorticoid therapy. Glucocorticoids inhibit the reabsorption of calcium in the GI tract. Hydorcortisone, 25 to 100 mg IV, can be given every 6 to 8 hours. Indomethacin, 25 mg PO every 6 hours, can also be given to reduce the calcium level. Surgery or irradiation therapy is required for PTH-producing neoplasms.

MAGNESIUM

The normal serum concentration of magnesium is 1.8 to 2.4 mg/dl or 1.5 to 2 mEq/l. The total body concentration of magnesium is about 2000 mEq, with 50 to 70% in the bone. Less than 1% is found in the ECF. Magnesium is needed for chlorophyll metabolism. Magnesium is needed for the metabolism of many enzymes and adenine triphosphatase (ATPase). Hypomagnesemia can cause cardiovascular, neuromuscular, and GI problems.

Hypomagnesemia

Hypomagnesemia can be caused by GI disorders, renal disorders, and endocrine disorders and can be drug induced. It is often found in patients with diarrhea, cirrhosis, and pancreatitis and also in malnourished patients and in patients with chronic hyperparathyroidism. Burns, sepsis, sweating, lactation, and hungry bone syndrome can all cause hypomagnesemia. Drugs such as digoxin, insulin, diuretics, aminoglycosides, cisplatin, and alcohol can cause hypomagnesemia. Endocrine disorders such as hyperparathyroidism, aldosteronism, and hyperthyroidism can be attributed to hypomagnesemia.

It is common for patients with diabetic ketoacidosis or patients with long-term hyperalimentation, who are not given supplemental magnesium, to develop hypomagnesemia.

Patients with hypomagnesemia present with muscular irritability and CNS symptoms of vertigo, ataxia, depression, and seizures. In alcoholics, hypomagnesemia can contribute to delirium tremens. In patients on digitalis, hypomagnesemia can contribute to cardiac arrhythmias.

The plasma level of magnesium is an unreliable gauge to diagnose hypomagnesemia or hypermagnesemia. Plasma levels do not reflect total body magnesium levels. Patients can present with Chvostek's or Trousseau's sign and increased neuromuscular irritability. If calcium levels are normal, these signs can suggest hypomagnesemia. On an ECG, the PR interval can be prolonged, the QRS complex widened, the ST segment depressed, the T wave inverted, and the QT interval prolonged.

When evaluating hypomagnesemia, always evaluate the potassium, calcium, and phosphate levels. Hypokalemia, hypophosphatemia, and hypocalcemia are often also present with hypomagnesemia.

Treatment of hypomagnesemia is directed at replacement of magnesium, which can be replaced either PO or IV. Magnesium can be given PO as 6 g/day of $MgSO_4$. In patients with alcoholism or delirium tremens, up to 8 to 12 g/day can be given. Magnesium can be given as 10 to 15 mEq (1.5 to 2 g) IV as $MgSO_4$ IV over 1 to 2 hours, then 4 to 6 g/day IV thereafter. Magnesium can also be given to a patient on hyperalimentation at 12 to 16 mEq (1.5 to 2 g) a day as total parenteral nutrition (TPN).

Deep tendon reflexes will start to disappear at 3 to 4 mEq/l.

Hypermagnesemia

Hypermagnesemia rarely occurs, but when it does, it is usually in patients with renal failure or in patients who have been taking antacids that contain magnesium. It can also be seen in patients with rhabdomyolysis, tumor lysis hyperparathyroidism, hypothyroidism, and dehydration. There is increased muscular weakness and deep tendon loss at levels above 4 mEq/l. At levels between 5 and 6 mEq/l, severe respiratory depression can occur. At levels of 8 to 10 mEq/l, cardiac conduction abnormalities and neuromuscular paralysis with hypotension, ventilatory failure, and even death can occur.

Treatment of hypermagnesemia is much like the treatment of hypercalcemia, consisting of diuretics, furosemide, and IV saline. Calcium gluconate can be used in severely symptomatic patients to control symptoms. If systems are severe, hemodialysis or peritoneal dialysis should be considered.

PHOSPHORUS

Eighty percent of phosphorus is in the bones. It is essential for energy metabolism as phosphocreatine and phosphates. The normal serum phosphorus levels are 3 to 5 mg/dl in adults and 4 to 7 mg/dl in infants. Phosphorus and calcium are inversely proportional.

Hypophosphatemia

Hypophosphatemia is rare, except when there is an excessive movement of PO_4 from the ECF into the cells, or oral intake is reduced, or there is excessive phosphate loss. Most commonly, patients on TPN, if phosphate is not replaced, will have hypophosphatemia. Patients on ephinephrine drips, given sodium bicarbonate or steroids can also develop hypophosphatemia. It is seen in patients with peptic ulcer disease who are taking antacids for a prolonged time. Metabolic or respiratory alkalosis can produce hypophosphatemia.

Hypophosphatemia causes depletion of adenosine triphosphate (ATP) in the platelets, white blood cells, and red blood cells. This causes impaired platelet aggregation and increased bleeding tendency. Red blood cells also become rigid spherocytes and impair capillary perfusion. 2,3-Diphosphoglycerate decreases and increases the affinity of hemoglobin to oxygen, thus reducing the PO_2 and the oxygen that are available for tissue use. Patients also have a decreased resistance to infection secondary to chemotaxis, intracellular killing, and phagocytosis impairment by macrophages.

Patients with hypophosphatemia can also present with CNS symptoms of circumoral and fingertip paresthesias along with an absence of deep tendon reflexes. Hyperventilation, anorexia, and mental obtundation are common at low levels. Patients can become very weak with respiratory depression and even require ventilator therapy. At decreased levels of phosphate, cardiac function is depressed and left ventricular stroke work can be impaired.

Treatment of hypophosphatemia is directed at good nutritional care. Patients need 7 to 9 mmol/day of phosphate as a dibase or monobasic phosphates. Remember that phosphate can cause a reduction in calcium, thus calcium should always be given with phosphate therapy.

Hyperphosphatemia

Hyperphosphatemia is usually seen in patients with renal disease or dysfunction. It is seen in patients with reduced renal excretion or in conditions that cause increased movement of phosphate out of the cells and into the ECF. It is also seen in patients who have an increased vitamin D intake or increased phosphate intake. It is often seen in association with hypomagnesemia and hypocalcemia and in patients with hypoparathyroidism.

Hyperphosphatemia in and of itself is not a problem. It is the associated renal failure that causes the problems along with the co-presence of hypomagnesemia and hypocalcemia. Therapy is directed at treatment of the underlying cause of hyperphosphatemia. Calcium phosphate should be restricted to less than 200 mg/day. Patients with normal renal function can be given acetazolamide, 500 mg every 6 hours, along with 1 to 2 liters of normal saline 0.9% every 4 to 6 hours. Aluminum carbonate or hydroxide 30 to 45 ml QID can also be given to decrease phosphate levels. If renal failure is present, then hemodialysis should be considered.

CHLORIDE

Chloride is an essential extracellular anion that is important in maintaining ECF volume, normal anion gap, and acid-base and potassium balance mechanisms. Chloride also maintains urine output and concentrations in the renal countercurrent mechanisms. The normal serum chloride is 96 to 108 mEq/l.

Chloride is transported by both passive and active mechanisms with either bicarbonate or sodium. It is absorbed in both the small and large intestines. There is a normal $Cl-HCO_3$ exchange in the small bowel. Parietal cells of the stomach secrete chloride plus hydrogen ions into the gastric fluids. Chloride is 90% excreted in the urine. Chloride is also excreted in the stool and in sweat. The main function of chloride is to concentrate urine in the kidneys. Reabsorption of chloride occurs passively with sodium in the renal tubule, except in the loop of Henle where chloride and sodium are reabsorbed actively. This active transportation establishes a transport gradient that is needed for the "countercurrent" urine-concentration mechanism. When ADH is absent, the "countercurrent" mechanism allows the kidney to absorb solute without water in the collecting ducts, which allows urine to be more dilute if needed.

Chloride is also essential for acid-base regulation in the plasma. There are reciprocal changes in chloride and HCO_3.

Hypochloremia

Hypochloremia signifies a chloride level of less than 95 mEq/l. It is usually caused by excessive use of loop diuretics and high gastric acid secretion, secondary to nasogastric suctioning or vomiting. Metabolic alkalosis is usually present when there is hypochloremia. Hydrogen and chloride are secreted into the gastric fluid by the gastric parietal cells when bicarbonate is created in the circulation. Hydrogen and chloride maintain an acid-base balance in the distal GI tract. When the patient is vomiting, there is a change in the acid-base balance and there is external loss of hydrochloric acid. In the presence of ECF, volume depletion and increased renal absorption of sodium and bicarbonate alkalosis is maintained. The normal process of the kidneys is to maintain fluid volume by conserving sodium over acid-base and potassium. This process is influenced by aldosterone. Aldosterone accelerates the exchange of sodium for potassium and hydrogen ions. If there is an abundance of chloride present, then the pattern is reversed and there is bicarbonate diuresis, which helps to correct the alkalosis.

A diagnosis is made by a history of diuretic therapy, vomiting, or nasogastric suctioning, along with chloride values, in the presence of metabolic alkalosis. If urine chloride levels are greater than 40 mEq/l, then hypochloremia is due to dilution. If urinary chloride levels are low, less than 10 mEq/l, then hypochloremia is due to chloride-responsive alkalosis.

Chloride-resistant metabolic alkalosis requires potassium and sodium chloride solutions IV. In chloride-responsive metabolic alkalosis, usually only IV sodium chloride is necessary. Give one fourth of the calculated chloride deficit as KCl and three fourths as NaCl. Total body chloride deficit is determined by multiplying 20% of the body weight by the serum chloride deficit:

$$(\text{kg} \times 20\%)\,(100 - \text{serum chloride}) = \text{deficit}$$

Hyperchloremia

Hyperchloremia is usually secondary to dehydration or excessive administration of sodium chloride. It can present as a normal anion gap metabolic acidosis. This is usually in conjunction with diarrhea or pancreatic fistulas. Patients on hyperalimentation can develop hyperchloremic metabolic acidosis secondary to the hyperalimentation amino acids which are given as chlorides or hypochloride. Patients who are hypernatremic are also usually hyperchloremic. These patients are usually in metabolic alkalosis with a normal anion gap.

When the sodium and chloride levels are both elevated, this usually means that the patient is dehydrated. When the chloride level is elevated and the sodium level is normal or low, then too much chloride has been given (e.g., in sodium chloride therapy or in hyperalimentation, when amino acids are given as hydrochlorides) or there has been an excessive loss of bicarbonate from the body.

A patient with an anion gap of less than 10 mEq/l in the presence of hyperchloremia has a condition that is usually secondary to nephrosis, hypoalbuminemia, or cirrhosis. Hypermagnesemia, hypercalcemia, lithium overdose, and multiple myeloma can all present with hyperchloremia.

If hyperchloremia is due to dehydration, then isotonic IV fluids should be given slowly without chloride. If hypotonic fluids are given, especially if given too quickly, cerebral edema can develop. If there has been an excessive loss of bicarbonate or excessive administration of chloride, then these conditions should be corrected.

HYPOTHYROIDISM AND MYXEDEMA COMA

Definition

Hypothyroidism is a chronic systemic disorder that is recognized as a progressive slowing of body functions secondary to decreased thyroid hormone. Myxedema coma is a life-threatening form of hypothyroidism. There are two types of hypothyroidism: primary and secondary.

Epidemiology

Myxedema coma usually occurs in the elderly female population with long-standing undiagnosed hypothyroidism. It occurs mainly in the winter and is usually precipitated by a physical or emotional event. The mortality rate for persons treated for myxedema coma is 50%.

Hypothyroidism is present in 0.1% of the male population and 1% of the female population. It is six to seven times more common in women older than 60 years of age than in men.

Pathology

The anterior pituitary gland regulates the release of thyroid-stimulating hormone (TSH), which stimulates the thyroid gland to release thyroid hormone. Thyrotropin-releasing hormone (TRH) is released by the hypothalamus, which stimulates the anterior pituitary gland to release TSH. The hypothalamus uses the level of TSH as a feedback mechanism to withhold or release TRH.

Primary hypothyroidism is caused by the intrinsic failure of the thyroid gland. Ninety-five percent of all hypothyroidism is due to primary failure. The most common cause of primary hypothyroidism in adults is the treatment of Graves' disease—the use of radioactive iodine for the treatment of hyperthyroidism. The second most common presentation occurs 12 to 15 months after surgery for hyperthyroidism. Primary hypothyroidism can take years to present after surgical therapy or radioactive iodine therapy.

Hashimoto's thyroiditis is an autoimmune thyroid disorder that can cause primary hypothyroidism. These conditions are the most common cause of goitrous hypothyroidism. This type of primary hypothyroidism is believed to be caused by an autoimmune destruction of the thyroid gland, which produces thyroid failure secondary to glandular atrophy. Lithium, phenbutazone, congenital causes,

Graves' disease, iodine deficiency, and antithyroid drugs have all been implicated as causes of primary thyroid failure.

In secondary hypothyroidism, disease or destruction of the pituitary gland or the hypothalamus can cause hypothyroidism. Five percent of hypothyroidism is caused by secondary failure. Causes of secondary failure include postpartum hemorrhage, pituitary tumors, infiltrative disorders, and sarcoidosis. The difference in primary and secondary failure is that primary failure involves failure of the thyroid gland, and secondary failure involves failure of the pituitary gland. In primary failure, the TSH level is high and the pituitary gland is working, whereas in secondary failure the TSH is low and the pituitary gland is diseased, but the thyroid gland is producing TSH.

Rarely, tertiary hypothyroidism occurs secondary to failure of the hypothalamus. In tertiary hypothyroidism, the patient responds to TRH administration, meaning that both the pituitary and thyroid glands are functioning.

Clinical Presentation/Examination

Commonly patients with hypothyroidism present with weakness, fatigue, constipation, cold intolerance, weight gain, and increased appetite. As the disease progresses, patients present with decreased hearing, muscle cramps, menstrual irregularities, and mental disturbances. In myxedema coma, the patient presents with dry, waxy skin; nonpitting skin with swelling of the subcutaneous tissues, and often a very puffy face. There can also be thinning of the eyebrows with scanty body hair. The patient's voice often changes and becomes deep and coarse. On examination, the patient's tongue is thickened.

The patient will have prolongation of the deep tendon reflexes. Paresthesias and ataxia can also be present. There is often constipation or fecal impaction.

There are often mental status changes including "myxedema madness" hallucinations, delusions, and psychosis. Cardiac changes include an enlarged heart, bradycardia, and a low-voltage ECG. Generally there is mild hypertension, and hypercholesterolemia and angina pectoris are often present. On ECG examination sinus bradycardia is the most common cardiac rhythm noted with low voltage, flatting or inversion of the T waves, and prolongation of the PR interval. Congestive heart failure is often noted as an underlying disease.

Bradycardia is the most common abnormality found in myxedema coma. If hypothyroidism has been long-standing, cardiomegaly may be seen on radiologic examination. Hypotension can be present from decreased synergistic effect due to thyroid hormone deficiency. The use of vasopressors are limited in the treatment of hypotension, secondary to the absence of thyroid hormone. Ventricular arrhythmias can occur secondary to the use of vasopressors and simultaneous administration of thyroid hormone.

CNS manifestations of myxedema coma are a direct result of the lack of thyroid hormone in the brain. On examination, patients can present with personality changes, psychiatric disorders, slow mentation, hallucinations, psychosis, or delusions. Intention tumors, cerebellar ataxia, nystagmus, and difficulty with coordinated movements may be present.

Patients can also present with abdominal distention secondary to ascites or paralytic ileus. Some are often found to have acquired megacolon. Patients are often malnourished secondary to poor food intake. They may also present with urinary retention.

The patient should be given a complete examination, especially at the neck to look for a surgical scar from prior thyroid surgery.

Diagnosis

The diagnosis is made by clinical presentation and history. TSH, T_3, and T_4 levels will help to make the diagnosis.

Laboratory Findings

A CBC, electrolytes, BUN, creatinine, cortisol level, cardiac enzymes, blood cultures, urinalysis, TSH, T_3, T_4, and T_3 RU (triiodothyronine resin uptake) should be drawn on each patient. Hyponatremia and hypochloremia are often present in the myxedema patient. The serum potassium can be variable. The serum cholesterol level is usually elevated. CPK, LDH, and SGOT levels can also be elevated.

If a lumbar puncture is performed, a common finding is that the CSF protein will be greater than 10 mg/dl with increased opening pressures of greater than 400 mm H_2O.

Treatment

Treatment of hypothyroidism is replacement of thyroid hormone as L-thyroxine at an average maintenance dose of 0.1 to 0.3 mg/day.

Treatment of myxedema coma consists of treating the underlying precipitating event and thyroid hormone replacement. The danger in treating myxedema coma is not recognizing it. Do not give phenothiazines for psychosis secondary to myxedema. β-Blockers can cause myxedema coma secondary to reduced thyroid hormone levels through conversion of thyroxine to triiodothyronine. Remember that the hypothyroid patient metabolizes medications slower than does the normal patient, thus drug dosages should be checked.

A patient who presents with hypothermia should be treated with gradual re-warming. If the patient is warmed too rapidly, peripheral vasodilation can occur and circulatory collapse can ensue. A normal or elevated temperature in a patient with myxedema coma can represent an underlying infection.

Hyponatremia and hypochloremia are often present in the patient with myxedema. Hyponatremia is usually secondary to a dilutional effect secondary to water retention. The hyponatremia is treated with water restriction. If the serum sodium level is less than 115 mEq/l, give hypertonic saline solution and furosemide until the level is corrected.

Good respiratory support is essential in the patient with myxedema. Patients with myxedema coma present with hypercapnia, hypoxia, and hypoventilation. Mechanical ventilation may be required in the first 48 hours of treatment.

If infection is present, appropriate antibiotics should be given. Hydrocortisone, 300 mg/day, should be given.

Thyroid hormone should be given slowly and cautiously. This hormone can be fatal to a euthyroid comatose patient. IV thyroxine is given at an initial dose of 400 to 500 μg slowly and then 50 to 100 μg IV daily. Some authors recommend no further thyroxine therapy after the loading dose for 3 to 7 days. Oral therapy can be started with once daily dosing at 100 to 200 μg/day.

Triiodothyronine at a dose of 12.5 to 25 μg every 6 to 8 hours can also be given in place of thyroxine. Triiodothyronine has a shorter half-life but has an more rapid onset of 24 to 36 hours.

Any patient with myxedema coma should be admitted to the ICU for treatment and good supportive care.

HYPOGLYCEMIA

Definition

Hypoglycemia is defined as a serum glucose of less than 50 mg/dl.

Epidemiology

Hypoglycemia usually occurs in insulin-dependent diabetics secondary to insulin therapy and accounts for 3 to 7% of insulin-dependent diabetes. It also occurs in patients who are on sulfonylureas and in toxic drug overdoses.

Pathology

Glucose is the only source of energy for the CNS. Hypoglycemia thus causes CNS depressant symptoms. Glucose hemostasis is maintained by the liver, adrenal glands, pancreas, and the pituitary gland, and anything that interferes with this homeostasis can cause hypoglycemia. Anything that interferes with glucocorticoid, glucagon, catecholamines, and growth hormone regulation can thus interfere with glucose homeostasis.

Glucose is metabolized in two states: feeding and fasting. In the feeding state, glucose intake stimulates the release of insulin and tissue uptake and storage. During the fasting state, decreased insulin levels mobilize the stored fuels from tissues. Glycogen in the liver is the major source of stored fuels. Triglycerides in the adipose tissue and protein tissue are the other two major sources of stored fuels in the body.

When glucose or food is taken in, a release of insulin from the pancreatic beta cells is promoted. Insulin promotes the uptake of glucose by the liver, which is transformed into glycogen, which is then stored in the liver. Insulin also inhibits the release of glucose by inhibiting glycogenolysis (the breakdown of glycogen to glucose). Insulin also inhibits the formation of glucose from precursors (gluconeogenesis). Insulin also causes decreased lipogenesis, thus increased energy stores, and enhances lipolysis in fat cells by promoting the uptake of amino acids into muscle protein and inhibiting proteolysis.

Initially, in the fasting state, stored glucose in the liver is utilized by glycogenolysis. After several hours the stored glucose (glycogen) is used up, and the fasting state ensues. In the fasting state, gluconeogenesis is the primary source of glucose metabolism. Muscle proteins, in the form of amino acids and alanines, are the primary source of glucose metabolism in the liver via proteolysis during the fasting state.

Triglycerides or free fatty acids along with glycerol are the major sources of glucose from stored fat tissue. Lipolysis metabolism is caused by low insulin levels along with the presence of growth hormone and epinephrine.

Clinical Presentation

A patient with hypoglycemia presents with adrenergic or sympathomimetic symptoms of pallor, tremulousness, diaphoresis, visual disturbances, palpitations, tachycardia, weakness, mental confusion, and lightheadedness. A patient with chronic CNS glucose deprivation presents with fatigue, memory loss, confusion, seizures, and coma. The patient's symptomatology is dependent on the patient's age and the patient's "normal" glucose level.

A patient who presents to the ED either has spontaneous hypoglycemia or induced hypoglycemia. In spontaneous hypoglycemia, hypoglycemia is secondary to reactive or postprandial hypoglycemia, diabetes mellitus, or idiopathic causes. A patient who has had a gastrectomy can present with dumping syndrome secondary to a rapid dilution of hyperosmolar load in the jejunum and presents with nausea, vomiting, weakness, palpations, dizziness, diarrhea, and gastric discomfort.

A patient with early diabetes can present with hypoglycemia 3 to 5 hours after ingestion of a meal. This initial episode lasts 15 to 20 minutes and can be the first sign of type II diabetes. A patient with idiopathic hypoglycemia can present 2 to 4 hours after a meal or after a change in mealtimes. The patient presents with sweating, lightheadedness, confusion, shakiness, and numbness.

Fasting hypoglycemia is the most common type of presentation in a patient who presents to the ED. Fasting hypoglycemia is often a sign of serious underlying organic disease. Fasting hypoglycemia occurs 5 to 6 hours after the patient's last meal. The patient is often difficult to arouse after a 24-hour or overnight fast.

Patients with islet cell tumors of the pancreas secondary to insulinomas present with confusion or abnormal behavior in 80% of cases. The tumor is usually a single small tumor. Of these patients, 10% will present with multiple tumors or multiple endocrine neoplasia type I, and 10% present with metastatic malignant insulinomas. Insulinomas present in women from 40 to 70 years of age, and these patients present with palpitations, sweating, weakness, blurred vision, and diplopia. Eighty percent present with confusion; 12% present with seizures; and 50% present with amnesia or coma. Symptoms are episodic, occurring irregularly, usually in the late afternoon or early morning before breakfast, and are often induced by exercise. These patients are often misdiagnosed before the insulinoma is found. Treatment involves excision of the tumor.

Mesenchymal tumors are often tumors of the thoracic or retroperitoneal areas, usually fibrosarcomas or mesotheliomas. Mesenchymal tumors are the most common nonpancreatic tumors that cause hypoglycemia. These tumors can reach the weight of 20 kg or more and grow very slowly. These patients present with weight loss, depressed cerebral function, profound hypoglycemia, and intrathoracic or intraabdominal masses. Epithelial tumors involving the liver adrenal glands also can cause hypoglycemia. Hepatic carcinomas are in a 4:1 ratio of men to women. Carcinoid tumors are slow-growing tumors that develop from the amine precursor uptake and decarboxylation (APUD) series and develop from various locations. They consist of a variety of active biologic substances.

There are many endocrine-related causes of hypoglycemia. Deficiencies in growth hormone, glucagon, and glucocorticoids can all cause hypoglycemia. Adrenal insufficiency, either primary or secondary, can cause hypoglycemia. Hypopituitarism, secondary adrenal insufficiency, has a very pronounced presentation, secondary to the concomitant growth hormone and glucocorticoid deficiencies. Thyroid hormone deficiency, especially when myxedema coma is present, can cause hypoglycemia.

When 80 to 85% of the liver function is impaired or destroyed, gluconeogenesis and glycogenolysis are severely impaired and thus severe hypoglycemia can occur. The HELLP syndrome (*h*emolysis, *e*levated, *l*iver, enzyme levels and *l*ow *p*latelet count) in preeclampsia or pregnancy can cause hypoglycemia. In children, kwashiorkor, meningitis, or sepsis can cause hypoglycemia.

Induced hypoglycemia is usually secondary to ingestion of salicylates, alcohol, sulfonylureas, or insulin. In children younger than 2 years of age, hypoglycemia is usually secondary to chronic salicylate ingestion or an acute drug overdose. In the adult population, most comas are secondary to insulin and sulfonylureas. Renal or hepatic disease and restricted carbohydrate intake are predisposing factors for hypoglycemia.

In the insulin-dependent diabetic, late or absent meals, emotional stress, exercise, low carbohydrate intake, alcohol ingestion, or errors or overtreatment in insulin therapy are major causes of hypoglycemia. Insulin-dependent diabetics can also develop Somogyi syndrome secondary to excess insulin therapy. These patients present with nocturnal hypoglycemia with rebound hyperglycemia. The patient with nocturnal hypoglycemia presents with nightmares, morning headache, seizures, night sweats, depression, lethargy, and hepatomegaly secondary to glycogen accumulation. A patient who has a true insulin overdose will present with nocturia, polyuria, and enuresis and a history of increased insulin dosing. Ketoacidosis, weight gain, excessive appetite, and mood swings are commonly noted in these patients. Often it is noted that the patient's insulin dose is greater than 1 unit/kg.

Insulin-dependent diabetics can also develop a "dawn phenomenon." There is an increase in serum glucose levels and hyperglycemia between 5:00 AM and 9:00 AM. This dawn phenomenon can occur in insulin-dependent patients, noninsulin-dependent patients, and patients who do not have diabetes. It is important to distinguish between the dawn phenomenon and Somogyi syndrome in each patient, because the treatment is very different for these conditions.

Sulfonylureas, first-generation agents (e.g., tolbutamide, chlorpropamide, tolazamide, and acetohexamide) and second-generation agents (glipizide and glyburide) can cause hypoglycemia. Chlorpropamide is the most dangerous secondary to its long half-life of up to 36 hours. Glipizide and glyburide have the greatest hypoglycemic effect per milligram. Sulfonylureas stimulate the release of insulin from the pancreas. The danger of sulfonylureas is their long half-life (up to 36 hours). Any patient with a sulfonylurea overdose should be admitted to the hospital. Hypoglycemia may not occur for 12 to 24 hours after ingestion. Sulfonylurea-induced hypoglycemia is often refractory to glucose therapy alone.

A patient with a salicylate overdose presents with hypoglycemia. The patient can present with convulsions, coma, or cardiovascular collapse. β-Blockers have also been attributed to hypoglycemia. Hypoglycemia can also present in patients who are on hemodialysis or who are receiving hyperalimentation.

Infants or children with hypoglycemia can present to the ED with increased irritability, convulsions, apnea, abnormal cry, bradycardia to an asymptomatic presentation, limpness, or coma.

Many drugs can induce hypoglycemia: sulfa drugs, haloperidol, chloramphenicol, dicumarol, manganese, monoamine oxidase inhibitors, oxytetracycline, disopyramide, quinine, phenylbutazone, pentamidine, pheothiazines, Kerola herbs, hypoglycine, and akee nuts. A history of any chronic or acute medication use or change in medications should be noted.

Examination

The patient should be given a complete examination, including a complete neurologic examination. As in any patient with altered mental status, a rectal examination should be performed to rule out a lower GI bleed as a cause of altered mental status.

Diagnosis

A diagnosis is made by a rapid Dextrostix in the ED or a serum glucose level below 50 mg/dl. A history of insulin or noninsulin diabetes, alcohol, sulfonylurea, or salicylate ingestion or other toxic ingestion should be obtained.

Laboratory Findings

All patients who present to the ED with altered mental status should have a CBC and electrolytes, including sodium, potassium, CO_2, chloride, BUN, creatinine, and glucose, drawn. An ABG should also be drawn if toxic ingestion or alcohol ingestion is suspected. If alcohol ingestion is suspected, obtain LFTs, including GGT, AST, ALT, total bilirubin, and amylase and lipase to rule out pancreatitis. Acetaminophen, aspirin, lithium, and other toxic drug levels or screens should be drawn as needed.

Artifactual hypoglycemia can be found when the lymphocyte or leukocyte count is markedly elevated over 60,000 mm^3. Artifactual hypoglycemia has also been reported in various leukemias and because of refrigerated blood samples or the addition of antiglycolytic agents in blood products (sodium fluoride).

Alcohol-induced hypoglycemia in alcoholics presents with elevated blood alcohol, mild acidosis, and ketonuria without glycosuria. This alcohol-induced hypoglycemia is secondary to the inhibition of gluconeogenesis during alcohol metabolism.

If transient hypoglycemia is suspected, a CSF glucose level can be obtained to evaluate this condition. The glucose in the CSF lags behind the serum glucose changes by 4 to 6 hours before the CSF glucose level becomes normal.

A 6-hour GTT can be performed to obtain levels, C peptides, insulin antibodies, and insulin levels to assist in determining the cause of the hypoglycemia.

Treatment

Any patient who presents to the ED with altered mental status or coma should be considered to be hypoglycemic. Two large-gauge IV lines of normal saline 0.9% should be started, and the patient should be placed on a cardiac monitor. The patient should also be placed on oxygen, and the aforementioned laboratory studies should be drawn. A Dextrostix should be done in the ED, and if the patient is hypoglycemic, glucose should be administered. If the patient is an alcoholic or has a history of alcohol ingestion or abuse, the altered mental status should be considered secondary to alcohol ingestion. Give thiamine, 100 mg IM or IV, then give 50 ml of 50% glucose. Naloxone (Narcan), 2 to 4 mg IV or IM should also be given to any patient with altered mental status. Remember that good cervical spine control is important in patients who are brought to the ED with altered mental status and a poor history of how they became unconscious. In alcoholic patients, remember never to attribute their altered mental status just to alcohol or hypoglycemia. Alcoholics get drunk, develop hypoglycemia, fall down, and hit their heads. Always have a high index of suspicion for an intracranial bleed in these patients.

In patients who have an overdose of sulfonylurea, give IV glucose 50 ml of 50% and diazoxide, 300 mg slow IV infusion over 30 minutes every 4 hours. Check the patient for hypotension.

Alcohol-induced hypoglycemia should be treated with thiamine, 100 mg IV or IM first, then 50 ml of 50% glucose.

For persistent hypoglycemia, an infusion of 5, 10, or 20% glucose solution can be started and continued for 4 to 6 hours until glucose levels normalize or are at least 100 mg/dl. If the patient is still hypoglycemic after 1 liter of glucose solution is given, give the patient 100 mg of hydrocortisone and 1 mg of glucagon, added to each liter of glucose. Glucagon is not effective in treating hypoglycemia in alcohol-induced hypoglycemia or in chronic alcoholics secondary to depleted glycogen stores. Glucagon can be given IV or SC in a dose of 0.5 to 2 mg. If glucagon is given IV, it should be given in continuous infusion secondary to its short half-life. If the hypoglycemia is refractory to these treatments, then a secondary cause of hypoglycemia should be considered.

LACTIC ACIDOSIS

Definition

Lactic acidosis can be a life-threatening event or can be a well-tolerated process. It is the most common form of metabolic acidosis. It is divided into type A and type B forms. The types are based on the oxygen supply to the tissues. In type A lactic acidosis, there is clinical evidence of hypoperfusion or hypoxia. In type B lactic acidosis, there are no signs of hypoxia. Lactic acidosis can occur in a wide variety of problems. Lactic acidosis is most often diagnosed when the anion-gap is determined on a patient with an underlying illness.

Epidemiology

The mortality rate for patients with type A lactic acidosis is approximately 80%. The mortality rate for patients with type B lactic acidosis is between 50 and 80%.

Pathology

Lactate is a byproduct of anaerobic glycolysis. In a 70-kg man, the normal lactate production is 1300 mEq/day with a normal serum lactate of approximately 1 mEq/l. Lactate is the immediate precursor of pyruvate. In normal metabolism, the body's lactate is disposed of by the liver and the kidneys by gluconeogenesis, which converts lactate back into pyruvate. The liver clears 50% of the lactate produced, and the kidneys clear another 30%. Hydrogen ions produced during the formation of lactic acid are utilized in the process of gluconeogenesis and help to maintain the acid-base balance of the body. Lactic acidosis is the imbalance between the rate of production of lactate by tissues in active glycolysis and the rate of utilization by the tissues in active gluconeogenesis.

Pyruvate plus NADH and hydrogen ions (H^+) are catalyzed by lactate dehydrogenase (LDH) into lactate and NAD. The normal ratio of this metabolic process is lactate:pyruvate ratio of 10:1. The production of lactate is a dead endpoint in metabolism. It must be metabolized back into pyruvate for gluconeogenesis for oxidation to CO_2 and H_2O via the Krebs cycle. Oxygen must be present as a cofactor to convert lactate back into pyruvate. The goal of this process is to produce energy in the form of ATP and to oxidize NADH to NAD. For each milliequivalent of lactic acid that is produced an equal amount of hydrogen ions and lactate is liberated. As the hydrogen ions are released, bicarbonate buffers the lactic acid and is consumed by utilization of lactate via gluconeogenesis or oxidation. However, as lactic acid production is increased and lactic acid utilization is decreased, the body's buffering system is overwhelmed. Excess hydrogen ions are present, and thus acidosis occurs.

Pyruvate is used in glycolysis and is formed by oxidation of glucose, and transamination, a process in which pyruvate can be derived from amino acids (alanine). Intracellular redox state is a factor in determining the concentration of lactate. Oxygen must be available at the tissue level for lactate to be reoxidized back into pyruvate. If oxygen is not available, such as in prolonged anaerobic conditions, lactate cannot be transformed back into pyruvate because of the lack of NAD. When NAD is not available for conversion, lactate accumulates.

The intracellular pH can determine the lactate concentration within the cystol of the cell. Changes in pH can affect intracellular enzymatic reactions and lactate:pyruvate ratios. A rise in the intracellular pH causes an increase in lactate concentration, and a decrease in intracellular pH causes a fall in the intracellular lactate concentration. As the serum pH decreases to below 7.0, the liver stops clearing lactate and starts producing lactate.

Clinical Presentation

Patients with lactic acidosis present with nonspecific presentations. They present with Kussmaul respirations or hyperventilation. They may present awake or in coma with or without abdominal pain. Hypotension is usually present in type A lactic acidosis.

Patients with type A lactic acidosis often present with cardiogenic, septic, hypovolemic, or hemorrhagic shock. Type A lactic acidosis is directly related to inadequate tissue perfusion secondary to a shock state and tissue anoxia, secondary to lactate and hydrogen ion accumulation. The decreased lactate clearance by the liver is caused by decreased splanchnic and hepatic artery perfusion and the ensuing hepatocellular ischemia secondary to the shock hyperfusion. Remember that as the pH approaches 7.0, the liver stops clearing lactate and starts producing lactate. Treatment of type A lactic acidosis is directed at treating the underlying cause.

Type B lactic acidosis involves all types of lactic acidosis in which no signs of tissue anoxia are present. There is no cardiovascular dysfunction, and no hypotension is present. Type B lactic acidosis is further divided into types B1, B2, and B3. Type B1 often occurs in association with other medical disorders, such as renal or hepatic failure or disease, diabetes, neoplasm, or infection. Cirrhosis and hepatic necrosis are often associated with type B1 lactic acidosis. Hodgkin's disease, leukemia, multiple myeloma, and Reye's syndrome are also associated with lactic acidosis.

Type B2 lactic acidosis is associated with the acidosis-induced form of chemical or toxic ingestion of drugs or toxidromes. Ingestion of ethanol is the most classic cause of lactic acidosis. Epinephrine, sorbitol, fructose, methanol, and salicylates are associated with lactic acidosis.

Type B3 is associated with inborn errors of metabolism and type I glycogen storage disease (glucose-6-phosphatase dehydrogenase [GGPD] deficiency) and hepatic fructose-biphosphatase deficiency.

Examination

The patient should be examined for underlying causes of lactic acidosis.

Diagnosis

A diagnosis of lactic acidosis is made by a lactate concentration of 5 to 6 mEq/l in the presence of metabolic acidosis and an arterial pH of less than 7.35. However, this can only be a presumptive diagnosis. Many other situations can raise the serum lactate level and include seizures, hyperventilation, vigorous exercise, and infusion of bicarbonate and saline. There is always an anion-gap acidosis present, but all other causes of the anion-gap metabolic acidosis must be excluded.

Type A lactic acidosis is defined as a clinically evident tissue anoxia secondary to hypoxia or shock. Type B lactic acidosis is defined as lactic acidosis in which there is no evidence of tissue anoxia.

Laboratory Findings

A CBC, electrolytes, BUN, creatinine, glucose, phosphate, uric acid, serum lactate level, LFTs, amylase, lipase, ABE, and a urinalysis should be performed on all patients with suspected lactic acidosis. Often there will be hyperphosphatemia and hyperuricemia present. The white blood cell count is often elevated. Hyperglycemia may be present if there is underlying liver disease.

Treatment

The primary focus on treatment of lactic acidosis is to treat the underlying cause of the lactic acidosis and to correct the accumulation of lactic acid. This is performed by correcting the causes of shock and by maintaining adequate ventilation. The restoration of fluid volume and renal and hepatic perfusion is essential. Vasopressors should not be used secondary to their ability to decrease tissue perfusion and worsen the current acidosis.

Sodium bicarbonate should be used to treat the lactic acidosis and should be used if the arterial pH is less than 7.0. It can be given by adding 3 to 4 ampules of $NaHCO_3$ (44 mEq/l) to 1 liter of 5% dextrose and water. This solution provides 132 to 176 mEq/l of bicarbonate. The correct dose of sodium bicarbonate that needs to be replaced can be determined by using the following formula:

$$HCO_3 \text{ deficit} = (25 \text{ mEq/l } HCO_3 - \text{measured } HCO_3) \times 0.5 \text{ (body weight in kg)}$$

Patients who have trouble tolerating massive fluid and sodium overloads, such as those with a history of congestive heart failure, can be treated with bicarbonate infusion, potent loop diuretics, or tris (hydroxymethyl) aminomethane (THAM).

Loop diuretics should be utilized to maintain a urine output at 300 to 500 ml/hr. Sodium and potassium levels should be monitored closely and should be replaced as needed. If the patient is oliguric, hemodialysis is required for the administration of sodium bicarbonate.

If the patient is an alcoholic, thiamine 100 mg IV or IM should be given. Thiamine is a cofactor for the enzymes that catalyze the first step in the oxidation of pyruvate. Numerous other treatments have been tried in the treatment of lactic acidosis, but all have been ineffective. These patients should be admitted to the ICU, and the underlying cause of the lactic acidosis should be aggressively treated with good respiratory ventilation, bicarbonate therapy, and the maintenance of adequate tissue perfusion.

NONKETOTIC HYPEROSMOLAR COMA

Definition

Hyperglycemia, hyperosmolality, and dehydration without ketoacidosis are present in nonketotic hyperosmolar coma. Nonketotic hyperosmolar coma, which is distinguished from diabetic ketoacidosis by the lack of the presence of serum ketones, is at the other end of the spectrum with regard to lipid metabolism in diabetic ketoacidosis.

Epidemiology

Nonketotic hyperosmolar coma is found most often in diabetics but can also occur in the nondiabetic patient. It is much less common than diabetic ketoacidosis. It usually occurs as the initial event in adult onset diabetes. Nonketotic hyperosmolar coma is found usually in the new-onset diabetic patient who is middle-aged or elderly, and it is often found in the nursing home patient or the mentally retarded patient and is insidious in onset.

Pathology

The exact explanation of why nonketotic hyperosmolar coma occurs is not fully understood. It is believed that the lack of ketosis is secondary to the acute extreme hyperglycemia. Acute hyperglycemia is unrecognized by the body's glucose metabolism. This is because the beta cells of the pancreas respond to stress, the cause of increasing the blood glucose levels, by releasing increasing amounts of insulin. The insulin stores become rapidly depleted, and the glucose level continues to rise rapidly unchecked. There are also increasing elevated levels of glucagon in the liver, and these also increase hyperglycemia. With the new-onset diabetic there is no supplemental insulin available, as with the diabetic who is taking insulin, so when the insulin stores are depleted, the patient's glucose level can rise unchecked to an extreme level higher than 1000 mg/dl.

It is believed that the reason why ketoacidosis does not occur is secondary to the low levels of free fatty acids in the presence of normal or low insulin, normal glucocorticoid, and normal growth hormone levels. During normal or higher concentration levels of insulin, in the presence of lower lipolytic hormone levels, the patient prevents ketosis. When lipolysis is prevented or absent, the precursors required for formation of ketone bodies are not released, and ketoacidosis does not develop.

Other investigators believe that the absence of ketosis is secondary to the intrahepatic oxidation of the incoming free fatty acids (FFAs). In the nonketotic patient, the prehepatic insulin levels are twice the posthepatic levels, and it is believed that the liver is "bathed" in insulin, thus preventing the formation of ketones.

The hyperglucose state causes an acute osmotic diuresis that causes fluid and electrolyte imbalances. When no insulin is present, the cell membrane is impermeable to glucose and water is drawn from the cell into the ECF compartment. After the maximum level of ADH excretion has been reached by the posterior pituitary gland, osmotic diuresis occurs. Serum osmolality is increased, and TBW is decreased. The average patient can lose 8 to 12 liters of body fluid.

Clinical Presentation

Often patients with nonketotic hyperosmolar coma present with a history of a major illness, unlike diabetic patients who present with a history of a minor illness as the precipitation of the event. Often the patient with nonketotic hyperosmolar coma has a history of gram-negative pneumonia, myocardial infarction, acute GI bleeding, acute cerebrovascular accident, acute pancreatitis, acute pyelonephritis, subdural hematomas, uremia, or peripheral vascular occlusion. These patients often present with a history of chronic cardiovascular or renal disease.

There is often a history of use of cimetidine, phenytoin, corticosteroids, mannitol, calcium channel blockers, propranolol, or immunosuppressive agents. Thiazide diuretics and diazoxide are well-known causes of nonketotic hyperosmolar coma. Patients will sometimes give a history of ingesting enormous amounts of sugar-containing fluids.

These patients present with acute neurologic changes. They present with confusion, stupor, drowsiness, or coma. As the serum osmolality increases, the mental status changes increase (>380 mOsm/kg). These patients present with hemisensory defects or hemiparesis, or both. Fifteen percent present with seizure activity. Eighty-five percent present with focal motor symptoms. Patients can present with a wide variety of neurologic complaints, including aphasia, hyperreflexia, positive plantar response, depressed deep tendon reflexes, and nuchal rigidity.

Patients present with significant dehydration, and often fever, hypotension, and tachycardia are present. Those with gram-negative pneumonia can present in shock. There is no fruity odor on the patient's breath, but shallow respirations, hyperpnea, and tachypnea are often present.

Diagnosis

A diagnosis is made by a blood glucose level greater than 800 mg/dl, usually over 1000 mg/dl, serum osmolality greater than 350 mOsm/kg, and negative serum ketones.

Laboratory Findings

A CBC, electrolytes, BUN, creatinine, glucose, serum ketones, LFTs, CPK, LDH, and osmolar levels should be drawn on every patient in whom nonketotic hyperosmolar coma is suspected. There is total body potassium loss secondary to the osmotic diuresis, and this loss is usually greater than in the patient with diabetic ketoacidosis. These patients can lose 400 to 1000 mEq of potassium.

Water loss is greater than sodium loss, thus the patient is usually hypernatremic, which results in hypovolemia and hypertonic dehydration. Serum sodium can range from 120 to 160 mEq/l. Remember that for every 100 mg/dl increase in serum glucose, the serum sodium will decrease by 1.6 mEq/l. A patient can also lose magnesium and phosphate secondary to osmotic diuresis.

The BUN is often elevated, and the ratio of BUN to creatinine can be 30:1. Often the CPK is markedly elevated secondary to the presence of rhabdomyolysis. The average osmolality level of a comatose patient is around 380 mOsm/kg.

Blood and urine cultures should also be obtained if an underlying infection is considered or if the patient is believed to be septic. On examination of the CSF, the glucose level in the CSF can be 50% of the serum glucose level.

Treatment

Any patient with an altered mental status should have two large-gauge IV lines placed with normal saline 0.9%. The patient should be placed on a cardiac monitor and given 2 liters of oxygen via nasal cannula. The aforementioned laboratory tests are drawn. A chest x-ray and an ECG should also be performed to rule out a precipitating cause of the nonketotic hyperosmolar coma.

The primary therapy for nonketotic hyperosmolar coma is correction of the electrolyte imbalance, rehydration, and reduction of the serum glucose level and the hyperosmolar state. The goal of this therapy is reduction of serum glucose to 250 mg/dl, a urine output of 50 ml/hr, and a reduction of serum osmolality to below 320 mOsm/kg in the first 36 hours of treatment. This is achieved by giving isotonic saline 0.9% or half-normal saline 0.45%. The fluid choice is made by the initial serum sodium level. If the serum sodium level is greater than 155 mEq/l, then a hypotonic solution should probably be used. The patient is usually 20 to 25% fluid depleted by 8 to 12 liters. Fluid should be given rapidly until the patient has a normal blood pressure and good urine output, and then the fluid should be slowed down. One way of replacing the water deficit is by giving 50% of the water deficit in the first 12 hours and then the remaining balance in the next 24 hours.

Potassium replacement should be at a rate that is no greater than 10 to 20 mEq/hr, and the patient should be placed on a cardiac monitor to watch for the development of hyperkalemia while the patient is receiving potassium. If the patient's magnesium level is low, then it should also be replaced.

Insulin should be given at a rate of 5 to 10 units/hr by an infusion pump. No priming dose is required. As the serum glucose approaches 250 mg/dl, glucose should be added to the IV solution. The IV insulin infusion, should not be abruptly terminated. SC insulin should be started while the patient is still on the insulin infusion.

The role of phosphate replacement is also controversial in nonketotic hyperosmolar coma as in diabetic ketoacidosis. It should be given with caution. Any patient with nonketotic hyperosmolar coma should be admitted to the ICU.

RHABDOMYOLYSIS

Definition

Rhabdomyolysis is a condition caused by injury to skeletal muscle that can lead to acute renal failure or to acute renal tubular necrosis. It can be caused by intrinsic muscle dysfunction (e.g., burns, trauma, genetic disorders, immunologic disorders, metabolic disorders, hyperthermia, drugs, infections, toxins, malignant hyperthermia, neuroleptic malignant syndrome, and conditions that cause tissue hypoxia such as sickle cell anemia or external compression etiologies).

Pathology

The skeletal muscles must have a normal functioning sarcolemma. The sarcolemma regulates myoglobin, aldolase, lactic dehydrogenase, glutamic oxaloacetic transaminase, creatinine phosphokinase, phosphorous, and potassium. The sarcolemma must also regulate sodium along with the sodium-potassium-ATPase pump. Concentration gradients regulate the intracellular and extracellular sodium and calcium ion shifts. Any trauma, drug, or metabolic abnormality that causes an increased intracellular sodium concentration or impairs the sodium-calcium exchange mechanism will elevate the intracellular calcium stores. The enzymatic proteases and proteolytics are present in the cytoplasm of the sarcolemma. It is the function of the proteases and proteolytics to myofibrillar proteins so they may be recycled into new or restructure proteins. The protease and proteolytic metabolism is dependent on the intracellular calcium levels. The more calcium present, the more disinhibited or active these enzymes become. When severe hypercalcemia is present in the cell, the increased enzyme activity can cause destruction to the cell itself.

It is believed that rhabdomyolysis is caused by direct membrane injury secondary to sodium pump dysfunction, a mismatch between the supply and demand of energy, and defective energy utilization, which leads to cellular membrane injury and sodium and calcium accumulation in the cell. Calcium accumulation in the cell, causes increased protease activity, followed by increased myofibrillar protein decomposition, then increased cell injury and eventually cell death and the release of myoglobin.

Clinical Presentation

Patients with acute rhabdomyolysis present with specific symptoms (e.g., trauma, heat injury, drug overdose). Patients can present with muscle weakness and tenderness, and swelling with discoloration of the skin; however, these symptoms are present only 4% of the time.

Patients present with four general types of complications secondary to acute rhabdomyolysis: (1) acute renal failure, (2) compartment syndrome, (3) DIC, and (4) metabolic complications; hyperkalemia;

hypocalcemia or hypercalcemia; hypophosphatemia or hyperphosphatemia; hyperuricemia; and hypoalbuminemia.

Patients can present with an acute compartment syndrome secondary to rhabdomyolysis. Ischemic changes can take place in as little as 2 to 4 hours. If the compartmental pressure exceeds 35 mm Hg, then a fasciotomy should be performed.

The main complication of rhabdomyolysis is acute renal failure. Up to 33% of patients with acute rhabdomyolysis will develop acute renal failure. Acute renal failure is secondary to decreased urine output, secondary to dehydration. The major cause of acute renal failure in the presence of rhabdomyolysis is acute tubular necrosis (ATN) with a decreased glomerular filtration rate (GFR). The ATN is secondary to increased renal vascular resistance, which causes the decrease in glomerular filtration rate and renal blood flow. The renal vascular resistance is increased by both afferent and efferent arterial vasoconstriction.

The diagnosis of ATN is made by the presence of odorless urine, with a specific gravity higher than 1.015, urine sediment; dirty brown, granular casts, urine osmolarity of less than 350 mOsm/l, osmolality, partial pressure osmolality ratio less than 1.1, urine sodium greater than 20 to 40 mEq/l, urine-plasma ratio of urea less than 4, urine-plasma ratio of creatinine less than 20. Acute renal failure can be diagnosed by:

$$\text{Renal failure index: } \frac{\text{UNa}}{\text{U/P creatinine}} > 1\text{--}2$$

There is also a tubular obstruction by myoglobin and broken-down muscle products. There is also probably some leakage of filtrate across the injured tubular cell membrane.

A patient with DIC presents with thrombocytopenia, hypofibrinogenemia, increased fibrin split products, and a prolonged PT interval. DIC is secondary to muscle necrosis and the liberation of activation substances for the injured cells, which induce the clotting of DIC.

Examination

The patient should be given a complete examination, including a neurologic examination and a rectal examination. A rectal temperature is required. Make sure to examine all extremities for compartment syndrome.

Diagnosis

A diagnosis is made by history of the following: trauma, metabolic disorders, drug abuse or use, toxin ingestion, hyperthermia or hypothermia, infections or intrinsic muscle dysfunction, elevated CK-MB five times greater than normal, elevated serum or urine myoglobin in the presence of acute renal failure or acute tubular necrosis, hyperkalemia, DIC, hyperphosphatemia, hypercalcemia, or hypoalbuminemia, or any combination of these findings.

Laboratory Findings

The serum or urine myoglobin levels are often used to diagnose rhabdomyolysis, but this test is unreliable in the case of rhabdomyolysis. The half-life of serum myoglobin is 1 to 3 hours and may be completely gone in as little as 6 hours. One hundred gm/dl are needed for staining the urine or serum for a diagnostic test.

The urine dipstick test is commonly used when the laboratory cannot obtain a serum or urine myoglobin level. This test is performed by dipping the urine with a urine dipstick. To check if the sample is positive for blood, the urine is spun and then examined. If no blood is found on microscopic examination, it is assumed that the positive dipstick test result was actually caused by the presence of myoglobin in the urine. For the result of the urine dipstick test to be positive, the serum myoglobin level must be at least 1.5 mg/dl or 100 g of muscle must be destroyed.

The creatinine phosphokinase (CK) level is more sensitive in the diagnosis of rhabdomyolysis. The CK-MB is specific for skeletal muscle and peaks within 24 to 36 hours of injury. A patient is considered to have rhabdomyolysis if the serum CK-MB level is five times the normal CK-MB value.

Hyperkalemia is secondary to the rapid destruction of muscle cells and the acute release of potassium into the plasma. As rhabdomyolysis worsens, renal failure occurs, and thus there is an even greater increase in the potassium level in the serum.

Hyperphosphatemia is secondary to the damaged cell leaking phosphorous into the plasma, much like what happens with potassium. Hyperphosphatemia causes a precipitation of calcium phosphate in soft tissues, eyes, and blood vessels, which can then lead to hypophosphatemia.

Hypocalcemia is seen in rhabdomyolysis secondary to calcium deposits in damaged cells. Do not give calcium to an asymptomatic patient with hypocalcemia because it can promote further cell injury. Hypercalcemia occurs later in the syndrome and is usually found in the presence of acute renal failure. It is also believed that there is an increased mobilization of calcium by the damaged cells as the syndrome progresses.

The release of intracellular purines from the damaged muscle cells causes hyperuricemia. There is usually an anion gap metabolic acidosis present with or without renal failure. Hypoalbuminemia is often associated with rhabdomyolysis, secondary to leakage of protein from damaged cells.

A CBC, electrolytes, calcium, magnesium, phosphorous, uric acid, CK, CK-MB, LDH, AST, ALT, GGT, ABG, and a urinalysis should be performed. If DIC is suspected, the fibrin and fibrin split products and PT and PTT should be drawn.

Treatment

Any patient who is believed to have rhabdomyolysis should have two large-gauge IV lines with normal saline started. The patient should be placed on the cardiac monitor and should get oxygen. A Foley catheter should be placed, and the aforementioned laboratory examinations should be performed.

The mainstay of therapy for acute rhabdomyolysis is the institution of large volumes of saline as rapidly as possible to prevent renal failure. A high volume of normal saline causes an increased tubular flow, which causes an increased excretion of substances that can injure or obstruct the renal tubules. The goal is to maintain urine flow at a rate of 200 to 300 ml/hr in the first 24 hours.

The urine should be alkalinized with sodium bicarbonate secondary to the toxic effects of myoglobin in an acidic urine, causing uric acid to crystallize.

Mannitol or furosemide should be given if acute renal failure or ATN is present, in the presence of decreased urine outflow, or if adequate urine outflow cannot be maintained. If the patient does not respond to therapy with fluids and diuretics, dialysis may be required. In cases of acute renal failure, patients may convert from oliguric renal failure to nonoliguric renal failure, which has a somewhat better prognosis.

DIC is treated with platelets, vitamin K, fresh frozen plasma, and heparin as needed (see the section on DIC).

Any patient with suspected rhabdomyolysis or compartment syndrome should be admitted to the hospital for treatment and observation.

THYROID STORM

Definition

Thyroid storm is seen in patients as a rare complication of hyperthyroidism. It is a condition of thyrotoxicosis that is acute and life-threatening.

Epidemiology

Thyroid storm is seen in patients with severe Graves' disease and is usually precipitated by a physical or emotional stressful event. Patients with undiagnosed Graves' disease are at the greatest risk for developing thyroid storm. Thyroid storm affects a person of any age, sex, or race equally.

Pathology

The exact cause of thyroid storm is still not completely understood. However, there is an acute production of excess thyroid hormone, which elevates T_3 and T_4, but thyroid storm can also occur without elevation of the thyroid hormones. If both thyroid hormones are acutely elevated, this suggests a causative ideology.

One theory is that there is acute adrenergic hyperactivity secondary to either patient sensitization by thyroid hormones or altered interaction between thyroid hormones and catecholamines. Norepinephrine and epinephrine levels are not increased during thyroid storm.

The second theory of thyroid storm is that there is an altered peripheral response to the thyroid hormone, which causes increased lipolysis and overproduction of heat. The excessive lipolysis is caused by catecholamine-thyroid hormone interaction, which results in excessive thermal energy and fever. This leads to exhaustion of the body's tolerance to heat and causes a decompensated thyrotoxicosis, which in turn causes an altered response to thyroid hormones rather than an acute increase in concentration.

Clinical Presentation

Patients who present to the ED in thyroid storm have usually had symptoms of hyperthyroidism for months or years. The majority have had symptoms for less than 24 months. There is usually a precipitating event that causes the thyroid storm. The most common cause of thyroid storm is surgery for hyperthyroidism. Pulmonary infection is the second most common cause of thyroid storm. In diabetics who are also hyperthyroid, diabetic ketoacidosis, hyperosmolar coma, and insulin-induced hypoglycemia are common causes.

Often the patients or family will give a history of the patients stopping the thyroid medication without or against the health care provider's advice. Alternatively, the patients intentionally overdose on the thyroid medication. Treatment of hyperthyroidism with radioactive iodide or iodinated contrast medium for radiologic testing can precipitate a thyroid storm. Pregnant patients with toxemia of pregnancy and patients with a pulmonary embolism or a vascular accident can precipitate thyroid storm.

A patient presents with symptoms of tachycardia, fever, diaphoresis, emotional lability, and increased CNS activity. Tachycardia ranges from 120 to 200 beats/min. Fever ranges from 38° C (100.4° F) to 41° C (105.8° F). CNS symptoms include anxiety, restlessness, agitation, manic behavior, psychosis, mental confusion, obtundation, and coma. CNS symptoms are present in 90% of all patients with thyroid storm.

Patients can present with a thyrotoxic myopathy that usually involves the proximal muscles. Of patients with thyroid storm, 1% will present with myasthenia gravis. These patients only partially respond to the edrophonium (Tensilon test). Patients can also present with hypokalemic periodic paralysis with thyrotoxicosis.

GI symptoms include a history of weight loss, diarrhea, and hyperdefecation, which heralds an impending storm and can be severe. Hepatomegaly and jaundice secondary to congestion of the liver or hepatic necrosis have been noted. Jaundice is a poor prognostic sign. During the thyroid storm patients can complain of nausea, vomiting, and cramping abdominal pain.

Cardiovascular problems are present in 50% of patients who present with thyroid storm, whether or not cardiac problems existed before the thyroid storm. Sinus tachycardia is the most common presenting rhythm in thyroid storm. Atrial fibrillation is the most common cardiac arrhythmia found in patients with thyroid storm. Premature ventricular contractions and complete heart block have also been noted. If pulmonary edema, congestive heart failure, and circulatory collapse occur, these are considered terminal events in thyroid storm.

Examination

The patient should be examined thoroughly to look for a precipitating event. The patient's neck should be examined to look for a surgical scar from recent thyroid surgery.

Diagnosis

The diagnosis of thyroid storm is made by the presence of marked tachycardia, a fever greater than 37.8° C (100° F), dysfunction of the GI system, CNS, or cardiovascular system, and exaggerated peripheral manifestations of thyrotoxicosis. These symptoms occur suddenly, but there may also be a prodrome prior to the thyroid storm.

In the elderly, an "apathetic" thyrotoxicosis may be found. It is frequently missed or misdiagnosed. These patients often present in coma. These patients often have a history of lethargy, slowed mentation, and placid apathetic facies. They are usually in their seventh decade of life. They present with blepharoptosis, exophthalmos, and staring facies, but lid lag is not usually found. There will be a history of weight loss and proximal muscle weakness.

Masked thyrotoxicosis refers to the condition of thyrotoxicosis in which one organ system dominates the illness. A high index of suspicion is required to diagnose this disease in older patients secondary to their apathetic response.

Laboratory Findings

A CBC, electrolytes, BUN, creatinine, glucose, LFT, cardiac enzymes, T_3, T_4, TSH, cortisol level, and urinalysis should be drawn on each patient with suspected thyroid storm. T_3 and T_4 levels are usually elevated. If radioactive iodine (RAI) is used, the uptake is very high during a thyroid storm. Some authors recommend a rapid 1- to 2-hour RAI uptake study after β-blockers have been started but before treatment with antithyroid medications and iodides. ^{99}Tc-pertechnetate as a rapid 15-minute dynamic flow study is recommended by other authors.

There is often a left-sided shift in CBC, and hyperglycemia is often present. One study found that patients with thyroid storm had low cholesterol values with a mean of 117 mg/dl.

Treatment

Thyrotoxicosis is a clinical diagnosis that must be recognized early and treated aggressively. Treatment is divided into five areas: (1) general supportive care, (2) inhibition of thyroid hormone synthesis, (3) retardation of thyroid hormone release, (4) blockade of peripheral thyroid hormone, and (5) identification and treatment of precipitating events.

1. IV fluid and electrolyte replacement is essential in the treatment. Treat the patient's fever with a cooling blanket and antipyretics. Aspirin should not be used during the thyroid storm, because salicylates increase free T_3 and T_4 levels secondary to decreased protein binding.

   Congestive heart failure should be treated with diuretics and digitalis. Atropine should be avoided, because it can counter the effects of propranolol.

   Hydrocortisone, 300 mg/day IV, should be given. Dexamethasone is also recommended in the treatment of thyroid storm, because it decreases the peripheral conversion of T_3 and T_4.

2. Antithyroid drugs propylthiouracil (PTU) and methimazole block the synthesis of thyroid hormone by inhibiting the organification of tyrosine residues. The action of PTU starts within 1 hour of administration, but it takes several weeks for complete therapeutic action. A dose of PTU is a 900- to 1200-mg initial loading dose, then 300 to 600 mg/day for 3 to 6 weeks PO.

   Methimazole can be used as an alternative therapy and should be given in a 90- to 120-mg initial dose, then 30 to 60 mg/day PO.

3. Iodide in a dose of 30 drops/day PO or sodium iodide, 1 g every 8 to 12 hours, can be given by slow IV infusion. It should be given at least 1 hour after the antithyroid medication has been given to prevent utilization of iodide by the thyroid in the synthesis of new hormone.

4. The blockade of peripheral thyroid hormone is achieved by adrenergic blocking with the use of β-blockers, such as propranolol at a rate of 1 mg/min with cautious increments of 1 mg every 10 to 15 minutes up to a total dose of 10 mg. Propranolol will control the cardiac and psychomotor manifestations usually within 10 minutes. The dose must be repeated every 3 to 4 hours. In children, a total dose of 240 to 320 mg/day may be needed. Patients with lung disease or heart block should be monitored very carefully when given a β-blocker. In patients with congestive heart failure, the risks and benefits of giving a β-blocker must be weighed.

   Reserpine and guanethidine can also be used as an alternative to propranolol. Guanethidine can be given at a dose of 1 to 3 mg/kg/day PO (50 to 150 mg) with an onset within 24 hours, but maximal effects may not be seen for days. Guanethidine depletes the catecholamine stores and blocks the release of catecholamine.

Reserpine also depletes catecholamine stores. It is given as an initial dose of 1 to 5 mg IM, then 1 to 2.5 mg every 4 to 6 hours. The therapeutic result of reserpine will be seen in 4 to 8 hours.

The average recovery time after initial therapy is 3 days or 1 to 8 days in duration. The underlying illness or disease must be vigorously looked for. These patients must be admitted to the ICU and monitored closely.

BIBLIOGRAPHY

Braunwald E, Isselbacher KJ, Petersdorf RG, et al (eds): Harrison's Principles of Internal Medicine, 11th ed. New York, McGraw-Hill, 1987

May HL, Aghababian RV, Fleisher GR (eds): Emergency Medicine, 2nd ed. Boston, Little, Brown, 1992

Rosen P, Barkin RM (eds): Emergency Medicine: Concepts and Clinical Practice, 3rd ed. St Louis, Mosby-Year Book, 1992

Schwartz GR, Cayten CG, Mangelsen MA, et al (eds): Principles and Practice of Emergency Medicine. Philadelphia, Lea & Febiger, 1992

Tierney LM, McPhee SJ, Papadakis MA (eds): Current Medical Diagnosis and Treatment, 33rd ed. Norwalk, CT, Appleton & Lange, 1994

Tintinalli JE, Krone RL, Ruiz E (eds): Emergency Medicine: A Comprehensive Study Guide, 3rd ed. New York, McGraw-Hill, 1992

Chapter 9

Neurologic Emergencies

ACUTE STROKES

Definition

A stroke is an acute loss of neurologic function of a specific region or side of a body attributed to a thrombotic, ischemic, embolic infarct or hemorrhage, which causes vascular compromise to a region of the brain.

Pathology

For the brain to function, the brain needs a constant supply of oxygen and glucose. If there is a decrease in blood supply to the brain, an ischemic event takes place.

An understanding of the blood supply of the brain is essential to understanding the stroke syndrome. Eighty percent of the brain is supplied anteriorly by the carotid arteries. The anterior blood supply supplies the deep gray matter structures, cortical areas, optic nerve, and retina. The vertebrobasilar system or the posterior system supplies the remaining 20% of the brain's blood supply. The posterior supply or vertebral arteries are branches off the subclavian arteries that enter the skull through the foramen magnum and combine near the pontomedullary junction to form the basilar artery. The posterior system supplies the brain stem, upper spinal cord, cerebellum, and parts of the deep gray matter. The anterior and posterior systems form to make the arterial circle of Willis.

The majority of strokes are caused by ischemic events secondary to a thrombotic occlusion of a vessel or an occlusion of a vessel secondary to an embolus from another site. Occlusion can also occur from external compression or from hemorrhage at the site or a mass lesion.

Thrombotic ischemia is usually secondary to atherosclerosis or vasculitis from giant cell arteritis or systemic lupus erythematosus (SLE). Any condition that increases the viscosity of blood can cause an ischemic event. Acute infections, such as syphilis or trichinosis, can cause an ischemic event. Takayasu's aortitis, aortic arch aneurysms, and arthritis of the cervical spine can cause cerebral ischemia. The most common cause of infarction is atherosclerosis from the internal carotid arteries caused by an embolism. Lacunar and small cystic infarcts are the most common form of cerebral infarctions.

A cerebral embolism is an acute occlusion of the intracranial vessels by a fragment of foreign substances originating from outside the brain. When the embolism reaches its end point in the vascular system, vascular stasis occurs and edema ensues, causing necrosis and death of the distal brain tissue. Embolisms can be made up of fat, air, and plaque. They are caused by fragments from endocarditis, infection, release of a fragment of a mural thrombus, secondary to atrial fibrillation and plaque from other arteries or veins. Transient ischemic attacks (TIAs) are usually secondary to showers of microemboli from plaques in the carotid vessels of the neck.

Risk Factors

Cerebrovascular accidents (CVAs) from thrombotic or embolic lesions occur in patients with prior TIAs, who have hypertension and evidence of atherosclerosis, cardiac abnormalities, diabetes mellitus, elevated blood lipids, smoking cigarettes, and a history of gout. TIAs are an early warning sign of impending stroke. Seventy percent of persons who have anterior circulation TIA will have another TIA or a CVA within 2 years. Aneurysm bleeding and spontaneous interparenchymal rupture are associated with a history of hypertension. Atherosclerosis has a direct correlation with CVAs and TIAs, especially if plaque is present in the carotid arteries. Bruits of the carotid arteries can be an early warning physical finding in the diagnosis of CVAs or TIAs. Carotid bruits are present in 90% of CVAs.

Patients with intermittent claudication of the lower extremities and angina pectoris are at a greater risk for a stroke. Patients with septal defects, valvular disease, thyroid disease, and chronic atrial fibrillation are at increased risk of having an embolic stroke. It has long been known that patients with diabetes are at an increased risk of stroke secondary to the ability of diabetes to accelerate hypertension, atherosclerosis, and peripheral vascular disease.

Clinical Presentation

Different strokes present with different symptoms based on the location of the CVA. Middle cerebral artery syndromes are usually secondary to an embolic event. These patients present with contralaterial hemiplegia, hemianesthesia with contralateral homonymous hemianopsia, and impaired conjugate gaze. The conjugate gaze will be opposite the lesion, and aphasia will dominate the involved side. Constructional apraxia and anosognosia of the nondominant hemisphere will be present. Arm involvement is usually greater than leg involvement. This syndrome is caused by an occlusion of the branches of the middle cerebral artery.

Posterior cerebral artery syndromes present with contralateral homonymous hemianopsia or quadrantanopsia, dyslexia without agraphia, memory loss, contralateral hemiparesis, ipsilateral third nerve palsy, contralateral hemisensory loss, and contralateral hemiplegia. This lesion is secondary to an event involving the posterior cerebral artery to the occipital cortex and the branches that supply the upper midbrain.

Transient global amnesia is caused by an acute ischemic event in the area of the hippocampus and amygdaloid. This syndrome occurs in patients who are older than 60 years of age. These patients present with an abrupt loss of the ability to recall recent events or record any new memories. Past memory is usually left intact. Speech is not affected, and the patient can perform complex tasks. Most patients recover completely, and this syndrome is believed to be a warning sign of future strokes.

Lacunar infarcts are microinfarcts of the deep gray matter and brain stem. There are four specific types of lucunar infarcts.

1. Patients presenting with a clumsy hand dysarthria syndrome secondary to a small lesion of the mid pons.
2. Patients presenting with ataxia and paresis in one leg secondary to a lesion in the pons or internal capsule.
3. A lesion of the thalamus that causes a pure sensory loss. The sensory loss is usually of the face, leg, and arm with no hemiplegia.
4. Patients presenting with pure motor hemiplegia secondary to a lesion in the pons or internal capsule present with paralysis of the face, leg, and arm. No sensory loss or aphasia is present. If left hemiplegia is present, parietal lobe findings are also present.

These patients almost always present with a history of hypertension. Therapy is directed at lowering blood pressure and aspirin therapy.

Patients with vertebrobasilar lesions present with ipsilateral ataxia, contralateral hemiplegia with sensory loss, ipsilateral horizontal gaze palsy with contralateral hemiplegia, internuclear ophthalmoplegia, vertigo, nystagmus, ipsilateral peripheral seventh nerve lesions, vomiting, deafness, and tinnitus. This lesion of the vertebrobasilar arteries is secondary to an embolic event or a narrowing of the artery secondary to atherosclerosis.

Basilar artery occlusion is secondary to an occlusion of the basilar artery and presents as a "locked in" syndrome. Patients present with quadriplegia and coma. The only motor function is upward eye gaze, which is secondary to a lesion of the tectal pons.

Patients with cerebellar infarcts present with a rapid downhill presentation. They will present with nausea, vomiting, mental status changes, dizziness, and nystagmus, and they will be unable to walk or stand if the midline cerebellar function is involved. If an acute bleed is found on a computed tomography (CT) scan or if a rapid downhill course is present, the patient will require emergency decompression of the posterior fossa.

A patient with a subarachnoid hemorrhage will present with the worst headache of his or her life without loss of consciousness. If untreated, the patient will progress to coma without lateralizing signs. The patient is usually 36 to 65 years of age. The subarachnoid hemorrhage is secondary to a rupture of a saccular aneurysm at a site of arteriolar bifurcation or branching. This patient will require a neurosurgical consultation.

Patients with hypertensive intracerebral hemorrhage present with several different presentations secondary to their location. The hemorrhage is secondary to damaged small vessels or small penetrating vessels of the brain. If the hemorrhage takes place in the putamen, the patient presents with hemianesthesia, contralateral hemiplegia, homonymous hemianopsia, hemineglect, and aphasia. Mental status changes with conscious depression will be present.

A patient with a pontine hemorrhage will present with pinpoint pupils, which are slowly reactive to light, and decerebrate posturing. The patient will rapidly progress to coma, and there will be a lack of normal oculovestibular reflexes when caloric testing is performed.

Patients with thalamic hemorrhage present with contralateral hemiparesis with contralateral hemianesthesia. The sensory loss will be greater than the motor deficit. Upward gaze is often restricted, or a skewed deviation of the eyes without a visual field defect is often present.

A patient who has a cerebellar hemorrhage will present with sudden dizziness and vomiting with marked truncal ataxia. The patient will be unable to walk or stand but will be alert and oriented. This patient will rapidly progress to a coma if not treated. Often there is an associated compromise of the ipsilateral pons, ipsilateral sixth nerve palsy, or parapontine gaze center abnormalities with fatal brain stem compression. A patient with this lesion will need immediate neurosurgical decompression.

The patient who presents with alternating symptoms has a lesion on one side that involves the cranial nerves on one side of the brain stem and sensory or motor problems on the opposite side of the body. This lesion must involve the descending tracts after they have left the cortex and the internal capsule and before they have decussated into the lower medulla.

Examination

The patient should be given a complete examination, including a neurologic examination. Vital signs are very important, especially the patient's blood pressure. The carotid arteries, temporal arteries, and abdomen should be examined for bruits. All pulses at the extremities should be palpated and checked for symmetry. The strength of the extremities should be noted, and a comparison of the left and right sides, upper and lower extremity strength, and sensory level should be annotated. The extraocular movement (EOM) of the eyes should be checked along with a good fundoscopic examination. The eyes will look toward the lesion (conjugate deviation) in a major hemisphere lesion and away from the lesion in a brain stem lesion. The main goal of the physical examination is to determine the location of the lesion and whether the lesion is secondary to an infarct or a hemorrhage. These findings will determine the type of treatment to be administered.

If aphasia and right-sided weakness are present, then the lesion must have a cortical component. If a true cortical sensory loss is present, the patient will have decreased two-point discrimination, stereognosis, or graphesthesia. If the patient has more loss of sensation on the face and arms than on the legs, then a middle cerebral artery lesion is suggested.

Always check EOMs. Remember that eyes will deviate toward the involved hemisphere and away from hemiparesis.

Subcortical lesions present with abnormal posturing, extremely dense sensory loss, and eye deviation to the side of the cortical lesion. If the left brain stem is involved, there will be right hemiplegia with cranial nerve palsies on the left side of the face. There will be abnormal cerebellar signs. The finger-to-nose and rapid alternating movement on the left side will be present. There will be weakness on the right side and nystagmus that is increased when the patient looks toward the side of the lesion.

There can be hearing loss, tongue deviation, and dysarthria. The patient will have trouble looking to the left. There can also be sensory loss on the right side of the body and sensory loss on the left side of the face.

A patient with a spinal cord lesion will present with paralysis on the same side as the lesion and loss of temperature and pain sensation on the opposite side of the lesion. Bowel or bladder problems are often present.

Left-sided hemiplegia is due to the fact that most people are dominant in the left hemisphere. The right hemisphere in most people controls the left side of the body. To test for left hemiplegia, test the nondominant or right hemisphere. If the patient fails to recognize or ignores the left side of his or her body or recognize his or her own body parts, then the left hemisphere is involved.

Diagnosis

A diagnosis is made by a history of hypertension, atherosclerosis, diabetes, clinical presentation, physical examination, CT scan of the head, and a lumbar puncture. A CT scan will visualize almost all supratentorial hemorrhages and most cerebellar hemorrhages. It will not detect small hemorrhages, and it will not see arteriovenous malformations and aneurysms in most cases. If the result of a CT scan is negative and the clinical presentation of the patient suggests a hemorrhage, then a lumbar puncture should be performed for examination of blood in the cerebrospinal fluid (CSF). Angiography is used to diagnose the presence of an arteriovenous malformation or aneurysm. Often serial CT scans or magnetic resonance imaging (MRI) will need to be performed. Pale infarcts can convert to hemorrhage when necrosis occurs. A negative result of a lumbar puncture does not rule out every intracerebral bleed. There are incidences in which the bleeding does not communicate with the subarachnoid space. If the CT scan shows blood secondary from hemorrhage, then a lumbar puncture is not required.

When a lumbar puncture is performed, the CSF is examined for red blood cells. The first and last tubes should be examined for red blood cells. If the first tube has red blood cells in the CSF, then the last tube should have none or a significant decrease in red blood cells for a normal or negative tap. If the CSF in the first and last tubes has the same or increasing red blood cell count, then it is positive for a bleed. If the bleed has been present for more than 6 hours, then the CSF should show xanthochromia.

Lumbar punctures are contraindicated in subdural hematomas, brain abscesses, mass lesions, and cerebellar hemorrhages. An MRI is more sensitive for small infarcts and pale infarcts.

Laboratory Findings

A complete blood count (CBC), electrolytes, prothrombin time (PT), partial thromboplastin time (PTT), blood urea nitrogen (BUN), creatinine, glucose, calcium, magnesium, cardiac enzymes, CPK, aspartate aminotransferase (AST), alanine transferase (ALT), lactic dehydrogenase (LDH), and urinalysis should be performed. A lumbar puncture should be performed when indicated.

Treatment

Any patient with a suspected CVA or TIA should be placed on a cardiac monitor and given 2 liters of oxygen via nasal cannula. The patient should have at least one intravenous (IV) line with normal saline started, and the aforementioned laboratory test should be drawn. An electrocardiogram (ECG) should be performed and also a CT scan or an MRI. A chest x-ray should also be performed to rule out infection.

The treatment for thrombotic and embolic strokes consists of aspirin therapy. TIAs and CVAs should be treated with aspirin. Aspirin has been shown to reduce anterior circulation TIAs and CVAs and also posterior circulation TIAs, but not posterior CVAs.

If the patient presents with hypertension, the blood pressure should not be lowered acutely unless it is above 130 mg Hg. Some authors suggest that a diastolic pressure of 120 mg Hg should not be lowered for 7 to 10 days after the stroke and then slowly to 100 mm Hg.

There is much controversy as to the use of anticoagulants in the treatment of a stroke. Some studies show that there is no increased benefit of heparin or warfarin over aspirin. Some treatment guidelines for heparin or warafrin are:

1. Treat crescendo TIAs with oral antiplatelet therapy if no surgical lesions are found on MRI or a CT scan.
2. If a stroke in progress is present, with a defined progressive neurologic involvement, and no mass or hemorrhagic lesion is present on CT or MRI, the patient should be treated with heparin.

There are current studies in the use of tissue plasminogen, strepokinase, and anisoylated plasminogen streptokinase activator complex (APSAC) for treatment of stroke, but these findings are still pending.

There is no evidence that vasodilators improve outcome, and they probably do harm in the acute stroke victim by causing hypoperfusion or an intracerebral "steal" syndrome. Corticosteroids and anticonvulsants have no benefit in treating strokes. A carotid endarterectomy is the most common surgical procedure performed for ischemic cerebrovascular disease.

The treatment for hemorrhagic stroke is quite different than for a thrombotic or embolic stroke. The mainstay of treating hemorrhagic stroke is to lower the blood pressure, if elevated, to a diastolic pressure of 100 to 110 mm Hg. The next therapeutic action is to treat the cerebral edema, which is almost always present with hemorrhagic stroke. Treatment is to prevent herniation. Progressive obtundation is often the cardinal sign of herniation. Cerebral edema is treated with mannitol or urea.

If the patient who is having a hemorrhagic stroke is on anticoagulant therapy, rapid correction of the clotting factors is necessary. Under no circumstances should a lumbar puncture be performed on a patient who is having a hemorrhagic stroke. Early neurosurgical consultation is required for such a patient. Nimodipine, a calcium channel blocker, is used at some institutions to prevent or reduce cerebral vasospasms. Nimodipine should be started within the first 72 hours of the stroke.

There is some controversy with regard to which patient to admit and who not to admit to the hospital. Often those patients with TIAs are sent home on aspirin therapy, and their work-up is performed on an outpatient basis. Any patient who is having a stroke in progress or who has underlying disease (e.g., diabetes) should be admitted to the hospital for observation and treatment.

BELL'S PALSY

Definition

Bell's palsy is a temporary paralysis of the seventh cranial nerve of unknown etiology.

Epidemiology

Bell's palsy affects males and females in equal numbers.

Pathology

Bell's palsy affects the motor fibers of the facial nerve, lacrimal gland of the eye, and stapedius muscle of the ear. The exact cause is unknown. Bell's palsy presents in three fashions. If Bell's palsy involves the nervus intermedius, taste sensation can be involved for the anterior two thirds of the tongue. If the lesion involves the forehead it has to be at the level of the nucleus of the brain stem, and sixth cranial nerve involvement is often present. If the forehead is not involved, then the lesion is a central seventh cortical lesion. The submaxillary and sphenopalatine ganglia, if involved, will affect the innervation of the salivary and lacrimal glands. If the stapedius muscle of the ear is involved, then hyperacusis to loud low tones will be present. The more proximal the lesion, the more involvement will be present.

The cause is believed to be secondary to swelling of the seventh nerve within the stylomastoid foramen secondary to a virus.

Clinical Presentation

A patient with Bell's palsy will present with an acute unilateral facial palsy that develops over 12 to 48 hours. If bilateral palsy is present, then the diagnosis of seventh nerve involvement with sarcoidosis should be considered. There is asymmetry of the patient's smile, less blinking of the eye, ptosis, and sagging of the lower eyelid. Bell's phenomenon involves the upper rolling of the eye when the patient attempts to close the lid. The corner of the mouth will droop, and there will be weakness of the platysma muscle, decreased lacrimation from the affected eye, and corneal drying. The patient will often complain of a vague numbness on the affected side prior to the onset of weakness. There is usually no sensory loss.

Examination

A complete neurologic examination should be performed, including a check of the corneal reflex. In true Bell's palsy, the corneal reflex should be intact.

Diagnosis

A diagnosis is made by clinical presentation and physical examination.

Laboratory Findings

There are no laboratory tests to rule in or rule out Bell's palsy.

Treatment

The mainstay of treatment is corticosteroids. Steroids decrease the duration of palsy and increase the speed of recovery. A dose of prednisone, 60 mg/day by mouth (PO) for 5 days then tapered by 5 mg/day over the next several days, is usually effective. The eye should be kept moist and protected and should often be taped down at night to prevent corneal drying.

BOTULISM

Definition

Botulism is a preformed toxin that is acquired from the organism *Clostridium botulinum*. This anaerobic gram-positive bacillus affects smooth and striated muscle. There are seven major toxins of botulism.

Toxins A, B, and E affect humans. Types A and B are usually from contaminated food. Type E is from fish products. There is also a form of infant botulism that is traced to the child ingesting raw honey.

Epidemiology

Botulism is acquired in the United States primarily by contaminated food sources or inadequately prepared food. Canned foods and honey are the main sources of botulism contamination. Wounds can also be infected with botulism.

Common foods sources are canned foods, potato salads, baked potato in foil, and garlic butter that is kept at near-incubation temperatures. IV drug users can also contract botulism from injecting at a contaminated wound site.

Pathology

Botulism is caused by the release of toxins by the *Clostridium* organism. These toxins inhibit the release of acetylcholine at the myoneural junction. The toxins do not affect the muscle fibers or the peripheral nerve itself. The botulism spores are very sturdy and can survive boiling for 2 hours or more. The toxin can be inactivated with boiling for 10 minutes at 80° C.

Clinical Presentation

The signs and symptoms of botulism appear within 24 to 48 hours after ingestion. Nausea, vomiting, and diarrhea are early signs of botulism. The first neurologic complaint is weakness of the eye and bulbar musculature presenting as diplopia, ptosis, and extraocular muscle weakness. A hypoactive gag reflex is often an early presenting complaint. Fixed and dilated pupils are often present. Dry mouth, dysarthria, and dysphagia are also presenting complaints. Other symptoms include a rapidly spreading weakness of the trunk and extremities with occasional involvement of the smooth muscles of the bladder and intestine. An acute ileus or urinary retention can also be the presenting complaint.

The classic presentation is one of symmetric, descending weakness with no sensory loss.

Children with infant botulism will present with failure to thrive, lethargy, and constipation that progresses to death. The presentation is often insidious.

Examination

The patient should be examined completely and should be given a neurologic examination. The patient's mental status remains good until just prior to death. Reflexes are normal or hypoactive.

Diagnosis

A diagnosis of botulism is made by finding the organism in the stool or serum or finding the spores in the contaminated food source.

Electromyograms may show decreased amplitude of muscle contraction after tetanic stimulation.

Botulism must be differentiated from Guillain-Barré syndrome, which is an ascending transverse myelitis that usually does not involve the eye musculature. A patient with Guillain-Barré syndrome will respond to the edrophonium chloride (Tensilon) test, whereas a patient with botulism will not.

Laboratory Findings

A CBC, electrolytes, BUN, creatinine, glucose, blood cultures, stool cultures with ova and parasites, and viral cultures should be performed on all suspected cases of botulism.

Treatment

Good supportive care and respiratory assistance are the mainstay of botulism therapy. Trivalent (A,B,E) antitoxin can be obtained from the local health department or the Centers for Disease Control and Prevention (CDC) in Atlanta. The trivalent antitoxin should be given as soon as the diagnosis of botulism is made.

DIPHTHERIA

Definition

Diphtheria is an infection caused by *Corynebacterium diphtheriae,* which presents as an acute peripheral muscle weakness, and as a respiratory, pharyngeal, or dermal infection.

Epidemiology

The *C. diphtheriae* organism is spread primarily by person-to-person contact. It is usually found in crowded indoor living areas. Diphtheria is rare in the United States secondary to the school-age immunization and booster programs.

Pathology

C. diphtheriae gives off an exotoxin that acts directly on the heart, kidneys, and nervous system. It is a club-shaped gram-positive bacillus organism. It affects primarily the skin and respiratory tract. The exotoxin acts to inhibit protein synthesis at the cell level, which affects all areas of the body but mainly affects the heart and central nervous system (CNS). The incubation period of diphtheria is 2 to 4 days but can range up to 8 days before signs of infection occur.

Clinical Presentation

Patients with diphtheria present with exudative pharyngitis, malaise, and fever. A patient can present with difficulty speaking secondary to soft palate involvement and changes in the voice. If the eye musculature is involved, the patient will present with ptosis, strabismus, extrinsic and intrinsic muscle weakness, and accommodation problems.

Severely ill patients present with symmetric flaccid weakness and paralysis of the extremities and absent deep tendon reflexes. Urinary retention is often present secondary to involvement of the musculature of the bladder. There may also be bowel involvement. There is usually no sensory loss.

A patient usually presents with fever, chills, sore throat, adenitis, nausea, vomiting, headache, nasal discharge, and in severe cases a "bull-neck," massive cervical edema.

Diphtheria can be limited to the nasal area. Bilateral or unilateral serous or serosanguineous discharge may be the only presenting sign, and the patient usually appears quite well.

A patient can present with cardiac problems that correlate with the degree of infection. Cardiac signs usually appear 1 to 2 weeks after infection and present as myocarditis. Cutaneous diphtheria is mostly found in the tropical regions of the world and presents as an ulcer with a gray membrane.

Examination

On examination, the patient's throat will have a gray-brown membrane covering the pharynx, with surrounding edema and cervical adenitis. The exudate is made up of leukocytes, erythrocytes, epithelial cells, fibrin, and bacteria that will cause a localized necrosis. Look for skin lesions. Always be sure to examine the nose for lesions.

Diagnosis

A diagnosis is made by culturing the *C. diphtheriae* organism from the nose, mouth, or serum.

Laboratory Findings

A CBC, electrolytes, BUN, creatinine, glucose, blood culture, throat culture, nasal culture, and urinalysis should be performed. If diphtheria is suspected, the cultures must be grown on Loeffler's or tellurite media plates. The cultures should be collected before the start of therapy with antibiotics. Thirty percent of cultures that will grow out *C. diphtheriae* will also grow out *Streptococcus.*

On the CBC, the white blood cell (WBC) count will usually be elevated, and the platelet count will be decreased. The urinalysis will show protein.

Treatment

A high index of suspicion is needed to diagnose diphtheria in the United States. Good supportive care is required. The equine serum diphtheria antitoxin should be given as soon as the diagnosis is made. The antitoxin is given as a 20,000- to 40,000-unit dose for pharyngeal or laryngeal involvement of less than 48 hours duration. A dose of 40,000 to 60,000 units is given for nasopharyngeal lesions, and 80,000 to 100,000 units are given for extensive disease or disease that has lasted for 3 days or more.

Erythromycin, 40 mg/kg/day, should be given IV for 14 days. Procaine penicillin G can also be given in a dose of 300,000 to 600,000 units intramuscularly (IM) every 12 hours for 14 days. Successful therapy is considered if the results of three successive cultures are negative.

Carriers of diphtheria should receive oral penicillin G or erythromycin for 7 days or benzathine penicillin G 600,000 to 1,200,000 units IM. A booster should be given every 5 to 10 years for diphtheria, tetanus, and pertussis (DTP), diphtheria and tetanus (DT), or tetanus-diphtheria (TD).

Any patient with suspected diphtheria should be admitted to the hospital for good supportive and respiratory care.

DIZZINESS AND VERTIGO

Definition

Dizziness is the term used to describe vertigo. Vertigo is the illusion of motion. Patients describe vertigo or dizziness as a whirling or spinning sensation. Syncope is the transient loss of consciousness with a rapid return to normal. Near syncope is often used to describe the impending loss of consciousness. Vertigo is described as central or peripheral.

Pathology

The pathophysiology of vertigo involves spatial orientation. Spatial orientation is regulated by the interaction among visual, labyrinthine, and proprioceptive systems. If any one of these systems is interrupted, the patient will complain of a disorder of sensation of position, spatial orientation, or motion.

The visual system interacts between the visual cortex, optic pathway, and eyes, which are all part of the visual-spatial orientation. The labyrinthine system is made up of the otoliths and the semicircular canals. The labyrinthine system is driven by changes in the movement of the head, which cause a change in the afferent vestibular nerve impulses. When there is an alteration of input from one of these systems, a perception of motion is noted. There are also proprioceptors in the joints and muscles of the limbs that regulate the body's sense of position.

The brain regulates the sensory input from the proprioceptors in the cerebellum, the brain stem, vestibular nuclei, the medial longitudinal fasciculus, the basal ganglia, the red nuclei, the cerebral cortex, and the temporal and parietal lobes. Vertigo can occur when one or all of the processes of these systems are interrupted. Metabolic, toxic, vascular, neuronal, or psychogenic changes can also affect these systems and thus cause vertigo.

As humans grow older, there are diminished labyrinthine hair cells, labyrinthine nerve fibers, diminished visual acuity, proprioceptive sensations, auditory sensations, and diminished integrative abilities of these systems.

Clinical Presentation

A patient with peripheral vertigo presents with an intense vertiginous or whirling feeling. Associated presenting symptoms include nausea, vomiting, sweating, diarrhea, alteration of blood pressure and pulse, and pallor. These symptoms are usually abrupt in onset, and the feeling of propulsion is very intense. In peripheral vertigo, the vertigo is influenced by changes in position and is made worse by certain positions more than others. Tinnitus is often present, and the nystagmus is fatigable. With peripheral vertigo, nystagmus is inhibited by ocular fixation.

Common causes of peripheral vertigo are vestibular neuronitis, labyrinthitis, and medications. Patients with vestibular neuronitis present with positional nystagmus and fullness in the affected ear or tinnitus. No hearing loss is present. Caloric vestibular testing is usually present in the affected ear. The exact site of the lesion is unknown but is suspected to be of viral origin. The symptoms are of acute onset, and the vertigo is made worse by certain head movements. Vestibular neuronitis can last for days or weeks.

True labyrinthitis is peripheral vertigo with hearing loss. Labyrinthitis is usually caused by a viral infection, but there are cases of bacterial labyrinthitis. If labyrinthitis is caused by a perilymphatic fistula, the patient will complain of positional vertigo that is exacerbated by sneezing, coughing, or straining, as with a bowel movement, with fluctuating hearing loss. Hennebert's sign is diagnostic for a perilymphatic fistula. It is performed by using a pneumatic otoscope. If subjective vertigo and nystagmus occur when air is blown on the tympanic membrane, it is a positive finding.

A common type of labyrinthitis is Meniere's disease. Meniere's disease presents with severe exacerbations of nausea, vomiting, prostration, and progressive deafness and tinnitus. Attacks of Meniere's disease run in clusters over time in which successive attacks of vertigo are less severe, but the deafness is progressive. The attacks progress over several minutes and last 30 minutes to 1 hour with profound diaphoresis. The attacks are believed to be caused by gross dilatation of the endolymphatic system of the inner ear. Meniere's disease presents equally in men and women in middle age.

Eighth nerve lesions also produce vertigo. They are usually secondary to acoustic schwannomas or meningiomas. The onset of vertigo is gradual and is usually preceded by hearing loss. Often the patient has an unsteady gait or ataxia secondary to involvement of the cerebellopontine angle.

Benign positional vertigo is a syndrome of symptoms that is usually brought on by a sudden change in posture or position. There is no associated hearing loss or tinnitus. It is more common in the elderly and usually lasts for seconds to minutes. Benign positional vertigo is thought to be caused by calcium carbonate crystals that have detached from the otoconia of the utricle and have fallen against the cupula of the posterior semicircular canal.

Numerous drugs can cause vertigo. Aspirin and aminoglycosides can produce vestibular neuroepithelial damage. Aspirin can cause tinnitus. Phenytoin can produce vestibular symptoms. Diuretics, non-steroidal anti-inflammatory drugs (NSAIDs), anticonvulsants, and cytotoxic agents can all cause vertigo.

Children younger than 3 years of age can develop benign paroxysmal vertigo. It occurs abruptly and is paroxysmal and self-limiting and can resolve spontaneously within months or years. The etiology is unknown.

Post-traumatic vertigo occurs after a cerebral concussion. There are two types: acute post-traumatic vertigo and post-traumatic positional vertigo. Acute post-traumatic vertigo occurs secondary to direct trauma to the labyrinthine system and presents with nausea, vomiting, and vertigo. Symptoms improve gradually and resolve in a few weeks.

Post-traumatic positional vertigo occurs days or weeks after the initial head injury and is precipitated by changes in head position. This type of vertigo resolves over months and is usually completely gone within 2 years of the injury.

A patient with central vertigo presents very differently than does a patient with peripheral vertigo. Symptoms of central vertigo are slow in onset and are not exacerbated by motion or by specific positional changes. There is no nausea, vomiting, diaphoresis, or pallor. The feeling of vertigo is less intense than in peripheral vertigo. Central vertigo is caused by disease of the cerebellum and brain stem.

A patient with central vertigo presents with signs of other brain stem pathology. Ataxia, dysphagia, dysarthria, facial numbness, diplopia, bilateral limb weakness, or bilateral visual blurring and oscillopsia are often present. The patient's hearing is unaffected, and tinnitus is absent.

The usual presentation is an acute onset of ataxia and vertigo, with or without nausea and vomiting or an acute headache. Sixth nerve palsy may be present with conjugated eye deviation to the side opposite to that of the hemorrhage. This patient is often unable to sit up, but the findings of the neurologic examination with the patient in the supine position will be normal. The patient describes the vertigo as occurring from side to side or from front to back.

Wallenberg's syndrome is a lateral medullary infarction that causes vertigo, ipsilateral paralysis of the soft palate, larynx, and pharynx, dysphonia, dysphagia, ipsilateral facial numbness and loss of corneal reflexes, ipsilateral Horner's syndrome, ipsilateral cerebellar asynergy, and hypotonia. Hiccups, nystagmus, nausea, and vomiting have been reported in sixth, seventh, and eighth nerve lesions. If present, there is contralateral loss of pain and temperature on the limbs and trunk.

Ependymomas of the fourth ventricle can cause brain stem symptoms. Multiple sclerosis (MS) can produce brain stem dysfunction and vertigo as a presenting complaint.

Psychogenic vertigo presents as a long-standing vertiginous feeling that is not caused by position or motion and presents without nausea and vomiting. Anxiety can produce vertigo characterized by disequilibrium. Disequilibrium is vertigo caused by a multiple sensory mismatch. Symptoms of disequilibrium syndrome can be increased at night secondary to decreased ambient light sources. Symptoms can be increased by unfamiliar situations or by the environment. Sedatives can also exaggerate or precipitate symptoms of disequilibrium syndrome.

Near syncope is a complaint of dizziness and is the feeling of impending syncope. All of the conditions that can cause syncope can cause near syncope. There are very few truly life-threatening causes of syncope. Syncope caused by an arrhythmia is of concern secondary to the likelihood of a recurrence of the arrhythmia.

Examination

Nystagmus is a to-and-fro movement of the eyes caused by injury to the vestibular system. It is described by the direction of the fast movement of the eyes. In peripheral vertigo, vestibular nystagmus or the rapid beating phase is away from the affected ear. A patient with peripheral vertigo will describe the spinning sensation in the direction of the fast component of the eye examination.

The three main causes of life-threatening syncope are arrhythmias, lack of glucose to the brain, and lack of oxygen to the brain. The physical examination, ECG, and laboratory examinations should be directed toward uncovering or eliminating these three causes of syncope.

Diagnosis

A diagnosis of syncope and vertigo is made by clinical presentation, history, and physical examination along with radiologic tests, an ECG, and laboratory tests.

Laboratory Findings

A simple CBC and electrolyte panel, including a BUN, creatinine, and glucose, will suffice to determine or rule in or out the metabolic causes of dizziness or syncope.

Treatment

All patients who present to the emergency department (ED) with vertigo, dizziness, near syncope, syncope, or altered mental status should have an IV line of normal saline started and should be placed on a cardiac monitor. The patient should be placed on 2 liters of oxygen and should have the aforementioned laboratory tests performed along with an ECG. A rapid glucose Dextrostix should be performed at the patient's bed side.

Antihistamines have been used for 40 years in the control of vertigo and dizziness. Antihistamines with anticholinergic properties work best on peripheral vertigo. Antihistamines work at the brain stem level, peripherally, centrally, and within the labyrinthine apparatus. Diphenhydramine, meclizine, promethazine, cyclizine, dimenhydrinate, atropine, and scopolamine can all be used in treatment of vertigo from a peripheral origin. The antimetics hydroxyzine and promethazine can be used in the treatment of vertigo. Diazepam, which is a sedative, works well on Meniere's disease. Chlordiazepoxide also works on peripheral vertigo. Calcium channel blockers such as flunarizine also work on peripheral vertigo. Remember that all medications that are used to control peripheral vertigo will worsen the symptoms of a patient with disequilibrium syndrome or ill-defined lightheadedness.

A CT scan or MRI is required if any focal neurologic abnormality is found on examination. A lumbar puncture will be required to rule out meningitis or a subarachnoid hemorrhage. All mass lesions, hemorrhage, and neoplasms will require a referral to a neurosurgeon. Any patient with a metabolic cause of vertigo should be admitted to the hospital until the electrolyte abnormality is corrected. Ensure a good follow-up plan for a patient discharged with the diagnosis of peripheral or central vertigo.

HEADACHES

Definition

Headaches can be caused by trauma, increased intracranial pressure secondary to a subdural or epidural hematoma, sentinel bleed, aneurysm, meningitis, viral or hepatic encephalitis, vascular (migraine) or tension headache, sinusitis, temporal arteritis (giant cell arteritis), brain abscess, pseudotumor cerebri, traction headache, postconcussive headache, trigeminal neuralgia, or idiopathic cranial neuralgia.

Epidemiology

Forty percent of the population have significant headaches. Ten percent will have chronic headaches.

Pathology

Pain from the area of the brain that causes an acute headache can come from sensors in the blood vessels, fat, muscle, skin, periosteum, dural arteries, falx cerebri, and large arteries of the brain's connective tissue. Remember that the arachnoid, the dura, and the pia mater are incapable of producing painful stimuli. Pain from the neck area is caused by dilatation, distention, tension, inflammation, or traction processes.

The underlying cause of migraines is the onset of vasoconstriction of the intracranial arteries, which reduces cerebral blood flow. Vaso-constriction causes an aura that is system-dependent and is based on where the vasoconstriction occurs. The vasoconstriction causes increased serotonin release, which increases interaction with tyra-mine, histamine, free fatty acids, prostaglandins, and bradykinins to produce a sterile perivascular inflammation. The serotinin levels are rapidly depleted, and then a rebound vasodilatation occurs, thus causing the headache secondary to the inflammation and distention.

Vascular headaches are often caused by a precipitating cause, such as chocolate, cheese, nuts, alcohol, air pollution, fatigue, perfumes, oversleeping, stress, vasodilators, or monosodium glutamate. In men-struating women, onset of their menstrual period can be a precipitat-ing event to a migraine.

There are four types of migraine headaches: (1) classic, (2) common, (3) ophthalmoplegic, and (4) hemiplegic. *Classic migraines* present with a sharply defined prodrome or aura. Fifteen percent of all mi-graine headaches are of this type. The prodrome or aura can last for up to 60 minutes prior to the onset of the headache. The aura is usually visual with scotomas, homonymous hemianopsia, or photo-phobia. The patient also presents with nausea, vomiting, and tingling in hands, feet, lips, mouth, or face as a prodrome. Mild aphasia can occur.

Common migraines have no sharply defined aura prior to the onset of the headache. These patients usually present with nausea, vom-iting, and throbbing unilateral pain. There is usually a family history of common migraines.

Ophthalmoplegic migraines are rare and present in young adults. They usually involve the third, fourth, or sixth cranial nerve. Oph-thalmoplegic migraines present with intense unilateral pain with a dilated pupil and the eye outwardly deviated with ptosis.

Hemiplegic migraines are rare. These patients present with unilat-eral motor or sensory symptoms of hemiparesis or hemiplegia. The symptoms can last longer than the headache, and this finding is a diagnosis of exclusion.

Cluster headaches are a form of vascular headaches seen predomi-nantly in adult males. These headaches come in clusters of severe ocular and retro-ocular pain, which lasts less than 2 hours and occurs several times a day in clusters for weeks or months.

The patient with a cluster headache presents with unilateral rhinorrhea, conjunctival injection, flushing of the forehead, and sweating. Horner's syndrome is often present. The patient will be holding the side of the head that is affected and will be rocking or pacing.

Toxic metabolic headaches are headaches that are caused by vasodilatation of pain-sensitive arteries. A lowered pain threshold is brought about by toxic substances. Foods containing tyramine, ripe cheeses, monosodium glutamate, and sodium can precipitate these headaches. These headaches can also occur when there is food or beverage withdrawal such as coffee, tea, cola, or alcohol hangover. Hypoglycemia, hypoxia, hypercapnia, indomethacin, oral contraceptives, and nitroglycerin are all causes of toxic metabolic headaches. Ascents to altitudes greater than 12,000 feet can also cause headaches. The most common cause of a toxic headache is a fever greater than 102° F.

Hypertension with a diastolic pressure greater than 130 mm Hg can cause a throbbing headache. The control of the blood pressure will resolve these headaches.

Traction headaches are headaches that are produced by traction, displacement of pain-sensitive structures, and direct pressure usually on blood vessels. Traction headaches can be divided into categories by their causes: mass lesion, subarachnoid hemorrhage, postlumbar puncture, postconcussive headaches, brain abscess, and pseudotumor cerebri.

Mass lesion headaches are caused by subdural or epidural bleeding. Subdural hemorrhage can be acute, such as with head trauma, or can be chronic, as in the elderly. Patients with an acute subdural hematoma present obtunded and often cannot complain of a headache. In the elderly, the traumatic event is often not remembered and the cause may be atraumatic.

Epidural hematomas present with a history of trauma with a brief period of unconsciousness, then consciousness with an onset of a headache. A patient will often present with a unilateral dilated pupil secondary to uncal herniation and a fracture through the middle meningeal groove with laceration of the middle meningeal artery.

Brain tumors will present with two different pain patterns. Tumors above the tentorium present with referred pain to the frontal region or vertex. Subtentorial lesions cause pain in the occipital area. Often the pain awakes the patient from sleep, and pain can be made worse by the Valsalva maneuver. Nausea and vomiting can be present, and focal neurologic changes may or may not be present.

Subarachnoid hemorrhage is caused by bleeding from an intracranial aneurysm. These patients present with the "worst headache of their life," and loss of consciousness may occur. In the younger age group, the bleed is usually from an arteriovenous malformation. On examination, meningismus may be present with the onset of vomiting, which is a sign of increased intracranial pressure. A CT scan should be performed, and if no bleed is noted, a lumbar puncture should be performed to check for blood in the CSF.

Pseudotumor cerebri (benign intracranial hypertension) is present in the obese young female who has amenorrhea or irregular menstrual periods. This patient will complain of nonspecific visual complaints with a severe headache. Papilledema will be present. On CT examination, slit-like ventricles are present without a mass effect.

Postlumbar puncture headaches are caused by leaking CSF. A patient presents with a bicranial, pulsatile, frontal headache that is made worse by standing up.

Temporal arteritis (giant cell arteritis) is a disease of inflammation. It involves the branches of the external carotid artery. The artery becomes infiltrated with lymphocytes, multinucleated giant cells, and plasma cells. It is often seen in women more than men in a 4:1 ratio. The woman is often older than 50 years of age. Often these women have polymyalgia rheumatica. They complain of a severe piercing or burning pain, which can be bilateral or unilateral and which usually occurs at night. The inflamed artery is enlarged, pulseless, and tender. A CBC and an erythrocyte sedimentation rate (ESR) should be performed. The ESR is usually greater than 50 mm/hr. A diagnosis is made from a piece of biopsied artery. The major complication of temporal arteritis is blindness.

Trigeminal neuralgia is an idiopathic neuralgia. It occurs more often in women than in men in a 2:1 ratio. These women are usually older than 50 years of age. Patients with trigeminal neuralgia present with unilateral, right-sided face pain in the third and second branches of the fifth cranial nerve. The pain is often of sudden onset; brief in duration, lasting for seconds or minutes; and often severe and lancing.

Often there are "trigger points" that exacerbate an episode. The upper eyelid, nasal labial fold, lips, certain facial movements, shaving in males, teeth brushing, or eating or drinking fluids can cause an acute attack.

Acute narrow-angle glaucoma can cause a piercing pain in and around the orbit of the affected eye. Nausea and vomiting are often present with acute narrow-angle glaucoma. The intraocular pressure will be elevated, the cornea will be edematous, and the pupil will be in the midposition. Decreased visual acuity will be present.

Other causes of headache include referred pain from the temporomandibular joint, iritis, optic neuritis, and eye strain.

Clinical Presentation

A patient who presents to the ED with a headache must be assessed as to whether he or she has a life-threatening cause of the headache. Three types of patients present to the ED with headaches: (1) the patient with chronic headaches (like migraines) who presents for pain control, (2) the patient who has never had a severe headache like this one before, and (3) the patient who has had headaches in the past and presents with a headache that differs from their usual one.

Always ask the patient whether this is the worst headache that the patient has ever had in his or her life. An easy way to determine this is to ask the patient how bad the headache is based on a scale of 1 to 10, with 10 being the worst headache of their life. It is important to determine the time of onset of the headache, the location of the headache, and the quality of the headache.

A sudden severe onset of a headache in a person who never has headaches is indicative of a serious anatomic process such as a subarachnoid hemorrhage. A history of headaches just prior to the onset of sexual intercourse or physical exercise is indicative of a subarachnoid hemorrhage. A history of any preceding events or changes in diet, drugs, or menstrual cycle is often helpful in determining the cause.

The location of the headache is also important. A headache that is gradual in onset at the same location and does not go away is suggestive of a mass lesion. Migraines are usually unilateral, and tension headaches are bilateral and circumferential in presentation.

Obtain a history of the quality of the headache. Always ask if the pain is shock-like, deep, or piercing. Throbbing headaches are usually vascular in nature like migraine headaches. Shock-like pain is seen in trigeminal neuralgia and fifth cranial nerve lesions. Deep, piercing, very intense, unilateral pain of rapid onset is seen in cluster headaches. Patients with vascular headaches present with nausea, vomiting, and anorexia.

Examination

A complete physical, mental, and neurologic examination should be performed on all patients who present with headaches. Vital signs are a great help in differentiating the type and severity of pain and headache. Tachycardia will be seen with severe pain, and hypertension is usually seen with subarachnoid hemorrhage. Always obtain the patient's temperature. Fever is seen with meningitis, encephalitis, and brain abscesses.

Always assess the patient's cranial nerves, and do a fundoscopic examination on every patient. On the fundoscopic examination, assess for papilledema, preretinal hemorrhages, exudates, and subhyaloid hemorrhages. Hypertensive encephalopathy will present with hemorrhages and exudates. Subarachnoid hemorrhage will present with preretinal or subhyaloid hemorrhages. Increased intracranial pressure will cause papilledema.

Always percuss and palpate the sinus and the scalp in the temporal areas. Tenderness over the temporal areas is indicative of temporal arteritis. Tenderness over the sinus area is indicative of sinusitis. If the patient tells you that palpation of the scalp area on examination makes the pain better, this is indicative of a tension or muscle traction headache.

Laboratory Findings

There are no specific tests to rule in or out headaches. If temporal arteritis is suspected, an ESR can be obtained. A CBC and blood cultures should be ordered if meningitis is suspected. A lumbar puncture can be performed to evaluate for infection of the CSF or to rule out a subarachnoid hemorrhage and to monitor CSF pressure.

Ancillary Tests

A CT scan can locate a mass lesion and is only 90% diagnostic in subarachnoid bleeds. An MRI is better for anatomic lesions.

Treatment

The treatment for migraine headaches is divided into four categories: general, abortive, acute, and preventive measures. In the ED, we generally treat the acute headache. There are numerous treatments for acute migraines. Give prochlorperazine (Compazine) 10 mg IV to control the nausea and vomiting. Often therapy with prochlorperazine alone will stop the headache. For treatment of the headache, give dihydroergotamine, 0.5 to 1.0 mg every 30 minutes for two doses. Meperidine hydrochloride (Demerol), 25 mg IV or 50 to 75 mg IM, or butorphanol tartrate (Stadol), 1 to 2 mg IV, can also be used for pain relief. Butorphanol tartrate also comes in a nasal form, which can be used to abort the headache or treat the onset of the headache. Ketorolac tromethamine (Toradal) is an NSAID that can be given as a 60-mg dose IM or a 30-mg dose IV for treatment of pain.

For the acute exacerbation of cluster headaches, the patient should be placed on 100% oxygen. Also 5 to 10% cocaine solution or 4% lidocaine solution can be placed into the ipsilateral nostril to abort the acute cluster headache.

The treatment of toxic metabolic headaches is the removal of the toxic substance and analgesia for pain.

Any patient with a headache secondary to a suspected mass lesion requires a CT scan or MRI and an immediate referral to a neurosurgeon.

A subarachnoid hemorrhage is treated by lowering the intracranial pressure and cerebral edema by hyperventilation and by elevation of the head of the bed by 30 degrees. Some neurosurgeons recommend the use of nimodipine to reduce arterial spasm. An urgent neurosurgical consultation is required.

Patients with suspected temporal arteritis should be treated on clinical presentation. A biopsy should not delay treatment. Treatment consists of long-term treatment with prednisone, an NSAID, and analgesia.

Pseudotumor cerebri is treated with steroids and repetitive lumbar punctures to relieve the pressure.

Postlumbar puncture can be treated with IV fluids, caffeine 500 mg IV, analgesics, or blood patch by anesthesiology. Often a short burst of prednisone, 60 mg/day for 5 days, will help to reduce the pain. The patient should be placed on bed rest for several days.

Postconcussion headaches are treated with an NSAID, and they are usually self limiting.

Trigeminal neuralgia is treated with analgesic medications. Outpatient therapy is treated with carbamazepine, 100 to 200 mg three times a day (TID). If this treatment fails, neurosurgical consultation is advised for progressive sectioning of the sensory nerve roots.

MULTIPLE SCLEROSIS

Definition

MS is a demyelinating disease that expresses itself as focal or patchy destruction of the myelin sheaths of the CNS, in the presence of an inflammatory process. Symptoms of MS wax and wane over a period of time and are referable to separate areas of the CNS.

MS is diagnosed as the presence of a predominantly white-matter disease involving two areas or more of the CNS, with two separate episodes or more, each lasting greater than 24 hours, and at least 1 month apart, in a progressive course over at least 6 months, with onset between the ages of 10 and 50 years.

Epidemiology

MS rarely develops before 20 years of age or after 50 years of age. Women develop MS 1.8 times more often than do men, and whites are twice as likely to develop MS as are blacks. There is a 15- to 20-fold likelihood that a first-line relative with MS will have a family member with MS. Only 30% of patients with MS develop a progressive course of the disease that predominantly involves the spinal cord. It is estimated there are 123,000 persons in the United States who have MS. The disease is uncommon in Asians. MS is more common in the northern and southern temperature latitudes than in the equatorial regions.

Pathology

It is believed there are numerous genetic and environmental causes or combinations of factors that cause MS. In MS, the conduction of the nerve impulses are slowed secondary to the presence of plaques. The plaques are scattered in areas of white matter in the CNS and are usually concentrated in the periventricular areas of the cerebrum, brain stem, spinal cord, and optic nerve.

Clinical Presentation

MS is known as the great imitator. MS can present in a variety of ways. The first episode presents with more than one sign or symptom in 55% of the cases. The first, or most common, presentation is optic neuritis in 10 to 30% of the cases. The most common complaint of optic neuritis is loss of central vision and pain with movement of the globe of the eye. Often a patient with known MS presents to the

ED with the complaints of an elevated temperature, a urinary tract infection, decubitus ulcers, or pneumonia as a complication of the neurologic lesions. Patients also present with complaints of nystagmus, vertigo, internuclear ophthalmoplegia, trigeminal neuralgia, Lhermitte's sign, ill-defined sensory symptoms, and diplopia secondary to sixth nerve paresis. A patient will often present with vomiting, nystagmus, and vertigo when the MS lesions are near or involve the vestibular complex.

If the lesions involve the spinal cord, in particular the corticospinal tracts, patients will present with upper motor neuron dysfunction presenting as clonus, hyperreflexia, spasticity, paresis, a Babinski response, and abnormal reflexes. If the patient's hand appears useless with no motor or sensory function, this dysfunction is secondary to a lesion at the lateral portion of the posterior column of the spinal cord. These patients will also lack two-point discrimination, vibratory sense, and joint position.

If spinothalamic tract involvement is present, the patient will have diminished pain and temperature sensation. If true cord lesions are present, the patient will complain of Lhermitte's sign: tingling down the back, into the legs, in an electric shock-like pattern.

A patient can present with dysautonomia of the gastrointestinal tract, vesicourethra, and sexual dysfunction secondary to lesions of the corticospinal tracts. Vesicourethral dysfunction can include the inability to store urine, empty the bladder, or a detrusor-external sphincter dyssynergia problem. The presence of a vesicourethral problem is a poor prognostic sign. There is an increased risk of death from pyelonephritis, septicemia, and hydronephrosis in patients with MS.

Five percent of patients with MS will present with cerebral MS, which presents as depression. If the patient presents with euphoria, this is a sign of widespread cerebral disease, dementia, and pseudobulbar palsy. Five percent of patients with MS will eventually have seizures.

Patients with MS can exacerbate their systems with exercise or any activity that will raise the body's temperature. Hyperthermia causes an increased blocking of a nerve impulse in the demyelinated nerve.

Examination

A good fundoscopic examination should be performed in any patient suspected of having MS. If optic neuritis is present, and if the lesion is anterior in the nerve, the optic disk will be swollen (papillitis) and may be indistinguishable from papilledema. If the lesion of demyelination is posterior, such as in retrobulbar optic neuritis, the disk will appear normal. As the disease progresses, optic nerve atrophy will occur and the disk will have an abnormal pallor. Optic neuritis can precede the onset of MS by 10 to 35 years.

Always check for diplopia and EOMs of the third, fourth, and sixth cranial nerves. If acute bilateral internuclear ophthalmoplegia is present in a young adult, secondary to a bilateral medical fasciculus, this finding is diagnostic of MS. This ophthalmoplegia is described as the presence of a coarse nystagmus when the patient attempts to gaze to one side. The abducting eye is unable to move beyond the midline, at which time a coarse nystagmus occurs, but convergence is preserved in most cases.

Always examine all of the cranial nerves, including the cranial nerve involving smell. Lesions of the brain stem usually affect the third, fifth, seventh, and eighth cranial nerves. If the fifth nerve is involved, there will be unilateral facial numbness, pain, or paresthesia. If the seventh nerve is involved, there will be a unilateral facial palsy with no change in taste. A patient can also present with tic douloureux–like symptoms of paroxysmal unilateral facial pain without sensory loss.

Diagnostic Tests

An MRI is the best test for imaging the lesions of MS. On MRI, there will be multiple discrete lesions on the supratentorial white matter, especially on the periventricular areas. The MRI is 70 to 90% specific for MS lesions. In a questionable lesion, gadolinium contrast can be used to enhance the lesion.

Evoked-response testing can be used to measure the electrical response to stimulation in a sensory pathway. It shows slowed conduction in the auditory, somatosensory, and visual areas. A slowed evoked response will be present 80% of the time in one of these areas.

Diagnosis

It may be impossible to diagnose MS in its early stages secondary to its multiple presentations and the changing clinical course of the disease. MRI should be performed on any patient suspected of having MS. A diagnostic lumbar puncture should be performed to evaluate the CSF for infection, protein level, and CBC level. WBC counts greater than 50 cells/mm^3 are rare in the CSF. WBCs, if present, are T lymphocytes. CSF protein will be increased in 25% of patients with MS. An increased level of immunoglobulin G (IgG) in the CSF is diagnostic for MS, secondary to an increased synthesis of IgG in the CNS. The sensitivity of the test can be enhanced by measuring the IgG and albumin in the CSF and by using a formula to determine the CSF IgG index:

$$\text{CSF IgG index} = \frac{\text{CSF IgG/CSF albumin}}{\text{Serum IgG/CSF serum albumin}}$$

An index greater than 0.77 is found in 80 to 90% of patients with MS.

Laboratory Findings

A CBC, electrolytes, BUN, creatinine, glucose, drug toxicology screen, liver function tests, culture of spinal fluid, human immunodeficiency

(HIV) test, rapid plasma reagin (RPR), or Venereal Disease Research Laboratory (VDRL) should all be performed.

Treatment

The main concern with a patient who presents to the ED with MS is to determine if the presenting symptoms are caused by MS or another illness or disease. Diseases that can mimic MS are SLE, myasthenia gravis, ankylosis, brain tumors, ulcerative colitis, thyroid disease, diabetes mellitus, scleroderma, migraines, Lyme disease, neurosyphilis, HIV, cobalamin deficiency, and cancer.

The primary reason why a patient with MS presents to the ED is secondary to his or her co-complaints of UTI or bowel or respiratory problems.

The treatment of MS is directed at slowing the progression of the disease, amelioration of an acute exacerbation, and relief of symptoms. If a patient with MS presents to the ED with an acute symptomatic exacerbation of MS, the patient should be given a pulsed IV dose of methylprednisone 500 mg for 5 days, followed by a tapered dose of oral prednisone for 3 weeks. Daily or alternate-day steroids should not be given as long-term therapy for symptoms of MS.

Azathioprine or cyclophosphamide are immunosuppressive medications that are used to slow the process of the disease. These drugs should only be given under the direction of the patient's neurologist.

The primary complaint that the health care provider in the ED will encounter in the patient with MS are urinary complaints. A urinalysis and urine culture should be performed on all patients with MS who present to the ED. If the post-voiding residual urine is greater than 100 ml or more than 20% of voided urine, the patient should probably be performing intermittent catheterization by clean technique to prevent infection. Often, the patient with MS who has an acute UTI will be asymptomatic. Any patient with MS who presents with a fever, back pain, or abdominal pain should be considered to have a UTI. Any patient with MS and a UTI should be ensured good follow-up. If follow-up is not ensured, the patient should be admitted to the hospital for treatment.

All patients with MS should be referred back to their primary neurologist for follow-up care.

MYASTHENIA GRAVIS

Definition

Myasthenia gravis is an autoimmune disease that causes a defect in the transmission of acetylcholine across the neuromuscular junction. The patient presents to the ED in a myasthenic crisis.

Epidemiology

Myasthenia gravis is a rare disease that can affect anyone from infancy to old age. There is a transient form of the disease found in neonates. Neonatal myasthenia gravis occurs from a passive transfer of antibodies from the mother to the neonate. The symptoms resolve as the antibodies clear from the neonate.

Pathology

When a neuromuscular junction is discharged, acetylcholine is released by the nerve endings and migrates across the junction to the acetylcholine receptor on the muscle membrane. When enough acetylcholine is bound, then muscle activity is initiated. In the presence of excess acetylcholine, acetylcholine esterase destroys any excessive acetylcholine present. Myasthenia gravis is a condition in which autoimmune antibodies are working against the acetylcholine receptors and prematurely destroy the receptors. This leaves the neuromuscular sites with fewer and fewer binding sites. Thus, there is a build-up of acetylcholine. Weakness and fatigue of muscles occur, secondary to the inability of the muscles to precipitate muscle contractions, secondary to the lack of acetylcholine esterase. For an unknown reason, there are often associated abnormalities of the thymus. Thymic hyperplasia or thymoma is often present.

Clinical Presentation

A patient with myasthenia gravis presents with skeletal muscle weakness and fatigue in which the weakness and fatigue increase with muscle use. The most common presenting symptoms are ptosis, diplopia, and blurred vision, often in just one eye. In severe disease, jaw weakness, dysarthria, and dysphagia can be the presenting complaints. If neck muscles are involved, the head can drop or droop forward. The weakness and fatigue are asymmetric, and limb muscles are more involved than are cranial muscles. Respiratory insufficiency can be present and can be fatal.

Examination

The patient should be given a complete examination, including a complete neurologic examination.

Diagnosis

A rapid bedside test for myasthenia gravis is the ice pack test. An ice pack should be applied to the affected eye. If the ptosis improves after moderate cooling with an ice pack to the eyelid, it is suggested that ptosis is caused by myasthenia gravis. A drug test using 1 to 2 mg of edrophonium may be given for muscle fatigue, and if improvement is seen, the diagnosis of myasthenia gravis should be entertained.

A history of use of cardiovascular drugs, antibiotics, hormones, and neurologic and psychotropic drugs should be obtained. β-Blockers, aminoglycosides, tetracyclines, thyroid hormone replacement medications, phenytoin, lithium, timolol, chloroquine, muscle relaxants, and steroids have all been linked to myasthenia gravis. If the patient is taking one of these medications, the medication should be stopped.

Laboratory Findings

No specific laboratory tests are available for myasthenia gravis.

Treatment

Patients present to the ED with two types of myasthenia crisis. The first presentation is one of acute muscle weakness secondary to inadequate acetylcholine-acetylcholine receptor action. The second presentation is one in which the patient's muscle fibers remain depolarized after firing or the patient is in cholinergic crisis, and this is secondary to overtreatment with acetylcholine esterase inhibitors. Patients with an acute cholinergic crisis present with muscarinic effects of small pupils, sweating, lacrimation, salivation, tachycardia, and gastrointestinal hyperactivity.

The immediate concern in both types of crisis is respiratory depression, secondary to chest wall muscle weakness. If the patient has acute muscle weakness, give edrophonium 1 to 2 mg IV. This will increase muscle tone if the patient is not already into crisis. If there is no change, give the patient 8 mg of edrophonium IV up to a total of 8 mg. This treatment can also be used as a test to diagnose myasthenia gravis. Any patient on a medication that can induce myasthenia gravis should discontinue the medication at once.

Acetylcholine cholinesterase inhibitors are the mainstay of treatment. A typical treatment is to give pyridostigmine, 60 mg every 4 to 6 hours. The dose range has not been established. In severe cases, prednisone can be given in a dose of 50 to 100 mg every other day.

A thymectomy should be performed if disease is present. This procedure has shown long-term benefits in the treatment of myasthenia gravis.

Patients with myasthenia gravis are resistant to succinylcholine and can take up to three to five times the normal dose to be effective in paralyzing a patient. Use 1.5 to 2 mg/kg of succinylcholine to paralyze a patient with myasthenia gravis.

THE NEUROLOGIC EXAMINATION

The neurologic examination should be systematic, and the examination should answer two questions: "Where is it?" and "What is it?" The former question refers to the location, cerebral hemisphere, brain stem, cerebellum, spinal cord, or peripheral nerve. The latter question refers to the historical mechanism by which the nervous system is compromised.

HISTORY

Always determine if the compromise or change in neurologic status was gradual or rapid in onset. Rapid changes are usually vascular in nature. An example of a vascular compromise is a TIA. A TIA is a warning of a pending stroke.

If you cannot obtain a history from the patient, obtain a history from the patient's family or health care provider. If there is a history of a progressive decline of mental status or neurologic function, then the compromising process is a chronic, degenerative disease or a chronic, dementing process. Patients with a history of a sudden decline of mental status over 2 to 3 days should be considered to have a subdural hematoma. Patients whose mental function fluctuates should be considered to have underlying metabolic, electrolyte, or drug-induced neurologic changes. In the elderly population, people often overmedicate themselves or are victims of dehydration or toxic metabolic conditions.

MS presents with rapid multiple focal, nebulous neurologic changes. The neurologic changes will not relate to a single anatomic site.

EXAMINATION

The neurologic examination should consist of a mental status examination, a cranial nerve examination, a motor and sensory examination, a complex motor or cerebellar examination, a gait or station examination, and an examination of deep tendon reflexes and plantar response.

Mental Status Examination

A mental status examination tests the patient's ability to relate to both the environment and to himself or herself. The patient's level of consciousness, or arousal level, should be tested. In most people, the right side of the brain is the nondominant side and is responsible for sound localization, spatial orientation, and body self-imaging. The left side of the brain, or dominant side for most people, is responsible for mathematical ability, speech, and communication skills.

In order to test the level of consciousness, test the patient's language ability by testing his or her grammar, word choice, and comprehension. Ask the patient to write a sentence, name objects, follow a written command, and read. Test the patient's memory by testing his or her past and recent memory. Use digit span testing repetition of three objects and serial sevens. Test new or recent memory by asking the patient to name three items, and then ask the patient to repeat those three items in 5 minutes. Amnesia is the inability to make new memory. To test higher memory, ask the patient to draw a clock and pentagons, and ask the patient to interpret proverbs, do calculations, and make judgments.

Cranial Nerve Examination

A cranial nerve examination is a test of cranial nerves II through XII, but mainly nerves II through VII.

I—*Olfactory,* involves smell.

II—*Optic,* involves vision and intact reception for pupillary response. Test with a vision chart and visual field testing.

III—*Oculomotor,* involves the levator, and palpebral muscles; the superior, inferior, and medial rectus muscles; and intact motor outflow for pupillary response. Check the midbrain and pontine function by testing EOMs.

IV—*Trochlear,* involves the contralateral superior oblique muscle connected with downward rotation of the eye. Test the midbrain and pontine function by checking EOMs.

V—*Trigeminal,* involves the sensory functioning of the ophthalmic, maxillary, and mandibular areas; also the anterior two thirds of the tongue (sensory). Test by placing a wisp of cotton on the cornea to check the cornea–reflex.

VI—*Abducens,* involves the lateral rectus muscle of the eye and eye movement laterally away from the midline. Check the midbrain and pontine function by testing EOMs.

VII—*Facial,* involves the motor movement of the three branches: frontal (forehead), maxillary (cheek area), and mandibular (jaw area). Test by asking the patient to smile and to show his or her teeth or have the patient squeeze the eyes tightly and then tell the patient to open the eyes against resistance. Also have the patient purse the lips together as to whistle. Upper motor neuron lesions are characterized by unilateral weakness of the lower half of the face, whereas peripheral lesions involve the entire half of the face.

VIII—*Acoustic,* involves the vestibular nerve connected with equilibrium and the cochlear nerve connected with hearing. Test both the vestibular and cochlear parts of the nerve for balance and hearing.

IX—*Glossopharyngeal,* involves the posterior half of the tongue (motor), middle ear sensation, and the parotid gland. Ask the person to stick out his or her tongue and watch for drift. The tongue will *drift toward the lesion.*

X—*Vagus,* involves the motor of the oral pharynx, epiglottis, and superior laryngeal nerve. Ask the person say "AA."

XI—*Spinal accessory nerve,* involves the motor nerve of the sternomastoid muscle and trapezius muscles. Test by asking the patient to shrug the shoulders.

XII—*Hypoglossal,* involves the motor movement of the tongue.

Motor Examination

A motor examination involves the testing of strength, muscle tone, and symmetry of tone. To test muscle tone, ask the patient to lie down and lift the patient's knee up quickly. If the patient drags the heel of the foot along the bed, there is normal tone. If the foot and leg come up as a unit, then there is increased tone. Another test is the pronator drift test. Ask the patient to stand with both arms raised and hands with the palms up and eyes closed. Look for a downward movement of one of the arms. You can also ask the patient to walk on his or her heels and toes. This action requires intact muscle tone and strength.

Sensory Examination

A sensory examination is conducted by first asking the patient to draw out or describe the area of sensory loss. If the patient presents with a stocking or glove pattern of decreased sensation, peripheral nerve lesions should be considered. If the patient presents with an upper extremity deficit with a cloak-like area across the chest, consider a spinal cord lesion secondary to syringomyelia. Central cord lesions of the cervical cord can also present with a cape-like distribution. Entire sensory loss below a central point is indicative of a spinal cord lesion.

Brown-Séquard's syndrome, which involves a lesion high in the CNS before entering the brain stem, has partial cord involvement and a mixed sensory presentation. The patient presents with complete sensation on one side of the body. If a patient presents with a facial finding on one side and a lower body finding on the other side—this is indicative of a brain stem lesion.

Complex Motor or Cerebellar Examination

A complex motor or cerebellar examination involves the Romberg test, which is used to test the patient's cerebellar coordination. Ask the patient to stand with arms to the side, eyes open, and feet together. If the patient has trouble standing with his or her eyes open, then the problem is related to cerebellar coordination. Ask the patient to stand in this manner and then close his or her eyes. If the patient has trouble standing in this manner with the eyes closed, and if the patient has no trouble standing in this manner with the eyes open, then there is a problem with sensation or an abnormal position sense. If a patient has a problem standing with the eyes closed, this is usually indicative of a posterior column function.

Gait or Station Examination

A gait or station examination is also an examination of the patient's cerebellar function. To test the patient's gait, ask the patient to walk and observe the patient's gait. If the gait is wide-based, then there is usually a cerebellar dysfunction. To test peripheral cerebellar function, use the finger-to-nose test. Ask the patient to touch the end of his or her nose with the index finger and then touch your index finger as rapidly as possible. If oscillation occurs a few inches from the target finger, then there is an abnormal peripheral cerebellar function. A patient who has trouble sitting up in bed without help usually has a midline cerebellar dysfunction or lesion.

Deep Tendon Reflexes and Plantar Response Examination

Deep tendon reflexes and plantar response examination is a test of the symmetry of reflexes. Abnormal symmetry is usually a finding of a lateralizing lesion high in the CNS. If there is a difference in reflexes between the upper and lower extremities, this is indicative of a spinal cord lesion. If the reflexes are depressed in only one extremity and all other extremity reflexes are symmetric, this suggests a peripheral nerve root lesion.

The Babinski reflex is a pathologic reflex indicative of the higher cortical centers of primitive stereotype responses. The Babinski reflex is elicited by stroking the lateral aspect of the foot with any metal object. The normal response is curving of the toes; fanning of the toes is abnormal. Be aware that a significant number of patients have a normal toe fanning response.

OTHER TESTS

Any patient with neurologic changes should have a CBC drawn to rule out anemia or a low hematocrit (HCT) and hemoglobin. They should also have a potassium, sodium, chloride, CO_2, BUN, creatinine, glucose, amylase, lipase, and liver function tests to include AST, ALT, gamma glutamyltransferase (GGT), total protein, and bilirubin drawn to rule out metabolic causes of neurologic changes. Remember that the primary cause of mental status changes or agitation in the ED is hypoxia. Always obtain a pulse oximetry or an arterial blood gas value on every patient who presents with mental status changes. Always get a history of thyroid problems, and, if present, obtain a thyroid panel.

SEIZURES AND STATUS EPILEPTICUS

Definition

Seizures are abnormal episodes of neurologic function caused by abnormal electrical discharge of the neurons in the brain. Epilepsy is a condition in which recurrent seizures occur. Seizures are divided into two categories: primary or idiopathic and secondary or symptomatic. Primary seizures are seizures that occur in persons in whom no underlying cause can be found to cause the seizure. Secondary seizures are caused by an identifiable neurologic condition.

Seizures are classified as grand mal, petit mal, and psychomotor. They are also classified by the League Against Epilepsy as generalized or focal seizures.

Epidemiology

Seizure or epilepsy affects 1 to 2% of the population. Ten percent of the population will suffer a seizure at least once in their lifetime. The mortality rate of true status epilepticus is 20%. Thirty to 70% of patients presenting to the ED with a seizure will have another seizure within 1 year.

Pathology

Generalized seizures are caused by electrical discharge originating deep in the brain and spreading outward until the entire cerebral cortex is simultaneously activated by this electrical discharge.

Clinical Presentation

Patients with generalized seizures present with a true abrupt loss of consciousness. They may have a seizure, jerking movements, or no motor movement of any kind. If there is a motor function deficit present, as in generalized seizure activity, it usually involves all four extremities. The motor function may manifest itself as myoclonic jerks, drop attacks, or clonic jerking of the body or extremities with or without tonic posturing. Patients with generalized seizures may complain of a prodrome that lasts for several hours prior to the seizure, including a feeling of tension, irritability, or isolated myoclonic jerks. Remember that true sensory auras are not present in generalized seizures.

Petit mal seizures last only for a few seconds with the patient presenting with the complaint or presentation as "out of contact" with the world. The patient does not respond to verbal communication and can stare without verbal response or have twitching of the eyelids. There is no loss of continence or involuntary movements in petit mal seizures. Petit mal seizures can occur 100 times or more a day. They are often found in school-aged children and are attributed to daydreaming by parents and teachers.

Grand mal seizures are the seizures that most people are familiar with. The patient becomes suddenly rigid with the onset of abrupt loss of consciousness. True auras do not occur, and there is usually no early warning sign. There is often urinary and bowel incontinence. The initial event will leave the patient cyanotic. The rigid phase, or tonic phase, is the first phase. After the tonic phase, the onset of the rhythmic clonic jerking ensues. The third phase will leave the patient flaccid and unconscious with deep rapid breathing. The fourth phase is a postictal phase in which the patient recovers from the attack and is awake but is "tuned out." The typical seizure lasts 60 to 90 seconds. Bystanders will often give a history of the seizure lasting much longer. The postictal phase can last from minutes to hours.

Focal or partial seizures are caused by an acute electrical discharge in a localized region of the cerebral cortex. Focal seizures can remain focal or can become generalized to encompass the entire cerebral cortex, thus becoming a generalized seizure. The presence of focal seizures often implies a focal structural lesion of the brain. Seizures localized to one extremity or side of the body originate from a lesion in the motor cortex. Patients with frontal lobe lesions present with tonic deviation of the head and eyes away from the side of the lesion. Patients with sensory cortex lesions present with sensory hallucinations, paresthesias, or numbness. Patients with occipital lesions present with flashing lights and distortions of vision. Patients with medial temporal lobe lesions present with olfactory hallucinations of smell. Patients with true auras present with focal seizures only, not generalized or petit mal attacks.

Temporal lobe seizures are complex partial seizures and present as focal seizures in which consciousness and changes in mentation occur. These seizures are also called psychomotor seizures and are quite common. These seizures present with bizarre symptoms that often have psychic components. Psychomotor seizures are often misdiagnosed as psychiatric problems. The main component of these seizures involves hallucinations, dream-like states, affective disorders, automatisms, visceral symptoms, and memory disturbances. The hallucinations can involve smell, taste, vision, or hearing. Objects can change shapes, color, and size, and changes in perception can occur. Déjà vu and jamais vu can occur.

Automatism movements are repetitive, purposeless movements of short duration. Patients can present with an affective disorder that mimics paranoia, depression, and rarely ecstasy or elation.

Examination

The patient should be given a complete examination, including a complete neurologic examination. An examination of the head for trauma should always be performed in a postictal patient. Examine the patient's extremities to rule out fractures or sprains. Pay particular attention to any focal changes of weakness or reflex changes or sensory changes.

Diagnosis

The key to diagnosing what type of seizures that the patient presents with is the history of the seizure. Migraine headaches, syncope, narcolepsy, cataplexy, hyperventilation syndrome, fugue states, rage attacks, TIAs, psychogenic seizures, and paroxysmal vertigo can all imitate seizure activity.

Questions to ask are: Did the patient have an aura? Was there motor movement, and how or where did it start? Was the patient postictal, and does he or she remember the postictal state? How did the attack start, and how did it end?

A CT scan should be performed on anyone who presents with his or her first seizure, especially in adulthood, to look for a structural lesion. This CT scan should be done both with and without contrast to rule out metastatic or primary tumors or vascular anomalies. If

MRI is available, it should be used instead of a CT scan. It is better at detecting subtle changes in the brain.

The electroencephalogram (EEG) is used to evaluate and diagnose the presence of epilepsy. The EEG records changes and can help to distinguish focal seizures from generalized seizures.

Laboratory Findings

There are no particular laboratory tests to predict or prove that an episode was a seizure. A CBC, electrolytes, BUN, creatinine, glucose, calcium, magnesium, and a toxicology screen should be obtained on anyone who presents with his or her first seizure to rule out metabolic causes of the seizure. If the patient is on anticonvulsant medication, a serum level should be drawn.

Treatment

Any patient who presents to the ED with a possible seizure should have two large-gauge IV lines of normal saline started, and the patient should be placed on 2 liters of oxygen via nasal cannula. The patient should be placed on a cardiac monitor and have a glucose check performed. The aforementioned laboratory examinations should be performed. The first problem in treating a patient presenting to the ED with a possible seizure is to determine if the patient really had a seizure. Remember that alcoholics fall down, strike their heads, then have seizures. Always perform a good physical examination, which should include a good neurologic examination and examination of the head for signs of trauma or alcohol abuse.

Try to determine the underlying cause of the seizure to include hypoglycemia, head trauma, metabolic acidosis, hyponatremia, and hyperosmolar states. Determine if the patient is on anticonvulsant medication and if the patient has been compliant with his or her medication regimen. Often the patient has run out of medication for several days or weeks or is trying to wean himself or herself off of the medications. Try to determine if the patient has used or increased use of alcohol, has had sleep deprivation, or changes in medication. Always determine if this is the patient's first seizure, or if this seizure is different from the patient's usual seizure.

If the patient is actively seizing upon arrival in the ED, use gentle restraints and protect the patient's tongue, extremities, and airway.

If this is the patient's first seizure, the work-up will be more extensive, especially if the onset of seizures is in adulthood versus a febrile seizure in a 9-month-old child or a patient with a long-standing history of seizures. There is controversy as to when one should be started on anticonvulsants after the first seizure. Thirty to 70% of patients who present to the ED with a seizure will have another seizure within 1 year. The decision to start a patient on anticonvulsant medication should be made along with the consent and consultation with the patient's primary care provider.

All adult patients with new-onset seizures require a head CT scan to rule out mass lesions or intracranial bleeding. Any patient who is having seizures due to withdrawal from alcohol should be treated accordingly and admitted to the hospital.

A patient presenting with status epilepticus, or seizure activity occurring every 20 to 30 minutes, must be treated aggressively. A patient can die of cardiovascular collapse, anoxia, renal failure, and trauma if not treated within 1 hour of onset of seizure activity. A permanent neurologic deficit can occur within 1 hour of the start of seizure activity if it is not controlled.

Patients in status epilepticus need good airway control. Treatment is in a stair-step manner. After the aforementioned safety net precautions are established, perform the following in a step-wise manner:

Give: Glucose, 25 to 50 g IV
　　　Thiamine, 100 mg IV

Give for seizure control:
　　　Diazepam, 5 mg IV; repeat every 5 minutes until 20 mg are given; *or*
　　　Lorazepam 5 mg IV until 0.1 mg/kg is given

Give after diazepam or lorazepam:
　　　Phenytoin 18 mg/kg IV at 25 mg/min

If phenytoin does not work give:
　　　Phenobarbital 100 mg/min IV to a total of 100 mg/kg or until the seizure activity stops

If this dose does not stop the seizure activity give:
　　　Phenobarbital 50 mg/min to a total of 20 mg/kg (including the previous loading doses)

If this dose does not work give:
　　　Phenobarbital 50 mg/min to a total of 30 mg/kg (including the previous loading doses)

If this regimen does not work, consider general anesthesia, a diazepam drip, or barbiturate coma. The major concern with barbiturate use is respiratory depression and hypotension.

Pancuronium and vecuronium are often useful in refractory status epilepticus. Both these drugs will stop the tonic-clonic movements and will assist in ventilating the patient. Remember that these drugs do not stop the abnormal neural activity. Patients in status epilepticus who are paralyzed will require EEG monitoring to determine when the neural seizure activity stops.

Most patients with a history of seizures can be sent home on the correct dose of anticonvulsant medication. A loading dose of their seizure medication can be given in the ED with good follow-up care.

Any patient with new-onset seizures, with a mass lesion, or intracranial bleed should be admitted to the hospital for further examination. All patients with seizures due to alcohol withdrawal should be admitted to the hospital for treatment.

COMMON ANTICONVULSANT MEDICATIONS

Phenytoin   300–400 mg/day, used for tonic-clonic and partial seizures

Carbamazepine   800–1200 mg/day, used for tonic-clonic and partial seizures

Ethosuximide   750–1000 mg/day, used for absence seizures

Phenobarbital   90–120 mg/day, used for tonic-clonic and partial seizures

Primidone   150–1000 mg/day, used for partial seizures

Valproic acid   750–1000 mg/day, used for myoclonic, absence, and partial seizures

BIBLIOGRAPHY

Braunwald E, Isselbacher KJ, Petersdorf RG, et al (eds): Harrison's Principles of Internal Medicine, 11th ed. New York, McGraw-Hill, 1987

May HL, Aghababian RV, Fleisher GR (eds): Emergency Medicine, 2nd ed. Boston, Little, Brown, 1992

Rosen P, Barkin RM (eds): Emergency Medicine: Concepts and Clinical Practice, 3rd ed. St. Louis, Mosby-Year Book, 1992

Schwartz GR, Cayten CG, Mangelsen MA, et al (eds): Principles and Practice of Emergency Medicine. Philadelphia, Lea & Febiger, 1992

Tierney LM, McPhee SJ, Papadakis MA (eds): Current Medical Diagnosis and Treatment, 33rd ed. Norwalk, CT, Appleton & Lange, 1994

Tintinalli JE, Krone RL, Ruiz E (eds): Emergency Medicine: A Comprehensive Study Guide, 3rd ed. New York, McGraw-Hill, 1992

Weiner HL, Levitt LD: Neurology for the House Officer, 2nd ed. Baltimore, Williams & Wilkins, 1978

Chapter 10

Gynecologic and Obstetric Emergencies

ABORTION

Definition

Spontaneous abortion is defined as the termination of the birth process prior to the 20th week of gestation. It is the expulsion of all or part of the products of conception with a weight of less than 500 g.

A complete abortion is the expulsion of all the products of conception. An incomplete abortion is the expulsion of some, but not all, of the products of conception. An early abortion occurs before the 12th week, and a late abortion occurs between the 12th and the 20th week. A threatened abortion is bleeding from the uterus before the 20th week, with or without uterine contractions and with or without expulsion of the products of conception. Inevitable abortion refers to bleeding of intrauterine origin, before the 20th week, with a dilated cervix with impending expulsion of the products of conception.

A missed abortion is when the fetus or embryo dies in the womb and the products of conception are not expelled before the 20th week. The products of conception are retained in the womb for 8 weeks or more. An infected abortion or septic abortion is one in which an infected abortion occurs with disseminated infection.

Epidemiology

Spontaneous abortion occurs in 15 to 40% of all pregnancies. The most common causes of spontaneous abortion are genetic defects of the embryo, ovulatory or endocrine deficiencies, and uterine anomalies. In 5% of women who have spontaneous abortions, they will have repetitive abortions. Most spontaneous abortions occur in the 8- to 9-week interval but can present up to 13 weeks.

An infected abortion occurs after the fetal contents of the uterus are expelled either spontaneously or by instrumentation of the uterine cavity by dilatation and curettage. Postabortal endometritis is usually secondary to instrumentation by unsterile catheters or by foreign objects used in an abortion.

Pathology

First-trimester abortions are usually caused by a gross anomaly of chromosome structure, mostly X monosomy, trisomy, polyploidy, abnormal formation of the placenta, congenital absence of the embryo, or localized anomaly of the embryo.

Second-trimester abortions are usually caused by shallow circumvallate implantations in the placenta, syphilis, or erythroblastosis.

Maternal factors that cause an abortion are maternal infections,

285

rubella virus, chlamydia, herpes simplex virus type 2 (HSV-2). *Mycoplasma, Toxoplasma gondii,* and cytomegalovirus, cardiovascular-renal hypertensive disease, systemic lupus erythematosus, hyperthyroidism, hypothyroidism, or diabetes mellitus.

Trauma either direct or indirect from a motor vehicle accident (MVA) or surgical trauma can cause an abortion.

Blood group incompatibility due to Rh, ABO, or Kell factors can also cause a spontaneous abortion. Folic acid antagonists, anticoagulants, lead poisoning, maternal hypoxia, or thalidomide are toxicologic causes of spontaneous abortions.

Clinical Presentation

Most patients who present with spontaneous abortions present with a history of minimal, intermittent, or continuous spotting that progresses to heavy bleeding then passage of clots and gestational tissue. Pain presents after the start of bleeding and is midline and cramping in nature. If the pain is severe and more unilaterally localized, consider an ectopic pregnancy or a ruptured ovarian cyst. The patient with postabortal endometritis will present with cramping pain, fever, nausea, generalized malaise, and continued bleeding.

Examination

An examination of the patient with a threatened abortion or a spontaneous abortion will be determined by the place on the continuum of the abortive process in which the patient presents. The patient with a threatened abortion will present with midline suprapubic tenderness with a closed os and minimal bleeding. If the patient presents in the abortive process, the patient's uterus will be firm and tender, with the os open with blood clots and with the products of conception present. After all products of conception have passed through the os, the uterus will be small and firm with the os closed.

The patient with postabortal endometritis will present on examination with a purulent discharge from the cervical os and hemorrhagic cervical discharge, and the uterus will be large, boggy, and tender. Adnexal tenders may be present along with a tender paremetrium or myometrium. There can be tenderness in the cul-de-sac. Uterine perforation has been reported.

Diagnosis

A diagnosis is made by history, positive result on a pregnancy test, physical examination, and ultrasound examination.

Laboratory Findings

All patients with a suspected abortion should have a complete blood count (CBC) with special attention to the hemoglobin and hematocrit, electrolytes, prothrombin time (PT), partial thromboplastin time (PTT), and quantitative and qualitative β-human chorionic gonadotropin (HCG) should be drawn. If bleeding is profuse, blood for type and crossmatch should be prepared. If significant bleeding has occurred, anemia will be present. If the white blood cell count is greater than 12,000 to 20,000 the diagnosis of septic abortion should be entertained. All aborting women should have their Rh factor typed. If the blood type is Rh negative, then the aborting woman should receive Rho (D) immune globulin (RhoGAM).

Treatment

All women who present to the emergency department (ED) with a history of pregnancy, missed menses, positive result on a pregnancy test with vaginal bleeding, and abdominal pain are presumed to have an ectopic pregnancy until proven otherwise. The patient's vital signs should be assessed for hypotension and tachycardia, and the patient's temperature should also be taken. You should establish your "safety net" of two large-gauge intravenous (IV) lines of normal saline or lactated Ringer's solution and draw laboratory measures with type and crossmatched blood, if the possibility of ectopic pregnancy is entertained.

A pelvic ultrasound should be obtained immediately, and an obstetric/gynecologic (Ob/Gyn) consultation should be ordered urgently. If a threatened abortion is the diagnosis, the patient is sent home with the instructions of bed rest, no intercourse, and no tampon use. She is to return to the ED if increased vaginal bleeding or products of conception occur or if the pain becomes unilateral.

In the case of an incomplete abortion, the os will be open and fetal contents may be present in the os. Immediate Ob/Gyn consultation is needed, and the uterine contents should be evacuated to prevent excess bleeding and the possibility of postabortal endometritis.

If the patient presents with a massive bleed and there are products of conception in the open os, the fetal contents should be gently withdrawn and the bleeding will abate.

All tissue that is recovered should be sent for histologic examination to be evaluated for hydatidiform molar pregnancy, ectopic pregnancy, chorionic villi, and the presence or lack of normal trophoblastic tissue.

The treatment of a postabortal abortion involves an Ob/Gyn consultation, admission to the hospital, and parenteral antibiotic therapy. Often redilatation and curettage are performed to prevent abscess formation and septic pelvic thrombophlebitis.

Any woman who is Rh negative should receive Rho(D) immune globulin, 300 μg intramuscularly (IM).

AMNIOTIC FLUID EMBOLISM

Definition

Amniotic fluid embolism is the release of amniotic fluid into the maternal circulation.

Epidemiology

The major cause of amniotic fluid embolism is oxytocics during labor. Amniotic fluid embolism is the leading cause of death in induced abortions. It also occurs in miscarriage and is rare during spontaneous abortions. Amniotic fluid embolism can occur with abdominal trauma or can be caused by an attempted amniocentesis. Ninety percent of patients with amniotic fluid embolism die secondary to the embolism. Nine percent of maternal deaths are caused by amniotic fluid embolism. Within the first hour 50% of these patients will die of cardiovascular collapse, and 80% will die within 4 to 5 hours.

Pathology

Amniotic fluid embolism is caused by the release of amniotic fluid into the maternal circulation during intense uterine contractions or during uterine manipulation. Abruptio placentae is also a cause of amniotic fluid embolism. The placenta separates from the uterine decidua basalis and the amniotic fluid embolism is released. A two-phase reaction occurs. The first phase lasts up to 30 minutes in which vasospasm, release of vasoactive substances, and mechanical plugging of vessels occur. The majority of this process takes place in the mother's pulmonary tree. Abrupt cardiopulmonary collapse occurs and is almost always fatal.

The second phase, if the patient survives the first phase, is dominated by the onset of pulmonary edema with left ventricular failure. This leads to acute respiratory distress syndrome (ARDS). Forty percent of the patients who survive to phase 2 die of secondary coagulopathy.

Clinical Presentation

The patient presents with sudden hypoxia, hypotension, and coagulopathy. Of these patients, 10% will have a seizure. Bleeding diathesis will occur in 10 to 15% of patients. The HELLP (*h*emolytic anemia, *e*levated *l*iver enzymes, and *l*ow *p*latelet count) syndrome of pre-eclampsia or abruptio placentae or idiopathic thrombocytopenic purpura should also be considered.

Examination

The patient should be given a complete examination, including a pelvic examination.

Diagnosis

A diagnosis is usually made on autopsy with the findings of squamous cells, fetal hairs, or debris in the maternal circulation.

Laboratory Findings

A CBC, electrolytes, arterial blood gas, PT, PTT, urinalysis (UA) with blood cultures, and a chest x-ray should be obtained.

Treatment

Amniotic fluid embolism is very rare. A high index of suspicion is indicated for proper diagnosis. It should be considered in any pregnant female who has had an abortion or is currently on oxytocics, or has had an amniocentesis, who becomes acutely hypoxic and hypotensive and has coagulopathy. The patient should be placed on 100% oxygen with ventilator support, aggressive fluid resuscitation, inotropic cardiovascular support, and anticipation and management of consumptive coagulopathy. The patient should be treated in the intensive care unit (ICU) with early Ob/Gyn consultation. A Foley catheter should be placed, and the patient's urine output should be monitored.

ECTOPIC PREGNANCY

Definition

An ectopic pregnancy is an extrauterine pregnancy in which a fertilized ovum is implanted in an area outside the uterine cavity.

Epidemiology

Ectopic pregnancies are the main cause of maternal mortality in the first trimester. There is a higher risk of a recurrent ectopic pregnancy in a patient who has had a previous ectopic pregnancy. Ninety-nine percent of ectopic pregnancies occur in the uterine tube. The incidence of occurrence is 1 in 100 pregnancies. Seventy-five percent are diagnosed before the 12th week of gestation. Forty percent of ectopic pregnancies occur in patients between the ages of 20 and 29 years. Ten to 20% of women with one ectopic pregnancy will have a second ectopic pregnancy, and 4 to 5% will occur in the other tube. One in 1000 ectopic pregnancies result in maternal death.

Pathology

Ectopic pregnancies can occur anywhere in the pelvic area.

1. Tubal
   a. Isthmic (25%)
   b. Ampullary (55%)
   c. Fimbrial (17%)
   d. Interstitial (2%): bilateral, distal with segmental absence of the tube
2. Uterine (rare): cornual, angular or in a uterine diverticulum, rudimentary horn, intramural
3. Cervical: rare
4. Intraligamentous: rare
5. Ovarian (0.9%): tubo-ovarian, abdomino-ovarian (secondary to abdominal pregnancy)

6. Abdominal (0.1%): primary, secondary, abdomino-ovarian, tuboabdominal
7. Associated with hysterectomy: rare
8. Combined with intrauterine pregnancy (1 in 1700 to 30,000 pregnancies)

Numerous factors can lead to an ectopic pregnancy. Tubal factors include a previous episode of salpingitis (50%). Chronic salpingitis will be found 50% of the time on histologic examination.

Congenital diverticula, accessory ostia, and atresia can all cause an ectopic pregnancy. Abnormal tubal anatomy due to exposure to diethylstilbestrol in utero, previous tubal or microsurgery, tubal ligation, or conservative treatment of unruptured tubal pregnancy, extrinsic adhesions, peritonitis, kidney transplant, diverticulitis, pelvic tumor, and endometriosis can all predispose a woman to an ectopic pregnancy.

Abnormal sperm counts or a high incidence of abnormal spermatozoa have been reported to be associated with ectopic pregnancies. Ovarian factors implicated in ectopic pregnancy include ovarian enlargement due to the use of clomiphene (Clomid) or menotropins (Pergonal).

Clinical Presentation

Only one fifth of patients with ectopic pregnancy present with pain and vaginal bleeding. Most have a history of amenorrhea or unusual vaginal bleeding. The pain usually presents with unilateral lower abdominal pain.

Pain alone is the presenting complaint in 99% of the cases. Forty-four percent of the women who present with ectopic pain will have generalized pain, and 33% will present with unilateral pain. Abnormal bleeding will be present in 75% of presenting women. Amenorrhea will be present in 68% prior to presentation. Syncope will be the presenting complaint in 37% of the cases.

Examination

On examination of the adnexae, the examination will reveal asymmetry of the adnexae with fullness and tenderness. An adnexal mass will be present in about half of the patients prior to rupture. At time of rupture, the patient may faint secondary to a vasovagal response to pain. The patient might comment that the intensity of the pain has somewhat subsided after rupture. The patient with a ruptured ectopic pregnancy can present with normal vital signs or frank hemorrhagic shock.

On examination, 71% of the patients will have a normal-sized uterus. There will be adnexal tenderness in 96% of the presenting patients. There will be a palatable adnexal mass in 53% of the cases.

The Adler sign is the presence of a "fixed abdominal tenderness" on turning the patient from one position to another.

Diagnosis

A diagnosis is made by a positive pregnancy test with a positive endovaginal sonography or a positive culdocentesis. The culdocentesis will be positive only if there is blood in the cul-de-sac (pouch of Douglas). An 18-gauge spinal needle on a 10-ml syringe is used to attempt to aspirate blood from the pouch of Douglas. If the blood does not clot, it is from intraperitoneal bleeding secondary to fibrinolysis of the bleeding ectopic pregnancy. If the blood clots, it is probably from a vessel puncture in the wall of the vagina. The cul-de-sac usually contains some straw-colored fluid and, if aspirated, can assist you in locating the cul-de-sac. If no blood is obtained and straw-colored fluid is aspirated, then you can be assured that you are in the cul-de-sac. The fact that no blood is aspirated from the cul-de-sac does not rule out an ectopic pregnancy, because it might not have ruptured as of yet.

Laparoscopy can be used to rule out an early unruptured ectopic pregnancy. If an ectopic pregnancy is noted on laparoscopy examination, then a laparotomy can be performed to remove the ectopic pregnancy.

Laboratory Findings

A CBC, PT, PTT, electrolytes, type and crossmatch of 6 to 8 units of blood with Rh determination, and a quantitative and qualitative analysis should be performed.

Treatment

The ED treatment of an ectopic pregnancy is a high index of suspicion for an ectopic pregnancy. If it is believed that a patient has an ectopic pregnancy, then obtain your "safety net" early. Two large-gauge IV lines of normal saline or lactated Ringer's solution should be started. The patient should be placed on oxygen, and a CBC for hematocrit evaluation (serial hematocrits should be drawn) and type and crossmatch 4 to 6 units of blood should be performed. An early culdocentesis or ultrasound should be performed. Continual evaluation and reevaluation of the patient's vital signs must be performed until a definitive determination of the cause of the patient's pain and bleeding is made.

An early Ob/Gyn consultation and an ultrasound or laparotomy are indicated.

FEMALE SEXUAL ASSAULT

Definition

Sexual assault or rape is carnal knowledge of the victim without the victim's consent through fear, force, fraud, or compulsion. There must be three components for rape to occur: (1) compulsion; (2) carnal knowledge; and (3) nonconsensual coitus. Seminal emission is not required to commit rape. Even slight penile penetration can be deemed rape. Rape has been divided into four degrees. In first- and third-degree rape, penetration must take place, which is defined as penetration of the assailant's penis, or any part of their body, into the anus or genital area. Second- and fourth-degree rape occur when intentional touching or fondling of the intimate parts of the victim or the coercion of the victim to fondle the assailant's intimate parts takes place. The woman is sodomized if there is unwilling oral or anal penetration.

Epidemiology

The exact number of rapes in the United States is unknown, but it is estimated that more than 500,000 rapes are not reported each year because of fear or shame. The median age of the rape victim is 15 to 26 years. Over half of the rape victims know their assailant. Eighty percent of rape victims are divorced, separated, or single. Only 2% of those charged with rape are convicted of rape in the United States.

Examination

The rape examination should be a prepared protocol. A trained emergency medicine physician, physician assistant, or Ob/Gyn physician should perform the examination. A protocol involving the local police, Social Work Service, or Rape Crisis Team should be mobilized. A standardized rape kit should be available.

The patient should not eat or drink anything, take any medications, change her clothes, or take a shower prior to presentation to the ED. She should not urinate or defecate. A consent should be granted before any examination is performed. This consent should include photography and the release of information to the proper authorities. If the victim is under age, the victim's parents or guardian should give consent before the examination.

The rape examination contains two major parts: (1) a history of evidence, and (2) a gynecologic and medical examination.

The history should include:

1. Who was the assailant?
2. Where was the assault?
3. What happened?
4. When did the assault happen?
5. What is the date of your last menstrual period (LMP)?
6. Do you use birth control?
7. When did intercourse occur prior to the assault?
8. Have you changed clothes, showered, or douched prior to arrival in the ED?
9. How many assaults were made and how many assailants were involved?

10. Was there use of restraints?
11. Were threats of violence made?
12. Did the victim lose consciousness?
13. Had the victim or assailant consumed alcohol in the past 24 hours?
14. What was the type of assault?
    a. Oral, anal, or vaginal penetration?
    b. Was there ejaculation on or in the body?
    c. Was a condom used?

Look for and document bruising, cuts, or lacerations on the entire body. Ensure that photographs are taken of these findings. Do a head-to-toe examination. You can use toluidine blue dye to identify small pelvic lacerations caused by traumatic intercourse. Samples of semen should be obtained before the application of toluidine blue dye, secondary to its spermicidal activity.

When the vaginal examination is performed, the speculum should be lubricated with water and not KY jelly. If the woman is a virgin, the condition of the hymen should be noted as: (1) present and intact, (2) hymen present and intact with old scarring, (3) hymen present and recently ruptured, or (4) hymen absent.

Laboratory Findings

Laboratory tests should include a pregnancy test, rapid plasma reagin (RPR) (Venereal Disease Research Laboratory [VDRL]), and human immunodeficiency virus (HIV). The anus, oral mucosa, vagina, and cervix should be cultured for gonorrhea and chlamydia. Other examination-directed laboratory tests and x-rays should be performed. A line of custody should be maintained in handling all specimens that go to the laboratory or to the police.

Treatment

Both the physical and psychological trauma should be addressed. The patient's physical safety should also be addressed at the time of discharge from the hospital. Is she safe from future assault by her attacker(s)?

Sexually transmitted diseases can be addressed in 48 to 72 hours when the results of the cultures are obtained. Some practitioners and patients prefer to begin treatment at the time of the patient's initial visit to the ED for "safety" concerns. The following regimens can be utilized:

1. Ceftriaxone 250 mg IM with doxycycline 100 mg by mouth (PO) twice a day (BID) for 10 to 14 days.
2. Spectinomycin, 2 g IM with doxycycline 100 mg PO BID for 10 to 14 days.
3. Ciprofloxacin 500 mg PO in one dose, with doxycycline 100 mg for 10 to 14 days.

All patients should be referred for final HIV, RPR (VDRL), gonorrhea, and chlamydial results and cultures.

The issue of possible pregnancy should be raised with the victim. Ninety to 95% of all conceptions result from a single act of intercourse between 120 hours before ovulation and 10 hours after ovulation. The date of the victim's last menses is very important in determination of the risk of pregnancy. A negative result on a pregnancy test should be obtained before any postcoital therapy is offered. If the patient requests postcoital therapy, the following regimens can be utilized:

1. Norgestrel and ethinyl estradiol (Ovral), 2 tablets initially and 2 tablets in 12 hours
2. Diethylstilbestrol in a 25-mg dose BID for 5 days
3. IV conjugated estrogen (Premarin) 50 mg once a day for 2 days
4. Conjugated estrogen 30 mg once a day PO for 5 days

The risk of contracting HIV should be addressed. If the victim believes that the rapist is HIV-positive, zidovudine (AZT) should be offered.

The psychological trauma of rape should be addressed. Ninety-nine percent of all physical trauma heals, but the psychological trauma can last for a lifetime. The psychological aspect of treatment should be addressed as soon as the patient arrives in the ED.

Reassure the patient that she is safe in the ED. Listen to the patient's ordeal. Tell the patient the truth. Do not be afraid to use the word rape when asking the patient about the history of the event. Discuss the psychological sequelae of rape. Ensure a psychological follow-up with Social Work Services or a Rape Crisis Center. Ensure an Ob/Gyn follow-up in 2 weeks for the victim.

GENITAL HERPES

Definition

Genital herpes is a sexually transmitted disease.

Epidemiology

Genital herpes is caused primarily by two antigenic groups: herpes simplex virus type 1 (HSV-1) and HSV-2. In earlier times, HSV-1 caused oral lesions and HSV-2 caused genital lesions. Eighty-five to 90% of genital herpes is caused by HSV-2.

Pathology

HSV-2 has an incubation period from 1 to 45 days. The mean time from infection to presentation is 5.8 days. After the initial presentation, the virus lives in the dorsal root of the sacral ganglia. When exogenous or endogenous stresses occur, the virus travels down the sensory nerve root to the lower genital area where it replicates and becomes symptomatic.

Clinical Presentation

Women present with painful lesions of the lower genital tract. Neonatal infections have a very high mortality and morbidity after passage through the birth canal. The initial infection is usually the most severe and lasts longer than recurrent infections. The ulcers will remain for 4 to 15 days and will usually heal completely in 21 days. The patient will complain of urethritis with severe dysuria. A patient can present with pharyngitis and secondary infection or with myalgias, headache, fever, and malaise. Complications of HSV-2 include aseptic meningitis, hepatitis, and autonomic nervous system dysfunction.

In recurrent episodes, the patient will complain of early numbness or tingling with an acute onset of pain. With recurrent attacks, the symptoms are usually milder and tend to be in the same location as previous episodes. With recurrent episodes, the symptoms last from 4 to 8 days and subside in 10 days.

Examination

On examination of the female genitalia, the lesions will be painful to palpation. The fluid-filled vesicles or papules will be well circumscribed and occasionally coalescent, and they will have shallow-based ulcers. Deep inguinal nodes and severe pelvic pain with lymphadenopathy will be present.

Diagnosis

The diagnosis is made by physical examination, Tzanck smear, or culture.

Laboratory Findings

Suspected lesions can be cultured for HSV. An intact vesicle can be unroofed and the fluid placed on a glass slide. A Tzanck smear with a Wright or Giemsa stain can be examined. If giant cells are present, the diagnosis of herpes is made.

Treatment

Acyclovir 200 mg PO five times a day for 7 to 10 days or until clinical resolution is given as a treatment. Acyclovir is not curative. Acyclovir decreases the severity and shortens the course of the disease. For patients with severe disease or complications, hospitalization is necessary and acyclovir 5 mg/kg IV every 8 hours for 5 to 7 days is required for resolution of the attack. Therapy should begin within 2 days of onset of symptoms to be most effective. Patients with recurrent episodes do not benefit much from the use of acyclovir.

For patients with chronic episodes, acyclovir 200 mg up to five times a day or 400 mg BID can be given to suppress outbreaks. Acyclovir should not be used in pregnant patients unless life-threatening hepatitis, pneumonitis, or encephalitis is present. A patient with HIV should be treated with the same initial dose as that given to a nonimmunocompetent patient.

EMERGENT PELVIC AND ABDOMINAL PAIN

True gynecologic and obstetric emergencies include:

1. Ruptured tubo-ovarian abscess
2. Ruptured ectopic pregnancy
3. Ruptured hemorrhagic ovarian cyst
4. Premature rupture of membranes
5. Pre-eclampsia and eclampsia
6. Preterm labor
7. Diabetes mellitus
8. Uterine perforation or rupture
9. Abruptio placentae
10. Placenta previa
11. Gestational trophoblastic disease (molar pregnancy)

Other causes of female pelvic pain include:

1. Pelvic inflammatory disease (PID)
2. Mittelschmerz (small amount of blood causing peritoneum irritation)
3. Menses
4. Endometriosis
5. Adnexal torsion
6. Ovarian cysts
7. Ruptured corpus luteum cyst
8. Vaginitis
9. Pelvic neoplasm
10. Foreign bodies or objects
11. Uterine leiomyoma

The approach to the female patient with abdominal pain is very simple. All female patients of child-bearing age are pregnant until proven otherwise. They have either a tubo-ovarian abscess, hemorrhage of an ovarian cyst, or an ectopic pregnancy until proven otherwise. These three conditions cause hemorrhage or death if not addressed promptly. The three aforementioned "true" gynecologic emergencies are not the only diseases that can cause abdominal pain or are a threat to the life in the female patient. Nongynecologic conditions that cause abdominal pain in the child-bearing years should be evaluated with a high index of suspicion, along with gynecologic causes of abdominal pain. Some causes of nongynecologic pain that should be considered in the diagnosis are:

Appendicitis	Gastric or duodenal ulcers
Lower lobe pneumonia	Cholecystitis
Colitis	Ileitis
Diverticulitis	Pancreatitis
Gastroenteritis	Pyelonephritis
Sickle cell crisis	Musculoskeletal pain
Myocardial ischemia	Pulmonary embolism
Aseptic necrosis of the femoral head	

Pain from pelvic organs can radiate to the upper and lower abdomen, back, thighs, buttocks, and perineum. Pathology from the uterine fundus, the adnexae, and the dome of the bladder will cause localized pain in the lower abdomen via the hypogastric nerve plexus. Pathology from the uterine segment, cervix, bladder, trigone, and rectum will cause pain in the back, perineum, legs, and buttocks via the second to fourth sacral nerve roots. Pain that is poorly localized is usually visceral or splanchnic pain from distended hollow viscous organs (fibroids, dysmenorrhea, or labor contractions) or the capsule of a solid organ (cysts) or the stretching of the round ligament or adhesions.

Sudden pain is usually caused by a vascular or ischemic insult or an acute irritation of the peritoneum of a large amount of blood. Gradual onset of pain usually means pain that is suggestive of a slow vascular leak or PID. Colicky pain suggests pain from a hollow viscous organ (gallbladder or uterus). A dull, throbbing pain is suggestive of chronic inflammation.

Always assume the worst when evaluating a female in child-bearing years. If a female presents with abdominal pain who is tachycardiac, hypotensive, diaphoretic, with a history of missed menses or has had amenorrhea for several months, assume an ectopic pregnancy or hemorrhage. Obtain your "safety net"—two large-bore IV lines with normal saline or lactated Ringer's solution. Place the patient on oxygen, and draw laboratory values to include CBC, electrolytes, PT, PTT, serum qualitative and quantitative pregnancy test, and type and crossmatch of blood for 6 units. Determine if the patient is Rh negative or positive. Examine the patient early, and perform ultrasound as soon as possible. It is most important to consult a gynecologist as soon as possible. A true hemorrhage from ectopic pregnancy is a "clinical" diagnosis, and the patient must be operated on immediately.

When evaluating a female in child-bearing years, always obtain the following important historical information:

- Ask the patient for the date of her LMP. Always ask if this was a "normal" period for this patient. Are the patient's periods always regular or irregular? If the patient states that her periods are always irregular, then the history of last menstrual period is of poor historical quality. If the patient states that her menses are regular, then this is an important piece of historical information. Obtain the first day or date of her last menses. Any female who is 4 weeks past her normal menses is presumed pregnant until proven otherwise. If the patient is bleeding, try to get a sense of how much the patient is bleeding. A soaked sanitary napkin holds approximately 20 to 30 ml of blood. Obtain a history of how many "soaked" sanitary napkins have been required over a specific period of time.
- A good rule is, if there is a history of amenorrhea for any length of time, followed by abdominal pain and vaginal bleeding, this is an abnormal pregnancy until proven otherwise. Ask the patient if she feels pregnant. Are her breast sore, or does she have morning sickness, weight gain, or leg edema?
- Obtain a history of past pregnancies: gravida (total prior pregnancies), para (live births), and abortions (spontaneous miscarriages or induced abortions). Obtain the history of each pregnancy—whether delivered by cesarean section or by vaginal delivery. Was the patient pre-eclamptic or eclamptic during any of the prior pregnancies? Was the delivered child premature or term delivery? Were there any complications at birth? Inquire about the reason for an induced abortion.
- Ask about the patient's sexual activity. Ask the date of last sexual intercourse and if contraception was used (i.e., birth control pills, diaphragm, prophylactic, intrauterine device, rhythm method, or prior tubal ligation).

When in doubt as to what your diagnosis is, obtain your safety net early and schedule an Ob/Gyn consultation as soon as possible.

HYPEREMESIS GRAVIDARUM

Definition

Hyperemesis gravidarum is the persistence of vomiting during pregnancy.

Epidemiology

Hyperemesis gravidarum usually occurs during the 8- to 14-week period of pregnancy and is more common in the younger, nulliparous females who are obese. Severe vomiting with weight loss, dehydration, and ketosis are present.

Pathology

Estrogen levels are often higher in patients with hyperemesis gravidarum. Several studies have shown that patients with hyperemesis have had a better fetal outcome than have those without hyperemesis. Persistent hyperemesis in the second trimester has been associated with molar pregnancies.

Clinical Presentation

The patient looks sick and is usually afebrile. The patient should have no abdominal pain. If abdominal pain is present, look for another diagnosis as the cause of the vomiting (i.e., appendicitis).

Examination

The patient should be given a complete examination, including a pelvic examination. Particular attention should be made to note the presence of costovertebral angle tenderness or abdominal tenderness. Remember that the appendix rises in the abdomen as the uterus enlarges. The appendix may be about the line of the umbilicus at 20 weeks. Perform a rectal examination on all patients with hyperemesis, especially those who present with diarrhea. Patients with hyperemesis gravidarum do not have diarrhea. The diagnosis is more likely to be gastroenteritis.

Diagnosis

Hyperemesis gravidarum should be a diagnosis of exclusion. Pyelonephritis, gastroenteritis, hepatitis, cholecystitis, or appendicitis should be ruled out before the diagnosis of hyperemesis gravidarum is made.

Laboratory Findings

A CBC, electrolytes, including calcium, magnesium, phosphorus, and a UA with urine culture should be obtained. Liver function tests should be obtained to look at the bilirubin and transaminase levels to rule out gallbladder disease or hepatitis. Ketones will often be present in the urine.

Treatment

The goal of the treatment of hyperemesis gravidarum is to stop the vomiting and to clear the urine of ketones. IV hydration with normal saline, lactated Ringer's solution, D5 normal saline (NS), or D5 lactated Ringer's (RL) should be used.

Phenothiazines and related antiemetics are Food and Drug Association (FDA) category C drugs, but there is little evidence of a risk to the fetus when these drugs are used for hyperemesis, especially when the sequelae of prolonged starvation and dehydration are considered.

Phenergan 12.5 to 25 mg IV or rectally can be used. Compazine, 5 to 10 mg IV or 25 mg rectally, can also be used. If vomiting cannot be stopped and ketones cannot be cleared, then the patient should be admitted to the hospital.

Patient teaching is very important in the patients who are sent home. The patient should take small, frequent meals to keep calorie intake up. Small frequent amounts of fluid should be taken hourly to prevent the recurrence of dehydration. The patient should be instructed to return to the ED if she is unable to keep food or fluid down.

OVARIAN CYSTS

Definition

A cyst is a fluid-filled sac containing semisolid material. There are two kinds of ovarian cysts—follicle and corpus luteum cysts (granulosa lutein and theca lutein)—that are both transient normal physiologic structures. Abnormal cysts are ruptured, hemorrhagic, or infectious in nature. Follicular cysts occur in the first 2 weeks of the menstrual cycle, and the corpus luteum cysts occur during the last 2 weeks of the menstrual cycle. Ovarian cysts can also be malignant, benign (dermoid or cystic teratoma), or endometriotic.

Epidemiology

An ovarian cyst can occur from puberty to menopause. Most follicle and lutein cysts resolve within 60 days of onset spontaneously.

Pathology

Follicle cysts represent the failure of the fluid in an incompletely developed follicle to be reabsorbed.

Granulosa lutein cysts are functional, non-neoplastic enlargements of the ovary. After ovulation the granulosa cells become luteinized, and this causes increased vascularization. Blood accumulates in the central cavity and the corpus hemorrhagicum. When the blood is reabsorbed, a corpus luteum cyst forms. If the corpus luteum cyst is persistent, local pain and tenderness can occur along with either amenorrhea or delayed menstruation followed by brisk bleeding after resolution of the cyst. When the cyst ruptures, torsion of the ovary is encouraged. Large amounts of bleeding from a ruptured corpus luteum cyst will cause hypovolemia. Most corpus lutein cysts resolve within 2 months without intervention.

Theca lutein cysts are usually bilateral and filled with clear to straw-colored fluid and are found in association with choriocarcinoma, gonadotropin, or clomiphene therapy or hydatidiform mole.

Clinical Presentation

A patient with a ruptured ovarian cyst presents with a history of a sudden, sharp, unilateral pain. There will often be a history of intercourse or exercise in association with the pain. The patient can present with orthostatic hypotension. A careful history of the LMP must be taken. A determination of the point in the cycle that the cyst ruptures can give a clue as to what kind of cyst has ruptured. Follicular cysts with extrusion of an ovum from the ovary occurs midcycle following a normal menses and may accompany slight vaginal bleeding. When pain is unilateral and the duration of discomfort is only a few hours to 2 to 3 days, it can be termed *mittelschmerz* pain. With mittelschmerz pain, the patient can present with nausea, malaise, and abdominal tenderness. If the patient is on anticoagulants when mittelschmerz occurs, life-threatening blood loss can occur.

A corpus luteum cyst ruptures just before menses. There is intraperitoneal bleeding that causes unilateral or bilateral abdominal pain.

An intraovarian hemorrhage can occur into a cyst or tumor. The onset of pain is usually sudden and unilateral. The pain is described as sharp, boring, or throbbing and increasing in severity as the mass expands prior to rupture.

The pain of an enlarging ovarian neoplasm is one of increasing pain and is described as a "fullness" secondary to stretching of supporting ligamentous structures. The patient often complains of increasing pelvic girth. Ascites is the presenting complaint in 30% of the women with the diagnosis of ovarian cancer.

Patients with a theca lutein cyst usually have very few symptoms. They present with a sense of "pelvic weight" and may describe the pain as aching. The cysts can range in size from 1 cm to several centimeters in size. Ruptured cysts cause intraperitoneal bleeding. Patients can present with symptoms of pregnancy, including hyperemesis or breast paresthesias.

Examination

On pelvic examination, there may be no or little tenderness of the ovary. A cystic mass can sometimes be palpated. Little or no peritoneal signs are found. If a careful history is taken, often a presumptive diagnosis of the kind of cyst can be made. The pain of a serous cyst will often subside rapidly. When a dermoid cyst or an endometrioma ruptures, the pain is prolonged secondary to a chemical peritonitis. Fever and ileus are often present.

With a corpus luteum cyst, the examination reveals peritoneal irritation and the pain can be localized or diffuse. Peritonitis and hemorrhagic shock depend on the size of the tear of the ovarian vessel.

On examination, the finding of a new or enlarging mass is suggestive of an intraovarian hemorrhage. The mass will feel tense and extremely tender.

The examination of a woman with suspected ovarian cancer will reveal a fixed, bilateral, solid mass, and this cancer is associated with pelvic nodularity. If the mass is less than 5 cm before ovulation or menstruation, it is usually benign.

Diagnosis

A diagnosis is made by history of the time of rupture of the cyst in the menstrual cycle and by pelvic ultrasound examination.

Laboratory Findings

A CBC, electrolytes, PT, and PTT should be drawn. Blood for type and crossmatch should be drawn if a ruptured hemorrhagic cyst is suspected. A UA with culture and sensitivity along with quantitative and qualitative β-HCG should be drawn. The Rh factor should be noted.

In theca lutein cysts, very high levels of chorionic gonadotropin can be present.

Treatment

Any patient who presents in child-bearing age with an acute onset of pain and vaginal bleeding should be assumed to have an ectopic pregnancy or a ruptured hemorrhage cyst of life-threatening nature until proven otherwise. You should establish your "safety net" with two large-gauge IV lines with normal saline or lactated Ringer's solution. The patient should be placed on 100% oxygen by facemask, and the aforementioned laboratory specimens should be drawn. An early pelvic ultrasound should be performed, and an early Ob/Gyn consultation should be made.

If a ruptured dermoid or endometrioma cyst is suspected, an exploratory laparotomy needs to be performed for diagnosis and for peritoneal irrigation to treat the chemical or hemorrhagic peritonitis.

In an uncomplicated ruptured serous cyst, the patients can be sent home with reassurance and pain medication. When symptoms are disturbing or painful, the re-establishment of the ovarian cycle may be therapeutic. A 5-day therapy of a daily injection of progesterone in oil, 5 mg IM or hydroxyprogesterone caproate 1.25 to 2.5 mg IM can be given. Clomiphene citrate (Clomid) 50 mg once a day PO for 5 days can also be given. These therapies are rarely indicated. Understand and explain the medicolegal aspects of the treatment and the association of fetal abnormalities with the use of progesterone therapy.

If a ruptured corpus luteum cyst is the diagnosis and unless acute hemorrhage is present, symptomatic therapy is all that is necessary. Remember, however, that there is increased risk of torsion of the ovary, and eccyesis may be present. Suspect an ectopic pregnancy. If a large corpus luteum cyst ruptures, a catastrophic event may take place. Be certain of your diagnosis before you send a patient home.

Intraovarian hemorrhage needs immediate surgical consultation. If surgery is delayed, the ovary can infarct or necrosis can occur. If the cyst ruptures, systemic toxicity or bleeding can occur.

With the diagnosis of theca lutein cysts, curettage should be performed if there is any question of retained products of conception, choriocarcinoma, or proliferative mole. Always consider intrauterine pregnancy with these symptoms. If normal menses resumes, the possibility of a bilateral ovarian neoplasm must be ruled out. These cysts usually disappear spontaneously following the destruction of the choriocarcinoma, discontinuation of gonadotropin therapy, or destruction of the molar pregnancy.

Any cysts that persists or grows for more than 60 days in a normal menstrual period should be further evaluated to rule out a neoplasm.

OVARIAN TORSION

Definition

An ovarian torsion is the twisting or turning of the ovarian pedicle, uterine tube, or broad ligament.

Epidemiology

Twenty percent of ovarian torsions occur during pregnancy, and they are uncommon in the normal adnexae. The torsion occurs most commonly in the first trimester of pregnancy but can occur in the second trimester. The right ovary is the most common ovary involved.

Pathology

Cystomas and benign cystic teratomas are the most common pathologic findings on postsurgical examination. The corpus luteum is predisposed to torsion secondary to increased vascularity and cystic formations during pregnancy, allowing the ovary polarity as it rises out of the pelvis.

Clinical Presentation

The patient with an ovarian torsion presents with unilateral ischemic pain, nausea, vomiting, and restlessness. The pain can be of slow onset, then intermittent, and can progress to severe pain. The pain often resolves spontaneously, only to recur later with increased pain.

Examination

The patient with an ovarian torsion can be very difficult to examine secondary to pain. The pain will be localized. A palpable adnexal mass will be felt on examination. Actual peritoneal signs will be absent unless bleeding or leakage of cystic fluid has occurred.

Diagnosis

A diagnosis is made by ultrasonography. Laparoscopy or laparotomy is needed for the final diagnosis and treatment.

Laboratory Findings

A CBC, electrolytes, and quantitative and qualitative β-HCG should be drawn along with PT, PTT, UA, and type and crossmatched blood if bleeding is entertained or if unstable vital signs are present. Check the patient's vital signs. Leukocytosis is rare.

Treatment

ED treatment is based on early suspicion of a torsed ovary determined by the history and physical examination. In early pregnancy, ectopic pregnancy must always be considered. Ruptured ovarian cysts, pyelonephritis, renal colic, and acute appendicitis must always be considered with unilateral lower abdominal pain. An early ultrasound and an early Ob/Gyn consultation should be the normal protocol.

PLACENTA PREVIA

Definition

Placenta previa is the implantation of the placenta over the lower uterine segment over the zone of effacement with or without the dilatation of the cervix, causing an obstruction to the descending part of the fetus.

Epidemiology

Placenta previa occurs in one in 200 births. Only 20% entirely cover the cervix. Ninety percent of the patients with placenta previa are parous. Approximately 55% of all spontaneous abortions involve placenta previa. Grand multiparas involved one in 20 placenta previas. The incidence of placenta previa increases with age, previous cesarean deliveries, and multiparity. Placenta previa accounts for 60% of perinatal deaths (gestational age < 36 weeks). Perinatal mortality is 15 to 20% with placenta previa.

Pathology

Placenta previa is believed to be caused by any one or a combination of:

1. Poorly vascularized endometrium in the corpus
2. Large placenta
3. Abnormal forms of placentation, such as a succenturiate lobe or placenta diffusa

4. Low cervical cesarean section scar triples the incidence of placenta previa
5. Rupture of poorly supported venous lakes in the decidua basalis, which have been engorged with venous blood
6. Mechanical separation of the placenta from the implantation site at the time of effacement and the dilatation of the the cervix at the time of labor or as a result of intravaginal manipulation by the examiner or placentitis.

Clinical Presentation

The patient with placenta previa will present with sudden, *painless,* profuse bleeding in the third trimester or spotting during the first or second trimester. Only 10% of the patients presenting with placenta previa present with cramping as an initial complaint. Painless vaginal bleeding is the hallmark of placenta previa. Hemorrhage from placenta previa usually occurs after 28 weeks and is of sudden onset, painless, and profuse. The blood is bright red and clots. The blood loss is not extensive; usually does not produce shock; and is almost never fatal. Spontaneous labor occurs in 25% of the patients with placenta previa in the next 2 to 4 days.

On examination, the uterus is soft, nontender, and relaxed, and no fetal distress is present. In abruptio placentae the uterus is tender and has increased tone, and cramping is present with fetal distress.

Examination

An ultrasound should be performed prior to a vaginal examination of the uterus to differentiate between placenta previa and abruptio placentae. Prior to a vaginal examination, your "safety net" should be obtained. Two large-gauge 14- or 16-gauge IV lines with normal saline or lactated Ringer's solution should be started. Type and crossmatched blood, 4 to 6 units, should be obtained. A CBC, electrolytes, PT, PTT, and qualitative and quantitative beta pregnancy tests should be drawn.

Diagnosis

Ultrasound of the uterus and placenta is the examination of choice to rule in or out placenta previa. Thirty percent of the time, during the middle of the second trimester, on ultrasound examination, the placenta will cover the internal cervical os. Serial ultrasounds are needed to diagnose placenta previa beyond the second trimester. The placenta implantations are usually carried to a higher station as the fetus grows.

Laboratory Findings

CBC, PT, PTT, electrolytes, type and crossmatch of 4 to 6 units of blood, and Rh type should be obtained.

Treatment

All patients with suspected placenta previa or abruptio placentae should have a "safety net." Two large-gauge IV lines of normal saline or lactated Ringer's solution should be started, and laboratory values should be drawn. Early consultation with Ob/Gyn should be obtained, and ultrasound should be performed before a pelvic examination is done.

The type of treatment is based on:

1. The duration of the pregnancy
2. The viability of the fetus
3. The amount of uterine bleeding
4. The presentation, position, and station of the fetus
5. The gravidity and parity of the patient
6. The status of the cervix
7. The status of labor—labor present or not present

With regard to the status of the fetus, the status of pulmonary maturity must be determined before the decision for early delivery is made. Before 36 weeks' gestation, tocolytics and blood replacement are often used. After 36 weeks' gestation, the benefits of additional maturity must be weighed against the risk of future hemorrhage and delivery of the fetus. This delivery is based on lung maturity. Cesarean section is the delivery of choice for placenta previa. Vaginal delivery is reserved for patients with low-lying implantation and cephalic presentation or a greater degree of placenta previa when there is little or no hope of salvaging the fetus.

Early ultrasound examination before pelvic examination and early Ob/Gyn consultation should be the rule for evaluation of placenta previa. Obtain a "safety net" at an early stage.

PRE-ECLAMPSIA AND ECLAMPSIA

Definition

Pregnancy-induced hypertension (PIH) or pre-eclampsia is defined as edema, hypertension, and proteinuria without seizure activity after the 12th week of pregnancy. There are two types of pre-eclampsia—mild and severe. Mild pre-eclampsia is defined as a systolic blood pressure greater than 20 mm Hg or a diastolic rise of 10 mm Hg in the first 32 weeks of pregnancy. The rise of blood pressure from the second trimester to full term should not be more than 15 mm Hg for both systolic or diastolic pressure. Severe pre-eclampsia is defined as a blood pressure greater than 160 mm Hg systolic or 110 mm Hg diastolic, recorded on two occasions at least 6 hours apart with the patient on bed rest, proteinuria exceeding 5 g in a 24-hour period or 3 to 4 + on dipstick testing, oliguria less than or equal to 500 ml in a 24-hour period, cerebral or visual disturbances, epigastric pain, pulmonary edema, or cyanosis.

Eclampsia or toxemia of pregnancy is defined as an acute onset of edema, hypertension, and proteinuria after the 12th week of pregnancy with seizures.

Epidemiology

Pre-eclampsia occurs in 8% of the general population. Black race, maternal age younger than 20 years of age or older than 35 years of age, nulliparity, multiple gestations, lower socioeconomic status, hydatidiform mole, diabetes, chronic hypertension, and underlying renal disease are all associated with pre-eclampsia.

Eclampsia occurs in 0.2 to 0.5% of all pregnancies or 1 in 300 deliveries. Eclampsia occurs after 12 weeks' gestation. Seventy-five percent of eclamptic seizures occur before delivery. Fifty percent of postpartum seizures occur within the first 48 hours of delivery, but postpartum seizures can occur up to 6 weeks after delivery. The perinatal mortality rate for PIH is 37.9 deaths per births, twice that of normotensive pregnancies.

Pathology

The exact cause of pre-eclampsia is unknown. Theories include compromised placental perfusion, rejection phenomenon, insufficient production of blocking antibodies, decreased glomerular filtration rate of the kidneys, altered vascular reactivity, decreased intravascular volume, disseminated intravascular coagulation (DIC), imbalance between prostacyclin and thromboxane, uterine muscle stretching causing ischemia, dietary factors, and genetic factors have all been postulated as the cause of pre-eclampsia. If pre-eclampsia is left untreated, fetal risks include uteroplacental insufficiency, stillbirth, or intrapartum fetal distress.

The theory of eclampsia is also controversial. Seizures have been attributed to platelet thrombi, hypoxia due to localized vasoconstriction, and foci of hemorrhage in the cortex.

Clinical Presentation

Both pre-eclamptic and eclamptic patients can present with serious retinal detachment, hemorrhage, and blindness. Pulmonary edema can occur, and cardiogenic or noncardiogenic shock can occur. Cerebral edema has not been verified in the pre-eclamptic or eclamptic patient.

Cardiovascular effects include hypertension and CVA. The patient with pre-eclampsia usually has normal clotting studies. The liver can develop chronic passive congestion and subcapsular hemorrhage. The characteristic renal lesion of pre-eclampsia is glomeruloendotheliosis.

The patient who presents eclamptic will usually not have an aura or prior notice of seizure activity. The seizure is usually tonic-clonic.

Examination

The patient should be given a thorough examination. A fundoscopic examination should be performed to document retinal hemorrhage. In the cardiac examination, a note should be made of any new murmur. The lung examination should include a check for pulmonary edema. The abdomen should be examined for liver tenderness. A fetal assessment should be performed and documented to include the fetal heart tone rate and the mother's feeling of movement of the fetus. A rectal examination should be performed to document bleeding. The grade of edema should be documented to include +1 to +4 and the site—the face or the upper or lower extremities.

Hyperactive reflexes are seen in 80% of the patients with eclampsia. Clonus will be present in half of those patients.

Diagnosis

A diagnosis is made based on blood pressure changes, proteinuria, edema, and associated symptoms to include visual disturbances, headache, upper abdominal pain, seizures, oliguria, hyperbilirubinemia, elevated liver enzymes, pulmonary edema, or signs of end-organ damage.

A form of severe PIH is the HELLP syndrome. The HELLP syndrome is present in 10% of patients with eclampsia. It is seen more frequently in white patients and, if not diagnosed, can lead to abruptio placentae. It can occur early in the pregnancy, and elevation of the blood pressure can be absent. It is often a missed diagnosis. It is often diagnosed as gallbladder pain, hepatitis, idiopathic thrombocytopenic purpura, or thrombotic thrombocytopenic purpura.

Laboratory Findings

Thrombocytopenia of less than 150,000 μl is found in 15 to 20% of patients with pre-eclampsia. Fibrinogen levels are usually elevated in the pre-eclamptic patient. If low fibrinogen levels are noted, this is associated with placental abruption and fetal demise. Fibrin split products are elevated in 20% of pre-eclamptic patients. Microangiopathic hemolytic anemia with or without signs of DIC may be seen. Hemoglobin and hematocrit may be elevated due to hemoconcetration or anemia secondary to hemolysis. Uric acid is usually elevated above 6 mg/dl. Alkaline phosphatase is elevated two to three times above normal. Urinalysis will show a hyaline cast and proteinuria. Twenty-four-hour urine studies for creatinine clearance and total protein should be performed for the pre-eclamptic patient. Liver function studies, uric acid, electrolytes, and serum albumin along with PT and PTT, fibrinogen, and thromboplastin time should be obtained in all pre-eclamptic patients. A baseline magnesium level should be drawn.

Treatment

A pregnant patient who presents to the ED with edema, headache, vision disturbances, abdominal pain, elevated blood pressure, or proteinuria is considered to be pre-eclamptic-eclamptic until proven otherwise. An IV line should be established, and fetal monitoring should be initiated. Hospitalization and early Ob/Gyn consultation should be the normal treatment for any patient with a blood pressure above 140/90 and signs of PIH. The goal of treating an eclamptic patient is to control the seizures and hypertension. The following management protocols should be performed.

1. If the patient is seizing in the ED, the patient should be treated with IV magnesium sulfate 6 g (20% solution) over 15 minutes. A magnesium drip of 2 g/hr IV should be started.

    OR

    The Parkland intramuscular protocol is:

    Magnesium sulfate 4 g (20% solution) IV/5 minutes

    plus

    Magnesium sulfate 10 g deep IM (3-inch needle) divided in both buttocks (50% solution), mixed with lidocaine

    Magnesium sulfate 2 g IV (20% solution) if seizures persist for more than 15 minutes after the above dose

    Magnesium sulfate 5 g IM every 4 hours, starting 4 hours later unless:

    a. Patellar reflexes are absent
    b. Respiratory depression is present
    c. Urine output is less than 100 ml in the prior 4 hours

    The goal of magnesium therapy is to control the seizures. Respiratory depression occurs at levels over 12 mg/dl. Loss of patellar reflexes occurs at levels between 8.4 and 12 mg/dl. Give calcium gluconate 1 g slow IV push if signs of hypermagnesemia occur.

2. Lower the patient's blood pressure slowly. Do not lower the patient's blood pressure too rapidly. Too rapid lowering of the blood pressure can cause uterine hypoperfusion. Antihypertensive treatment is initiated only if the diastolic blood pressure remains above 110 mm Hg after the initiation of magnesium sulfate. Control of the hypertension should be obtained by using:

    a. Hydralazine 5 mg IV and then repeated in doses of 5 to 10 mg every 20 minutes until the blood pressure is below 110 mm Hg.
    b. Sodium nitroprusside can also be used on a short-term basis in view of the risk of thiocyanate toxicity.
    c. Nitroglycerin can also be used. It is safe for the fetus and is a primary venous vasodilator.

The treatment of mild pre-eclampsia includes bed rest and delivery of the baby. The patient can be sent home or hospitalized. If the patient is sent home, the patient's urine must be tested daily for proteinuria and the patient's blood pressure must be monitored several times a day and with a physician follow-up twice weekly.

SEXUALLY TRANSMITTED DISEASES AND PELVIC INFLAMMATORY DISEASE

Definition

PID is a generalized term used to describe a multitude of subacute, acute, recurrent, or chronic infections of the female organs. It can involve any part or all of the ovaries, oviducts, adnexae, and uterus and can lead to a septic presentation. Complications of acute salpingitis include pelvic peritonitis, severe pelvic cellulitis, infertility, and intestinal adhesions or obstruction. If the peritoneal surfaces around the liver become infected and inflamed, a localized pelvic peritonitis can occur called Fitz-Hugh–Curtis syndrome.

Epidemiology

There are more than 2.5 million visits for acute salpingitis with 250,000 hospitalizations and 150,000 surgical procedures in the United States for female pelvic infections. PID is the most common serious infection in the United States in reproductive age women. Fifteen percent of asymptomatic gonococcal cervical infections will develop acute salpingitis. Only one third of the patients with PID will have a fever higher than 38° C (100.4° F).

Pathology

PID or salpingitis is a polymicrobial disease. It can be caused by a single agent or by multiple agents, including *Chlamydia, Neisseria gonorrhoeae, Bacteroides, Peptostreptococcus, Peptococcus,* and *Escherichia coli.*

Clinical Presentation

Acute salpingitis usually has an onset after menses and is associated with vaginal discharge, lower abdominal pain, or pelvic pain. The patient may be febrile with systemic manifestations of headache, malaise, and lassitude. There can be pelvic peritonitis present. The pain is usually bilateral and is insidious in onset. The patient may complain of pelvic pressure with back pain radiating down both legs. The swelling of the infected tubes causes lower abdominal pain. Nausea with or without vomiting can occur.

Risk factors for PID include:

1. A history of previous gonococcal salpingitis
2. Frequent sexual activity with multiple partners
3. Adolescence
4. Use of intrauterine devices

A history of recent dilatation and curettage, endometrial biopsy, tubal insufflation, cautery, or cryotherapy of the cervix can predispose a female to endometritis or salpingitis.

Examination

On examination, the patient with acute salpingitis will have exquisite tenderness of the involved organs. There will be a purulent discharge from the vagina and the cervical os. Always examine the periurethral (Skene) and Bartholin glands for discharge of pus. The cervix will be very tender upon manipulation. If a culdocentesis is performed, cloudy peritoneal fluid is often noted. This fluid is a "reaction fluid" to the infection. It may contain leukocytes with or without gonococci organisms.

If an abdominal upright and flat plate of the abdomen are performed, an ileus might be noted. If a pelvic abscess or ectopic pregnancy is considered, a pelvic ultrasound should be obtained.

Diagnosis

A diagnosis in the ED is presumptive without the results of a culture. A definitive diagnosis is made only after cultures have grown an organism in 48 to 72 hours.

Laboratory Findings

A CBC, electrolytes, blood culture, *N. gonorrhoeae* and chlamydia cultures should be performed. Gram-negative intracellular diplococci are seen on a smear of cervical or periurethral gland exudates. Leukocytosis with a shift to the left is often present. An HCG should be obtained on every patient to determine pregnancy status.

Treatment

All patients who present with a suspected tubo-ovarian abscess; a temperature greater than 38° C (100.4° F); pregnant; nausea or vomiting that prevents the patient from taking PO antibiotics; upper peritoneal (Fitz-Hugh–Curtis) syndrome; intrauterine device; or failure to respond to antibiotics in 48 hours should be admitted to the hospital.

The Centers for Disease Control and Prevention (CDC) Recommended Treatment for Acute PID-1989* follows:

---

*Adapted from MMWR (Suppl) 38, 1989.

Outpatient
>   Cefoxitin 2 g IM plus probenecid 1 g PO *or*
>   Ceftriaxone 250 mg IM *or* equivalent cephalosporin
>> *followed by*
> Doxycycline 100 mg PO BID for 10 to 14 days *or*
>   Tetracycline HCl 500 mg PO QID for 10 to 14 days

Inpatient
>   Recommended regimen A
>   Cefoxitin 2 g IV every 6 hours *or*
>   Cefotetan 2 g IV every 12 hours
>> *plus*
>   Doxycycline 100 mg every 12 hours PO or IV for 48 hours
>   Doxycycline 100 mg BID for 10 to 14 days after discharge from hospital

Recommended regimen B
>   Clindamycin 900 mg IV every 8 hours
>> *plus*
>   Gentamicin loading dose IV or IM (2 mg/kg), followed by a maintenance dose of 1.5 mg/kg every 8 hours for 48 hours
>   Doxycycline 100 mg BID for 10 to 14 days after hospital discharge
>   Clindamycin 450 mg PO QID continued for 10 to 14 days

Patients who are sent home after IM ceftriaxone and PO doxycycline therapy should have a follow-up in 48 hours with their primary care physician or an Ob/Gyn physician or should be told to return to the ED if nausea, vomiting, increased abdominal pain, fever, or back pain with radicular pain occurs.

TOXIC SHOCK SYNDROME

Definition

Toxic shock syndrome (TSS) is a acute, febrile illness characterized by diffuse desquamating erythroderma, mucous membrane hyperemia, vomiting, diarrhea, pharyngitis, and myalgias. It can progress to multisystem dysfunction and hypotension. There is a classic peeling of the soles of the feet and the palms and digits of the hands.

Epidemiology

TSS was first described in 1978 by Todd. The first description was of seven children with *Staphylococcus aureus* infections. The first episode of TSS in women was diagnosed in 1981 in menstruating women who were using tampons.

There were 351 cases of TSS in 1988 as reported by the CDC. TSS is seen in menstruating women from 15 to 24 years of age. TSS has been also associated with burns, nasal packing, abrasions, and abscesses.

Pathology

TSS is associated with the *S. aureus* organism. Sixty-seven percent of the organisms are phage I type, and 25% are nontypable. *Streptococcus pneumoniae, Pseudomonas aeruginosa,* and group A streptococci have been associated with a clinically indistinguishable TSS-like disease. Vasodilatation and fluid movement of serum proteins and fluids from intravascular to extravascular spaces occur with TSS, causing acute hypotension.

Clinical Presentation/Examination

A patient may present with a fever, chills, headache, vomiting, nausea, and diarrhea with massive vasodilatation. An acute onset of hypotension, edema, oliguria with low central venous pressure present later in the syndrome at time of hospitalization. Muscle weakness and tenderness with abdominal pain are often present. Pharyngitis and strawberry tongue with conjunctival hyperemia and vaginitis can be present.

A patient will present with nonmeningeal central nervous system (CNS) symptoms: confusion, agitation, somnolence, disorientation, and seizures. Diffuse organ pathology will be present. The patient will present on their third to fifth day of menses.

On the fifth to the 10th day, a generalized pruritic maculopapular rash develops in 25% of hospitalized patients. The secondary rash is a diffuse blanching erythrodermal rash that fades in 3 days, and then a full-thickness desquamation of the palms of the hands and the soles of the feet occurs on days 6 to 14 of hospitalization. Hair and nail loss can occur in up to 50% of the hospitalized patients. ARDS and ventricular arrhythmia have been reported.

Diagnosis

The CDC criteria for the diagnosis of TSS follow. All criteria must be present for the diagnosis of TSS:

1. A temperature higher than 38.9° C (102° F)
2. A systolic blood pressure less than 90 mm Hg, an orthostatic decrease of systolic blood pressure by 15 mm Hg, or syncope
3. Rash (diffuse, macular erythroderma) with subsequent desquamation, especially on the palms and soles of the feet
4. Involvement of three of the following organ systems clinically or by abnormal laboratory tests:
    a. Gastrointestinal: Vomiting and profuse diarrhea
    b. Musculoskeletal: Severe myalgias or twofold increase in creatine phosphokinase
    c. Renal: Increase in BUN and creatinine twice the normal values; pyuria without evidence of infection
    d. Mucosal inflammation: Vaginal, conjunctival, or pharyngeal hyperemia
    e. Hepatic involvement: Hepatitis with a twofold elevation of

bilirubin, serum glutamic-oxaloacetic transaminase (SGOT), and serum glutamic-pyruvic transaminase (SGPT)

   f. Hematologic: Thrombocytopenia less than 100,000 platelets/mm³

   g. CNS: Disorientation without focal neurologic signs

5. Negative serologic tests for Rocky Mountain spotted fever, leptospirosis, measles, hepatitis B surface antigens, fluorescent antinuclear antibody, VDRL, and monospot; and negative blood, urine, and throat cultures

Laboratory Findings

A CBC, electrolytes, calcium, magnesium, PT, PTT, blood and urine cultures should be performed. Vaginal cultures for gonorrhea (GC), chlamydia, and *Streptococcus* should be performed.

Hypocalcemia, hypophosphatemia, hyponatremia, hypokalemia, and metabolic acidosis can be seen. Liver function abnormalities are common. Red blood cell casts can be seen with azotemia. Acute renal failure secondary to acute renal tubular necrosis can be seen. Leukocytosis with lymphocytopenia can be seen.

Treatment

The mainstay of treatment of TSS is aggressive fluid replacement in the presence of hypotension. Fresh frozen plasma may be required. Dopamine is the vasopressor drug of choice. Whole blood transfusions are often needed. Thrombocytopenia will require platelet transfusions.

Many authors recommend vaginal irrigation with a saline and povidone-iodine solution.

Antibiotic therapy should include an antistaphylococcal penicillin or a cephalosporin with beta-lactamase stability.

1. Oxacillin or naficillin, 1 to 2 g every 4 hours
2. Cefazolin 2 g every 6 hours
3. Trimethoprim-sulfamethoxazole, vancomycin, or rifampin can be used in methicillin-resistant strains of *Streptococcus*

The use of methylprednisolone 30 mg/kg may reduce the severity of the illness.

All patients should be admitted to the ICU, and an infectious disease specialist should be consulted.

TUBO-OVARIAN ABSCESS

Definition

Tubo-ovarian abscess formation usually occurs following an acute episode of salpingitis and is seen as a recurrent infection superimposed on chronically damaged adnexae. Enlarging purulent exudate may cause the rupture of the abscess with resultant fulminating peritonitis. The abscess may also leak slowly and form a secondary abscess in the cul-de-sac.

Epidemiology

Tubo-ovarian abscesses often occur in association with the use of an intrauterine device. The typical patient who presents with a tubo-ovarian abscess is a young low-parity female with documented previous pelvic infections. With proper treatment, the current mortality rate should be less than 5%.

Pathology

A tubo-ovarian abscess can occur in the presence of tuberculosis or actinomycosis. The abscesses are usually polymicrobial and occur bilaterally. An unruptured tubo-ovarian abscess can present like an ovarian cyst, unruptured ectopic pregnancy, uterine leiomyoma, hydrosalpinx, or preappendiceal abscess.

Clinical Presentation

Patients with a tubo-ovarian abscess may be asymptomatic, and the mass may be discovered during a routine examination, or the patient may present with septicemic shock. The symptoms of the patient who is symptomatic are that the patient will present with 1 or 2 weeks of nausea, vomiting, fever, tachycardia, and lower abdominal or pelvic pain. The patient usually presents 2 weeks after her menses. In uncomplicated acute salpingitis, the patient presents shortly after the onset or cessation of menses. Tenderness in all four quadrants can be present. A patient with a ruptured tubo-ovarian abscess will present with signs and symptoms of a surgical abdomen. The patient can present in septic shock with disorientation, tachypnea, oliguria, and hypotension.

Examination

A culdocentesis can be performed to evaluate the cul-de-sac for pus, but a culdocentesis should be performed with extreme caution secondary to the possibility of rupturing or lacerating a pelvic abscess. If performed in the presence of a ruptured tubo-ovarian abscess, gross pus will be withdrawn from the cul-de-sac on culdocentesis. On pelvic examination, the patient's adnexae, uterus, and cervix will be very tender to the point that a good examination will be difficult to perform.

Diagnosis

A diagnosis is made with the history, ultrasonography examination, and culdocentesis.

Laboratory Findings

A CBC, blood cultures, PT, PTT, electrolytes, and UA with urine cultures should be performed. GC and chlamydia cultures of the cervix should be performed. On kidney, ureter, and bladder, (KUB) or acute abdominal series, an adynamic ileus will be noted.

Treatment

A tubo-ovarian abscess is a true gynecologic emergency. The threat of an unruptured tubo-ovarian abscess is that it will rupture. A ruptured tubo-ovarian abscess is a surgical emergency, and an immediate Ob/Gyn consultation is necessitated. The ruptured tubo-ovarian abscess can cause septic shock, intra-abdominal abscesses, septic emboli, and renal, lung, and brain abscesses.

Treatment of an unruptured tubo-ovarian abscess is immediate hospitalization, with the patient placed in the semi-Fowler position, with continuous vital sign and urinary output monitoring, nasogastric suctioning, and administration of IV fluids that contain sodium. Several combinations of IV antibiotics are recommended:

1. Penicillin G and chloramphenicol
2. Penicillin G plus metronidazole or clindamycin plus an aminoglycoside
3. Cefoxitin or cefamandole plus clindamycin, metronidazole, or chloramphenicol
4. Moxalactam or cefotaxime with or without clindamycin, metronidazole, chloramphenicol, or an aminoglycoside

If, during the course of the treatment, there is any suspicion of leakage or rupture or if the patient is not responding to antibiotic therapy, a laparotomy is mandatory.

A ruptured tubo-ovarian abscess is a true life-threatening catastrophe requiring immediate medical therapy followed by an immediate laparotomy. A central line should be placed to monitor the patient's central venous pressure. Administration of oxygen by facemask should be performed. Replacement of IV fluids to maintain a urine output greater than 30 ml/hr should be maintained. Methylprednisone succinate 15 to 30 mg/kg is given as an IV bolus immediately and is repeated every 4 to 6 hours for four doses.

The patient is taken to the operating room and a total hysterectomy and a bilateral salpingo-oophorectomy are usually performed. The abscess is dissected from adjacent structures. IV antibiotics are given to the patient for several days.

VULVOVAGINITIS

Definition

Vulvovaginitis is an acute vaginal infection caused by many different organisms.

Epidemiology

Vulvovaginitis can be caused by many organisms, such as *Trichomonas, Gardnerella,* and *Candida albicans.* Herpes simplex virus and local contact vulvovaginitis or vaginal foreign bodies can all cause vulvovaginitis. Atopic vaginitis can occur in virgins and in postmenopausal women. Bacterial vaginosis has been linked to premature rupture of the membranes and premature delivery.

Pathology

The normal female vagina has a thick vaginal epithelium. This epithelium contains large amounts of glycogen, which protects the vaginal mucosa. The glycogen causes the normal flora to consist of lactobacilli and acidogenic corynebacteria to form lactic and acetic acid. The normal vaginal pH is 3.5 to 4.1. When there is a lack of estrogen, progesterone results in an atopic vagina. This acidic environment discourages the growth of pathogenic bacteria. The pH just before menarche and menopause is 6 to 7.

Alkaline secretions from the cervix before and during menses or semen predispose the vagina to infection. There are very few nerve endings in the vagina, thus the patient is asymptomatic until the vagina and the vulva are heavily involved with the infective organism.

Candida vaginitis is the most common cause of vaginitis. It constitutes the normal flora for up to 50% of all females. As long as normal flora remain in balance, there will be no overgrowth of *Candida.* Antibiotics, loss of normal glycogen stores, diabetes mellitus, pregnancy, use of birth control pills, the postmenopausal female vaginal mucosa, or an increase in the pH of the vagina will cause an overgrowth of *Candida.*

Trichomonas vaginalis is caused by a flagellated protozoa that may live in the paraurethral glands for many days or months before a diagnosis is made. *Trichomonas* can live for many hours in hot tubs, urine, tap water, and swimming pools and on toilet seats.

Acute bacterial vaginosis is usually caused by *Gardnerella, Haemophilus,* and *Corynebacterium,* which are nonspecific organisms. Acute bacterial vaginosis is caused by an alteration of the normal vaginal microflora that promote the synergistic growth of the aforementioned organisms.

Clinical Presentation

The female with *C. albicans* will present with dysuria or dyspareunia, vaginal pruritus, leukorrhea, vulvar edema, and erythema and will complain of a thick "cottage cheese" discharge. Patients with recurrent vaginal *Candida* should be evaluated for predisposing causes, including diabetes, chronic use of antibiotics, pregnancy, or HIV. Male sexual partners should be examined for candidal balanitis.

T. vaginalis is asymptomatic in up to 50% of the patients who have this infection. It is almost always a sexually transmitted disease. Patients with *Trichomonas* have the classic gray or yellow vaginal discharge that is malodorous and is described as "frothy." The patient will complain of vulvovaginal fullness, intense or mild, and intermenstrual or postcoital spotting. Ninety percent of males who are infected are asymptomatic.

Women with acute bacterial vaginosis will present with mild pruritus and copious vaginal discharge with a "fishy" odorous vaginal discharge.

Examination

The patient with *Candida* will present on examination with vulvar erythema and edema. Vaginal erythema will be present in 20% of the patients. A "cottage cheese" discharge will be present.

The patient with *T. vaginalis* will present on examination with a frothy gray or yellow to green discharge with the classic strawberry cervix on gynecologic examination. The strawberry cervix (punctate hemorrhages) will only be seen 20% of the time on examination. Vaginal vault erythema will be seen in 80% of the presenting cases.

Women with bacterial vaginosis will present on examination with mild vaginal erythema and a thin, frothy gray-white vaginal discharge.

Diagnosis

A diagnosis of vaginal *Candida* is made by microscopic examination of vaginal secretions on a potassium hydroxide slide. Pseudohyphae or budding yeast will be found.

A diagnosis of *T. vaginalis* is made by a vaginal pH greater than 4.5 and a microscopic examination of vaginal vault secretions. Many polymorphonuclear leukocytes and motile pear-shaped, flagellated *Trichomonas,* which are slightly larger than the leukocytes, will be seen on microscopic examination.

For the diagnosis of acute bacterial vaginosis to be made the CDC states that the following criteria must be present:

1. Homogeneous discharge
2. A pH of discharge greater than 4.5
3. A positive amine odor test
4. The presence of clue cells

Gram-negative rods are found in 40% of asymptomatic women and children who have no prior sexual contact. Males can harbor the organisms and be asymptomatic. On a wet mount saline slide, on microscopic examination, the pathognomonic clue cells will be noted. Clue cells are clusters of bacilli clinging to the surface of epithelial cells.

Laboratory Findings

A normal saline and potassium examination of vaginal fluid should be performed with every pelvic examination. The vaginal pH should also be checked in each patient with nitrazine paper. Cultures for GC and chlamydia should be performed on all females with vulvovaginitis. A UA with a urine culture should also be obtained on each patient presenting with the symptoms of vulvovaginitis. Any patient who presents with any suspected sexually transmitted disease should have a RPR (VDRL) and HIV drawn to complete the work-up.

Treatment

C. albicans is treated with 3 to 7 days of miconazole nitrate, clotrimazole, or butoconazole intravaginally.

The treatment of *T. vaginalis,* in the nonpregnant patient, is accomplished by giving the patient 2 g of metronidazole (Flagyl) PO in a one-dose treatment. If the 2-g dose fails, 500 mg of metronidazole PO BID for 7 days can be given to the nonpregnant patient. Metronidazole has an Antabuse-like reaction that will cause vomiting. Alcohol should be avoid for at least 24 hours after the last dose of metronidazole. Pregnant patients with severe symptoms who are after their first trimester can be treated with 2 g of metronidazole after gynecologic consultation. The safe use of metronidazole in the first trimester has not been established and therefore it should not be given. Both male and female sexual partners should be treated to prevent reinfection.

The CDC does not recommend treatment of asymptomatic females who have bacterial vaginosis. For symptomatic females, metronidazole 500 mg BID PO for 7 days is recommended. The male sexual partner should also be treated. If it is necessary to treat the pregnant patient, clindamycin 300 mg PO BID is given for 7 days in the first trimester of pregnancy.

ABRUPTIO PLACENTAE

Definition

Abruptio placentae is defined as the early separation of the placenta from the site of implantation on the uterus before delivery of the fetus.

Epidemiology

Abruptio placentae occurs in 1 in 500 to 750 deliveries. Approximately 30% of all third-trimester bleeding, after 26 weeks, is caused by abruptio placentae. Fetal mortality rates range from 50 to 80%. Morbidity of live births, hypoxia, birth trauma, and prematurity range from 40 to 50%.

Pathology

There are two types of abruptio placentae presentations. The concealed form (20%) is when the bleeding is confined to the uterine cavity. The complications are often severe or fatal secondary to the complete separation of the placenta with no bleeding through the cervix into the vagina.

The external form (80%) in which the hemorrhaging blood drains through the cervix and the placental detachment is more likely to be incomplete than complete. Complications are often less severe and less life threatening with the external form of abruptio placentae.

Several causes of premature placental separation are suggested. Local vascular injury at the site of attachment leads to vascular rupture into the decidua basalis, causing bleeding and hematoma formation and thus separation. Also suggested as the cause of an acute abruptio placentae is an acute rise in uterine venous pressure transmitted to the intervillous space. This results in engorgement of the venous bed and in separation of the placenta.

Trauma or a sudden decompression of the uterus with the delivery of the first twin or rupture of the membranes in hydramnios can cause traction on the placenta and thus rupture.

After one episode of abruptio placentae, there is a 10 to 17% increased risk of a second occurrence of abruptio placentae. If hypertension is present, either chronic hypertension or PIH, there is a 2.5 to 17.9% incidence of placental separation.

Other predisposing factors to abruptio placentae include:

Advanced maternal age	Uterine distention
Multiple pregnancies	Hydramnios
Diabetes mellitus	Leiomyomas
Alcohol consumption	Tobacco use
Possibly maternal type O blood	Trauma
Rapid amniotic fluid loss	Abnormally short cord

Clinical Presentation

There must be a high index of suspicion to diagnose abruptio placentae. Thirty percent of separations are small and produce few or no symptoms. Large separations can produce abdominal pain and uterine irritability. Hemorrhage can be either visible or concealed.

Patients can present with DIC, hypovolemic shock, fetal distress, or uterine tetany. Eighty percent of patients will present with vaginal bleeding, and two thirds will present with uterine tenderness with or without abdominal pain or back pain. One third of patients presenting with abruptio placentae will present with high-frequency contractions, and half will present with hypertonus.

Examination

The vaginal examination of a patient with suspected abruptio placentae is to be performed with extreme caution. Without an ultrasound examination, the differentiation of abruptio placentae from placenta previa cannot be made. A pelvic examination can turn a simple placenta previa into a fatal event. Before a vaginal examination is performed, your "safety net" should be obtained. Two large-gauge 14- to 16-gauge IV lines and type and crossmatched blood, 6 to 8 units, should be readily available along with an immediate Ob/Gyn consultation. If there is a high index of suspicion of abruptio placentae or placenta previa, the Ob/Gyn physician should be physically present when the pelvic examination is performed and the operating room should be readily available for immediate cesarean section. If time permits, an ultrasound should be done before the pelvic examination is performed.

Diagnosis

The diagnosis is assumed in any female who presents with hemorrhage, uterine spasm, and fetal distress in the third trimester. Early ultrasound and consultation with an obstetrician are indicated.

Laboratory Findings

Obtain a CBC, electrolytes, PT, PTT, type and crossmatch 6 to 8 units of blood, and determine Rh type. If DIC is considered, obtain a peripheral blood smear; look for schistocytes; and order fibrinogen and fibrin split products.

A quick test for DIC is to place a venous sample of blood into a test tube every hour. If the blood fails to clot in progressive blood samples, then there is a deficiency of fibrinogen and platelets.

Treatment

If abruptio placentae is diagnosed with severe hemorrhage and the patient is in danger, the membranes should be ruptured to minimize the possibility of DIC or amniotic embolus. Internal monitoring should be obtained to provide information on uterine tonus and contractions and the status of the fetus. This should be done in consultation with an obstetrician.

Two large 14- to 16-gauge IV lines should be started with normal saline or lactated Ringer's solution. The patient should be placed on oxygen. Type and crossmatched blood should be obtained for 6 to 8 units. Fresh whole blood is the blood of choice, because it contains all necessary factors. Packed red blood cells can also be used but they do not contain clotting factors. Platelets can be used to counteract clotting deficiencies.

Fibrinogen is rarely indicated. If there is no active bleeding the fibrinogen deficiency may resolve spontaneously in a few hours. Do not give fibrinogen based on laboratory values. Cryoprecipitate is the best choice after whole blood for fibrinogen replacement but should be given only when needed secondary to the chance that fibrinogen products can be converted to a fibrin emboli. The initial dose of fibrinogen is 4 to 6 g, but DIC may require 20 to 24 g of fibrinogen.

Heparin should be administered to block conversion of prothrombin to thrombin, reducing the consumption of coagulation factors. There are risks to the use of heparin in the treatment of acute placental separation not in DIC. Heparin can cause bleeding problems at the time of delivery or cesarean section and postoperative hemorrhage. It should not be used without consultation of an obstetrician. Aminocaproic acid (Amicar) should not be given, because it interferes with the mechanism of fibrinolysis.

Be aware of the possibility of uterine apoplexy, the loss of myometrial contractility secondary to extensive infiltration of the myometrial wall with blood. Thus a prompt cesarean section is indicated if severe abruptio placentae is diagnosed. If uterine apoplexy is severe, a hysterectomy is indicated.

MASTITIS AND BREAST ABSCESS

DEFINITION

Mastitis is the engorgement, inflammation, and infection of the breasts of postpartum females. An abscess is a localized, encapsulated infection of the breast.

ETIOLOGY AND EPIDEMIOLOGY

Mastitis usually occurs 5 days or longer post partum in the primiparous nursing female. It can also occur in females who are weaning their babies from breast milk. Often, the mother acquires the infection while in the hospital and can pass the infection on to her infant.

PATHOLOGY

Mastitis is usually secondary to a coagulase-positive *Staphylococcus aureus* organism.

CLINICAL PRESENTATION AND DIAGNOSIS

Women with mastitis present with painful erythematous lobules in an outer quadrant of the breast. This is usually noted in the second or third week of puerperium. The infection may be limited to the subareolar region of the breast, or it may involve an obstructed lactiferous duct and surrounding breast tissue. The female presents with high fever, nausea and sometimes vomiting, and a very warm, tender, engorged breast. A breast abscess is an inflamed area with some degree of fluctuation.

LABORATORY FINDINGS

A CBC, electrolytes, BUN, and creatinine test results should be obtained. A urinalysis with culture findings should also be considered if urinary symptoms are present. A blood culture should be obtained if the nursing female appears septic or has a very high temperature. The presence of the antibody-coated bacteria in the milk indicates infectious mastitis. If the nursing infant has recurring infections, or if the mastitis is bilateral or recurring, he or she may harbor the *S. aureus* organism and reinfect the mother.

TREATMENT

Mastitis is treated by the application of local heat. If no fissures are present, breast-feeding should be continued. If fissures are present on the nipple, milk engorgement should be relieved with a breast pump. A well-fitted brassiere is needed for relief of pain.

Antibiotic treatment is directed toward penicillinase-producing bacteria, which are usually the causative organisms. Cephalosporin, methicillin sodium, cloxacillin, and dicloxacillin can all be used to treat mastitis. If mastitis is not treated properly, it can develop into a breast abscess. If a breast abscess is present, it should be incised, drained, and cultured. When a breast abscess is present, breastfeeding should be discontinued. Phenergan or Compazine suppositories should be given along with oral antibiotics at hospital discharge to prevent nausea and vomiting. If the patient appears septic, is in severe pain, or has refractory nausea and vomiting, she should be admitted by the OB/GYN service for nausea and vomiting control and intravenous antibiotic therapy. Any female with a breast abscess should also be considered for hospital admission. If the mastitis is bilateral or recurrent, the mother's infant should be referred to pediatrics to rule out streptococcal infection.

PREVENTION

To prevent the recurrence of mastitis, the mother should be instructed in meticulous breast hygiene. If there is a breast fissure, a nipple shield should be worn to protect the nipple and to allow the infant to still breast-feed.

BIBLIOGRAPHY

Braunwald E, Isselbacher KJ, Petersdorf RG, et al (eds): Harrison's Principles of Internal Medicine, 11th ed. New York, McGraw-Hill, 1987
Cark SL, Cotton DB, Hankins P (eds): Critical Care Obstetrics, 2nd ed. Boston, Blackwell Scientific Publications, 1991
Cunningham FG, MacDonald PC, Gant NF (eds): Williams Obstetrics, 18th ed. Norwalk, CT, Appleton & Lange, 1989
Hamilton GC, Sanders AB, Strange GR, Trott AT (eds): Emergency Medicine: An Approach to Clinical Problem-Solving. Philadelphia, WB Saunders, 1991
May HL, Aghababian RV, Fleisher GR (eds): Emergency Medicine, 2nd ed. Boston, Little, Brown, 1992
Pernoll ML (ed): Current Obstetric and Gynecologic Diagnosis and Treatment, 7th ed. Norwalk, CT, Appleton & Lange, 1991

Rosen P, Barkin RM (eds): Emergency Medicine: Concepts and Clinical Practice, 3rd ed. St Louis, Mosby-Year Book, 1992

Schwartz GR, Cayten CG, Mangelsen MA (eds): Principles and Practice of Emergency Medicine, 3rd ed. Malvern, PA, Lea & Febiger, 1992

Tintinalli JE, Krone RL, Ruiz E (eds): Emergency Medicine: A Comprehensive Study Guide, 4th ed. New York, McGraw-Hill, 1996

Chapter 11

Oncologic and Hematologic Emergencies

ACUTE BLEEDING DIATHESIS

Definition

Acute bleeding disorders are divided into four main classes: (1) coagulation factor disorders, (2) platelet disorders, (3) vascular bleeding, and (4) fibrinolysis.

Pathology

Coagulation factor problems are secondary to either an intrinsic or extrinsic pathway problem. When tissue is injured, both pathways are activated to produce an insoluble clot. Coagulation factor problems are mainly bleeding problems of the large vessels from hemophilia or sodium warfarin therapy.

The intrinsic pathway consists of factors VIII, IX, XI, and XII, then factors I, II, V, X, and XIII (common pathway). The intrinsic pathway is phospholipid dependent and is represented by the partial thromboplastin time (PTT). The PTT will be affected by deficiencies of factors VII, IX, and XI. The PTT is also affected by heparin. The normal PTT is 25 to 35 seconds.

The extrinsic pathway involves tissue thromboplastin and factors VII to X, then the common pathway factors V, II, I, and XIII. This pathway is represented by the thrombin time (PT) factors II, I, and XII and is not affected by heparin. Calcium must be present with thromboplastin for the extrinsic pathway to work. The PT is normal in hemophilia patients. It will be elevated in liver disease, warfarin therapy, or vitamin K deficiency. The common pathway is factors X, V, II, I, and XIII. The normal PT is 10 to 12 seconds.

When heparin is given it affects or inhibits thrombin and factor X, thus a heparin overdose will affect both the PT and PTT, factor X being common to both pathways. Sodium warfarin affects or depresses factors II, VII, IX, and X.

When tissue is injured, platelets release adenosine 5'-diphosphate (ADP) at the injury site. Platelet factor II and phospholipids are then released to catalyze the clot. A low platelet count in lieu of injury will cause small vessel bleeding or purpura.

Vascular bleeding is caused by a defect in the supportive connective tissue or the blood vessel wall secondary to inflammation. There are several intrinsic causes of vascular bleeding. The chronic use of steroids or increased vascular friability secondary to old age or senile purpura is the major cause of smaller vessel bleeding. Telangiectasia of the skin and mucous membrane (Osler-Weber-Rendu disease), prolonged traumatic bleeding, perifollicular bleeding, scurvy, and purpura (petechiae) are all causes of vascular bleeding. This increased bleeding reaction can be caused by allergic reactions to drugs, immune disease, scurvy, and vasculitis. In vascular bleeding, there will be prolonged bleeding times and a positive tourniquet test. The PT, PTT, and platelet counts will be normal.

Fibrinolysis is seen when there is an excessive or exaggerated hemostatic conversion of plasminogen to plasmin. This process cleaves fibrin polymers into fibrin degradation (split) products and acts to lyse thrombi. This exaggerated process causes an increased bleeding by altering other coagulation factors by inducing an accelerated consumption of clotting factors. This exaggerated consumption is one cause of disseminated intravascular coagulation (DIC).

Diagnosis

The diagnosis of a bleeding disorder is determined by the PT, PTT, fibrin, fibrin split product count, platelet count, and history of prior bleeding, hemophilia, or trauma.

Laboratory Findings

A platelet count PT, PTT, fibrin, fibrin split product count, and factor counts should be drawn in patients who are believed to have bleeding problems.

BLOOD TRANSFUSIONS

BLOOD COMPONENTS

Blood is made up of noncellular and cellular components. Plasma protein fraction (PPF), fresh frozen plasma (FFP), albumin, and cryoprecipitate are noncellular components of blood. Red blood cells (RBCs), platelets, and white blood cells (WBCs) are the components of cellular blood.

Whole blood is stored with citrate-phosphate-dextrose (CPD) or citrate-phosphate-dextrose-adenine (CPDA-1) at 4° C (39.2° F) and has no functioning granulocytes. Within 24 hours of storage of whole blood, only 50% of the platelets and factor VIII are functional. Within 72 hours, both factor VIII and platelets have degraded to negligible amounts. In 3 to 5 days factor V is 50% degraded, and in 4 to 6 days there is increased hemoglobin affinity for oxygen. At 6 days, there is decreased RBC viability and deformity. After the fifth day, ammonia, hydrogen, and potassium concentrations rise, and platelets, fibrin, and leukocytes microaggregate. By adding CPD to the whole blood, the shelf-life is increased to 21 days. If CPDA-1 is added, the shelf-life is increased to 35 days.

Packed red blood cells (PRBCs) are prepared and stored at a hematocrit no greater than 80 and have a shelf-life of 21 to 35 days.

PRBCs are used to replace volume lost by hypovolemia along with crystalloid solutions. PRBCs are excellent for rapid volume replacement. The advantages of using PRBCs are: (1) reduced volume overload; (2) decreased citrate, ammonia, and organic acids versus increased with whole blood; and (3) reduced risk of alloimmunization secondary to less antigens present in the PRBCs.

Platelets are used in trauma patients, surgery patients, and patients with thrombocytopenia in abnormal bleeding conditions. One unit of packed platelets will increase the platelet count by 4000 to 8000 in a 70-kg man.

Washed RBCs have a very short half-life of 24 hours. Washed RBCs are used in patients with known allergic reactions to plasma antigens, platelets, and granulocytes.

Fresh frozen plasma (FFP) contains all noncellular coagulation factors. ABO matching is required before use. FFP is used to correct significant deficiencies of clotting factors.

Cryoprecipitate is plasma that has been frozen and then rethawed. It is rich in factor VIII and fibrinogen. Cryoprecipitate does not require ABO crossmatching. Cryoprecipitate is used to replace bleeding factors in hemophilia.

Albumin is a "salt poor" preparation that is hyperoncotic to plasma and is available in a 5% buffered solution and a 25% iso-oncotic solution. A 12.5-g (25 ml) ampule has the oncontic effect of 1 unit of FFP. It contains between 130 and 160 mEq of sodium.

TRANSFUSIONS

A blood transfusion should be administered through large-gauge IV tubing with a Y device so that warmed normal saline can be infused at the same time as the blood. Glucose or calcium-containing solutions should not be used at the same time as a transfusion is being performed. All blood should be transfused through a micropore filter (20- to 40-μm pore size). Blood should always be warmed prior to administration. Cold blood can precipitate hypothermia. Pressure infusion devices can be used, but they should not be inflated to greater than 300 mm Hg.

All blood should be type specific and should be crossmatched when possible. It only takes an extra 5 minutes to type and crossmatch blood versus to type and screen the blood unit. In an emergency when blood is required immediately, you can use type O blood. Rh-positive O blood should be given to males, and Rh-negative blood should be given to females. Only PRBCs should be given to either male or female patients, and type-specific crossmatched PRBCs should be given as soon as possible. Most military studies were based on Rh-positive blood, and most civilian studies were based on the use of Rh-negative blood. The universal donor blood in civilian practice is Rh-negative blood.

Autotransfusion is the reinfusion of the patient's blood by collecting the blood from the thorax or peritoneal cavity after cell washing and antibiotic administration.

A *massive blood transfusion* is when 50% of the patient's blood is transfused in a 24-hour period or when 50% is transfused at one time. Massive blood transfusions have many complications, including adult respiratory distress syndrome (ARDS), hypothermia, hypocalcemia, citrate toxicity, and coagulopathies.

TRANSFUSION REACTIONS

There are four types of transfusion reactions: (1) allergic, (2) febrile, (3) delayed, and (4) hemolytic. Allergic reactions are seen in rapid uncrossmatched blood transfusions. They are usually seen the IgA-deficient recipient who has a history of numerous allergies. If an allergic reaction occurs, the transfusion should be stopped immediately and epinephrine, fluids, and antihistamines should be given along with good supportive care.

Febrile reactions are the most common reaction. Patients develop chills, malaise, and fever. They can progress to respiratory distress and hypotension. If a febrile reaction occurs, the transfusion should be stopped and a search for RBC destruction should take place for antibody mismatch.

A hemolytic blood transfusion reaction is an intravascular hemolysis and is the most serious of all reactions. It is often due to a mismatch of the patient's blood specimen for type and crossmatch or inapproperate labeling of the given blood unit. Rapid destruction of transfused RBCs take place secondary to an antibody-mediated reaction. When the RBCs are destroyed there is a release of free hemoglobin, which causes hemoglobinuria, hemoglobinemia, elevation of bilirubin, and depletion of haptoglobin. Anesthetized patients will develop hypotension. Patients who are awake will complain of low back pain, shortness of breath, fever, chills, and a burning sensation at the site of the blood transfusion.

Patients with a hemolytic reaction develop hemoglobin in the urine, free hemoglobin in the blood serum, a direct and indirect Coombs test, and coagulation. A rapid screen for hemolytic reaction is to centrifuge a complete blood count tube. If the color of the centrifuged blood is pink, it suggests free hemoglobin at levels of 50 to 100 mg/dl. If the centrifuged blood is pale brown, the hemoglobin concentration is at a level below 20 mg/dl.

The treatment of a hemolytic reaction is to immediately discontinue the transfusion. Give 80 to 100 mg of furosemide to increase the renal cortical blood flow. Very large amounts of normal saline should be utilized to increase urinary outflow at 0.5 to 1 ml/kg hr.

Delayed reaction can be seen several days after the transfusion. It will be diagnosed as a decrease in hemoglobin. This reaction is secondary to the transfused RBCs becoming coated with nonagglutinating antibodies and being removed by tissue-bound macrophages in the spleen. Fluid administration and re-determination of the transfusion compatibility and a check for the presence of undetected antibodies are the cornerstones of treatment.

HEMOPHILIA

Definition

Hemophilia is a disorder of the intrinsic clotting pathway and is divided into three types: (1) hemophilia A or classic hemophilia, (2) hemophilia B or Christmas disease, and (3) von Willebrand's disease.

Epidemiology

Hemophilia is primarily a hereditary bleeding disorder. In hemophilia A, only 50% of patients have a family history of hemophilia. In hemophilia B, there is a 75% family history of hemophilia. von Willebrand's disease is an autosomal dominant disease with variation in expression.

Pathology

Hemophilia A is a sex-linked disorder caused by a deficiency in factor VIII. Classic hemophilia is divided to three classes based on factor VIII activity: (1) severe, less than 2% activity; (2) moderate, 2 to 5% activity; and (3) mild, 5 to 30% activity. In hemophilia A, the PT is normal; the PTT is elevated; and factor VIII-C is decreased. The von Willebrand factor antigen (vWF:Ag) and ristocetin platelet aggregation (vWF activity) are both normal. The bleeding time is normal, and factor IX is normal in hemophilia A.

In hemophilia B, there is a deficiency in factor IX. There are mild, moderate, and severe forms of hemophilia B. Clinically, hemophilia B is indistinguishable from hemophilia A. Hemophilia B presents with a normal PT, factor VIII-C, vWF:Ag, vWF activity, and bleeding time. Hemophilia B will have an increased PTT and decreased factor IX.

von Willebrand's disease is a disorder of factor VIII coagulation activity and immunologic activity of the vWF:Ag and vWF aggregation. In von Willebrand's disease, the PT and factor IX are normal. The VIII-C, vWF:Ag, and vWF activity are decreased. The PTT and bleeding times are increased.

Clinical Presentation

Patients present in various ways, depending on the type and severity of bleeding disorders. They can present in adulthood with a history of minor or recurrent bleeding episodes. Profuse or serious bleeding often occurs after a major trauma, tonsillectomy, dental extractions, or pregnancy. Women will present with a history of easy bruising and excessive menstrual blood flow.

Adults frequently present with hematuria after exercise. Bleeding after circumcision is often a presenting complaint in the infant. Children will present with hemiarthroses and muscle hematomas after walking or sports activity.

Hemophilia patients with retroperitoneal hematomas present with groin pain at the insertion of the psoas muscle secondary to hemorrhage into the facial planes.

Examination

The patient should be given a complete examination, including a rectal examination to rule out gastrointestinal bleeding and a funduscopic examination to rule out retinal hemorrhage. Examine the spleen and liver very carefully. Evaluate all joints while looking for edema, warmth, and pain. Chronic inflammation will leave fibrous adhesions and joint ankylosis.

Diagnosis

A diagnosis is made by a family history, clinical presentation, PT, PTT, VIII-C, vWF:AG, vWF activity, bleeding times, and factor IX levels.

Laboratory Findings

A PT, PTT, vWF:AG, vWF activity, factor VIII-C, factor IX, and bleeding times should be drawn. A CBC, electrolytes, BUN, creatinine, glucose, liver function tests, and urinalysis should also be performed.

Treatment

Treatment is guided toward the specific type and severity of hemophilia disease. If a patient presents with an unknown type of hemophilia, FFP contains all types of coagulation factors.

Each milliliter of normal plasma contains 1 unit of factor activity. The average person contains 40 ml/kg of plasma. Each 40 units/kg of factor VIII will raise the factor VIII level by 100%. The normal dose of FFP is 10 to 15 ml/kg and will raise factor VIII by 20 to 30%.

Desmopressin acetate affects renal water conservation and is a synthetic analogue of the natural hormone arginine vasopressin. It is an antidiuretic hormone that can raise the factor VIII level.

I-deamino-(8-D-arginine)-vasopressin (DDAVP), an analogue of vasopressin, can also raise factor VIII activity rapidly within 30 minutes with a maximal effect in 90 minutes to 2 hours. It is given at a dose of 0.4 µg/kg over 10 to 15 minutes. The patient's blood pressure must be monitored carefully. Some patients will develop hypertension. The most common complaint is facial flushing. DDAVP will raise factor VIII levels by 300 to 400% and is usually adequate for hemostasis. It works best on patients with hemophilia A and von Willebrand's disease type 1. DDAVP is not effective in moderate hemophilia and type IIB von Willebrand's disease.

Cryoprecipitate at one time was the choice of treatment for mild classic hemophilia and von Willebrand's disease. It is used less today secondary to the potential for transfusion-transmitted viral diseases, but it can still be used if blood products are properly screened. Cryoprecipitate contains 50 to 100 units of factor VIII per bag.

Lyophilized concentrates of factors II, VII, IX, and X are used to treat factor IX deficiency. There are about 20 units/ml of factor IX in each bag.

Ice packs and ace wraps can be applied to areas of acute hematomas and hemorrhage sites. Appropriate analgesia should be administered. If there is an acute or chronic inflammation, synovitis, hematuria, or acute hemarthrosis present, steroids can be used in a dose of 1 mg/kg/day.

Specific Treatment

With hemophilia A or factor VIII deficiency, treat a minor exacerbation with 18 units of factor activity per kg. In moderate exacerbations, give 26 units of factor activity. In severe exacerbations, give 35 units of factor activity. After the bolus, give 10 units/kg every 8 to 12 hours for minor hemorrhage, 14 units/kg every 8 to 12 hours for mild hemorrhage, and 18 units/kg every 8 to 12 hours for 7 to 10 days for severe hemorrhage.

Patients with hemophilia B or Christmas disease secondary to a factor IX deficiency who have minor exacerbations should receive 25 units of factor activity per kg. A patient who has a moderate exacerbation should be given 35 units of factor activity, and a patient with a severe exacerbation should be given 45 units of factor activity bolus. The patient should then be given 5 units/kg every 12 to 24 hours for minor hemorrhage, 8 units/kg every 12 to 24 hours for moderate hemorrhage, and 10 units/kg every 12 hours for severe hemorrhage, for 7 to 10 days.

Cryoprecipitate contains approximately 80 units of factor VIII per bag. Heat-treated concentrates will have the values of factors VIII and IX. FFP contains 1 unit of factor IX or factor VIII per milliliter.

All patients with an acute hemophilia exacerbation should be referred to their hematologist within 72 hours.

SICKLE CELL ANEMIA

Definition

Sickle cell anemia is a chronic disease with acute exacerbations of sickling deformity of the RBCs, which limits the RBCs from passing through the microvasculature. It occurs in three types: (1) sickle cell anemia (homozygosity) Hb SS, (2) sickle cell trait (heterozygosity) Hb AS, and (3) doubly heterozygous (heterozygous for S, heterozygous for another abnormal hemoglobin).

Epidemiology

Sickle cell anemia affects 8% of the black population in America. It is an autosomal dominant inherited trait. Most patients with sickle cell disease present between the ages of 6 months and 15 years.

Pathology

Sickle cell disease is a biochemical abnormality that causes the RBCs to sickle. This sickling is the result of the substitution of B_6 valine for glutamic acid in the hemoglobin chain. This substitution causes the susceptibility of deoxygenated sickled hemoglobin to polymerize and aggregate, which induces the RBC deformity.

When the RBC is sickled, it is unable to pass through the microvascular and thus thrombosis and hemolysis occur. This event produces infarction, ischemia, chronic hemolytic anemia, and multisystem compromise.

Sickle cell anemia (Hb SS) is the most severe form of sickle cell disease. These patients have an increased susceptibility to infection, especially pneumococci and *Salmonella*. They also have diminished reticuloendothelial phagocytic and splenic function. They also have defective polymorphonuclear and granulation mobility and thus have increased risk of infection. The most severe infections occur in the Hb SS type of sickle cell anemia secondary to 75 to 95% of circulating hemoglobin in the sickled form. Sickle cell crisis occurs most often in the Hb SS patients secondary to disseminated microcirculatory thrombosis causing an acute pain crisis.

Hb AS, sickle cell trait, presents when one parent has the sickle gene and the other parent has the normal hemoglobin A gene. The patient will have both hemoglobin A and S in variable proportions. Only 50% of the circulation hemoglobin will sickle, and severe vasoocclusion and hemolytic manifestations do not usually occur.

Doubly heterozygous anemia expresses itself as Hb SC, Hb SB thalassemia, Hb SD, and Hb S-fetal persistence. This type of disease can present from asymptomatic disease to severe systemic complications.

Clinical Presentation

Any black child who presents with unexplained bone pain, anemia, jaundice, severe hemolytic anemia, or recurrent left upper quadrant pain should be considered to have sickle cell anemia.

Patients with doubly heterozygous disease may not present until late in the second or third decade of life. Hb SC disease can cause complications secondary to bone marrow infarction and fat emboli.

Patients can present with ischemic leg ulceration, respiratory insufficiency with cor pulmonale, congestive heart failure, progressive renal insufficiency, and nephrotic syndrome. Priapism is common in males with sickle cell crisis. Patients with acute sickle cell crisis present with back, abdominal, chest, tibia, and periarticular pain.

Examination

The patient should be given a complete examination with particular attention to tenderness over the liver and spleen. Examine the patient's back for costovertebral tenderness as a sign of renal involvement. Also perform a fundoscopic examination to rule out retinal hemorrhage. Perform a complete neurologic examination. Often in sickle cell patients neurologic changes can be subtle secondary to chronic organic brain syndrome.

Diagnosis

To diagnose double heterozygous disease, hemoglobin electrophoresis is required to distinguish this disease from sickle cell disease. Sickle cell disease is diagnosed by family history and electrophoresis.

Laboratory Findings

A complete blood count (CBC), PT, PTT, reticulocyte count, electrolytes, blood urea nitrogen (BUN), creatinine, liver function tests, cardiac enzymes and urinalysis should be drawn. In homozygous sickle cell disease, significant anemia and chronically elevated reticulocyte counts will be seen. Hemolytic anemia is usually present secondary to chronic bone marrow stimulus, thus the platelet counts and leukocytes are chronically elevated. The definitive test for sickle cell disease is demonstrating sickle hemoglobin by electrophoretic separation.

A rapid test for homozygous or double heterozygous sickle cell disease in the ED is microscopic examination of a peripheral blood smear. Irreversible sickled cells will be seen on examination of a peripheral blood smear. In Hb AS, cells can un-sickle when exposed to oxygen on a peripheral smear, therefore this is a poor test for Hb AS but a good test for Hb SS disease.

Patients with acute sickle cell crisis present with an exaggerated hemolytic process with a dramatic fall in the hemoatocrit and reticulocyte counts with aplastic crisis and jaundice. Crisis often accompanies an acute infection, which suppresses the bone marrow. Folic acid deficiency can also exacerbate sickle cell crisis. In children a life-threatening exacerbation of sickle cell disease can be associated with pancytopenia and a very painful swollen liver and spleen.

Many rapid sickle tests are available for testing for sickle cell anemia (e.g., Sickledex SickleScrene).

Treatment

Sickle cell crisis is a clinical diagnosis. The crisis is treated with oxygen, IV saline rehydration, correction of acidosis if present, and liberal use of analgesics. An aggressive attempt should be made to find the underlying cause of the exacerbation (e.g., pneumonia, kidney infection), and it should be treated appropriately with antibiotics.

Priapism is treated with ice compresses, liberal analgesia, and immediate urologic consultation. Hematuria can be a sign of obstruction at the ureteropelvic junction, especially if flank pain is present, and should be treated with copious fluid and analgesia. If a patient's single joint is swollen, it can be attributed to septic arthritis, osteomyelitis, hemiarthrosis, gout, and aseptic necrosis. In acute sickle cell crisis usually more than one joint is swollen and red. If joint edema is monoarticular, infection must be considered and arthrocentesis should be considered to rule out infection.

It is very common for the sickle cell patient to return several times in the first 72 hours during an acute pain crisis. Schedule a consultation and admit the patient early for fluid therapy and analgesia, especially in the use of Hb SS patients with infection.

BIBLIOGRAPHY

Braunwald E, Isselbacher KJ, Petersdorf RG, et al (eds): Harrison's Principles of Internal Medicine, 11th ed. New York, McGraw-Hill, 1987

Hamilton GC, Sanders AB, Strange GR, et al (eds): Emergency Medicine: An Approach to Clinical Problem-Solving. Philadelphia, WB Saunders, 1991

Kravis TC, Warner CG, Jacobs LM (eds): Emergency Medicine: A Comprehensive Review, 3rd ed. New York, Raven Press, 1993

May HL, Aghababian RV, Fleisher GR (eds): Emergency Medicine, 2nd ed. Boston, Little, Brown, 1992

Rosen P, Barkin RM (eds): Emergency Medicine: Concepts and Clinical Practice, 3rd ed. St Louis, Mosby-Year Book, 1992

Schwartz GR, Cayton CG, Manglesen MA, et al (eds): Principles and Practice of Emergency Medicine, 3rd ed. Philadelphia, Lea & Febiger, 1992

Tintinalli JE, Krone RL, Ruiz E (eds): Emergency Medicine: A Comprehensive Study Guide, 4rd ed. New York, McGraw-Hill, 1996

Chapter **12**

Orthopedic Emergencies

BASIC PRINCIPLES OF ORTHOPEDIC INJURIES

Definition

Patients can suffer fractures from falls, direct trauma, and motor vehicle accidents. The age of the patient, the underlying medical problems, and whether the injury is open or closed all determine the therapy.

Fractures are described by their location, whether they are open or closed, simple or comminuted, their position, displacement, and angulation. Valgus denotes a deformity in which the described part is angled away from the midline of the body. Varus denotes the angled deformity in which the angulation of the part is toward the midline. Fractures are described as either transverse, oblique, spiral, or comminuted.

Fractures in children differ from those in adults. Children's bones are softer and more resilient than are those of adults, and their bones can sustain greater forces and more incomplete fractures. In children, greenstick fractures, or incomplete fractures of long bones, are very common. The long bone bows with incomplete angulation. A torus fracture is an incomplete fracture, or a buckling or wrinkling of a bone's cortex.

Of most concern in children with fractures are those involving the epiphyses or cartilaginous centers at or near the end of children's growing bones. The cartilaginous portion of the epiphyses is not seen on radiographic examination. Injuries to the epiphyses may result from either compressive or shearing forces. In children, epiphyseal injuries are quite common, whereas sprains are rare. It is common for an inexperienced practitioner to label an epiphyseal injury as a sprain.

Epiphyseal injuries are commonly classified by the Salter-Harris classification. In Salter-Harris type I, there is a slip in the provisional calcification. Often this injury is very subtle and will require comparison views. There are no germinal layer disturbances in type I fractures. Any child with pain, edema, and a negative x-ray result should be treated as having a Salter-Harris type I injury, and the area should be x-rayed again in 10 days.

Salter-Harris type II fractures involve the metaphysis, and often the epiphyseal plate has also slipped. There is no germinal layer involved, thus there are no growth disturbances in type II injuries. Type II fractures involve a slip of the growth plate plus a fracture through the epiphysis involving the articular surface. Type III fractures involve the germinal layer and thus have a potential for growth disturbances. Type IV fractures involve the metaphysis and the growth plate, and these fractures have a high rate of growth disturbances. Type V fractures involve a crush injury to the epiphyseal plate. These injuries are often difficult to diagnose on a plain film. There is usually a growth disturbance in type V injuries.

All Salter-Harris fractures require a referral to an orthopedic surgeon for treatment and follow-up.

Examination

With any fracture, a good vascular and neurologic examination must be performed and documented. Soft tissue must be examined along with range of motion and strength. A good rule to live by in orthopedics is that pain over a bone implies a fracture until proven otherwise.

Another rule is to splint the patient where he or she lies. Do not perform a reduction until you have obtained a radiogram, unless there is neurologic or vascular compromise. Probably no circular casts should be applied to any sprained or fractured extremity in the emergency department (ED). Almost all injuries will swell, and if the extremity is in a circular cast this can act as a tourniquet. Sugar-tong or posterior gutter casts should be the normal treatment for splinting in the ED. Any patient who presents to the ED in a cast with pain, pallor, paresthesia, pulselessness, or paralysis is assumed to have neurovascular compromise, and the cast should be bivalved or removed entirely.

Early referral to an orthopedic surgeon for even trivial bony deformities should be the norm. When in doubt, consult in the ED early.

ORTHOPEDIC TRAUMA TO THE KNEE

Definition

The knee can suffer injury to the tibial spines, tuberosity, femoral condyles, patella, tibial plateaus, ligamentous and meniscal injuries and tears, knee dislocation, and osteochondritis dissecans.

Epidemiology

Most injuries to the knee are related to sports, motor vehicle, or industrial accidents.

Examination

The examination of the knee is divided into five parts: the history of the event, observation, inspection, palpation, and stress testing. The history or mechanism of how the injury occurred is very important. Often the history can reveal the diagnosis. Important questions to ask are: Did the patient hear a pop or a snap? Did the knee swell immediately after the injury? Could the patient bear weight after the injury? Is there a prior history of injury or surgery of the knee?

The patient should be observed for limping, guarding, weight bearing, sitting, extension of the leg, and muscular development upon entering the room. The manner in which the patient sits and stands should also be noted.

The inspection of the knee starts at the hip and ends at the ankle. The leg should be inspected for ecchymosis, edema, effusion, patella location, masses, and muscle mass, or the patient could be asked about trauma, warmth of the skin, and erythema.

The entire leg should be palpated, and areas of tenderness should be noted. The knee should be examined in flexion, extension, and during range of motion for tenderness, strength, and sensation.

The knee should be stressed to determine the stability of the anterior cruciate ligament (ACL), posterior cruciate ligament (PCL), lateral collateral ligament (LCL), medial collateral ligament (MCL), and patellar ligament. The patient should be able to fully extend the knee. The Lachman or anterior drawers should be performed. The femoral condyles, tibial spines, and tuberosity should be palpated for pain. The proximal head of the fibula should be examined.

The meniscus should be examined at the medial and lateral joint lines. The McMurray test can be utilized to examine the meniscus of the knee.

Diagnosis

Fractures of the patella can be secondary to a direct blow to the patella, a fall on a flexed knee, or forceful contraction of the quadriceps muscle. There are three types of patellar fractures: transverse, comminuted, and avulsion. All of the fractures can be open or closed.

The treatment of a nondisplaced patella fracture is immobilization for 6 weeks with a cylinder cast. The patient should bear weight with crutches. If the patellar fracture is displaced, the patella will probably require open reduction and fixation. Comminuted fractures require surgical removal of the smaller fragments or all of the fragments and suturing of the quadriceps tendon and patellar ligaments. Any open fracture of the patella requires débridement and irrigation.

Femoral condylar fractures can involve the supracondylar, condylar, intercondylar, and distal femoral epiphyseal areas. Condylar fractures are usually secondary to falls or direct blows to the knee. On examination the knee will be painfully swollen with rotation, deformity, and shortening. The treatment of these fractures depends on the type of fracture and injury and whether the fracture is displaced or nondisplaced. The ipsilateral hip should also be examined to ensure that there is no associated hip fracture. The space between the first and second toes should be examined for neurologic sensory status. The deep peroneal nerve can sometimes be injured with a condylar fracture, and the web space between the first and second toes is the best area to examine for sensation of the deep peroneal nerve.

Fractures of the tibial tuberosity and spines are common with a cruciate ligament injury. Fractures of the tibial spine are usually secondary to a force directed against the flexed proximal tibia in an anterior or posterior direction, which causes an incomplete avulsion of the tibial spine, with or without displacement, or a complete fracture of the spine. On examination there is a positive Lachman sign and hemiarthrosis, and the patient is unable to extend the knee fully.

The treatment for nondisplaced or incomplete fractures of the tibial spine is closed reduction. Complete reduction will require open reduction.

Fractures of the tibial plateau are common in the elderly. These fractures are caused by a direct force that drives the femoral condyles into the articulating surface of the tibia. Individual or bilateral condyles can be fractured. The lateral plateau is the more commonly fractured plateau. Nondisplaced tibial plateau fractures are treated with a long leg cast, whereas displaced fractures are treated with open reduction and elevation of the bony fragment.

ACL, PCL, LCL, and MCL injuries are usually secondary to direct trauma or adduction, flexion, internal rotation of the femur on the tibia, hyperextension, and anteroposterior (AP) displacement of the knee. Any of these forces can cause a strain or complete rupture of any one of these four ligaments. An evaluation of stability by stress testing is the mainstay of testing these four ligaments. The LCL and MCL are tested by valgus and varus stress to the medial and lateral sides of the knee. Valgus stress will test the MCL, and varus stress will test the LCL. The knee should be flexed at approximately 30 degrees when valgus and varus stresses are applied. Any unilateral opening greater than the other knee, without a good endpoint is suggestive of a collateral ligament strain or tear.

The ACL and PCL are tested by the Lachman test, pivot shift test, and anterior drawers sign. The anterior drawers sign is performed by placing the hip in flexion at a 45-degree angle and the knee at a 90-degree angle. The tibia is then displaced forward from the femur. A displacement of greater than 6 mm compared with the other knee is suggestive of an ACL tear.

The Lachman sign is performed by placing the knee in 20 degrees of flexion and by stabilizing the femur. The examiner then places anterior force on the tibia, attempting to displace the tibia forward. If the tibia is displaced more than 5 mm, this is suggestive of an ACL tear.

The pivot shift test is performed by placing the patient in the supine position with the hip flexed at 45 degrees. The examiner then lifts the heel and, with the opposite hand, grasps the knee with the thumb behind the fibular head. The examiner then internally rotates the ankle and knee and applies valgus force to the knee at the same time that the knee is flexed. If there is anterior subluxation of the tibia, then an ACL tear is present.

The PCL can suffer an ipsilateral injury or can also be injured when the ACL is damaged. To examine the knee for a PCL tear, a posterior drawers sign is performed. Force is applied to the tibial tubercle, and the tibial tubercle is displaced posteriorly. If there is posterior movement or sag, then this is suggestive of a PCL tear.

Meniscal tears are diagnosed by the McMurray test. Usually in an acute injury to a meniscus you will not be able to perform this test secondary to pain.

A patient who presents to the ED with a knee dislocation presents with tremendous ligamentous disruption and possible vascular compromise and neurologic injury. The knee should be reduced as soon as possible with orthopedic and vascular consultation.

Patellar dislocation is usually secondary to a twisting injury on the extended knee. The patella is usually displaced laterally over the lateral condyle. Reductions are performed by hyperextending the knee, flexing the hip, and sliding the patella back into place. If the patella is recurrently dislocated, the patient should be referred to an orthopedic surgeon for surgical intervention.

Children with knee injuries are often limited to fractures and not ligament injuries. Often the major knee injury to a child is a femoral epiphysis separation along the anterior or coronal plane. Anterior separation is secondary to hyperextension. Coronal separation is secondary to abduction and adduction of the knee. The patient presents with circumferential tenderness of the knee. A Salter-Harris fracture of the femur, tibia, or fibula is also quite common.

Children between the ages of 8 and 15 years often suffer intercondylar eminence fractures of the tibia secondary to a fall from a bicycle. This can cause an intercondylar eminence to be avulsed from the tibia. The patient will have a painful swollen knee with a positive Lachman test. These patients should be followed by an orthopedic surgeon.

Always remember that any child who presents with knee pain can have hip pathology causing the knee pain, and the child should have a complete hip examination.

All fractures, sprains, strains, ligament injuries, or tension injuries should be referred to an orthopedic surgeon for a follow-up evaluation and care.

ACUTE BACK PAIN

Definition

The spine is made up of seven cervical vertebrae, twelve lumbar vertebrae, and five lumbar vertebrae. There are five sacral nerves that exit from the sacrum.

There are eight paired cervical spinal roots in the cervical spine that exit from intervertebral foramina. The atlas of C1 supports the occipital condyles and the axis of C2. There are seven fascial planes of muscles in the neck. The dorsal nerve is the sensory part of the spinal cord. The ventral root is the motor root of the spinal cord. Thus if the ventral root is compressed, then painless weakness will occur. If only the dorsal root is compressed, only pain, without weakness, will occur.

The ligament structures of the spine consist of the anterior longitudinal ligament, posterior longitudinal ligament, ligamentum flavum, intraspinal ligament, supraspinal ligaments, intratransverse ligaments, and costotransverse ligaments.

Acute back pain can be caused from trauma to the vertebrae, prolapse of disks, osteoporosis, spurs, nerve entrapments, and numerous other pathologies leading to weakness, pain, and bowel or bladder problems.

Clinical Presentation/Examination

The patient should undress completely for the back examination. It is often very helpful to watch the patient get undressed to evaluate the patient's range of motion. If possible watch the patient walk from the waiting room to the examination room. This will give you some idea of the patient's true gait and disability. Always ask if there is pain, weakness, numbness, and in what distribution is the presentation. Are there associated bowel or bladder problems? What was the patient doing when the pain occurred? Is there radicular pain? Has the patient ever had back pain before, and is the distribution the same as before? Are there any associated symptoms (e.g., visual, auditory, pharyngeal-laryngeal symptoms)? Was the onset of pain slow or sudden? Does the pain wake the patient up during the night?

Check for flexibility of the neck and thoracic and lumbar spine. The neck should be checked for pain and range of motion. When there is ipsilateral neck pain that radiates into the shoulder or arm, a radicular component is present (Spurling's sign). When the head is moved to one side and there is ipsilateral neck pain on the side of movement, there is zygoapophyseal joint irritability. If there is contralateral neck pain with neck movement, then there is probably a ligamentous or muscular source of pain.

The thyroid gland should be palpated for enlargement or tenderness, and the carotid and subclavian arteries should be auscultated for bruits. The neck should be examined for lymphadenopathy. The posterior neck should be palpated. The pain of occipital neuralgia can be reproduced by palpating the occipital notch. If occipital neuralgia is present, this will produce scalp numbness and a burning dysesthesia in the occipital nerve distribution.

The first cervical rib is located directly behind the angle of the mandible, and the transverse process of the atlas is between the angle of the mandible and the mastoid process. The hyoid bone is at the level of C3. The thyroid cartilage is anterior to C4.

Always ask the patient if he or she has dysphagia or vocal hoarseness. Dysphagia can be secondary to pharyngeal edema or retropharyngeal hematomas. Vocal hoarseness can be secondary to the stretching of the larynx, with associated edema of the sternocleidomastoid muscles and carotid sheaths. If the patient complains of vertigo, tinnitus, ear and eye pain, visual aberrations, and headache, this is termed Leiou-Barré syndrome.

The temporomandibular joint should always be checked when performing a neck examination. Crepitus over the joint with weakness of the temporalis muscle is indicative of joint dysfunction.

The radial and ulnar pulses should always be evaluated with a back examination, especially when upper arm weakness or paresthesia is a presenting complaint. If the radial pulse is reduced with passive shoulder abduction in association with a bruit over the subclavian artery, this suggests thoracic outlet syndrome.

A complete neurologic examination is necessary on every patient. No back examination is complete without a rectal examination to check for tone or masses.

Any patient with lower lumbar pain should have an abdominal examination performed. If the lower lumbar pain is not easily determined or if pelvic pathology is considered, a pelvic examination should be performed on the female patient. Straight leg raises (SLRs) should always be performed. Pelvic tilts should be done, and an examination for a positive Patrick sign (loss of hip internal rotation with medial groin pain) should be performed.

The patient should be asked to walk on his or her heels and toes. If the patient cannot walk on his or her heels, this suggests an L5 radiculopathy, and the inability to walk on the toes suggests an S1 root involvement. Problems with squatting or rising are indicative of quadriceps weakness and thus an L4 compromise. Weak hip flexion suggests L3 involvement. The inability to extend the great toe suggests L5 involvement. Calf pain suggests S1 involvement.

A positive SLR involves the reproduction of sciatic pain when the hip is flexed and the leg is straightened at the knee (placed in extension). The "strum" sign is performed when the hip and knee are in flexion and the sciatic nerve is plucked behind the knee. If this procedure reproduces pain in the back, this sign is pathognomonic for a herniated disk. The crossed straight leg raise (CSLR) is positive when the contralateral leg is elevated, which produces sciatic pain in the symptomatic leg. A positive CSLR is suggestive of a herniated disk with an impacted nerve root.

Diagnosis/Specific Back Pain Etiologies

Pain bilaterally in the upper extremities is usually secondary to C6 spinal radiculopathies. Biceps tenderness is usually secondary to an acute subdeltoid bursitis.

A patient with a cervical soft tissue injury often presents with a history of an automobile accident, sports injury, or an accidental fall. The patient often complains of "whiplash" with very few objective findings. The new, more correct term for this injury is *acceleration flexion-extension neck injury.* Head-on injuries with extension of the neck produce ventral tears and hemorrhages in the sternocleidomastoid muscles and ruptures of the anterior longitudinal ligament and

Nerve Root	Disk Space	Reflex Tested	Sensory Distribution	Motor Distribution
C1–C2	C1–C2		Scalp	Deltoid, biceps, and spinati
C5	C4–C5	Biceps	Thumb and shoulder	Biceps, deltoid, pronator teres, and wrist extensors
C6	C5–C6	Biceps and brachioradialis	Index finger, thumb, and lateral forearm	
C7	C6–C7	Triceps	Forearm and middle finger	Pronator teres and triceps
C8	C7–T1	Triceps	Little and half-ring finger	Flexor carpi ulnaris, triceps, and hand intrinsics
L1	L1–L2	Cremasteric	Back to trochanter and the groin	Hip flexion
L2	L2–L3	Cremasteric and abductor	Back and anterior thigh to the level of the knee	Hip flexion and abduction
L3	L3–L4	Patellar	Back, upper buttock to anterior thigh, medial lower leg	Hip flexion, hip abduction, and knee extension
L4	L4–L5	Patellar, gluteal	Inner calf to medial foot and the first two toes	Knee extension
L5	L5–S1	Tibial posterior	Lateral lower leg, dorsum of the foot, first two toes	Toe extension and ankle dorsiflexion
S1	Sacral foramina	Ankle and hamstring	Sole, heel, and the lateral edge of the foot	Ankle plantar flexion and knee flexion
S2	Sacral foramina	None	Posterior and medial upper thigh	Ankle plantar flexion and toe extension
S3	Sacral foramina	Bulbocavernosus	None	None
S4	Sacral foramina	Bulbocavernosus	None	None
S5	Sacral foramina	Anal	None	None
C1	Tip of the coccyx	Anal	None	None

ventral parts of the annulus fibrosis. When the patient is rear-ended, this produces injury to the dorsal area of the spine, particularly injury to the annulus fibrosis and hemorrhage to the paraspinal muscles.

A patient with an acute cervical disk herniation presents with acute radiculopathy, myelopathy, or both. Neck stiffness, occipital neuralgia, and pain are present. Posterior ruptures of the cervical disk present with progressive myelopathy. Posterolateral herniations present with cervical radiculopathy. The most common cervical herniation is the C5–C6, C6 nerve root on the right side, and the C6–C7, C7 nerve root on the left side. The patient presents with the appropriate dermatome pattern into the correct finger and myotome pain pattern. If long-lasting, the patient will present with the appropriate atrophy and weakness in the innervation muscles.

The patient often presents to the ED for pain management of chronic degenerative disk disease secondary to cervical spondylosis or osteoarthrosis. Pain is secondary to a narrowing of the disk spaces, spurs off ligaments, and nerve compressions. Spurs can produce Horner's syndrome and vertebrobasilar symptoms.

Thoracic spine complaints are rarer than are cervical and lumbar complaints. They are usually secondary to trauma. The most commonly fractured area of the thoracic spine is the T10–T12 vertebrae. These fractures are usually seen in female patients older than 65 years of age secondary to osteoporosis. These patients present with severe pain without myelopathy. A metastatic malignancy should always be considered in the elderly with pathologic fractures without trauma. Thoracic herniated nucleus pulposus (HNP) accounts for less than 1% of all HNPs.

A patient who presents with acute thoracic pain in a unilateral dermatome radicular pattern should have herpes zoster or diabetic thoracic radiculopathy considered in the differential diagnosis.

The most common back complaint is lower lumbar pain. Lumbosacral pain can be caused by diverticulitis, a kidney or bladder infection, a disorder of the pancreas, a gallbladder disorder, endometriosis, pregnancy, ectopic pregnancy, gastrointestinal (GI) bleeding, appendicitis, or chronic pelvic pain other than musculoskeletal pathologies.

Lower lumbar pain that is made worse by ambulation can be secondary to peripheral vascular disease. Parasagittal brain tumors and thoracic root lesions can also cause back pain. Neurofibromata can also cause lower lumbar pain secondary to compression of a nerve root. Thoracic nerve root lesions are usually worse at night while the patient is reclining and are improved when the patient is in the standing position. A patient can also present with an S1, tibial nerve entrapment, in the tarsal tunnel, behind the medial ankle malleolus, which can present as lumbosacral pain.

Laboratory Findings

Laboratory examinations are usually of little help in the diagnosis of back pain. An erythrocyte sedimentation rate (ESR) and a complete blood count (CBC) may be helpful along with a rheumatoid factor in differentiating the causes of back pain. Any female with lower lumbar pain should have a urinalysis and a pregnancy test performed if in child-bearing years.

Radiographs

Any patient with a history of trauma, especially to the cervical spine, should have radiographs taken of the spine. If a compression fracture is suspected, radiographs should be taken. Without a history of trauma in most cases, x-rays of the spine are of little help in the diagnosis of acute back pain.

Magnetic resonance imaging (MRI), computed tomography (CT), and myelography can be used to determine if a fracture or HNP is present.

Electromyography (EMG) and *nerve conduction velocity (NCV)* are used to evaluate degrees of progressive motor impairment or to determine the level of neural compromise. Cervical spinal evoked potential can be used to determine cervical spinal myelopathies and thoracic outlet syndromes.

Treatment

The majority of cervical, thoracic, and lumbar pain can be treated with nonsteroidal anti-inflammatory drugs and pain medications (e.g., indomethacin, naproxen, ibuprofen) on an outpatient basis. Early bed rest with ice and heat applied to the affected area for 24 to 72 hours is the key to early recovery. Physical therapy is essential for recovery from injuries at work. All patients should be followed up in 72 hours to evaluate if the pain is decreasing and to determine if further testing is required.

ANKLE INJURIES

Definition

Ankle injuries can involve sprains, strains, dislocations, fractures from inversion or eversion injuries, external force injuries, and direct trauma. Injuries can occur from sports injuries, automobile accidents, industrial accidents, or falls. By far the most common type of injury to an ankle is a sports-related injury.

Epidemiology

Malleolar fractures account for 30% of all ankle fractures. Lateral malleolar fractures are the most common fractures, whereas bilateral malleolar fractures are rare. Men fracture the malleolus 1.5:1 more often when compared with women. The mean age of a person who fractures an ankle is 39 years of age.

In children, tibial malleolar fractures account for 14 to 15% of all fractures. The medial malleolus is more commonly fractured than is the lateral malleolus in children. The Salter-Harris description of fractures is the most commonly used tool for describing ankle fractures in children.

Anatomy

The ankle consists of three bones: the talus, the tibia, and the fibula. The ankle is a hinge joint. The talus forms the supporting body for the tibia and fibula, with the talus being wider anteriorly than posteriorly. The talus bears the majority of the stress during a twisting injury during dorsal flexion. In plantar flexion, there is more play secondary to the wider space that the talus occupies. Most twisting injuries occur in plantar flexion. Eversion injuries occur during dorsiflexion, and inversion injuries occur during plantar flexion.

There are three groups of ligaments that connect the bony structures together. The medial side of the ankle is supported by the deltoid or medial collateral ligament. It has both deep and superficial fibers. The fibers originate from the broad, short, and strong medial malleolus with the superficial fibers running in a sagittal plane inserting on the navicular and the talus. The deep fibers run horizontally and insert on the medial surface of the talus.

The ankle is supported laterally by the anterior talofibular, calcaneofibular, and posterior ligaments. They insert as they are named.

The tibia and fibula are held together by ligaments of syndesmosis. They consist of the interosseous ligament, the anterior and posterior tibiofibular ligaments, and the inferior transverse ligament.

The muscles of the ankle consist of four separate compartments. The anterior compartment consists of the tibialis anterior, extensor digitorum longus, and extensor hallucis longus. This compartment is involved in dorsiflexion. The medial compartment consists of the flexor digitorum longus, tibialis posterior, and flexor hallucis longus. This compartment contributes to inversion. The posterior compartment consists of the soleus and gastrocnemius muscle. This compartment provides plantar flexion. The lateral compartment consists of the peroneus longus and brevis muscles. This compartment contributes to eversion and plantar flexion.

The foot's blood supply consists of the iliac, femoral, and popliteal arteries. The entire foot is innervated by branches of the sciatic nerve.

Radiographs

The minimum radiographs for any ankle injury are an AP view with the ankle in 5 to 15 degrees of adduction, a true lateral that includes the base of the fifth metatarsal, and an internal oblique at a 45-degree angle.

In ankle sprains on radiographs, the talar tilt test can be performed to evaluate medial or lateral ligamentous systems for stability. A talar tilt test x-ray is positive if there is greater than 5 degrees of talar tilt.

If the talar tilt is greater than 25 degrees, there is an extreme injury to the ligaments on that side of the ankle. A difference of 5 to 10 degrees of talar tilt between ankles is suggestive of an injury to the ligament.

A good rule to live by is that pain over a bone indicates a fracture until proven otherwise. Another rule is that if it hurts to walk on, it is a fracture until proven otherwise. You cannot over-x-ray!

Clinical Presentation

A patient with an ankle injury will present with a history of an inversion or eversion injury or a fall. The patient will complain of painful weight bearing, edema, ecchymosis, or deformity.

Examination

The entire leg should be uncovered prior to the examination. The ankle starts at the knee, thus the knee should also be visualized. The ankle is examined for gross deformity, edema, and ecchymosis. The proximal fibular head should be palpated for tenderness. The entire shaft of the tibia should be palpated. The bony landmarks of the entire ankle should be palpated. The proximal head of the fifth metatarsal should be palpated. The ankle should be put through gentle range of motion to evaluate stability and to determine which positions cause and relieve pain. The ankle should be examined for instability by performing ankle anterior and posterior drawers tests.

A neurologic and vascular examination should always be documented during the examination of every extremity. The dorsalis pedis and the tibialis anterior pulse should be evaluated along with two-point discrimination. Ligament stability should always be documented along with range of motion, weight-bearing ability, amount of edema, and size of ecchymosis.

ANKLE SPRAINS

The most common ankle sprain is secondary to laxity of the anterior talofibular ligament. This can be assessed by the anterior drawers test. It is secondary to repetitive inversion injuries. An anterior drawers test is positive if there is movement of the talus by 3 mm or more. If more than 1 cm of movement is present, then there is a significant injury and the ankle is unstable.

MCL injuries by themselves are rare in adults. Usually both the MCL and the LCL are injured. To examine the ankle for an MCL injury, stress the ankle with a medial-to-lateral force that is simply a talar tilt sign.

Talofibular syndesmotic ligament injuries are a continuation of an ankle injury that involves the interosseous ligaments at the distal tibial and fibula. This injury is secondary to hyperdorsiflexion and an eversion injury. The talus is pushed superior against the fibula and tibia and displaces the fibula laterally by tearing or rupturing the interosseous ligament. The patient will prefer to walk on the toes. The injury will often be nonspecific. There will be tenderness over the anterior and posterior ligaments with some tenderness over the medial malleolus secondary to an associated MCL injury.

Ankle sprains are classified by first-, second-, and third-degree sprains. First-degree sprains consist of stretching or microscopic tearing of a ligament, causing local tenderness and minimal swelling. Usually weight bearing is possible, and x-rays are normal. Ankle sprains are treated with rest, ice, compression, and elevation (RICE) and anti-inflammatory agents. Aggressive range-of-motion exercises after ice massage work well with first-degree sprains. Usually plaster casting or splinting is not necessary.

Second-degree sprains involve partial tearing of a ligament with painful weight bearing. There are no bony abnormalities. There is usually minimal ligament function on examination. Second-degree sprains are treated as first-degree sprains with immobilization and non–weight bearing with crutches and RICE. Often a walking cast for 2 weeks, followed by a hinge cast for 2 weeks, will shorten the healing process.

A third-degree sprain involves the complete rupture of a ligament. The patient will not be able to bear weight, and there is often an obvious deformity. On x-ray, there is often an abnormal relationship of the talus to the mortise. There is controversy as to whether to treat third-degree sprains with conservative therapy, casting for 4 to 6 weeks, or with surgical therapy. All third-degree sprains should be treated with RICE, splinting, anti-inflammatory agents, crutches, and pain medication, and the patient should be referred to an orthopedic surgeon.

ANKLE FRACTURES

Fractures are caused by forces acting on the bones, ligaments, and muscles of the ankle. Avulsions are caused by injuries in which the ligament is stronger than the bones. Usually most malleolar fractures are transverse malleolar fractures or small chip or pull-off fractures of the malleolus below the joint line. If the talus shifts during injury, it can strike the opposite malleolus and can cause an oblique fracture, often on the side of the bone that was subjected to the compression force. Ligamentous injuries that occur with fractures have a more serious prognosis than has the fracture itself.

The Wilson classification of ankle fractures is often used to describe the mechanism of injury and fracture site. An external rotation force is associated with abduction, causing medial and lateral injury. A pull-off or transverse fracture of the medial malleolus or rupture of the deltoid ligament occurs. As the forces continue, the anterior tibiofibular ligament is ruptured. The talus then impacts on the fibula and fractures it. The posterior tibial tubercle fractures, and the interosseous, posterior inferior tibiofibular, and inferior transverse ligaments are torn.

In abduction injuries, the injury is caused by medial-to-lateral injury without the rotatory component. There is a transverse or pull-off fracture of the medial malleolus or rupture of the deltoid ligament, the latter of which is the rarer of the two. There is either a fracture of the fibula below the syndesmotic ligaments or a rupture of the syndesmotic ligaments. If the ligaments rupture before the fibula fractures, the fibula fractures near the junction of the middle and distal third of the fibula. The shaft of the fibula must be x-rayed to ensure that this fracture has not occurred.

Adduction force initiates lateral-to-medial forces, causing the lateral collateral ligament to rupture, or causing a pull-off or a transverse fracture of the lateral malleolus. If the force is continued through the ankle, the talus impacts on the medial malleolus, resulting in a spiral fracture.

Vertical compression fractures are injuries associated with other forces in the production of ankle fractures. This fracture is dependent on the position of the talus in the mortise at the time of the injury. On a radiogram, there will be a small fracture of the anterior or posterior lip of the tibia due to ligamentous pull-off or larger vertical fractures through the articular surface of the tibia. There is often communication with both anterior and posterior fractures.

Treatment of all ankle fractures involves stabilization, RICE, splinting, pain medication, anti-inflammatory agents, and a referral to an orthopedic surgeon for a follow-up visit. The goal of the orthopedic surgeon is to restore the talus in the mortise, return the joint line parallel to the ground, and ensure a smooth articular surface.

ANKLE DISLOCATION

The ankle joint can bear five times the body's weight during ambulation. The talus is trapezoidal, semicircular on its upper surface, and flat on its medial and lateral sides. In active dorsiflexion the foot and the fibula rotate externally on the oblique outer articular surface of the talus. When weight bearing occurs, the fibula descends and provides stability to the ankle mortise. When a dislocation of the talus occurs, there is displacement of the talar dome from the mortise, and this usually occurs in association with a fracture of the component of the mortise.

Posterior dislocation of the talus is more common, resulting from forces driving the entire foot backward, usually when the foot is plantar flexed at the ankle joint. Anterior dislocations are secondary to the talus being displaced forward at the ankle joint, usually when the ankle is dorsiflexed. The anterior lip of the tibia is frequently fractured by this mechanism. There is always extensive soft tissue and ligament damage with ankle dislocations.

All ankle dislocations should be immediately reduced after radiograms have been taken. If there is vascular or neurologic compromise, immediate reduction should be performed prior to radiograms being taken. To reduce an ankle dislocation, the knee is flexed to reduce tension on the Achilles tendon. Traction is applied to the foot down-ward, and the force is applied to the opposite direction that caused the injury. This can often be achieved by elevating the patient's bed and hanging the patient's ankle off of the end of the bed so that traction can be applied by pulling down on the ankle, with force applied in the opposite direction of the injury. After the ankle has been reduced, do not let go of the ankle until it has been splinted with a plaster cast, because it can go out again. Always do another x-ray after a reduction, and check the patient's vascular and neurologic status. An orthopedic referral is necessitated.

COMPARTMENT SYNDROMES

Definition

Compartment syndromes are secondary to skeletal or muscle injury secondary to trauma, infection, electrical injury, hyperthermia, hypo-thermia, snakebites, toxins, arterial embolism, polymyositis, seizures, cerebrovascular accidents (CVAs), or drug overdose. Early diagnosis must be made. If the diagnosis of compartment syndrome is missed, this can have devastating results with muscle, function, or limb loss. Compartment syndromes can also be caused by burn eschars, compression of the compartment, a pneumatic pressure garment, overexertion, and shin splints. Alcoholics are also at a higher risk for compartment syndromes secondary to limb compression while they are passed out in a prone or supine position.

Pathology

Compartment syndromes are secondary to increased pressure in a closed space or compartment, which compromises the flow of blood through closed tissue spaces and nutrient capillaries in the muscles and nerves. The normal pressure in an extremity compartment is usually less than 10 mm Hg. Any pressure greater than 20 mm Hg is considered to be high.

The anterior and posterior upper extremity compartments are at increased risk for compartment syndromes. The anterior compart-ment contains the biceps-brachialis muscle and the ulnar, median, and radial nerves. The posterior compartment contains the triceps muscle. The forearm compartment contains the volar and dorsal compartments. The volar compartment contains the wrist and finger extenders. The hand and thenar compartment contains the intrinsic muscles of the thumb and the little finger. The interosseous muscles of the hand are in their own compartment.

The buttocks contain three compartments: (1) the tensor muscle of the fascia lata, (2) the gluteus medius and minimus, and (3) the gluteus maximus.

The anterior thigh compartment contains the quadriceps groups, and the posterior thigh contains the hamstring group of muscles and the sciatic nerve.

The most common site of a compartment syndrome are the four fascial compartments in the lower leg in the peroneal, anterior, deep, and superficial posterior areas.

Clinical Presentation

A patient with a compartment syndrome of the lower leg presents with paresthesias and pain with passive toe and foot movement of the involved compartment. The next most common complication to a lower extremity injury is a compartment syndrome seen 24 to 48 hours after the injury secondary to swelling in the injured compartment.

The volar and dorsal compartments of the forearm and the interosseous muscles of the hand can also be affected. Upper extremity compartment syndromes will present like lower extremity compartment syndromes with painful passive flexion or extension of the fingers, wrist, or elbow with paresthesias.

Examination

There will be abnormal light touch or decreased or widened two-point discrimination. On examination of the extremity, the compartment will be tense, indurated, and erythematous.

By the time that a distal pulse is reduced in an extremity, muscle necrosis has occurred. An ischemic muscle hurts, and this pain is exacerbated by active muscle contractions and passive stretching of the muscle.

Diagnosis

To diagnose a compartment syndrome, one must have a high index of suspicion. Complete muscle, vascular, and neurologic death can occur in 4 to 6 hours. The diagnosis of an acute compartment syndrome is made by using a Wick catheter or an 18-gauge needle to measure the compartment pressure with a saline manometer. Normal compartmental pressure is 0 to 8 mm Hg. Any pressure greater than 30 mm Hg is considered to be a compartment syndrome. An emergency fasciotomy is indicated.

Laboratory Findings

A creatine phosphokinase (CPK), urine myoglobin, or serum myoglobin sample should be drawn on any patient who is considered to have a compartment syndrome. Rhabdomyolysis is often present. The CPK will normally be greater than 20,000 if a compartment syndrome is present. Renal functions, blood urea nitrogen (BUN), and creatinine should be also monitored.

Treatment

Treatment of compartment syndromes is based on the compartment pressures. Pressures between 15 and 20 mm Hg can be watched and measured. If the pressure is above 20 mm Hg, an orthopedic or surgical consultation should be standard practice. Pressures between 30 and 40 mm Hg are generally considered to be a basis for an emergency fasciotomy in the operating room.

ELBOW INJURIES

Definition

Injuries to the elbow are usually secondary to a fall on an out-stretched hand. They can be condylar, supracondylar, or epicondylar. The elbow can also be dislocated. A good neurologic and vascular examination with early reduction of fractures and dislocations is the normal practice with early orthopedic referral.

Anatomy

The elbow is made up of the lower or distal humerus and the proximal ends of the ulna and radius. The distal end of the humerus tapers into two columns of bone or the medial and lateral condyles. Between the condyles, an area of thin bone is formed, called the coronoid fossa. The proximal nonarticular parts of the distal humerus are called the epicondyles. A supracondylar ridge is formed just proximal to the epicondyles. The condyles and epicondyles serve as areas of attachment from the muscles of the forearm. The wrist extensors originate from the lateral epicondyles, and the wrist flexors originate from the medial epicondyle. The trochlear, the articular surface of the medial condyle, articulates with the deep trochlear notch of the ulna formed by the olecranon interiorly and posteriorly, and the coronoid process anteriorly. This articulation of the olecranon and coronoid allows the hinged flexion and extension of the elbow joint.

The lateral condyle articulates with the capitellum, which articulates with the radial head of the radius. The capitellum and radial head articulation allow the forearm to supinate and pronate.

The major ligament of the elbow is the annular ligament which, along with the radial collateral ligament, holds the radial head in place. The ulnar collateral ligament and the anterior capsule add stability to this joint.

The upper arm is divided into the anterior and posterior compartments. The anterior compartment contains the biceps brachii, the brachialis, and the coracobrachialis. The anterior compartment also contains the median, ulnar, and musculocutaneous nerves. The anterior compartment also contains the brachial artery. The posterior compartment contains the triceps brachii muscle and the radial nerve.

Examination

As with any injury, the history of the event that caused the injury is very important. Always document if the patient is right- or left-handed and if there was a prior assault to the injured extremity. Examinations of the extremities must include a neurologic, vascular, range of motion, soft tissue, ligamentous, and muscular examination. All of these items should be documented on the chart. Capillary refill or radial or ulnar pulses should be evaluated. Two-point discrimination in all three nerve areas of the hand, the medial, radius, and ulnar nerve areas should be documented. The ability of the patient to touch, with good strength (5/5) in all fingers by the thumb should be documented. Fanning of the fingers and the ability to flex and extend all fingers at all metacarpophalangeal (MP), proximal interphalangeal (PIP), and distal interphalangeal (DIP) joints should be evaluated. Good 5/5 flexion and extension at the wrist should be evaluated. The patient should be able to make an "OK" sign and abduct and adduct all fingers against resistance, both together and separately against resistance. The thenar and hypothenar areas of the hand and the muscles of the forearm should be visually inspected for size and presence of atrophy. You can never overexamine or overdocument a hand injury!

Clinical Presentation

The majority of elbow injuries are secondary to falls. *Supracondylar fractures* are fractures that occur proximal to the epicondyles of the humerus. The majority of these fractures are seen in children younger than 15 years of age. Supracondylar fractures are classified as either injuries of flexion or extension.

Extension supracondylar fractures are secondary to a fall on an outstretched hand with the elbow locked in extension. The force causes a posterior displacement of the distal fragment of the humerus. The danger of this fracture is that there is angulation of the proximal fragment into the antecubital fossa, in which the brachial artery and median nerve lie, endangering both structures. The triceps muscle also adds pull on the proximal fragment.

Treatment depends on the type of fracture, angulation, and displacement. One third will have little or no displacement. These fractures are treated acutely with just splinting. The other two thirds will require an orthopedic consultation secondary to displacement.

Intercondylar and transcondylar fractures are often seen in adults with elbow injuries and are secondary to a direct upward blow with the elbow in flexion. Transcondylar fractures have a fracture line that passes through both condyles within the joint capsule. Intercondylar fractures are Y- or T-shaped and will have variable degrees of separation of the condyles from each other. Nondisplaced fractures are treated with a posterior splint, immobilization, and casting with a referral to an orthopedic surgeon. Displaced fractures require surgical fixation.

Condylar fractures involve both articular surfaces and the nonarticular epicondylar surfaces of the distal humerus. The lateral trochlear surface is often involved. Nondisplaced fractures are treated with splinting and an orthopedic referral. Displaced fractures greater than 3 mm require surgical fixation.

Epicondylar fractures are common in children and usually involve the apophyses. Medial epicondylar fractures involve an avulsion fracture with a posterior dislocation in patients younger than 20 years of age. Repetitive valgus stress, such as baseball throwing, will cause an avulsion of the epicondyle. Any direct blow to the epicondyle can also cause a fracture. Minimally displaced fractures are treated with a posterior splint. These patients should be splinted with the elbow and wrist flexed and the forearm in pronation. If the epicondyle is displaced greater than 3 to 5 mm, then surgical treatment is required. These patients should be referred to an orthopedic surgeon.

Olecranon fractures are usually secondary to a fall or a direct blow to the olecranon. The triceps will pull the proximal fragment of the ulna proximately. Treatment involves ice, immobilization, and early range of motion with an orthopedic referral.

There are three types of radial head fractures. On radiograph, a positive fat pad sign is considered a radial head fracture until determined otherwise. A type I fracture is a nondisplaced fracture and is treated with aspiration of the hemiarthrosis, immobilization, and early range of motion within 24 to 48 hours.

Type II fractures have marginal displacement and are treated with ice and immobilization. If the patient does not improve and is still having pain, radial head excision is considered. Type III radial head fractures are comminuted fractures and require radial head excision.

Elbow dislocations require immediate reduction secondary to the possibility of neurologic or vascular injury associated with these fractures. It takes a large amount of force to dislocate an elbow. There is usually an associated fracture with a dislocation. The injury is often caused by a fall on an outstretched hand. These dislocations should be reduced as soon as possible, and an orthopedic referral will be required.

FOOT INJURIES

Definition

Foot fractures involve the calcaneus, talus, midfoot, metatarsal, phalanges, and fractures of the base of the fifth metatarsal.

Epidemiology

Most injuries to the foot are soft-tissue injuries rather than fractures or dislocations. The talus and the calcaneus are the most common bones involved in fractures and dislocations. Industrial accidents are the most common causes of foot injuries, and 65% occur from trauma. Fractures and injuries are uncommon in children secondary to the extraordinary resilience of children to traumatic foot events.

Anatomy

The foot contains 26 bones, including the metatarsals, the tarsal bones, and the phalanges. The midfoot contains the cuboid bone, three cuneiform bones, and the navicular bone. The hindfoot contains the talus and the calcaneus. The hindfoot and midfoot are separated by the Chopart joint, and the forefoot is separated from the midfoot by the Lisfranc joint.

Foot Fractures

The calcaneus is the most commonly fractured bone of the tarsal bones (60% of all tarsal fractures). Calcaneal fractures are divided into two types: (1) processes or tuberosity fractures, or (2) fractures involving the body of the calcaneus. Both types of fracture are usually caused by compression. The fracture site will be swollen and painful, and ecchymosis will be present. The patient will be unable to bear weight on the foot.

A large percentage of calcaneal fractures are associated with other fractures. Lumbar fractures have a 10% fracture association, and there is a 26% associated fracture rate with other extremity injuries. Any patient with a calcaneal fracture should have a complete orthopedic examination of the arms, hips, back, knees, legs, and ankles.

Standard films often show the fracture. All calcaneal fractures require a CT scan to determine the extent of the fracture and to determine the plan of care. The goal of treatment is to restore the normal anatomy of the calcaneus. There is often poor optimal treatment when dealing with calcaneal fractures. All calcaneal fractures should be referred to an orthopedic surgeon.

Talus fractures are the second most common talus bone foot fracture, and these fractures are relatively uncommon. The talus is usually fractured secondary to hyperextension. The talus is mostly covered with articular cartilage, and the blood supply is tenuous and enters by way of the ligamentous capsule supporting the bone. Therefore, fractures of the talus (especially of the neck) are associated with body dislocations and may cause avascular necrosis of the bone.

A patient with a talar fracture will present with severe pain and is unable to bear weight. There is edema and point tenderness at the fracture site. The calcaneus should be x-rayed, and if a fracture is noted, a CT scan should be performed to define the fracture and assist in the choice of treatment.

Simple talar, nondisplaced fractures or avulsion fractures can be immobilized, placed in ice, and elevated, and the patient should be sent for an orthopedic follow-up. If the patient has a fracture of the neck or body or fracture dislocation of the talus, an immediate orthopedic consultation should be made.

Midfoot fractures often involve multiple fractures secondary to direct trauma. The midfoot is the least mobile part of the foot. It involves articulations of five tarsal bones and their metatarsal articulations and supporting ligaments. Most injuries of the midfoot involve subluxations and dislocations.

The most common midfoot fracture is the Lisfranc (tarsometatarsal) foot fracture. There can be three types of Lisfranc fractures. The first type is one in which all five metatarsals are displaced transversely. The second type is an isolated dislocation of the first or second metatarsal displaced transversely. The third type is the divergent type in which sagittal and transverse displacement of the metatarsals occurs. Lisfranc fractures occur with direct or indirect trauma of the foot. Longitudinal force causes an AP compression on a plantar-flexed foot while the foot is trapped under the wheel of a car or while a horse stirrup immobilizes the foot. The most common radiologic sign is separation between the base of the first and second metatarsals, which suggests subluxation.

Treatment of a Lisfranc fracture is complicated and requires amputation through the Lisfranc joint. The major complication is compromised circulation with subsequent necrosis of the foot. All patients with Lisfranc fractures should be referred for an orthopedic consultation.

Metatarsal fractures usually occur involving the second and third metatarsals secondary to their anatomic configuration and their relatively fixed position. The first, fourth, and fifth metatarsals are relatively mobile and can sustain greater stressors.

Metatarsal fractures are divided into neck and shaft fractures, with pull-off fractures of the base of the fifth metatarsal being the most common fracture (a ballet dancer's fracture). Dancer fractures are secondary to plantar flexion and inversion, which causes the peroneus brevis tendon to pull off a portion of the bone where it inserts.

Almost all metatarsal fractures can be treated conservatively with splinting, casting, ice, and analgesics followed by a short leg cast for 3 to 6 weeks.

Stress fractures are seen in patients who have increased their exercise, walking, running, or marching quickly. Pain will appear before cortical stress reaction is noted on an x-ray. The patient presents with an insidious history of painful weight bearing or walking that is getting progressively worse. If the results of x-rays are negative and pain persists, the foot should be x-rayed in 2 to 3 weeks to check for a stress reaction of the bone. Stress reactions or fractures are treated with rest, non–weight bearing with crutches, and a gradual increase in walking, running, or marching over 2 to 3 months.

Phalangeal fractures are usually a direct result of trauma to the phalanx. Phalanges can be fractured or dislocated. The patient will present with pain, deformity, swelling, and ecchymosis. If the phalanx is subluxated or dislocated, then it should be reduced. Most phalangeal fractures can be treated with ice, elevation, and dynamic splinting. Fractures of the great toe should be referred to a podiatrist or an orthopedic surgeon.

INJURIES TO THE FOREARM AND WRIST

Definition

Injuries to the forearm, wrist, and hand can be devastating. Aggressive treatment to save tissue and function should be the normal practice. Injuries can occur from falls, lacerations, crush injuries, burns, and puncture wounds.

Anatomy

The forearm is made up of the radius and ulna, which are connected by a fibrous interosseous membrane with fibers running obliquely from a proximal origin on the radius to a distal insertion on the ulna. There are three muscle groups in the forearm: the pronator teres, the pronator quadratus, and the supinator.

The wrist is made up of the carpal bones, the distal ends of the ulna and radius. The distal end of the ulna is covered by a triangular fibrocartilaginous complex that separates the triquetrium distally. The radius articulates distally with the scaphoid and lunate bones.

The carpal bones of the wrist are arranged in two rows. The proximal bones from the radial side include the scaphoid-navicular, lunate, triquetrium, and pisiform. The distal row consists of the trapezium, capitate, and hamate. Both rows lie in a frontal plane arch. The long scaphoid bone bridges both rows of carpal bones of the wrist. The scapholunate joint is the most common site of injury in the wrist.

The ligaments of the wrist are arranged in three arcades of fibers, two of which are volar and one is dorsal. All three of these arcades originate at the radial styloid. The most common injury to the radial styloid is a Hutchinson fracture, which is an unstable fracture. The wrist is supplied by the radial and ulnar arteries and is innervated by the radial, median, and ulnar nerves.

Examination

As with any injury, the history of the event that caused the injury is very important. Always document if the patient is right- or left-handed and if there was a prior injury to the injured extremity. All extremity examinations involve a neurologic, vascular, range-of-motion, soft tissue, ligamentous, and muscular examination. All of these items should be documented on the chart. Capillary refill or radial or ulnar pulses should be evaluated. Two-point discrimination in all three nerve areas of the hand—the medial, radius, and ulnar nerve areas—should be documented. The ability of the patient to touch, with good 5/5 strength, all fingers by the thumb should be documented. Fanning of the fingers and the ability to flex and extend all fingers at all MP, PIP, and DIP joints should be evaluated. Good 5/5 flexion and extension at the wrist should be evaluated. The patient should be able to make an "OK" sign, adduct and abduct all fingers against resistance both together and separately against resistance. The thenar and hypothenar areas of the hand and the muscles of the forearm should be inspected for size and presence of atrophy. You can never overexamine or overdocument a hand injury!

Clinical Presentation

Injuries to the forearm are often secondary to a fall on an outstretched hand. Midshaft ulnar and radial fractures are usually secondary to direct blows. Fractures of the radial frequently occur at the junction of the middle and distal third of the radius. The ulna is usually fractured by a direct blow to it or as excessive pronation or supination is applied to the bone. On radiographic examination, the fractures to the ulna or radius are commonly displaced secondary to the total amount of force that is required to fracture these bones and the pulling of the associated muscles. The degree of angulation, displacement, and shortening is important in evaluating and treating the fracture.

Treatment of distal radial and ulnar fractures is dependent on the rotation or axial displacement and on the angulation of the bone at the fracture site. Nondisplaced fractures are placed in a sugar-tong splint and are referred to an orthopedic surgeon for follow-up and casting for 6 to 8 weeks. Closed displaced fractures are treated with closed reduction usually with the help of a hematoma block and finger traps traction.

A special fracture of the ulna is a Monteggia fracture dislocation of the proximal ulna. There is an accompanying radial head dislocation. This injury is often secondary to a direct blow to the posterior aspect of the ulna or a fall on the forearm. The patient will present with pain, a shortened forearm, and a palpable radial head in the antecubital fossa. The angle formed by the ulnar fracture generally points in the direction of the radial head dislocation. The radial head should align with the capitellum on the radiograph. If it does not, then the radial head is dislocated. Complications include paralysis of the posterior interosseous branch of the radial nerve, nonunion, recurrent dislocation, and subluxation of the radial head. An orthopedic consultation is necessitated.

Distal radial fractures are very common. A distal fracture of the radius with volar angulation is classified as a Colles fracture, secondary to a fall on an outstretched hand. The radius is fractured at the metaphysis, and the distal fragment of the radius is displaced dorsally. The ulnar styloid will be fractured in 60% of the cases when a Colles fracture is present. On a radiograph, the Colles fracture is described as a silver fork deformity.

Closed nondisplaced Colles fractures should be splinted and referred to an orthopedic surgeon for follow-up and casting. Displaced Colles fractures require closed reduction. A hematoma block or a regional Bier block should be performed prior to reduction. The fracture is reduced with finger trap distraction and pressure applied to the dorsal fragment. The distal fragment is displaced volar and pronated onto the proximal fragment. A sugar-tong splint is applied, and the patient is referred to an orthopedic surgeon.

A Smith fracture is the opposite of a Colles fracture. It is usually secondary to a direct blow to the dorsum of the hand with the hand flexed. There is pain and edema at the fracture site and angulation if displaced. Closed reduction as in a Colles fracture, only with opposite pressure against the distal fragment, is the usual form of reduction.

A Galeazzi fracture dislocation is the opposite of a Monteggia fracture. It is secondary to a direct blow to the back of the wrist or fall on outstretched hand. The shaft of the radius is fractured at the union of the middle and distal third of the radius, with a subluxation or dislocation of the distal radioulnar joint. The ulnar head will be very prominent, and the ulna will be displaced dorsally. An orthopedic consultation is necessitated.

A Barton fracture is secondary to an extreme force during which the wrist is in fixed dorsiflexion, with an accompanied pronating force. It involves the articular surface of the distal radius. It can involve the dorsal or volar aspect of the radius. The volar fracture is more common than is the dorsal fracture. These fractures require an orthopedic consultation, and often open reduction is necessary.

Wrist or *carpal injuries* usually result from falls. The most common in order of injury of the carpal bones are the scaphoid, dorsal chip, and lunate bones. The most common site of a scaphoid fracture is the middle third of the bone. The more proximal the fracture, the greater is the risk of avascular necrosis. On radiographs the fracture site may not be readily seen. Ten percent of navicular fractures will not be seen acutely on radiographs. A patient may present with pain in the "snuff box" area of the wrist, edema, and throbbing pain. Snuff box tenderness over the navicular is indicative of a fracture, and a splint should be applied. Another radiograph should be taken in approximately 14 days. All navicular fractures require an orthopedic referral to treat and follow the patient's injury for nonunion or avascular necrosis.

The scapholunate dislocation and rotatory subluxation of the scaphoid are also common. These injuries involve the ligaments that support the scaphoid, and this injury is secondary to forceful hyperextension of the wrist. A scapholunate dislocation refers to a diastasis or separation between the scaphoid and the lunate. When the ligaments are completely torn, the scaphoid slides into palmar flexion, thus a rotatory subluxation is present. On a radiograph, the scaphoid will be shortened and a dense, ring-shaped image around its distal perimeter is present. The injury necessitates a referral to an orthopedic surgeon for either open or closed reduction.

Dorsal chip fractures are the second most common carpal fracture and usually involve the triquetrium. The patient presents with tenderness and edema over the ulnar aspect of the wrist. Often on radiograph the acute fracture will not be seen; however, if present, this fracture is best seen on the lateral film. If a patient presents with a history of a fall on an outstretched hand and has volar tenderness of the wrist, he or she should be placed in a volar splint in the neutral position and referred to an orthopedic surgeon.

Lunate fractures are usually secondary to a fall. The lunate lies next to the navicular and articulates with the distal radius. The lunate articulates with two thirds of the surface of the radius and is important for pivot of all the carpal bones in the proximal row. The patient presents with tenderness over the lunate fossa, which is located just distal to the rim of the radius, directly at the base of the long finger metacarpal. If fractured the wrist would be placed in a thumb spica, and the patient would be referred to an orthopedic surgeon to evaluate and follow for avascular necrosis or Kienböch's disease.

Perilunate dislocations are usually secondary to falls. On a radiograph, the dislocated lunate remains in normal alignment with the radial head. The rest of the carpal bones are dislocated dorsally or volarly. This is best seen on the AP and lateral radiographs. The patient should be referred to an orthopedic surgeon for reduction by finger trap traction and immobilization.

The lunate can dislocate by itself without other associated fractures or dislocations. Dislocation of the dorsal lunate is best seen on a lateral radiograph. Volar dislocations involve displacement of the lunate in the volar direction. All lunate dislocations should be referred to an orthopedic surgeon for reduction.

When in doubt as to whether a fracture is present, splint the injury, and refer the patient to an orthopedic surgeon after a thorough neurologic and vascular examination has been performed.

HAND INJURIES

Definition

Hand injuries can be quite devastating. The hand is a dynamic, intricate mechanical instrument that allows humans to perform daily functions.

Anatomy

The hand is made up of bones, joints, intrinsic and extrinsic muscles, tendons, and ligaments. The carpal bones are arranged in two rows. The metacarpals and phalanges articulate with the distal row of carpals. The three phalanges to each finger—the proximal, middle, and distal—are divided by the DIP, PIP, and MP joints.

The extrinsic flexor system is made up of the flexor pollicis longus, flexor carpi radialis, palmaris longus, flexor carpi ulnaris, flexor digitorum superficialis, and the flexor digitorum profundus.

The extrinsic extensor system is made up of six compartments through which the extrinsic tendons pass. The first compartment contains the abductor pollicis longus and the extensor pollicis brevis. The second compartment contains the extensor carpi radialis longus and the extensor carpi radialis brevis. The third compartment contains only the extensor pollicis longus. The fourth compartment contains the extensor indicis proprius and the extensor digitorum communis. The fifth compartment contains only the extensor digiti minimi, and the sixth compartment contains the extensor carpi ulnaris.

The intrinsic muscle consists of five groups in the hand. The largest groups are the thenar and hypothenar groups. The other three small groups are the abductor pollicis, the lumbricals, and the interosseous muscles.

The innervation of the hand is by the radial, median, and ulnar nerves. The hand is supplied with blood by the ulnar artery and the radial artery, which anastamose in the hand by forming the superficial and deep palmar arches.

Examination

As with any injury the history of the event that caused the injury is very important. Always document if the patient is right or left handed and if there was a prior injury. All extremity examinations involve a neurologic, vascular, range of motion, soft tissue, ligamentous, and muscular examination. All of these items should be documented on the chart. Capillary refill or radial or ulnar pulses should be evaluated. Two-point discrimination in all three nerve areas of the hand (the medial, radius, and ulnar nerve areas) should be documented. The ability of the patient to touch, with good 5/5 strength, all fingers with the thumb should be documented. Fanning of the fingers and the ability to flex and extend all fingers at all MP, PIP, and DIP joints should be evaluated. Good 5/5 flexion and extension at the wrist should be evaluated. The patient should be able to make an "OK" sign, and abduct all fingers against resistance both together and separately against resistance. The thenar and hypothenar areas of the hand and the muscles of the forearm should be inspected for size and presence of atrophy. The Allen test can be performed to evaluate the integrity of the vascular supply of the hand. The patient should also close the hand. All of the fingertips should point to the thenar part of the palm. If they do not, there is probably rotation of the phalanx secondary to a fracture. You can never overexamine or overdocument a hand injury!

Clinical Presentation

Fractures to the middle and proximal phalanx are common. They are either open or closed, intra-articular, transverse, oblique, commuted, or spiral. The joint can also be dislocated.

Transverse fractures without rotation are splinted, and a referral is made. Oblique fractures are usually unstable and require reduction and stabilization by an orthopedic surgeon. Any fracture with rotation should be referred to an orthopedic surgeon. As little as 10 degrees of rotation can be disabling. Condylar fractures usually require open reduction.

Metacarpal fractures of the second through the fifth metacarpals are divided into four anatomic areas based on fracture sites: the head, neck, shaft, and base. Fractures of the metacarpal head are often severely comminuted and heal poorly. They should be splinted, and the patient should be referred to an orthopedic surgeon within 72 hours.

Metacarpal neck fractures are secondary to direct force. The most common fracture to the metacarpal neck is the "boxer's" fracture of the fifth metacarpal, secondary to a punch. These fractures usually angulate dorsally secondary to the pull of the interosseous muscles. Fractures of the second and third metacarpals are more serious than are fractures of the fourth and fifth metacarpals. All angulation should be eliminated at the second and third metacarpal neck. Any angulation can be a devastating deformity of these two fingers. The fourth and fifth metacarpals can accept 255 degrees of angulation without loss of movement. Ideally there should be no more than 15 to 20 degrees of angulation of the fourth and fifth metacarpals.

Metacarpal shaft fractures can also produce malrotation and dorsal angulation. No amount of rotation is acceptable with metacarpal shaft fractures. They must be reduced to preserve function. They should be splinted, and the patient should be referred to an orthopedic surgeon.

Fractures of the base of the metacarpals are isolated intra-articular fractures. Fractures at the base of the second and third metacarpals are rare and have little clinical significance. This fracture at the base of the fifth metacarpal is associated with a subluxation of the metacarpal-hamate joint. These fractures require surgical reduction.

Bennett's fracture, a fracture at the base of the thumb metacarpal, is of significant importance. Bennett's fracture involves the carpometacarpal joint and disrupts the joint at the volar base. This type of fracture requires open reduction and fixation, and the patient should be referred to an orthopedic surgeon.

Dislocations of the MP, DIP, and PIP joints are common occurrences in the ED secondary to sports injuries. DIP dislocations are almost dorsally dislocated secondary to direct trauma. They can be easily reduced after a digital nerve block and then placed in a splint for 10 to 21 days. A post-reduction film should be taken to ensure that there is no pull-off fracture of the distal phalanx at the extensor insertion site.

The PIP joint is the most commonly dislocated joint in the fingers. It has bilateral collateral ligaments, a fibrocartilaginous volar plate, and a dorsal extensor expansion that provides ligamentous support. The joint must always be evaluated for collateral ligament rupture, and thus instability or a partial avulsion of the volar plate of the

PIP. A hyperextension injury can cause a volar plate injury. These dislocations can easily be reduced after a digital nerve block. They should be re-examined and re–x-rayed after reduction for stability. If unstable, they should be referred to an orthopedic surgeon for evaluation and treatment. Treatment is controversial. Some authors treat these injuries conservatively, whereas others advocate surgical repair.

Metacarpophalangeal ligamentous injuries are common in skiers. The thumb is the most commonly injured MP joint. The joint consists of two collateral ligaments: the ulnar colateral and the radial colateral ligament. This is also called a "gamekeeper's thumb." The injury is caused by forced radial deviation or abduction to the MP joint of the thumb, which causes a partial or complete tear of the ulnar collateral ligament. There is an avulsion fracture at the volar base of the proximal phalanx, which tears the joint capsule and the volar plate. Disruption of the ligament without a fracture can also take place. To diagnose ligament injuries, stress radiographs should be performed on the individual joint. If there is more than 30 degrees of subluxation in a radial direction, compared with the joint in the other hand, without a good endpoint, then there is a complete tear. Often regional anesthesia or a block must be given to perform good stress examination secondary to pain. Treatment consists of surgical repair of complete ruptures. Partial tears are treated by a thumb spica cast for 3 to 6 weeks. It is very important not to miss a complete ligament rupture. A complete rupture renders the thumb unstable, and the patient will have difficulty pinching with the thumb and index finger.

Tendon injuries most commonly occur with lacerations to the hand. They are easily recognizable with a good hand examination. Extensor tendon injuries must be explored. They are divided into five zones. Zone I injuries include injury from the distal phalanx to the proximal interphalangeal joint and involve disruption of a distal insertion of the central slip of the finger, which often causes a mallet finger deformity if the injury is not treated. Closed mallet finger injuries are treated with mild hyperflexion for 6 to 8 weeks with a volar splint. These patients should be referred to an orthopedic surgeon for follow-up.

Zone II injuries involve the PIP joint and have a poor prognosis. These injuries result in a buttonhole boutonnière deformity with flexion of the PIP joint and forced extension of the distal joint over time. Closed injuries are treated with splinting in extension for 4 weeks of the PIP, whereas the DIP and MP joints are left mobile. The patient should do intermittent range-of-motion exercises.

Zone III injuries involve disruption of the common extensor tendon and hood as well as the extensor tendons across the dorsum of the hand. Closed injuries of this zone do well, but there can be an associated injury to the sagittal band of the extensor hood, which later results in slippage of the extensor tendon and finger drift to one side. These injuries are treated by repair of the tendon with 4–0 or 5–0 nonabsorbable sutures. The tendon is splinted with the extensor mechanism relaxed and with the wrist extended 30 degrees beyond the neutral position. The MP joint is flexed at 15 degrees, and the IP joint is slightly flexed for 6 weeks.

Zone IV injuries occur in the area of the dorsum of the wrist. The patient is often able to extend the involved MP joint if the injury is proximal. At the wrist, the proximal ends of the lacerated tendons retract and may be difficult to locate. These lacerated tendons require a consultation with an orthopedic surgeon and repair. Often adhesions will be present after treatment secondary to the lie of the tendon in the fibrous canals of the wrist.

Zone V injuries involve the tendons of the forearm and require repair in the operating room.

Flexor tendon injuries can be devastating. Each finger should be tested individually. If the tendons are lacerated, they should be repaired by an orthopedic surgeon or a hand surgeon.

High-pressure injections with liquids or gases can be threatening to the limbs. Pressures from 2000 to 12,000 psi can inject substances into the hand at a velocity of a rifle. The severity of the injury is determined by the pressure, the type of fluid, and the location. Upon presentation, the hand is pale, swollen, and increasingly painful at the injury site. Injected material can cause vascular insufficiency by direct pressure or indirectly by inducing an intense inflammatory response and marked swelling. All high-pressure injuries require an orthopedic consultation for surgical débridement and broad-spectrum antibiotic therapy.

Soft-tissue injury to the fingers and hand are quite common. Partial amputation of the fingertip is divided into three zones; zone I, the fingertip distal to the bony phalanx; zone II, between the distal end of the lunula and the end of the phalanx; and zone III, proximal to the distal end of the lunula.

Treatment with distal finger amputations is quite controversial. The length of the thumb is always preserved. In children, as much of the finger should be preserved as possible. All zone II and zone III amputations should be referred to an orthopedic surgeon or a hand surgeon.

Infections of the hand can be quite devastating secondary to the fibrous compartments of the hand. *Staphylococcus aureus* and β-hemolytic streptococci are the most common pyogenic organisms causing infections in the hand, but most infections are polymicrobial. Human bites are of special concern. "Fight bites" have a high rate of infection and should be referred to an orthopedic surgeon for irrigation in the operating room. An individual's occupation can give you a clue as to what organism is infecting the hand. Dentists and dental hygienists develop herpetic whitlow; fishermen and seafood handlers develop the *Vibrio* species, *Aeromonas hydrophila,* and *Mycobacterium marinum.* Gardeners who are stuck with thorns can develop sporotrichosis. Intravenous (IV) drug users develop gram-negative bacterial infections.

The treatment of any soft-tissue hand infection starts with a complete vascular and neurologic examination. All open draining wounds should be cultured. The antibiotic of choice should be a broad-spectrum antibiotic with penicillinase-resistant penicillin, such as dicloxicillin or nafcillin, or a first-generation cephalosporin. Usually hand infections require more than one antibiotic, such as cefazolin and penicillin. Diabetic patients with a hand infection should be also treated for gram-negative rods with an aminoglycoside and a second- or third-generation cephalosporin.

A *paronychia* is an infection of the lateral nail fold. If the infection extends over the soft tissue of the proximal nail, then it is termed an eponychia. *S. aureus* is the most common infecting organism in paronychial infections.

Treatment of paronychial infection is incision and drainage of the abscess with a No. 11 blade directed away from the nail bed and matrix, under the nail after a digital block has been performed. The patient should be instructed to apply hot soaks. The nail should be immobilized, and the patient should be placed on penicillinase-resistant penicillin, dicloxacillin, or a first-generation cephalosporin with follow-up in 1 to 2 days. Effective pain control medication should also be given.

A *felon* is an infection to the distal fingertip involving the pulp of the finger. The patient will present with severe pain and destruction of the soft tissue if the infection is not treated. All felons require an incision through the septae of the distal finger secondary to the strong, fibrous septae that bind the skin to the bone and provde stability to the finger during grasping. It is at this location that pockets of pus form. A longitudinal incision is made along the ulnar aspect of digits II and IV and the radial aspect of digits I and V. After the incision is made, the wound should be packed. The packing should be left in place for 48 hours. The finger should be splinted to the wrist. In 48 hours, the packing should be removed, and warm soaks should be applied.

Tenosynovitis must not be missed on examination. It is an infection that spreads along the course of the tendon sheath. As the pressure in the sheath grows secondary to the infection, the pressure can occlude the tenuous circulation and cause necrosis. If not treated aggressively, the infection can spread to the midpalmar space or the thenar or hypothenar spaces.

There are four cardinal signs of tenosynovitis: (1) tenderness along the course of the flexor tendon, (2) symmetric swelling of the finger, (3) pain on passive extension, and (4) flexed posture of the finger. Treatment consists of immediate surgical drainage and a high dose of antibiotics, immobilization, and elevation.

HIP AND FEMUR TRAUMA

Definition

The hip is a ball-in-socket joint comprising the acetabulum and the proximal femur. The proximal femur, 2 to 3 inches below the lesser trochanter of the femur, is included in the hip. Hip dislocations can occur either anteriorly, posteriorly, or centrally. Children have several different diseases secondary to the presence of an epiphysis.

Epidemiology

Hip fractures occur in the young population secondary to direct trauma. Hip fractures occur in the elderly, postmenopausal female with osteoporosis secondary to a fall. Children can suffer from congenital or traumatic pathology.

Anatomy

The femur is the strongest and longest bone in the body. The two femurs extend obliquely from the pelvis medial to the knee. The functions of the hip are weight bearing and movement.

The intertrochanteric line marks the junction of the femoral neck with the femoral shaft. A fibrous capsule surrounds the joint on all sides and gives support. The capsule attaches around the acetabulum proximally and runs to the intertrochanteric line distally on the anterior surface. Posteriorly, the capsule falls short of the intertrochanteric crest and inserts on the neck of the femur.

The hip is supplied by nutrient vessels of the obturator, medial femoral circumflex, and superior and inferior gluteal arteries. The major nerves of the hip are the femoral nerve and the sciatic nerve.

Clinical Presentation

Hip fractures are classified as femoral head fractures, femoral neck fractures, trochanteric fractures, intertrochanteric fractures, and subtrochanteric fractures.

Femoral head fractures are rare, and they usually occur with hip dislocations. Shear fractures of the superior aspect of the femoral head are associated with anterior dislocations, and shear fractures of the inferior femoral head are associated with posterior dislocations. The pain is attributed more to a hip dislocation than to a fracture. An orthopedic surgeon must be consulted for reduction and anatomic reduction of the fracture fragment.

Femoral neck fractures occur in older adults and are more frequent in women than in men. The fracture is secondary to minor trauma with torsion of the patient's femur, with the presence of osteoporosis or osteomalacia. Femoral neck fractures are classified by the fragments present and by displacement. A patient with a fracture without displacement may walk with some limping but will be unable to completely bear weight on the injured hip. Displaced fractures are painful. The patient will be unable to ambulate and will complain of limited range of motion. Upon palpation, there will be no extracapsular head movement. There will be slight external rotation, shortening, and abduction of the injured leg. On radiographs, the patient should be told to internally rotate the hip so that the best possible view of the femoral neck can be obtained. If a stress fracture is suspected, the hip should be x-rayed again in 10 to 14 days if pain is still present or a CT scan should be performed. Displaced fractures will need internal fixation or a prosthetic replacement. There is some controversy as to whether all nondisplaced fractures require fixation. There are significant complications of femoral neck fractures including avascular necrosis, infection, and pulmonary embolism.

Trochanteric fractures are divided into greater and lesser trochanteric fractures. Greater trochanteric fractures are usually secondary to avulsion at the insertion of the gluteus medius. Greater trochanteric fractures are usually seen in the 7- to 17-year-old population secondary to a true epiphyseal separation. In adults, the fracture is secondary to an avulsion with comminution.

The patient presents with hip pain when walking and pain upon palpation of the greater trochanter. There is also controversy as to whether conservative treatment or internal fixation should be performed.

Lesser trochanteric fractures are secondary to an avulsion of the iliopsoas muscle. These fractures are usually seen in the young athletes. A patient will complain of pain during flexion and internal rotation. Treatment usually involves bed rest and pain medications with gradual weight bearing.

Intertrochanteric fractures are secondary to falls in the presence of osteoporosis. It is believed that rotation and direct trauma cause the fracture. The patient presents with swelling and pain with any movement of the hip or weight bearing. The extremity will be externally rotated and shortened. Intertrochanteric fractures are further classified as stable or unstable. Stable fractures are fractures in which the medial cortices of the neck and femoral fragments abut. Unstable fractures will need internal fixation.

Subtrochanteric fractures are seen in the 40- to 60-year-old patient with osteoporosis and in younger people who have suffered kinetic energy trauma through the femur. A subtrochanteric fracture is often an extension of a intertrochanteric fracture. These fractures are classified as stable or unstable, as defined by the bony contact of the medial and posterior femoral cortices.

A patient can suffer a large blood loss and hypovolemic shock from these fractures. The fracture should be immobilized with a traction splint, and an orthopedic consultation should be made for internal fixation.

Hip dislocations are usually secondary to trauma. Ten percent of all hip fractures are anterior, secondary to automobile accidents. Anterior dislocations are secondary to a blow to the back while squatting. The force abducts the femoral head out of the anterior capsule, tearing the capsule. On a radiograph, the femoral head will be inferior and medial to the acetabulum. The best view will be a lateral view. Treatment involves early reduction by strong in-line traction while flexion and internal rotation is performed. General anesthesia is often required to perform this maneuver.

Posterior hip dislocations account for 80 to 90% of all hip dislocations. Posterior dislocations are caused by force applied to a flexed knee, directed posteriorly. On examination, the hip will be shortened and internally rotated and abducted. On a radiograph, it must be determined that there is no inferior femoral head fracture. The hip is reduced by in-line traction with gentle flexion to 90 degrees and then gentle internal-to-external rotation (the Allis maneuver). The Stimson maneuver can also be used to reduce the hip. There is sciatic nerve injury in 10% of patients with posterior hip dislocations. Avascular necrosis is increased in proportion by the time the hip was dislocated.

Congenital hip dislocations in children occur in one in every 1000 children and are often seen in the firstborn. It occurs six times more often in females than in males. The diagnosis of congenital hip dislocation is made by the Ortolani test or the Barlow test. If while performing the Ortolani test the femoral head subluxes, a palpable and audible click may be heard. If the femoral head subluxes, the child requires an orthopedic consultation.

Legg-Calvé-Perthes disease is most often found in males between 5 and 9 years of age. This disease is an idiopathic avascular necrosis of the femoral head. It presents insidiously with the symptoms of a painful limp. On examination there will be decreased range of motion and spasm. On a radiograph, there will be necrosis, reabsorption, and regeneration of bone in different stages. These patients should be referred to a pediatric orthopedic surgeon.

A slipped capital femoral epiphysis occurs in adolescents and preadolescents between the ages of 10 and 16 years. It is four times more common in males than in females and is bilateral in 20 to 49% of the cases. A slipped capital femoral epiphysis occurs in the male with Fröhlich's obesity body type, with underdeveloped genitalia, and in tall, rapidly growing adolescents.

A patient presents with an insidious onset of groin discomfort, which develops into hip stiffness and a limp. Often the primary complaint is knee pain secondary to a referred pain from the hip. On a radiograph, the initial radiograph may be normal. A slipped epiphyseal plate posteriorly is best seen on a lateral film. The patient should be referred to an orthopedic surgeon for traction and surgical fixation.

Children younger than 4 years of age present with a septic hip or septic arthritis. Septic arthritis is the most common finding in an infant with a painful hip. Hematogenous seeding is the most common mode of infection. The most common organism that causes a septic hip in an infant is group B *Streptococcus. S. epidermidis* and *Haemophilus influenzae* are the most common organisms that can occur in the first 2 years of an infant's life.

Children with septic arthritis present with a limp or painful weight bearing. Infants will be fussy and will cry when they are held. They will be irritable due to having a fever and will feed poorly. On examination, there will be decreased or painful range of motion. The child will lie with the hip flexed, abducted, and externally rotated. The result of blood cultures will be positive in 50% of the cases with an increased ESR. If a septic hip is suggested, the patient will require an immediate orthopedic consultation.

Any fracture of the midshaft of the femur will require a referral for possible placement of a rod into the femur by an orthopedic surgeon.

Examination

The patient should be completely unclothed from the waist down to evaluate the hip and check for shortening of the leg or internal or external rotation. A complete vascular and neurologic examination should be performed. A rectal examination should also be done.

Radiographs

All hip fractures should be evaluated with a low AP pelvis and a cross-table lateral of the injured hip. The hip should not be "frog-legged." Inlet or tilt views can be performed.

Laboratory Findings

Any patient with a hip fracture should have a CBC, prothrombin time (PT), partial thromboplastin time (PTT), electrolytes, glucose, and urinalysis with culture; also, 6 to 8 units of blood should typed and crossed.

Treatment

Any patient with a suspected hip fracture should have a "safety net" established. Two large-gauge IV lines of normal saline 0.9% should be established, and the patient should be placed on oxygen. The patient should also be placed on a cardiac monitor and have the aforementioned laboratory tests performed. Airway, breathing, and circulation (ABC) take precedence over the treatment of a hip fracture.

A Foley catheter should be placed after the integrity of the urethra has been established. A rectal examination should be performed on every patient, and a bimanual examination should be performed on any female. A complete neurologic examination should be done along with a complete vascular examination. A diagnostic peritoneal lavage should be performed if there is abdominal tenderness, but remember that it is a poor test for retroperitoneal bleeding or a hematoma.

Definitive treatment of a fracture is based on the type of fracture and whether the fracture is stable or unstable. An elderly person with a hip fracture should be admitted to the hospital secondary to the large number of complications associated with hip fractures in patients in this age group.

INFECTIONS OF THE BONES AND JOINTS

Definition

Infections of the bones and joints can occur in any age group or race. Infection of the bones is often called osteomyelitis, which means "inflammation of the marrow of bone." The most commonly used classification of osteomyelitis is the Waldvogel classification. Hematogenous osteomyelitis is when blood-borne bacteria are deposited in the bone. This occurs most commonly in children and in adults with vertebral osteomyelitis.

The next classification is a contiguous-focus osteomyelitis that occurs when the adjacent soft tissue is contaminated or infected. This infection is secondary to an abscess, cellulitis, or enteric infection.

The next type of infection involves osteomyelitis secondary to direct inoculation of bacteria into the bone from trauma, open fractures, surgery, or implantation of a surgical prosthesis.

Osteomyelitis secondary to vascular disease is seen mainly in the diabetic with foot problems and in patients with severe peripheral arterial disease.

A patient can also acquire chronic osteomyelitis. This is usually seen in the immunocompromised patient or in the diabetic patient.

Infection of the joints or septic arthritis is secondary to hematogenous migration of bacteria into a joint. Inoculation can be from an open fracture, puncture wound, or joint aspiration.

Epidemiology

Septic arthritis is seen in patients with diabetes mellitus, sickle cell disease, and acquired immunodeficiency syndrome and also in alcoholics, drug abusers, chronic corticosteroid users, and in patients with pre-existing joint disease.

Pathology

S. aureus is the most common organism that causes osteomyelitis in all age groups except neonates. In neonates, group B streptococci is the major cause of osteomyelitis. In children younger than 5 years of age, *H. influenzae* is a major cause of septic arthritis but is uncommon in osteomyelitis. *Neisseria gonorrhoeae* accounts for 50% of all cases of septic arthritis in sexually active adults. Gram-negative bacteria account for the majority of bone and joint infections in the elderly.

Clinical Presentation

A patient with osteomyelitis presents with pain in the affected bone or joint. In children, often the most common presenting complaint is a limp and a warm or tender joint. Fever is not always present. Anorexia, fever, malaise, fatigue, or headache may or may not be present. The patient does not always appear ill or to have a systemic infection. Osteomyelitis is most commonly found in the metaphyses of long bones. It is often difficult to determine if the infection is in a long bone or in a neighboring joint.

Laboratory Findings

CBC, electrolyte, glucose, ESR, and blood culture tests should be obtained on any patient with suspected septic arthritis or osteomyelitis. The white blood cell (WBC) count is usually no greater than $15,000/mm^3$ in a patient with osteomyelitis. The ESR will be elevated in 90% of the patients with a septic joint or osteomyelitis and is usually elevated to a mean of 70 mm/hr. An ESR of less than 15 mm/hr will be present in only 8% of the patients with osteomyelitis. The ESR will fall as the infection is cleared.

Radiographs

Radiographs in the early stages of osteomyelitis are rarely helpful. Before a lesion can be seen on a plain radiograph, 30 to 50% of the bone mineral must be lost. By 28 days of infection, plain films will be positive in 90% of cases. A periosteal reaction is an early sign of osteomyelitis. On plain films, there will be lucent lytic area of bone. In late stages of osteomyelitis, the lytic lesion will be surrounded by dense, sclerotic bone, and sequestration may be noted on a plain film. Always examine the surrounding soft tissue for swelling, distorted facial planes, and altered fat interfaces, all of which can be clues to early development of osteomyelitis.

The gold standard for diagnosing osteomyelitis is a radionuclide skeletal scintigraphy scan (or bone scan). A bone scan can detect infection in a bone within 49 to 72 hours of infection.

A CT scan can be used to detect and define areas of possible infection in bones that have a complex anatomy and are difficult to visualize on plain films or on a bone scan. MRI is being used more and more for the detection of osteomyelitis and is much better at defining changes in soft tissue than is a CT scan or a bone scan.

Treatment

The treatment of osteomyelitis involves a combination of both antibiotic and surgical therapy. Antibiotic therapy should involve first-generation cephalosporins and penicillins secondary to the low pH of bones. Aminoglycosides do not work well in the low pH of bones. The antibiotic of choice should cover *Staphylococcus,* and the patient should be treated with a penicillinase-resistant penicillin (e.g., nafcillin) or a first-generation cephalosporin. All patients with osteomyelitis should be referred to an orthopedic surgeon for follow-up and definitive care.

Septic arthritis and joint infections require a consultation with an orthopedic surgeon. The joint will require aspiration, and the fluid will require a laboratory evaluation for color, cell count, lactic acid level, Gram stain, and synovial fluid and glucose ratio. All aspirated fluid must be cultured. The same organisms that cause osteomyelitis also cause septic arthritis. Septic arthritis is treated as if the patient has osteomyelitis, i.e., with the same organism-specific antibioties.

LOWER EXTREMITY ORTHOPEDIC INJURIES

Definition

The lower extremity bony structures consist of the tibia and the fibula. The tibia is the most commonly fractured lower extremity bone and is the most common long bone fracture. Lower extremity fractures can be open or closed. There is a high complication rate with fractures of the tibia.

Anatomy of the Lower Extremity

The tibia and fibula are connected by the interosseous ligament, and the surrounding soft tissue is divided into three compartments. The anterior compartment consists of the tibialis anterior, extensor digitorum longus, extensor hallucis, and peroneus tertius muscles. The anterior tibial artery and the deep peroneal nerve run through the anterior compartment. There is not much space for swelling in this compartment, and this is where a compartment syndrome most commonly occurs.

The lateral compartment consists of the peroneus brevis and peroneus longus muscles and the superficial peroneal nerve. The superficial peroneal nerve can be injured when a fracture of the superior fibular shaft or the neck of the fibula occurs.

The posterior compartment consists of the soleus, gastrocnemius, tibialis posterior, flexor hallucis longus, and flexor digitorum longus muscles. The posterior tibial nerve and the posterior tibial artery are located in the posterior compartment.

Clinical Presentation/Examination

Both lower extremities should be examined for edema, ecchymosis, pain upon passive flexion or extension of muscle groups, the presence and intensity of pulses, and capillary refill. A good neurologic examination should be done, including a two-point discrimination test. Obvious deformity and crepitance are definite signs of a fracture. The leg should be examined for valgus or varus rotation.

AP and lateral x-rays of the lower extremity are the minimal x-rays to be performed in evaluating the lower extremity for trauma. Remember that the lower leg starts at the knee and ends at the ankle, thus any tenderness of either the knee or the ankle should be evaluated and x-rays should be taken.

Treatment

The treatment of any lower extremity injury is immobilization and monitoring the neurovascular status of the extremity. If a soft tissue injury is present, the tissue should be as well maintained as possible. If there is an abrasion or an open fracture, tetanus prophylaxis and antibiotic coverage should be standard treatment. Open wounds should be copiously irrigated with saline.

If there is vascular or neurologic compromise from a fracture or dislocation, the fracture should be reduced or repositioned until revascularization is accomplished. The most common complication associated with a fracture of the lower extremity is secondary infection, which occurs 24 to 48 hours after the injury. The next most common complication to a lower extremity injury is a compartment syndrome, which is seen 24 to 48 hours after the injury secondary to swelling in the injured compartment. The most common sites of a compartment syndrome are the four fascial compartments in the leg in the peroneal, anterior, deep, and superficial posterior areas. The volar and dorsal compartments of the forearm and the interosseous muscles of the hand can also be affected.

Compartment syndromes are secondary to skeletal or muscle injury secondary to trauma, infection, electrical injury, hyperthermia, hypothermia, snakebites, toxins, arterial embolism, polymyositis, seizures, CVA, or drug overdose.

To diagnose a compartment syndrome, one must have a high index of suspicion. Complete muscle, vascular, and neurologic death can occur in 4 to 6 hours.

A patient with a compartment syndrome of the lower leg presents with paresthesias and pain with passive toe and foot movement of the involved compartment. There will be abnormal light touch or a decreased or widened two-point discrimination. On examination of the lower extremity, the compartment will be tense, indurated, and erythematous.

A CPK, urine myoglobin, or serum myoglobin should be drawn on any patient who is considered to have a compartment syndrome. Rhabdomyolysis is often present. The CPK will normally be greater than 20,000. Renal functions, BUN, and creatinine should be also monitored.

The diagnosis of an acute compartment syndrome is made by using a Wick catheter or an 18-gauge needle to measure the compartment pressure with a saline manometer. Normal compartment pressure is 0 to 8 mm Hg. Any pressure greater than 30 mm Hg is considered to be a compartment syndrome. An emergency fasciotomy is indicated.

Achilles tendon ruptures involve the partial or complete rupture of the Achilles tendon. The superior portion of the Achilles tendon is formed by the distal ends of the soleus and gastrocnemius muscles. An examination of the Achilles tendon should be part of every ankle examination. Often, an Achilles tendon rupture is diagnosed as an acute sprained ankle.

Achilles tendon ruptures occur secondary to an acute forceful dorsiflexion of the ankle. They can also be lacerated or ruptured secondary to a direct blow. A patient will present with a history of an audible snap or pop and the immediate onset of pain, which is described by the patient as if someone was kicking him or her in the calf. On physical examination, the patient's calf will be tender and swollen. A palpable defect will be noted 2 to 6 cm proximal to the insertion of the Achilles tendon into the calcaneus.

The patient will be unable to plantar flex the foot. Active plantar flexion does not rule out an acute Achilles tendon rupture. The Thompson test is performed by compressing the patient's calf while the patient is lying on the abdomen with the knee flexed at 90 degrees. If the foot does not plantar flex, then there is an Achilles tendon rupture.

Partial tears are usually treated with casting in a toe-down position for several weeks without weight bearing. Complete tears need surgical repair by an orthopedic surgeon.

Fibular fractures by themselves are rare. The most common area of fracture is at the ankle. Midshaft or proximal fractures of the fibula often do not require immobilization and can be treated with conservative therapy. If casted, they usually only need treatment with a short leg walker for 2 to 3 weeks.

A patient can present with a gastrocnemius rupture or calf strain. A patient who falls with forceful dorsiflexion of the ankle or sudden push-off during athletic events, such as tennis or basketball, can cause a full or partial rupture of the medial head of the gastrocnemius at the musculotendinous junction. The patient presents with localized pain to the medial midcalf with ambulation and standing on tiptoes. The Thompson sign will be negative, and swelling and ecchymosis will be present. Treatment involves ice, elevation, and anti-inflammatory agents with use of crutches for approximately 1 week.

Children with tibial or fibular shaft fractures present with a deformity of the leg and pain on weight bearing. These injuries are usually secondary to a twisting motion or to indirect trauma. Tibial metaphyseal fractures and Salter-Harris fractures are common. All pediatric fractures should be referred for follow-up.

PELVIC TRAUMA

Definition

Pelvic trauma usually occurs secondary to falls or motor vehicle accidents. Hemorrhage is always a threat to any patient with a pelvic fracture. Internal organ injury can be massive in a clinically stable patient. All internal organs, including the bladder, uterus, adnexae, colon, and small bowel, as well as vascular and neurologic systems must be evaluated thoroughly in any patient with pelvic trauma.

Epidemiology

Pelvic fractures account for 3% of all fractures. Automobile accidents account for 60% of all pelvic fractures, and falls account for 30%. The mortality rate for pelvic fractures is approximately between 6.4% and 19%. A patient who presents to the ED with a pelvic fracture and who is hypotensive has a 42% to 50% mortality rate.

Anatomy

The pelvis consists of a ring-like structure with the right and left innominate bones, the sacrum, and coccyx. The innominate bones are made up of the ischium, the ilium, and the pubis, which fuses at the acetabulum. The pelvic ring provides the lower abdominal contents with some protection from injury. It also serves as a place of attachment for muscles and tendons. The posterior ligaments provide mechanical support, and disruption is a significant cause of pelvic instability after an injury. There is a considerable vascular network with major arteries and veins running through the pelvis, all of which can be injured during a traumatic event.

The iliopectineal, or arcuate, line divides the pelvis into upper and lower parts. The upper pelvis is part of the abdomen, and the lower pelvis is the true pelvis. The iliopectineal line is also part of the femorosacral arch and the subsidiary tie arch; the bodies of the pubic bones and the superior rami support the body in an erect position. The weight-bearing forces transmitted by sitting are supported by the ischiosacral arch and by its ties to the pubic bones, inferior pubic rami, and the ischial rami. When trauma occurs to the pelvis, the first ties to fracture are the symphysis pubis, pubic rami, and just lateral to the sacroiliac joint.

There are five joints in the pelvis that allow some movement. The lumbosacral, sacroiliac, and sacrococcygeal joints and the symphysis pubis allow some movement.

The ball-in-socket joint of the hip, the acetabulum, is divided into three parts: the iliac portion, or the superior dome portion, which is the weight-bearing surface of the hip; the inner wall, made up of the pubis, which is relatively thin and is easily fractured; and the posterior acetabulum, which is derived from the thick ischium.

The nerve supply of the pelvis is derived from the lumbar and sacral plexuses. The bladder also lies in the bony pelvis behind the symphysis and can be easily traumatized. The sigmoid and descending colon, rectum, and anus all lie in the bone pelvis and can be injured during a traumatic event.

Clinical Presentation/Diagnosis

There are four types of pelvic fractures. A *type I pelvic fracture* involves individual bones without a break in the pelvic ring. Type I fractures are stable fractures and make up one third of all pelvic fractures. Most type I fractures can be treated with bed rest and good pain control, because most of these fractures are very stable. There are several types of type I fracture.

Fracture of a single ramus of the pubis or ischium is usually seen in an elderly patient secondary to direct trauma from a fall. A patient presents with the ability to ambulate but with localized pelvic pain. A lateral film should be taken to distinguish a pubic bone fracture from a femoral neck fracture. These fractures heal without complication.

An avulsion of the anterior superior iliac spine is secondary to an avulsion of a piece of bone by the violent contraction of the sartorius muscle. A patient will present with localized pain, edema, and painful flexion and abduction of the thigh. On a radiograph, there will be minimal displacement of the anterior superior iliac spine. Usually no treatment is necessary.

Fractures of the coccyx are usually seen in women secondary to direct violence to the coccyx from a fall. The patient presents with pain, painful defecation, and ecchymosis of the sacral region. On rectal examination, palpation of the coccyx will elicit pain. Usually no treatment is necessary beyond pain control.

Avulsion fractures of the anterior inferior iliac spine occur when the rectus femoris muscle is violently contracted. A patient presents with sharp groin pain, painful and difficult ambulation, and inability to flex the hip. On an AP radiograph, there will be downward displacement of the fragment; however, this fragment must be differentiated from the epiphyseal line of the acetabulum.

Ischium body fractures are secondary to violent external trauma against the ischium. The patient presents with localized pain of the hamstring with movement. On a radiograph, the fracture of the body or the tuberosity of the ischium can be seen. It is often in a butterfly pattern on the PA film. Pain medication is usually the only treatment that is necessary.

An avulsion fracture of the ischial tuberosity is secondary to a hamstring contraction and is seen in youths whose apophyses are not united. The patient will present with acute or chronic pain while sitting or upon flexing the thigh with the knee extended. On rectal examination, the tuberosity will be tender. Radiographs will show a detachment of the apophysis from the ischium with minimal displacement. The apophysis closes between the ages of 20 and 25.

An acute sacral fracture is usually secondary to massive trauma and is associated with massive pelvic injuries. Direct posterior-to-anterior forces produce a transverse fracture. On rectal examination, there will be pain and movement at the fracture site. These fractures require an immediate orthopedic evaluation and internal organ evaluation.

An iliac wing fracture or a Duverney fracture is secondary to direct trauma to the iliac crest. The patient will present with pain, edema, and tenderness over the iliac wing. The patient will have severe pain and problems with ambulation. The Trendelenburg sign will be present. The internal organs should be evaluated by a CT scan, and an orthopedic consultation should be standard procedure.

A *type II pelvic fracture* involves a single break in the pelvic ring. This fracture consists of little or no displacement and is usually treated with bed rest and pain medication. One fourth of these patients will have soft tissue injuries, visceral injuries, genitourinary injuries, or hemorrhage; thus they should be evaluated by a CT scan.

Fractures near the subluxation of the symphysis pubis are secondary to direct trauma to the symphysis pubis. This injury, although rare, can also occur during or after childbirth. The patient presents with severe pain with some external rotation to the affected side. On examination, compression will produce displacement and pain. Ecchymosis is usually absent. On radiograph there will be subluxation, fracture, or dislocation. Subluxation will occur in either coronal or sagittal planes. If dislocated, the midline will overlap by superoposterior or inferoanterior displacement of one articulating surface in relation to the other. Sacroiliac joint disruption or genitourinary injuries are common with these fractures.

Fractures of the two rami ipsilaterally are secondary to direct trauma to the femur, which carries the force into the rami as the usual cause. On examination there will be ecchymosis and pain with motion. Often a hematoma can be palpated, and pain will occur on flexion, abduction, external rotation, or hip extension. On a radiograph, there will be no or minimal displacement.

A fracture near the sacroiliac joint or subluxation of the sacroiliac joint is secondary to direct trauma from behind or being struck from behind and laterally. The patient presents with localized pain and pain on ambulation. Pain can be reproduced with compression maneuvers. Often the posterior iliac spine appears more prominent on the traumatized side. On a radiograph the sacrum, pelvis, and sacroiliac joint can be noted. A CT scan should be taken to determine the extent of the fracture.

A *type III pelvic fracture* of the pelvis involves a double break in the pelvic ring. This fracture is unstable and requires an orthopedic consultation and treatment.

Multiple pelvic fractures are secondary to severe trauma and have a high incidence of internal organ damage. All multiple pelvic fractures require a CT scan. Usually treatment is conservative; however, if the ilium is fractured, adequate reduction is necessitated.

A Malgaigne fracture or a double fracture of the superior or inferior rami, or dislocation of the symphysis in association with a sacral or iliac fracture or sacroiliac joint dislocation, is secondary to direct trauma. The patient presents with crepitance, swelling, contusion, and decreased range of motion on examination. There will be fragment movement with compression. The ipsilateral leg will appear shortened. There is often associated internal organ injury. Sacroiliac joint reduction is difficult and may result in chronic pain.

Straddle fractures, or double vertical fractures, or dislocation to the pubis are secondary to direct trauma to the arch or lateral compression of the pelvis secondary to a fall. The patient presents with pain, edema, deformity, and swelling. The fracture is usually treated conservatively, but underlying genitourinary trauma is often present.

A *type IV acetabular fracture* is usually associated with an automobile accident. There are often many other pelvic injuries present with type IV fractures. There are four anatomic types of type IV fractures.

Posterior fractures are secondary to direct trauma to a flexed knee and hip. Complications can include sciatic nerve injury and femoral fractures. On a radiograph, a posterior acetabular fracture with a posterior hip dislocation is seen.

Ilioschial column fractures are seen when there is direct force to the knee with the thigh abducted and flexed. On a radiograph, a large medially displaced fragment with central dislocation of the femoral head will be noted. There is often injury to the sciatic nerve.

Transverse fractures of the acetabulum are secondary to lateral or medial forces over the greater trochanter, or forces acting posteriorly to anteriorly on the posterior pelvis with a flexed hip. On a radiograph, there will be a central hip dislocation.

Iliopubic column fractures are secondary to lateral forces to the greater trochanter with the hip externally rotated. On a radiograph, there will be external hip rotation; the ilioischial line will be disrupted; and the anterior lip will be fractured.

Radiographs

An AP radiograph and a lateral radiograph of the pelvis should be the minimal radiographs performed in the trauma room for a possible fractured pelvis. If the hip is also considered fractured, it should not be "frog-legged." The pelvis must be moved as little as possible until the type and severity of injury are determined. Stabilization takes priority over obtaining radiographs.

The symphysis pubis is normally less than 5 mm wide. A small offset of 1 to 2 mm on the left or right side is a normal variant. An overlapping symphysis is abnormal. The sacroiliac joint is normally 2 to 4 mm wide. A fracture of the fifth lumbar transverse process often accompanies a sacroiliac joint disruption or a vertical sacral fracture and is a clue to a posterior arch injury.

Specialized films of the pelvis can be used to obtain greater detail of the pelvis. The inlet and the tangential projection can be obtained. The inlet view is performed by taking a 30-degree caudal angulation of the beam. The beam is angled 60 degrees to the plate and is perpendicular to the pelvic inlet. This view helps to determine if there is a posterior arch or inward displacement of the anterior arch.

The tangential projection is the opposite of the inlet view, where the beam is directed cephalad. This view can help to determine if there is a sacral fracture or a displacement of the sacroiliac joint.

A CT scan of a fractured pelvis should probably be done to define the fracture and to check for internal organ damage.

Examination

Remember that the pelvis is a ring. If there is one fracture of the ring, always look closely for a second fracture.

Laboratory Findings

CBC, PT, PTT, electrolyte, glucose, liver function tests, amylase, lipase, and urinalysis with culture should be performed. A minimum of 6 to 8 units of blood should be typed and cross matched. If there is the possibility of bladder rupture or bowel perforation, blood cultures should be taken.

Treatment

Any patient with a suspected hip fracture should have a "safety net" established. Two large-gauge IV lines of normal saline 0.9% should be established, and the patient should be placed on oxygen. The patient should also be placed on a cardiac monitor, and the aforementioned laboratory tests should be performed. The ABCs take precedence over the treatment of a pelvic hip fracture.

A Foley catheter should be placed after the integrity of the urethra has been established. A rectal examination should be performed on every patient, and a bimanual examination should be done on any female. A complete neurologic examination should be performed along with a complete vascular examination. A diagnostic peritoneal lavage should be done if the patient has abdominal tenderness; however, this is a poor test for retroperitoneal bleeding or a hematoma.

A CT scan should probably be performed on any pelvic fracture to evaluate internal organ injury and to determine the extent of the pelvic fracture. Remember that AP films do not demonstrate the posterior aspect of the sacroiliac joints. Also remember that a diagnostic peritoneal lavage will not demonstrate a retroperitoneal hematoma, thus a CT scan needs to be performed to rule out a retroperitoneal hematoma. Pelvic fractures, like all fractures, are treated only after the patient has been stabilized.

SHOULDER

Definition

The shoulder consists of the clavicle, scapula, humerus, and three joints: the sternoclavicular, glenohumeral, and acromioclavicular joints. All of these bones or joints can be injured.

Anatomy

The clavicle is an S-shaped bone that acts as a bony strut; supports the upper extremity; and keeps the upper extremity away from the chest wall. The clavicle articulates with the sternum medially and the acromion process laterally. The sternoclavicular joint articulates the sternum with the shoulder. The sternoclavicular joint is stabilized by the anterior and posterior sternoclavicular ligaments and the interclavicular and costoclavicular ligaments.

The acromioclavicular joint forms part of the articulation between the upper extremity and the axial skeleton. It is a diarthrodial joint between the lateral end of the clavicle and the medial aspect of the acromion process. The joint is stabilized by the anterior, posterior, superior, and inferior acromioclavicular ligaments.

The scapula is a flat triangular bone that forms the posterior aspect of the shoulder girdle. The scapula consists of two processes, three angles, and three borders. The body of the scapula lies flat against the posterior ribs. The superior and inferior spine of the scapula give rise to the supraspinatus and infraspinatus muscles. The teres minor and major muscles give rise from the posterior aspect of the lateral border of the scapula. The superior border of the scapula gives rise to the coracoid process, where the biceps, coracobrachialis, and pectoralis minor muscles attach. The suprascapular nerve runs through the suprascapular notch.

The glenohumeral articulation is a diarthrodial ball-and-socket joint. The stability of the joint is dependent on the associated muscles and ligaments. The shoulder is formed by synovial capsules. A synovial membrane extends from the glenoid fossa to the humeral head. Two extensions of the synovial membrane are present. These synovial membranes extend medially to form the subcapularis bursa and laterally to envelope the long head of the biceps. The anterior capsule is thickened to form the superior, middle, and inferior glenohumeral ligaments. Superiorly, the capsule is protected by the acromial process and is strengthened by the coracohumeral ligament.

Clinical Presentation

Clavicle fractures occur secondary to trauma. Clavicle fractures account for 5% of all fractures. The clavicle is the most commonly fractured bone at birth. It is very commonly fractured in children with a history of a fall on an outstretched hand. Clavicle fractures are divided into three types. A fracture of the proximal third is usually a result of a direct blow to the anterior chest or clavicle. This fracture is quite rare.

Fractures to the middle third of the clavicle are secondary to an indirect force applied to the lateral aspect of the shoulder, which results in a shearing fracture proximal to the attachment of the coracoclavicular ligament. This fracture accounts for 80% of all clavicle fractures.

Fractures of the distal third of the clavicle comprise 15% of all clavicle fractures. This fracture is secondary to a direct blow to the top of the shoulder. The distal fractures are also classified into three subtypes by Neer and Rockwood. Type I fractures are undisplaced fractures with intact coracoclavicular ligaments. Type II fractures are associated with displacement and separation of the coracoclavicular ligaments from the proximal fragment. Type II fractures involve the articular surface and are frequently overlooked. The fracture is treated with a figure-of-eight bandage or clavicle strap.

Fractures of the scapula are quite rare. They are usually seen in young men and account for only 1% of all fractures. A considerable amount of force must be exerted to fracture a clavicle. Associated injuries are present in 75 to 98% of all cases of scapula fractures. First rib fractures, hemopneumothorax, pneumothorax, or pulmonary contusion are often present. Often the pneumothorax is delayed 2 to 3 days after injury, therefore the patient should be admitted to the hospital or close follow-up is required.

There are three types of scapula fractures. Type I fractures involve the body and spine. Type II fractures involve the acromion or coracoid processes. Type III fractures involve the scapular neck and glenoid fossa.

Scapular fractures are usually treated with conservative therapy. Ice, immobilization, analgesia, and an orthopedic consultation are usually all that is needed in the treatment of scapular fractures. Usually the associated injuries are more life threatening and should be aggressively looked for and treated.

Proximal humerus fractures account for 4 to 5% of all fractures and are commonly seen in elderly women with osteoporosis who fall. The humerus commonly fractures along old epiphyseal lines. There are basically four fracture lines of the proximal humerus. The articular surface or the anatomic neck, the greater tuberosity, the lesser tuberosity, and the humeral shaft or surgical neck. The proximal humerus can also suffer anterior and posterior fracture dislocations. A segment is considered displaced if the angle is 45 degrees or more and is separated by 1 cm of space or more. Thus fractures are minimally displaced or can have two-part displacement, three-part displacement, or four-part displacement.

Treatment of minimally displaced fractures (80 to 85% of all fractures) consists of ice packs, immobilization, and sling-and-swathe for a few days with early range of motion and an orthopedic consultation. Any two-, three-, or four-part displaced fractures or fracture dislocations should be referred to an orthopedic surgeon for treatment.

Humeral shaft fractures are often associated with radial nerve paralysis. The radial nerve is usually stretched, resulting in neuropraxia. The nerve is rarely truly lacerated. If the radial nerve paralysis has an onset immediately following the injury, the prognosis for return of the nerve is good. The extension of the wrist, thumb, and fingers should be documented prior to manipulation of the arm.

Treatment of the fracture without nerve involvement involves placing the arm in a coaptation splint, hanging cast, or another device for external immobilization. Fractures of the humerus are frequently associated with delayed union, and a referral should be made to an orthopedic surgeon for treatment and follow up.

Sternoclavicular joint injuries are rare and are secondary to signifi-cant forceful injuries. The sternoclavicular joint can be dislocated anteriorly or posteriorly. The patient will present with the injured extremity foreshortened and supported against the trunk by the oppo-site arm. The joint area will be swollen and painful when the shoul-der is moved. If the joint is dislocated posteriorly, there is usually more pain, hoarseness, dysphagia, dyspnea, or weakness, or paresthe-sias are present in the upper extremity. A thorough neurologic exami-nation should be done, and the superior mediastinal and thoracic structures need to be examined carefully.

Injuries to the sternoclavicular joint are graded in three types. Type I is a mild sprain secondary to stretching of the sternoclavicular and costoclavicular ligaments. Ice, immobilization, and anti-inflammatory medications are required for treatment. Type II injuries involve sub-luxation of the joint either anteriorly or posteriorly and involve a rupture of the sternoclavicular ligament. The costoclavicular ligament remains intact. Treatment is with a figure-of-eight splint and anti-inflammatory agents. A type III injury to the sternoclavicular joint involves a complete rupture of the sternoclavicular and costoclavicu-lar ligaments. In persons younger than 25 years of age, this injury is often a Salter type I injury.

Type II anterior dislocations can be reduced in the ED. A rolled sheet is placed between the patient's shoulders while the patient is in the supine position. Traction is applied to the arm in extension and abduction and inward pressure is applied to the medial end of the clavicle. Even after reduction, secondary to ligament ruptures, this joint is unstable. Type III injuries require an orthopedic referral. There is also a 25% associated injury rate with posterior dislocations to the intrathoracic and superiomediastinal structures. The underly-ing structures will require an evaluation.

An acute *acromioclavicular joint* occurs primarily in males and also as a result of falls or direct trauma to the shoulder. The external forces drive the scapula downward and medially to produce a rupture of the acromioclavicular capsule and ligaments. The trapezius and deltoid attachments are followed by a rupture of the coracoclavicular ligament. There are three types of injuries. A type I injury is a sprain of the joint without ligament rupture. A type II injury involves an associated disruption of the acromioclavicular ligaments. The joint space will be widened, and the clavicle displaces slightly upward. Type II injuries involve complete disruption of the acromioclavicular ligaments, coracoclavicular ligaments, and muscle attachments. The joint space will be wide, and the clavicle will be displaced upward. A type IV injury involves an inferior displacement of the clavicle inferiorly.

Treatment of type I and type II acromioclavicular joint injuries involve ice, immobilization, and anti-inflammatory agents with a follow-up referral to an orthopedic surgeon. Type II injuries are con-troversial. Some authors recommend conservative versus operative therapy. Application of ice, immobilization, and an orthopedic referral are necessitated in type II injuries.

Shoulder dislocations are very common in young males. They can occur anteriorly (95%) or posteriorly (5%). Anterior dislocations are caused by the head of the humerus being placed under marked abduction and external rotation, causing the tearing of the anterior capsules and glenoid labrum with dislocation of the humeral head anteriorly. The humeral head rests in a subcoracoid, anterior position. On a radiograph, the humeral head will be in a subcoracoid position. If there is any question as to whether the shoulder is dislocated or regarding the type of dislocation, axillary or tangential scapular views can be taken to confirm the diagnosis. On a radiograph, always look for an avulsion of the greater tuberosity. If there has been a tear in the glenoid labrum, a Bankart lesion may be present. If a Bankart lesion is present, the glenoid labrum does not reattach to the glenoid rim during the healing process. This increases the likelihood of recurrent shoulder dislocations. There is a high incidence of redislocation in males younger than 30 years of age. After the second shoulder dislocation, the patient should be referred to an orthopedic surgeon for surgical repair.

Posterior dislocations are rare. The most common cause of a posterior shoulder dislocation is a tonic-clonic seizure. The seizure causes a violent internal rotation of the humerus. These dislocations are also common in patients who have received an electrical shock. On radiograph, a true AP film of the scapula will not show overlapping of the humeral head at the glenoid. The best radiograph for evaluating a posterior dislocation is an axillary view. On examination the patient will not be able to passively externally rotate the arm. There will be prominence of the humeral head posteriorly and a relatively flat shoulder anteriorly.

There are several ways to reduce an anterior dislocation. The treatment of an anterior dislocation should be closed reduction. For a successful reduction, the patient must be completely relaxed. Adequate analgesic therapy is mandatory.

The Stimson or hanging weight method is atraumatic. The patient is placed in the prone position with a weight suspended from the wrist, not held in the hand. This is the most atraumatic way of reducing a posterior dislocation. With good relaxation, the shoulder will relocate in 2 to 3 minutes.

The traction-countertraction method can also be used. Traction is applied along the arm while the countertraction is applied by an assistant using a folded sheet wrapped around the chest.

The forward elevation maneuver of Cooper and Milch can also be used. The arm is initially elevated 10 to 20 degrees in forward flexion and slight abduction. Forward flexion is continued until the arm is directly overhead. Abduction is then increased, and outward traction is applied to complete the reduction.

The external rotation method of Leidelmeyer is another safe technique. The patient is placed in the supine position, and the involved arm is slowly and gently adducted to the side. The elbow is flexed to 90 degrees, and slowly external rotation is applied to achieve reduction.

Posterior dislocations can be reduced in the ED, but often general anesthesia and an orthopedic consultation are required for relaxation and reduction. Traction involves axial traction in line with the humerus, gentle pressure on the posteriorly displaced head, and slow gentle rotation.

Rotator cuff tears are secondary to indirect force applied to the shoulder. Injury to the rotator cuff involves the tendinous insertions of the subscapularis, supraspinatus, infraspinatus, and teres minor muscles. All of these muscles control internal and external rotation of the shoulder and initiate abduction. The tendinous insertions attach to the lesser and greater tuberosities of the shoulder.

The amount of force extended on the shoulder is very important in regard to the extent of the shoulder injury. In patients older than 50 years of age, the rotator cuff has degenerated and is stiffer and takes less force to tear. A rotator cuff tear in the elderly can prevent active abduction of the shoulder. In the younger population, greater force is required to tear the rotator cuff.

A patient with a rotator cuff tear presents with pain and has trouble abducting the shoulder at the glenohumeral articulation; however, the patient can shrug the shoulder. The patient will only be able to abduct at the thoracospacular area.

A rotator cuff tear can be diagnosed in the ED by infiltrating a local anesthetic into the area of tenderness of the shoulder. If the patient can abduct the shoulder in the absence of pain after a local anesthetic is applied, then the patient does not have a rotator cuff tear. If the patient cannot abduct the shoulder with active abduction but can in passive abduction, then the patient may have a rotator cuff tear.

On radiographs, the bony areas of the shoulder will be normal. If a calcified tendon is present, then bursitis or calcified tendinitis is the cause of the pain.

The gold standard for a rotator cuff tear is an arthrogram with dye extravasation from the shoulder joint. Treatment for small rotator cuff tears is physical therapy. Larger tears need surgical treatment.

BIBLIOGRAPHY

Brandenburg RO, Fuster V, Giuliani ER, et al (eds): Cardiology Fundamentals and Practice. Chicago, Year Book Medical Publishers, 1987

Braunwald E, Isselbacher KJ, Petersdorf RG, et al (eds): Harrison's Principles of Internal Medicine, 11th ed. New York, McGraw-Hill, 1987

Connolly JF: The Management of Fractures and Dislocations: An Atlas. Philadelphia, WB Saunders, 1981

Crenshaw AH: Campbell's Operative Orthopaedics, 7th ed. St Louis, CV Mosby, 1987

Hamilton GC, Sanders AB, Strange GR, et al (eds): Emergency Medicine: An Approach to Clinical Problem-Solving, Philadelphia, WB Saunders, 1991

Kravis TC, Warner CG, Jacobs LM (eds): Emergency Medicine: A Comprehensive Review, 3rd ed. New York, Raven Press, 1993

May HL, Aghababian RV, Fleisher GR (eds): Emergency Medicine, 2nd ed. Boston, Little, Brown, 1992

Rockwood CA, Wilkins KE, King RE (eds): Fractures in Children. Philadelphia, JB Lippincott, 1984

Rosen P, Barkin RM (eds): Emergency Medicine: Concepts and Clinical Practice, 3rd ed. St Louis, Mosby–Year Book, 1992

Schwartz GR, Cayton CG, Manglesen MA, et al (eds): Principles and Practice of Emergency Medicine, 3rd ed. Philadelphia, Lea & Febiger, 1992

Tintinalli JE, Krone RL, Ruiz E (eds): Emergency Medicine: A Comprehensive Study Guide, 4th ed. New York, McGraw-Hill, 1996

Turek SL: Orthopedics Principles and Their Applications, 4th ed. Philadelphia, JB Lippincott, 1984

Chapter **13**

Pediatric Emergencies

THE PEDIATRIC PATIENT: AN OVERVIEW

The most important realization about pediatric patients is that "they are not just little people." The child, especially under 6 months, markedly differs from an adult or even from an older child. Their anatomy and physiology differ from those of an older child or an adult.

Newborns, up to 6 weeks, are very demanding. The child bonds with the mother, father, and other children in the family during this first 6 weeks.

At 6 weeks of age, the child responds more to sounds, actions, faces, and light. The child starts to respond to sound in a pleasurable environment.

Between 4 months and 9 months, the infant grows by leaps and bounds. The infant goes from lying to sitting up and even to standing with support. The infant responds with facial expressions and sounds to different stimuli. The infant reaches for objects and must explore everything. The infant also tastes and touches every object. The infant starts to say "Dada" and "Mama" by the age of 9 months.

At 1 year to 18 months, the infant is on the threshold of walking and thus increased exploring. The infant's mobility and independence increase. The infant's vocabulary starts to increase to several single words.

From 18 months to 3 years, the child's mobility increases dramatically. The child learns to climb, ride a tricycle, jump, and kick. The child wants to be part of every activity and enjoys listening to stories.

At 4 to 8 years of age, the child makes improvements on performing complicated tasks. He or she learns to balance and play catch with a ball and wants to participate in group sports and activities. Hand-eye coordination and speed improve. Language goes from single words to sentences of multiple words. The child is now very independent and wants to dress himself or herself.

THE APPROACH TO THE CHILD IN THE ED

The ED can be a very scary place for both the child and the parent. The family may have to wait for a long time, and this creates frustration for both the child and the parent. People wearing white coats can be very scary to some children who have already had numerous visits to the physician. White coats represent "pain" or "shots" to many children.

If possible, separate quiet rooms designed for pediatric patients should be available. A calm, caring, concerned attitude toward both the child and the patient should be the norm. Remember that the child is there because someone brought him or her to the ED! It is

385

not the child's fault that he or she is here. Listen to what the adult who brought the child to the ED is saying. Ask, "What brings you to the emergency department today?" Ask in a caring and concerned voice. Remember that the family usually doesn't want to be there. Does the family have a primary care physician? When was the last time that the child was seen by the primary care physician? Has the child received all of his or her immunizations? Was the child born at term, premature, or late? Was the delivery normal? Did the mother have a cesarean section or a vaginal delivery, and did she have a single or multiple deliveries? Is the mother or the father present, and is this the first child of the parents? Are any of the other children at home who are also ill? Who is the primary care provider (e.g., grandmother, mother, father)? What has changed in the last 24 hours in the child's behavior? Is the child eating and drinking? Does the child have diarrhea? Are there any social concerns? Does the person who brought the child to the ED suspect child abuse, and if so, why? Has the child lost any weight?

The point here is to determine why the child and adult have really come to the ED. Do not judge the answer. Accept the explanation, and address the concerns of both the child and the parent as justifiable.

The vital signs should include the pulse, blood pressure, respirations, and rectal temperature, and pulse oximetry should be taken on every child. Remember that an infant younger than 3 months of age who has a temperature higher than 100.4° F is septic until proven otherwise. Note any allergies, prior hospitalizations, and whether the child had a prior hospital admission. If this was the case, determine for what illness or disease was the child admitted. What medications, if any, is (or was) the child taking, including over-the-counter medications? Antipyretics should be initiated in any child who has a fever higher than 39° C. Acetaminophen 15 mg/kg PO is the drug of choice.

The most common complaints of patients presenting to the ED with a child are:

1. Feeding problems, spitting up, vomiting
2. Not gaining weight
3. Crying or irritability
4. Intestinal colic
5. Diarrhea
6. Constipation
7. Rapid breathing, cough, or shortness of breath
8. Noisy breathing or stridor
9. Blue spells or cyanosis
10. Eye problems, discharge, redness, or drainage
11. Diaper rash
12. Thrush
13. Fever
14. Child abuse

15. Ear infections
16. Sore throat

Be flexible in your examination. Listen to what the child and adult are really trying to tell you. Remember that when in doubt of your diagnosis, consult pediatrics early and often. No one will ever blame you for setting up an early consultation. If someone does find fault, then that person doesn't understand the process of disease in children.

ABDOMINAL PAIN

Definition

Abdominal pain is the great imitator in children. Abdominal pain can be pathologic for infection, inflammatory, congenital, endocrine, or metabolic etiology. It can come from peritonitis secondary to a ruptured viscus or from urinary, genital, gastrointestinal (GI), pulmonary abdominal wall, systemic disease, or skin pathology.

Epidemiology/Pathology

In the infant population, abdominal pain is usually caused by acute gastroenteritis. Hirschsprung's disease, incarcerated hernia, intussusception or volvulus are also common in this age group.

In preschool children, constipation, appendicitis, acute gastroenteritis, pneumonia, viral syndrome, urinary tract infections (UTIs), or trauma are common causes of abdominal pain in the child.

In school-aged children, acute gastroenteritis, trauma, UTIs, and appendicitis and in the female child pelvic inflammatory disease (PID) and gynecologic problems (including ectopic pregnancy and torsion of an ovary) must be considered. Inflammatory bowel diseases such as Crohn's disease and ulcerative colitis can present for the first time in this age group.

A patient with a black widow spider bite can present with abdominal pain. Children with sickle cell disease often present with abdominal pain. Acute rheumatic fever will have a component of abdominal pain, and herpes zoster can also present as abdominal pain before vesicles present on the skin.

Males with testicular torsion can present with abdominal pain. Wilms' tumor, Henoch-Schönlein purpura, and neoplasms, including leukemia, neuroblastoma, and lymphoma, can present with abdominal pain. A patient with endocrine disease such as diabetes, diabetic ketoacidosis (DKA), porphyria, uremia, hypothyroidism, and hyperparathyroidism can present with abdominal pain.

Patients with true GI disease such as Meckel's diverticulum, volvulus, laceration of the liver or spleen secondary to trauma, and mesenteric infarct can all present with abdominal pain. In older children, peptic ulcer disease, esophagitis, or pancreatitis can present with some form of abdominal pain.

In older females, mittelschmerz, dysmenorrhea, an ovarian cyst, or a threatened abortion along with an ectopic pregnancy should be considered as a cause of abdominal pain.

Clinical Presentation

Peritonitis presents with tenderness of the abdomen, guarding, and rebound tenderness. The abdomen with an intestinal obstruction is often distended and will have high-pitched sounds upon examination. Sudden onset of abdominal pain is often a clue to intussusception, perforation, ovarian torsion, or ectopic pregnancy. Colicky pain is related to the biliary tree, uterus, fallopian tube, pancreatic duct, or intestinal pathology. An insidious onset of pain is often related to appendicitis, cholecystitis, or pancreatitis.

Children are notorious for presenting with abdominal pain and having a diagnosis of pneumonia. This referred pain is from diaphragmatic involvement. Pleurisy, pancreatitis, peritonitis, gallbladder disease, and disease of the spleen or a subphrenic abscess can all cause chest pain or abdominal pain. Pain in the right shoulder in gallbladder disease is the classic presentation of referred pain.

Kidney stones or renal disease often refer pain to the testicle or labia. Often acute appendicitis refers pain to the testicle. Rectal disease or retroperitoneal hematoma, pancreatitis, or uterine pathology can refer pain to the back.

Examination

All patients should have vital signs taken and a complete examination. The initial treatment and urgency of treatment are guided by the presentation of the patient. A 15-year-old female who had her last menstrual period 6 weeks ago and who has a blood pressure (BP) of 70/50 and a pulse of 120 beats/min is treated differently from a 7 year old who has had nausea, vomiting, and diarrhea for 3 days and has a BP of 110/70 and a pulse of 160 beats/min. When in doubt with abdominal pain, establish an intravenous (IV) access and a "safety net." Apply oxygen, draw laboratory values, and place the patient on a cardiac monitor. Be prepared for the worst, and keep re-evaluating the patient. A complete examination should be performed including a rectal examination to evaluate for blood. A pelvic examination should be performed if PID, ectopic pregnancy, ovarian torsion, appendicitis, or an infectious process is considered.

Laboratory Findings

A complete blood count (CBC) should be ordered to rule out infection and to evaluate hemoglobin and hematocrit. An evaluation of liver function tests (LFTs) should be done along with amylase and lipase if biliary pathology is considered. Abdominal x-rays (supine and upright) along with a posteroanterior (PA) and lateral chest x-ray should be ordered if bowel obstruction or pneumonia is considered. A urinalysis along with electrolytes should be ordered. Often diabetes is present with abdominal pain. Gonorrhea and chlamydia cultures should be obtained in sexually active females. Urine human chorionic gonadotropin (hCG) or serum β-hCG should be ordered to determine pregnancy status in all menstruating females. An intravenous pyelogram can be utilized to evaluate the urinary system for renal stones or congenital abnormalities. Ultrasound can be used to evaluate the kidneys and the female reproductive system. Computed tomography (CT) scanning can be used for an evaluation of abdominal pathology in trauma patients.

Treatment/Diagnosis

The treatment and diagnosis are guided by the differential diagnosis and by the presentation of the patient. The differential diagnosis will be guided by the patient's age and by the most likely cause of abdominal pain in this age group. Remember to consult a specialist early and often, and always establish a safety net early!

BACTEREMIA, SEPSIS, AND MENINGITIS

Definition

Bacteremia, sepsis, and meningitis are separate diagnoses but are interrelated on the continuum of bacterial invasion and infection. *Bacteremia* is defined as a positive blood culture with fever in a child who has no other symptomatology. *Sepsis* is defined as bacteremia with additional focal findings. *Meningitis* is defined as bacterial invasion or infection of the meninges. If bacteremia is not properly treated, it can lead to sepsis or meningitis.

Epidemiology

Bacteremia occurs in the 6- to 24-month age group predominantly. Sepsis in the neonate and infant younger than 3 months of age can present with either hypothermia or fever. There is an increased risk of sepsis in children who have sickle cell disease, sickle cell trait, immunodeficiency disease, in children who have had chemotherapy, or exposure to meningococcus or hyposplenism secondary to removal for sickle cell disease or hemoglobin disorders. Sepsis or meningitis can occur as a secondary infection from acute otitis media or from sinus infection. Contamination by vaginal or fecal material at the time of birth or contamination of the nasopharynx in older children are sources of infective organisms.

Children with ventriculoperitoneal shunts can also present with meningitis. They can present with headache, ventriculitis, nausea, malaise, and minimal fever.

Pathology

The organisms that are most likely to cause bacteremia are *Streptococcus pneumoniae* (60 to 80%) and *Haemophilus influenzae* (10 to 30%). *Neisseria meningitidis, Salmonella,* and group A streptococci also cause bacteremia.

In the neonate and infant younger than 3 months of age, the most common organisms causing sepsis are group B streptococci and *Escherichia coli.* From 3 to 24 months sepsis is usually caused by *H. influenzae, N. meningitidis* and *S. pneumoniae. Salmonella, Staphylococcus aureus,* and *Streptococcus* A are less common causes of sepsis in this age group. In children who are hyposplenic or who have sickle cell disease or sickle cell trait, the most common causes of sepsis or bacteremia are *S. pneumoniae* and *Salmonella.* There is a 400-fold increased risk of pneumococcal septicemia in children younger than 5 years of age and a fourfold risk of *H. influenzae* and septicemia in children younger than 9 years of age with sickle cell disease.

Meningitis in children is caused by *H. influenzae, S. pneumoniae, N. meningitidis, E. coli,* and group B streptococci. In neonates in the first month of life, *E. coli* and group B streptococci are the most common causes of meningitis. After the first 3 months of life, *H. influenzae* is the most common organism followed by *N. meningitidis* and *S. pneumoniae.*

Enterovirus, mumps, herpes simplex virus, California equine encephalitis virus, St. Louis equine virus, and Western equine virus can also cause meningitis.

Clinical Presentation

Children with bacteremia or sepsis can present with hypothermia or fever. Tachycardia is one of the first signs of bacteremia or sepsis. Hypotension, cold or clammy skin, lethargy, or coma can all occur as the initial presentation. Hemorrhagic skin lesions can be present in sepsis.

The symptoms of meningitis vary with the age of the child. The neonate might present with the complaint of poor feeding, decreased or increased activity, vomiting, decreased appetite, or poor sucking or rooting in breast-fed babies. Babies who are not easily consolable by cuddling or whose irritability increases when cuddled show possible signs of meningeal irritation secondary to meningitis. A bulging fontanelle is a late sign of increased intracranial pressure. The child with sepsis or meningitis can present with hypothermia or fever. Any child younger than 3 months of age with a fever higher than 100.4° F is septic until proven otherwise.

Sepsis or meningitis can present as a febrile seizure. The patient can present in shock. If the child has decreased activity, doesn't care what is done to him or her, is not easily cuddled, has increased irritability, doesn't cry, or looks toxic or sick is considered toxic until proved otherwise.

Cerebral edema with increased intracranial pressure and herniation, disseminated intravascular coagulation (DIC), subdural effusion, and empyema are all complications of meningitis.

Diagnosis/Laboratory Findings

A child younger than 24 months of age with a fever of 102.9° F (39.4° C) and a white blood cell count (WBC) greater than 15,000, or a polymorphonuclear neutrophil (PMN) count greater than 9000, and no focal site of infection or a child who appears toxic, should have a blood culture drawn to rule out bacteremia. If sepsis or meningitis is considered, a CBC, serum electrolytes, blood culture, and lumbar puncture should be performed. Stool samples for botulinum toxin testing and also clostridial and *Salmonella* cultures should be taken. A chest x-ray and urine culture should also be performed. If purpuric skin lesions are present, they should be lanced and a Gram's stain obtained. The WBC count will almost always be elevated, and the hemoglobin and hematocrit will be normal. If neutropenia is present, an overwhelming infection should be considered. DIC can be present and is reflected by the prothrombin time (PT) and partial thromboplastin time (PTT). If inappropriate antidiuretic hormone secretion is present, the sodium level may be lowered.

In meningitis, the lumbar puncture for cerebrospinal fluid (CSF) analysis by a Gram's stain and culture is the cornerstone of diagnosis. CSF should be analyzed for cell count, differential blood cell count, Gram's stain, protein, and glucose. (See the CSF analysis chart.) Cultures for tuberculosis or fungi should be taken if indicated.

If a child presents with a ventriculoperitoneal shunt, the shunt should be aspirated in consultation with a neurosurgeon. If a child with a ventriculoperitoneal shunt has CSF showing a WBC count above 100 cells/mm^3, there is a 90% chance of infection.

Treatment

Children with suspected bacteremia who look well enough to go home should receive ceftriaxone (Rocephin) 50 mg/kg intramuscularly (IM) or IV and should then be given amoxicillin 50 to 100 mg/kg three times a day (TID) or amoxicillin/clavulanate 50 mg/kg TID. The child should have a follow-up re-evaluation in 24 hours and the results of the blood culture should be determined. If a follow-up visit cannot be ensured, the child should be admitted to the hospital. Any child with a positive blood culture on follow-up should be admitted to the hospital if he or she is still symptomatic.

Children with suspected sepsis should receive ampicillin 150 to 200 mg/kg/24 hr every 4 to 6 hours IV and gentamicin 5 to 7.5 mg/kg/24 hr every 8 hours or ampicillin (as already mentioned) with cefotaxime 150 mg/kg/24 hr every 6 hours IV or cefuroxime 100 to 200 mg/kg/24 hr every 6 to 8 hours IV.

It has been suggested that in older children, because of the increased incidence of *H. influenzae,* chloramphenicol 100 mg/kg/24 hr should be used instead of gentamicin. If the infant is septic and *Salmonella* is suspected, chloramphenicol 100 mg/kg/24 hr should be added. Anemia should be treated with packet red blood cells, platelets, or fresh frozen plasma if a bleeding disorder is present. Shock should be treated with 20 ml/kg of normal saline (NS) and 5% dextrose.

If the child with meningitis presents with signs of cerebral edema (an infrequent complication) or herniation or focal neurologic signs, the child should be:

1. Hyperventilated to maintain a $Paco_2$ at 25 mm Hg
2. Given mannitol 20% solution at 0.5 to 1 mg/kg/dose every 4 to 6 hours IV
3. Given a diuretic—furosemide (Lasix) 1 mg/kg/dose every 4 to 6 hours IV
4. If seizures occur give:
   a. Diazepam (Valium) 0.2 to 0.3 mg/kg/dose every 5 to 10 minutes *or*
   b. Lorazepam (Ativan) 0.05 to 0.15 mg/kg/dose IV
   c. If seizures continue, give a loading dose of phenobarbital or phenytoin.

The use of steroids in meningitis is somewhat controversial. The administration of steroids has been shown to reduce the incidence of hearing loss and to produce a more rapid improvement in the opening CSF pressure and cerebral perfusion. Steroids will also decrease meningeal inflammation and reduce the patient's elevated temperature in the first few days of illness. Dexamethasone 0.6 mg/kg/24 hr every 6 hours IV for 4 days or 16 doses is used as steroid therapy.

Any health care provider, day-care contact or family member who has encountered a patient with *N. meningitidis* should receive chemoprophylaxis with rifampin. Children should receive 10 mg/kg/dose every 12 hours by mouth (PO) for four doses. Children younger than 1 month of age should receive 5 mg/kg/dose every 12 hours PO for four doses. Adults should receive 600 mg/dose every 12 hours PO for four doses.

Prophylaxis for exposure to *H. influenzae* type B disease in households or day-care settings in which the child is younger than 2 years of age and is in contact with an infected person 25 hr/wk or more should be treated. Prophylaxis should also be considered if two or more cases of *H. influenzae* type B disease occur in a day-care setting in a 60-day period. Give rifampin 20 mg/kg/dose (maximum of 600 mg/dose) every 24 hours for four doses. In children younger than 1 month of age, 10 mg/kg/dose every 24 hours for four doses should be used.

A child with viral meningitis should be admitted to the hospital.

Viral meningitis still requires supportive therapy. If herpes meningitis is considered, acyclovir therapy should be given. Aggressive management is usually required for herpes meningitis.

Cerebrospinal Fluid Analysis		
	Bacterial	**Viral**
Cell count	>500	<500
Cell type	80% PMN leukocyte	PMN leukocyte initially, then lymphocyte later
Glucose (mg/dl)	<40	>40
Protein (mg/dl)	>100	<100
CSF/blood glucose (%)	<40	>40
Gram's stain	Positive	Negative
Bacterial culture	Positive	Negative

BRONCHIOLITIS

Definition

Young children do not get bronchitis as adults do. They are afflicted with bronchiolitis. Bronchiolitis is an acute lower respiratory infection that produces lower inflammatory obstruction of the small airways and causes reactive airway disease.

Epidemiology

Bronchiolitis occurs in children younger than 2 years of age, and the highest incidence is in children younger than 6 months of age. The rates of attack from bronchiolitis are as high as 11.4% during the first year of a child's life.

Pathology

In 90% of the cases, bronchiolitis is caused by respiratory syncytial virus (RSV). Parainfluenza, influenza, and adenovirus are other less common causes of bronchiolitis. Bronchiolitis is primarily an inflammatory process with variability of bronchoconstriction. Asthma is primarily a bronchoconstrictive disease with secondary inflammation.

Clinical Presentation/Examination

Children with bronchiolitis usually first have an upper respiratory tract infection. Later on, an acute onset of tachypnea greater than 60 breaths/min with diffuse wheezing occurs. The child usually appears fairly well. Otitis media or viral pneumonia may accompany the tachypnea of bronchiolitis. The child will present with a poor feeding history, fever, rhinitis, cough, dyspnea, and irritability. Conjunctivitis and coryza can also be present.

On physical examination, the child will have nasal flaring, costal retractions with or without wheezing, and tachypnea. Remember that apprehensiveness, anxiety, and fatigue are all signs of hypoxia. Children with bronchiolitis will often present with dehydration secondary to the rapid respiratory rate and decreased fluid intake. Children younger than 6 months of age can present with apnea.

Asthma, pneumonia, foreign bodies, and pneumothorax can all mimic bronchiolitis. Asthma usually occurs in children younger than 1 year of age. Pneumonia produces wheezing and an elevated temperature. Heart failure, cystic fibrosis, vascular rings, toxic ingestions, metabolic acidosis, or smoke inhalation can all resemble bronchiolitis.

Diagnosis

The diagnosis is made by clinical presentation and by physical examination.

Laboratory Findings

On CBC examination, the WBC count is usually normal. In bacterial pneumonia, the WBC count is elevated. A blood culture, urine culture, CBC, and chest x-ray should be performed on every child younger than 6 months of age. An arterial blood gas (ABG) is indicated to evaluate respiratory distress, if present.

X-ray Findings

On the chest x-ray, the lungs will be hyperinflated and the diaphragm will appear flat on the anterior view.

Treatment

If the child is tachypneic, cyanotic, or hypoxic, oxygen should be administered. β-Agonists via a nebulizer should be given.

1. Albuterol (0.5% solution) (Proventil, Ventolin) 0.03 ml (0.15 mg)/kg/dose with 2 ml of 0.9% NS can be administered every 2 to 4 hours.
2. Terbutaline (0.1% solution) (Brethine) 0.03 mg (0.03 ml)/kg/dose with 2 ml of 0.9% NS can be administered every 2 to 4 hours.
3. Oral albuterol (2 mg/5 ml), 0.1 to 0.15 mg/kg/dose every 6 to 8 hours PO for outpatient treatment.
4. Children with a respiratory rate above 60 breaths/min and who present with fatigue, respiratory distress, hypoxia, or hypercapnia or who cannot keep food or fluids down should be hospitalized. If the results of the ABG show a PaO_2 less than 50

mm Hg or a Pa_{CO_2} greater than 50 mm Hg, the child is a candidate for intubation and admission to the hospital.

5. Aerosolized ribavirin has been shown to shorten the course of bronchiolitis in children who have RSV.
6. In children with bronchopulmonary dysplasia, IV immunoglobulins can reduce the number of hospitalizations.
7. Hydration with IV fluids is essential.
8. When in doubt that the child will get a follow-up visit or will show signs of improvement, consult specialists at an early stage and admit the child to the hospital.

CARDIOPULMONARY ARREST

The underlying condition in children is usually a pulmonary problem that causes circulatory collapse. The respiratory collapse is usually secondary to an obstruction or to hypoxia, which leads to cardiac arrest. Respiratory arrest usually precedes cardiac arrest. The child will usually be tachypneic, then bradypneic, then apneic. Cardiac decompensation follows, leading to a decreased cardiac output, hypotension, and then shock. Cyanosis, mottling, cool skin, and capillary refill time greater than 2 seconds will occur.

An upper airway obstruction and a lower airway disease can be caused by:

Epiglottis	Foreign bodies
Suffocation	Trauma
Croup	Strangulation
Pneumonia	Near-drowning
Smoke inhalation	Bronchiolitis
Asthma	Aspiration
Infection	

Narcotics, sedatives, tricyclics, and antidysrhythmics can cause respiratory depression. Sepsis, meningitis, encephalitis, hypoglycemia, hypocalcemia, and hyperkalemia can also cause cardiopulmonary arrest.

APPROACH TO THE CHILD IN CARDIOPULMONARY ARREST

- Establish unresponsiveness.
- Call for help.
- Place the patient in a supine position.
- Open the airway, and get the child in the "sniffing" position (if there is no concern of neck injury).
- Assess breathing, rate, depth, and movement. Is there stridor or wheezing? Is there a foreign body in the airway? If so, give five back blows in infants younger than 1 year of age; then give five

chest thrusts at the site of the chest compressions. If the child is older than 1 year of age, perform the Heimlich maneuver or abdominal thrusts. If the child is unconscious, ventilate the child, and keep attempting to dislodge the foreign object.

- Assess the child's cardiac function. What is the pulse rate and BP? Assess pulses at the brachial or femoral areas, if child is younger than 1 year old. Use the carotid pulse in older children.
- What caused the arrest (as earlier)?
- Is the patient in shock and, if so, what kind of shock—hypovolemia, cardiogenic shock, or distributive shock?
- Is there an electrolyte, acid-base disturbance, coagulopathy, cardiac tamponade, pneumothorax, or electromechanical dissociation?
- Is the patient breathing properly, and are the IV lines working?
- All children should receive oxygen at 3 to 6 l/min. Some oxygen and proper airway management can help greatly to resuscitate a child.
- If IV resuscitation is required secondary to hypovolemia, give a 20-ml/kg bolus of NS.
- If the fluid bolus is successful, maintain IV rates to correspond with fluid requirements:
    For older children, give NS 0.9%.
    For a newborn on day 1, give D10W at 3 ml/kg/hr.
    For a newborn on day 2, use D10/.25 NS at 4 ml/kg.
    For the first 10 kg, give 4 ml/kg/hr.
    For the next 10 kg, give 2 ml/kg/hr.
    Then give 1 ml/kg/hr for each kg over 20 kg.

Normal intravascular volume is about 80 ml/kg. IV access is the desired access for fluids. If an IV line cannot be placed, an intraosseous needle can be used. A bone marrow needle or a spinal needle with a stylet can also be used. Insert the intraosseous needle, bone marrow needle, or spinal needle perpendicularly into the proximal anterior tibia, midline on the flat surface, 2 to 3 cm below the tibial tuberosity. When there is lack of resistance and the needle stands by itself, attempt bone marrow aspiration. If marrow can be aspirated and fluid runs smooth, a crystalloid fluid or medications can be infused. Central venous catheters can be inserted into the internal jugular or femoral veins.

If the child needs intubation, remember to use an appropriate bag size. The tidal volume should be about 10 ml/kg. Bags for neonates contain 250 to 300 ml; bags for infants and children contain 550 to 600 ml.

1. Preoxygenate the child with 100% oxygen by facemask for 3 minutes.
2. Take the cricoid pressure.
3. If the child is younger than 10 years of age, give atropine 0.02 mg/kg.
4. Give lidocaine 1.5 mg/kg IV (especially in the presence of a head injury), then wait for 2 minutes.

5. Pretreat the patient with D-tubocurarine 0.05 to 0.07 mg/kg/dose IV or pancuronium (Pavulon) 0.01 to 0.03 mg/kg, 3 minutes before succinylcholine, to decrease muscle fasciculations.
6. Use as sedation agents:
    Fentanyl 3 μg/kg IV (best for head injury) *or*
    Thiopental 3 to 5 mg/kg IV *or*
    Midazolam 0.1 mg/kg IV (maximum of 4 mg)
      Ketamine 1 mg/kg IV (best for asthma or respiratory distress problems)
7. Paralytic agents:
    Succinylcholine 1.5 mg/kg IV
    Vecuronium 0.1 to 0.3 mg/kg IV (best for head injuries)
8. After intubation, to keep patient paralyzed, you can use:
    Pancuronium 0.1 mg/kg IV as needed
    Vecuronium 0.1 to 0.3 mg/kg IV

Drugs such as atropine, epinephrine, lidocaine, and naloxone can be administered through the endotracheal (ET) tube. The dose of epinephrine should be increased by 10 times for ET tube administration, followed by 1 to 3 ml of NS.

The following drugs are used in pediatric cardiopulmonary arrest:

1. Oxygen, if child is in arrest 100% oxygen on full, ventilate with an Ambu bag that is appropriate for age. Remember that oxygen and good airway control are usually all that is needed to correct acidosis.
2. Epinephrine
    Initial dose for asystolic or pulseless arrest: 0.01 mg/kg (0.1 ml/kg of 1:10,000) IV or intraosseous. The dose via the ET tube is 0.1 mg/kg of 1:1000 epinephrine.
    High dose of epinephrine, second dose, use 0.1 mg/kg of 1:1000.
    Second high dose, third total dose, 0.2 mg/kg of 1:1000.
    A continuous infusion dose of epinephrine at 20 μg/kg/min can be effective.
3. Atropine
    Initial dose of 0.02 mg/kg/dose (minimum dose of 0.1 mg dose, a maximum dose of 2 mg) can be used for bradycardia or heart block to increase vagal tone and atrioventricular (AV) node conduction. Atropine can be given IV or via ET.
4. If the child is normovolemic and shock persists, use dopamine at 5 to 20 μg/kg/min IV.
    Laboratory tests should consist of CBC, electrolytes, ABG, blood urea nitrogen (BUN), creatinine, calcium, and phosphorus.
    A chest x-ray should be taken.
    A nasogastric tube should be placed.
    An electrocardiogram (ECG) and continuous cardiac monitoring should be performed. A urinary catheter should be placed.
    A type and crossmatch of blood should be taken if appropriate.

Pediatric Ventricular Fibrillation and Ventricular Tachycardia Without a Pulse

Unresponsive, apneic, pulseless
Start cardiopulmonary resuscitation (CPR); continue until the pulse returns, except to check the pulse or to shock
ECG shows ventricular fibrillation or ventricular tachycardia without a pulse
Defibrillate at 2 joules (J)/kg
Check the pulse
If no pulse, defibrillate at 4 J/kg
Check the pulse
If no pulse, defibrillate at 4 J/kg
If no pulse, continue CPR, start an IV
Epinephrine 0.01 mg/kg (1:10,000); repeat every 3 to 5 minutes as needed (PRN)
Lidocaine 1 mg/kg
If no pulse, defibrillate at 4 J/kg, 30 to 60 seconds after medications
Check the pulse
(If converts, start a lidocaine drip at 20 to 50 µg/kg/min)
Epinephrine 0.1 to 0.2 mg/kg (1:1000)
Lidocaine 1 mg/kg
If no pulse, defibrillate at 4 J/kg, 30 to 60 seconds after medications
Check the pulse
Epinephrine 0.1 to 0.2 mg/kg (1:1000), repeat IV push PRN
Lidocaine 1 mg/kg
Consider bretylium 5 mg/kg via rapid IV push
If no pulse, defibrillate at 4 J/kg 30 to 60 seconds after medications
Check the pulse
If no pulse, bretylium 10 mg/kg via rapid IV push
If no pulse, defibrillate at 4 J/kg, 30 to 60 seconds after medications

Ventricular Tachycardia with Pulse (Unstable)

Oxygen
Cardiovert at 0.5 to 1.0 J/kg synchronized
(may give lidocaine first)
Check the rhythm
If still in ventricular tachycardia, cardiovert at 1.0 J/kg
Check the rhythm
If still in ventricular tachycardia, cardiovert at 2 to 4 J/kg

Check the rhythm
If still in ventricular tachycardia, lidocaine 1 mg/kg IV push
Cardiovert, then check the rhythm
If still in ventricular tachycardia, bretylium 5 mg/kg slow IV push
Check the rhythm
If still in ventricular tachycardia, cardiovert

Bradycardia

If secondary to hypoxia and ischemia or a neonate
Oxygenate and ventilate; give chest percussions if indicated
Epinephrine 0.01 mg/kg; repeat every 3 to 5 minutes PRN
If primary
Oxygenate and ventilate; give chest compressions if indicated
Atropine 0.02 mg/kg, minimum of 0.1 mg (1 ml)
Repeat every 5 minutes PRN
(Maximum single dose in a child is 0.5 mg; adolescent 1 mg)
Epinephrine 0.01 mg/kg; repeat every 3 to 5 minutes PRN
External pacemaker or epinephrine or isoproterenol drip

Supraventricular Tachycardia—Unstable

Synchronized cardioversion, 0.5 to 1 J/kg
If patient is digitalized, give lidocaine, 1 mg/kg, before cardioversion
If IV available, may use adenosine, 0.1 mg/kg rapid IV bolus
If no effect, double the adenosine dose (maximum single dose of 12 mg)

Electromechanical Dissociation

Continue CPR until pulse returns despite presence of rhythm
Epinephrine 0.01 mg/kg (1:10,000)
Repeat epinephrine 0.1 to 0.2 mg/kg (1:1000) every 3 to 5 minutes PRN
Consider pneumothorax, cardiac tamponade, hypovolemia, pulmonary embolism, severe hypoxia, or acidosis

Asystole

Unresponsive, apneic, pulseless
Start CPR; continue until pulse returns, except to check the pulse
Intubate, ventilate, start IV
ECG shows asystole

Box continued on following page

Epinephrine 0.01 mg/kg (1:10,000)
Repeat epinephrine 0.1 to 0.2 mg/kg (1:1000) every 3 to 5 minutes, PRN
Repeat ½ dose every 10 minutes or by ABG
Check the pulse
Atropine
Consider a pacemaker

CONSTIPATION

Definition

Constipation can be divided into congenital, intoxication, dietary, intrapsychic, or psychogenic causes. In older children, constipation is usually due to dietary or functional causes. In the neonate, constipation is usually caused by anatomic problems. Constipation is defined as the regular passage of firm or hard stool in small amounts or the passage of hard masses at long intervals. Social, cultural, and familial factors all influence the course of constipation.

Epidemiology

All children can become constipated. The key to the diagnosis of constipation lies in finding the cause and determining if constipation is simple or long-standing or if there is constipation with encopresis. Constipation is very prevalent in the mentally retarded and in those conditions associated with motor deficits and hypothyroidism.

Pathology

Congenital constipation can be caused by myelomeningocele, neurologic problems, including a degenerative central nervous system (CNS), Hirschsprung's disease, atresia of the colon or rectum, and meconium plug syndrome in association with cystic fibrosis.

Dietary causes include an excessive intake of cow's milk and an introduction of solid foods (e.g., yellow vegetables or cereals) at too early an age. Lack of adequate fecal bulk and roughage can cause inadequate peristaltic stimulus, thus causing constipation.

Intoxication constipation is caused by the excessive use of suppositories or enemas. This overuse of suppositories and enemas causes changes in the normal peristalsis of the bowel. Calcium channel blockers, antihistamines, diuretics, codeine-containing substances, and diphenoxylates (e.g., Lomotil) can all cause intoxication constipation.

Intrapsychic constipation is caused by difficulty in toilet training and voluntary retention secondary to habit. Intrapsychic constipation can be caused by remembrance of the pain secondary to an anal fissure. Intrapsychic constipation is caused by an attempt to avoid a painful event.

Psychogenic constipation is caused by environmental problems and stress in the parent-child relationship. When psychogenic constipation is present, encopresis can also be present. Encopresis is a liquid stool that forms around the fecal impaction. The child has liquid stools and prefers to soil himself or herself rather than pass a large mass of stool. Encopresis is often a sign of an underlying emotional disturbance.

Metabolic and endocrine causes of constipation include hypothyroidism, hypokalemia, and hypercalcemia.

Clinical Presentation

Infants younger than 6 months of age will often become red-faced and the infant's legs will be drawn up to the abdomen. This is often interpreted as constipation, even though the stool is quite soft.

Between the ages of 6 and 12 months, infants may become flushed and draw their legs up, acting as if they are in great pain and having difficulty passing a large amount of stool. What the infant is actually doing is attempting to withhold the stool.

Examination/Diagnosis

A complete examination should be performed on all children. When the diagnosis of constipation is questioned, an abdominal x-ray can be performed. A rectal examination should be performed and evaluated for blood.

Treatment

Simple constipation in infants can be treated by adding 1 to 2 teaspoons (tsp) of Karo syrup to each 8-oz bottle. In children 4 months or older, strained pears, peaches, apricots, or other fruit can be used. Apple juice is an excellent treatment for constipation. Do not use rectal suppositories in this age group.

In older children, prune juice diluted with soda to improve the taste is an excellent choice when treating children for constipation. Prunes, figs, raisins, celery, lettuce, and beans are all excellent choices in increasing the fiber and bulk of the stool. You can use apple juice in this age group also for treatment of constipation.

In older children, docusate sodium (Colace) 5 to 10 mg/kg/24 hr can be given every 6 to 12 hours PO for 5 to 7 days. Maltsupex ½ to 2 tsp/day twice a day (BID) PO can also be used.

Milk of magnesia 1 ml/kg/dose BID PO; castor oil (Castoria) 1 to 2 tsp if younger than 5 years, 2 to 3 tsp if older than 5 years; or senna (Senokot) 1 to 2 tsp if younger than 5 years, 2 to 3 tsp if older than 5 years can also be used.

Mineral oil can be used as a stool softener in a dose of 1 to 2 ml/kg BID PO.

Do not give honey to infants secondary to the increased risk of botulism.

Long-standing constipation or constipation in the mentally retarded or older child has to be aggressively addressed. Manual fecal disimpaction is often necessary. Hypertonic phosphate enema (Fleet) 30 to 60 ml/10 kg/dose can be given to the pediatric patient, and 120 ml/dose can be used for the adolescent. Docusate sodium 100 mg can be added to each enema.

Mineral oil at 1 to 2 ml/kg/dose, with a maximum dose of 120 ml/dose BID for 2 to 7 days in orange juice can be used. Docusate sodium 5 to 10 mg/kg/24 hr can be used to keep the stool soft. These children need a referral to rule out psychological causes for constipation.

DEHYDRATION

Definition

There is considerable difference in the fluid and electrolyte metabolism between children and adults. Children have a higher metabolic rate than do adults. Their turnover of fluids and electrolytes is three times faster than that of adults. Dehydration is usually divided into mild (<5%) 50 ml/kg of body weight, moderate (10%) 100 ml/kg of body weight, and severe (>15%) 150 ml/kg of body weight. The total body water (TBW) of a newborn is approximately 70 to 75% of the infant's total body weight. In prepubertal children, the TBW is approximately 65%. Dehydration is also classified as isotonic, hypotonic, or hypertonic, based on the serum sodium level.

Children are, however, better at compensating for fluid loss because of their ability to constrict peripheral blood vessels, thus redistributing blood flow centrally. When treating dehydration in children, the type of dehydration (i.e., isotonic, hypotonic, or hypertonic), the degree of dehydration (<5%, 10%, >15%), acid-base balance, and total body potassium loss must all be taken into consideration in the treatment of dehydration. In children, unlike adults, electrolytes and fluid loss can occur very rapidly and can become severe in a short time. The normal circulating blood volume is 80 ml/kg in children and can be used to determine fluid loss secondary to dehydration.

Epidemiology

The loss of fluid and electrolytes through environmental changes or GI loss are the main two causes of dehydration in children. Fluid and electrolytes are normally lost through the urine (55 to 60%), sweat, stool, and insensible water (40 to 45% including the lungs) loss.

The majority of children (70 to 80%) present with isotonic (isonatremic) dehydration (serum sodium of 130 to 150 mEq/l). With hypotonic (hyponatremic) dehydration, the child presents with a serum sodium of less than 130 mEq/l. In hypotonic dehydration, the sodium deficit is greater than the total water deficit. Water is shifted into the cells because of the low serum sodium; thus plasma volume decreases. CNS symptoms can occur with hypotonic dehydration and the child usually appears very ill, with shock occurring more rapidly than in isotonic dehydration. Seizures or coma can occur if the serum sodium is less than 120 mEq/l. Hypotonic dehydration usually occurs when the child is given sodium-poor fluids, such as tap water, in an attempt to rehydrate the child at home.

Hypertonic (hypernatremic) dehydration occurs when the serum sodium is greater than 150 mEq/l. Hypertonic dehydration occurs when free water intake is inadequate. If hypernatremia is present, a dehydration of at least 10% is present. It can occur when baking soda is given in water to the child as a home remedy for dehydration or when infant formulas are not prepared properly. In hypertonic dehydration, water is moved from intracellular areas to extracellular areas, thus causing swelling. Brain damage occurs in infants and children secondary to this type of dehydration.

Clinical Presentation/Examination

Complete vital signs should be taken, including pulse, respirations, rectal temperature, and blood pressure. Mild dehydration (5%) will present with dry mucous membranes and good skin turgor. The child will still be urinating with a urine specific gravity (SG) less than or equal to 1.020. The arterial pH will be 7.40 to 7.30. The BUN and creatine should be normal.

Moderate dehydration (10%) will present with dry oral mucous membranes, mildly reduced skin turgor, a depressed anterior fontanel, sunken eyeballs, tachycardia, sometimes orthostatic hypotension, and possibly hyperpnea. Oliguria will be present with an SG of more than 1.030. The BUN will be elevated, and the arterial pH will be between 7.30 and 7.00.

Severe dehydration (>15%) will present with oliguria and anuria, with a very high BUN and an SG higher than 1.035. The arterial pH will be less than 7.10. Physical signs of severe dehydration include dry oral mucosa, reduced skin turgor, tachycardia, orthostatic hypotension, sunken eyeballs, a depressed anterior fontanel, and hyperpnea.

In children who present with hypertonic hypernatremia, dehydration will be present with dry, rubbery skin, or doughy skin, lethargy alternating with hyperirritability to stimuli, hyperreflexia and increased muscle tone, seizures, and coma.

Diagnosis/Laboratory Findings

The BUN will be elevated in moderate and severe dehydration. It should decrease by 50% in the first 24 hours with proper therapy. If the BUN does not fall, you should consider hemolytic-uremic syndrome. A CBC should be performed. The potassium deficit must be determined. Large losses of potassium occur with severe diarrhea or with overuse of diuretics, or when chloride is lost secondary to metabolic acidosis. Remember that the serum potassium only makes up 2% of the total body potassium content. Usually when the sodium deficit is corrected, the potassium deficit will correct itself. Potassium replacement should not be started until there is adequate urine output. If serum potassium is still deficient, add potassium to IV solutions at 20 mEq/l.

Metabolic acidosis occurs secondary to chloride and bicarbonate losses in the stool secondary to diarrhea, increased production of ketones secondary to carbohydrate starvation, and hypovolemia. These losses lead to lactic acid production and decreased glomerular filtration rate (GFR), brought on by poor tissue perfusion due to hypovolemia. Always evaluate the anion gap when evaluating dehydration. Propylene glycol, methanol, salicylates, and aspirin can all cause an anion gap metabolic acidosis, with vomiting, dehydration, coma, seizures, lactic acidosis, and uremia. Don't miss the signs of an overdose!

Treatment

If the child is in shock, the prevention of circulatory failure takes precedence. A weight should be obtained on all children prior to the start of fluid resuscitation. The largest bore IV should be started as soon as possible. A CBC, electrolytes, including calcium, magnesium, and phosphorus should be obtained. A urine specimen should be obtained for culture and sensitivity and to measure urine output. If the child is believed to be septic or to have bacteremia or meningitis, blood cultures should be obtained. An ABG should also be obtained if the child appears severely ill to determine if acidosis is present, and if so what kind.

If the child is in shock, regardless of the type of dehydration, the child should receive a fluid bolus of 20 ml/kg of isotonic crystalloid. Either 0.9% NS or lactated Ringer's solution should be given. Avoid a bolus of glucose-containing fluid, because this can cause hyperglycemia. If the child is in severe shock, a 50-ml syringe can be used to deliver fluid at a faster rate through a three-way stopcock.

If the child is known to have pulmonary, renal, or cardiac disease and the amount of sodium in the fluid is a concern, a 10 ml/kg bolus of 5% albumin or fresh frozen plasma can be utilized as a resuscitation fluid. Hypoglycemia is treated with D25W 0.5 to 1 g/kg (2 to 4 ml/kg). After each bolus, the child's vital signs, skin turgor, capillary refill, mental status, and urine output should be re-evaluated.

If the serum HCO_3 is less than 10 or the pH is less than 7.0, you should consider giving sodium bicarbonate. Add 1 mEq/kg to the first liter of IV fluid over 1 hour. Do not correct the serum bicarbonate too rapidly. If the bicarbonate level is corrected too rapidly or if too much bicarbonate is given, alkalemia can occur.

When a child requires IV therapy for more than a few days, caloric requirements must also be maintained. A child's caloric metabolic needs can be determined by the following guidelines:

From 0 to 10 kg, 100 cal/kg/24 hr *plus*
From 10 to 20 kg, 50 cal/kg/24 hr *plus*
From 20 to 70 kg, 20 cal/kg/24 hr

Normal water requirements are equal to 100 ml per 100 calories expended. Thus the following formula can be used to determine daily water maintenance needs:

100 ml/kg for 0 to 10 kg + 50 ml/kg for each kilogram between 10 and 20 kg + 20 ml/kg for each kilogram over 20 kg = daily fluid needs divided by 24 will give you the hourly rate.

Sodium requirement of 3 mEq/kg/day
Potassium requirement of 2 mEq/kg/day

An IV solution containing 5% dextrose in 0.2 or 0.25 NS with 20 mEq KCl/l can be utilized to fulfil the aforementioned requirements (D5 0.25 NS or D5 0.2 NS) in children. In newborns, 10 g/100 ml of IV fluid should be used.

The correction of isotonic dehydration, 5% or less, can usually be performed with only oral rehydration. This can usually be achieved by giving the child small, 5-ml doses of Rehydralyte, Lyten, Pedialyte, or Ricelyte. This can be achieved by giving the parent a 5-ml syringe and slowly administering small 5-ml doses of fluid. If IV therapy is needed, the amount of fluid replacement can easily be determined. Remember that we classify dehydration by 5%, 10%, and more than 15%. Daily maintenance fluid is 100 ml/kg from 0 to 10 kg, 50 ml/kg from 10 to 20 kg, and more than 20 ml/kg/day for each kilogram over 20 kg. The amount of fluid deficit can be determined by **multiplying the percentage of dehydration by the weight of the child.** Therefore, if a child weighs 9 kg and is 10% dehydrated, the child's fluid deficit is 900 ml. An initial bolus of 20 ml/kg (180 ml) is given. The remaining fluid deficit is given as follows:

900 ml − 180 ml = 720 ml
Half of the remaining fluid deficit (rest of fluid to be given) (720 ml) is given over the next 8 hours (360 ml)
The remaining half is given over the next 16 hours (360 ml)
This fluid deficit (900 ml) is added to the maintenance fluids for this patient (<10 kg) of 100 ml/kg/day

In the first 8 hours, the patient would receive 45 ml/hr dose plus the maintenance rate of 37 ml/hr or a rate of 82 ml/hr for the first 8 hours, then 22 ml/hr deficit, for the next 16 hours and 37 ml/hr maintenance dose for a 16-hour rate of 60 ml/hr.

In hypotonic dehydration, which is usually hypovolemic dehydration caused by GI loss, rehydration can be achieved by giving a child a bolus of 0.9% NS, then starting the child on D5W 0.9% NS with 20 mEq KCl/l. If severe hyponatremia (<120 mEq/l) is present, a hypertonic solution of 3% saline should be used to raise the serum sodium to > 125 mEq/l at 4 ml/kg over 10 minutes. The serum sodium should be re-evaluated after each bolus. Half of the remaining sodium deficit should be corrected over the next 8 hours. In patients in whom the TBW is increased with hyponatremia, a fluid restriction is necessary. Excess TBW can be calculated by:

$$\text{Present TBW (l)} = \text{weight (kg)} \times 0.6$$

$$\text{Desired TBW (l)} = \frac{\text{weight (kg)} \times 0.6 \times \text{measured Na}^+ \text{ (mEq/l)}}{\text{Desired Na}^+ \text{ (mEq/l)}}$$

$$\text{Water excess (l)} = \text{present TBW} - \text{desired TBW}$$

Sodium is usually corrected to 125 mEq/l.

If the child is moderately or severely symptomatic, furosemide 1 mg/kg/dose can be used to diurese excess free water. If the child is diagnosed with syndrome of inappropriate antidiuretic hormone (SIADH) and is 8 years of age or older, demeclocycline can be administrated in patients in whom water restriction has not worked.

Hypertonic dehydration (hypernatremia) is treated by giving the patient free water. Rehydration should not be performed too rapidly. Serious neurologic complications, including seizures, can occur if free water is given too rapidly. If hypotension is present, 20 ml/kg of D5W 0.9% NS or D5W lactated Ringer's should be given during the first hour. The goal of rehydration in hypernatremic dehydration is to correct the water deficit over 48 hours.

- If serum sodium is greater than 175 mEq/l, decrease serum sodium by 15 mEq/l/24 hr.
- If serum sodium is less than 175 mEq/l, the replacement of water deficit should decrease serum sodium by half during the first 24 hours.

D5W 0.2% NS is the fluid of choice. An approximation of water loss can be determined by the serum sodium concentration. If serum sodium is 175 mEq/l, the water deficit is 50 ml/kg, 90 ml/kg of serum sodium is 160 mEq/l and 140 ml/mEq/l. Approximately 4 ml/kg of free water for each 1 mEq/l of sodium is needed to lower a serum concentration below 145 mEq/l in a 48-hour period.

In mild dehydration in which the child is taking fluid in the ED and there is good follow-up, the child can be sent home with the following instructions:

- Clear liquids should be given for the next 12 to 24 hours.
- Do not give the child tap water, rice tea, boiled milk, Kool-Aid, baking soda, milk, cheese, ice cream, or butter.
- Give child Rehydrate, Lytren, Pedialyte, Ricelyte, Gatorade, defizzed cola in children younger than 2 years old or ginger ale.
- Give the child soy formula instead of cow's milk if younger than 1 year of age (e.g., Isomil, ProSobee, or Soylac).
- Give parents a 5-ml syringe, and tell them to give 5 ml slowly as tolerated.

- Limit apple juice, because it is hyperosmolar and can increase diarrhea.
- Advance the diet when the child is keeping liquids down. Give dry toast, bananas, and strained carrots.
- Return to the ED or call your primary care health care provider:
  If vomiting or diarrhea increases.
  If the child is unable to keep any fluid down.
  If diarrhea or vomiting does not improve in 24 hours.
  If blood or mucus is found in or on stool.
  If the child has decreased urination in the first 8 hours after discharge from the ED; if the child's diapers are not wet; if lethargy occurs; if the child has no tears when crying; if the child becomes increasingly irritable; or if weight loss occurs.

THE CHILD WITH FEVER

Fever has different meanings in different age groups. In the neonates and infants younger than 3 months of age, a fever is 100.4° F (38° C). In infants 12 weeks or older, a fever is a temperature higher than 101.3° F (38.5° C). Fever in an adult or a teenager is any temperature higher than 98.6° F (37° C). Always be conservative in your interpretation of fever, especially in children younger than 3 months of age. It is usually the fever that is the key to illness in this age group. Fever is usually a sign of either a viral, chlamydial, rickettsial, parasitic, or bacterial infection in any age group. However, stroke, malignancy, collagen vascular disease, acquired immunodeficiency syndrome (AIDS), thyrotoxicosis, familial dysautonomia, acute myocardial infarction (AMI), toxic ingestion/drug-induced temperature, such as aspirin or CNS injury can all lead to an increase in temperature.

Hyperpyrexia is a temperature greater than 105.8° F (41° C). This is usually a sign of severe underlying disease. Children with temperatures this high will sometimes have seizures, and these seizures are sometimes the presenting complaint to the ED. In children, meningitis and Kawasaki disease must always be considered with hyperpyrexia.

With a temperature higher than 102.2° F (39° C), occult bacteremia should be considered, whereas temperatures higher than 107.6° F (42° C) are most often of a noninfectious origin. Head injury, heat stroke, malignant hyperthermia, or accidental ingestion of psychotropic drugs are causes of temperatures higher than 107.6° F.

Fever of unknown origin (FUO) is a term used to describe a fever that lasts longer than 14 days and has an unknown etiology. If several illnesses cannot be documented as back-to-back illnesses, neoplasms, Hodgkin's disease, systemic lupus erythematosus, Kawasaki disease, inflammatory bowel disease, and mononucleosis should all be considered. Travel history is also important in FUO. Malaria should be considered in children who are from or who have traveled to a tropical region where malaria is endemic.

In recognizing occult bacteremia, the mnemonic "the rule of two's," should be used:

Children younger than 2 years of age
Rectal temperature greater than 102° F
Peripheral WBC count greater than 20,000
A 20% risk of occult bacteremia

This mnemonic has been adjusted. There are many children with *H. influenzae* and *N. meningitidis* who will have a WBC count of 15,000.

The appearance of the child is very important, no matter what the child's temperature. If the child looks sick, the child is probably too sick to go home! Remember that the child who is active, wants to be held, interacts with the environment, plays, wants to explore his or her world, and takes food readily, is probably well enough to go home. On the other hand, the child who lies on the examination table, makes poor eye contact, doesn't care if he or she is held, and does not want to eat (no matter what this child's temperature is) is a sick child.

Any child who has a rectal temperature higher than 102° F and who is younger than 2 years of age and has a WBC count of more than 15,000 should have a blood culture performed and should be treated for possible occult bacteremia.

One of the scariest presentations for patients to the ED is a child who has had a febrile seizure. The patients will have very real concerns about what caused this seizure. Between 2% and 5% of all children will have a febrile seizure before the age of 5. Febrile seizures are uncommon after 5 or 6 years of age. Look for another cause.

The seizures rarely last longer than 15 minutes and are usually tonic-clonic in nature. These seizures usually peak between 8 and 20 months.

Meningitis is a real concern in children who have had a febrile seizure. The criteria set forth in a Johns Hopkins University study can predict those children who are more likely to have meningitis:

1. Younger than 18 months of age
2. Seizures in the ED
3. Focal seizures
4. Children who have been to their physician's office in the last 48 hours

Again the behavior and appearance of the child is very important. Children who are playful, nontoxic looking, and interact well with their environment usually do not have meningitis and, therefore, do not require a lumbar puncture.

Petechiae in a febrile child can be caused by otitis media, streptococcal pharyngitis, RSV, general viral illnesses, Henoch-Schönlein purpura, Rocky Mountain spotted fever, or acute leukemia. But by far the most life-threatening presentation of petechiae and fever is meningococcal sepsis. This diagnosis must not be missed. *N. menin-*

gitidis is the most common organism for meningococcal sepsis. True meningococcal sepsis will have a poor prognosis if it is not treated aggressively. DIC and shock will eventually occur.

Physical Examination in a Febrile Child

Look at the child and determine if he or she looks sick. Is the child playful? Does the child want to be held or does the child just lie on the examination table?

Take the vital signs yourself. A rectal temperature is the best. Is the child tachycardiac out of proportion to fever? If so, this could be a sign of septicemia, primary cardiac conditions, dehydration, myocarditis, or pericarditis. Take the child's respirations. Is the child tachypneic? This could be a sign of pneumonia, laryngotracheitis, or bronchiolitis.

Does the child have meningismus? This is an unreliable sign in a child younger than 12 months, but it is very reliable in a teenager. Does the child have a positive Kernig sign (painful extension of the knee while the hip is flexed) or a positive Brudzinski sign (reflex of the hip and knee when the neck is flexed)?

Laboratory Examination

- WBC count less than 5000 or greater than 15,000
- Erythrocyte sedimentation rate (ESR), greater than 30 mm/hr will help to differentiate occult bacteremia from a localized infection, septic arthritis, PID, osteomyelitis, collagen vascular disease, or inflammatory bowel disease.
- Blood cultures should be performed on all children younger than 2 years of age who have a temperature higher than 102° F, with a WBC count greater than 15,000 or who look sick.
- A catheterized urine sample with culture should be taken: Often a small child will be unable to tell you if he or she has dysuria, polyuria, or urgency.
- A stool sample should be taken if the child has diarrhea and also a smear to look for fecal leukocytes. Stool cultures should also be obtained if *Shigella, Salmonella, Campylobacter,* or any other bacterial organism is considered.
- A chest x-ray is taken if the child has wheezing, rales, or unexplained tachypnea. Remember that a child will sometimes present with abdominal pain with pneumonia, bronchitis, bronchiolitis, or pericarditis.

Admission criteria for a child younger than 8 weeks of age

1. Any child younger than 8 weeks of age with a fever higher than 100.4° F needs to be admitted to the hospital to rule out septicemia. A CBC, blood cultures, urine culture, lumbar puncture, chest x-ray, and electrolytes should be performed prior to the child's admission to the hospital. Common infections in this age group are:

    a. Occult bacteremia
    b. Pneumonia
    c. Aseptic meningitis
    d. UTI
2. The common organisms of infection in infants younger than 4 weeks of age are:
    a. *E. coli* (second most common)
    b. *Listeria monocytogenes*
    c. *H. influenzae*
    d. group B *Streptococcus* (most common)
    e. *N. meningitidis*
    f. *S. pneumoniae*
3. In the neonate, choices of antibiotics are:
    a. Ampicillin 200 mg/kg/day
    b. Gentamicin 7.5 mg/kg/day
4. In infants older than 4 weeks, there is an increased frequency of *H. influenzae.*
5. Infants older than 4 weeks should receive:
    a. Ampicillin 200 mg/kg/day
    b. A third-generation cephalosporin:
       ■ Cefotaxime 150 mg/kg/24 hr every 6 hours *or*
       ■ Cefuroxime 100 to 200 mg/kg/24 hr every 6 to 8 hours
    c. Chloramphenicol 100 mg/kg/day should be given to older children or to children in whom *Salmonella* infection is considered.
6. The infant older than 1 month who does *not* appear toxic, and has a WBC count less than 15,000 with normal urine, a normal chest x-ray, and a normal lumbar puncture is at low risk for infection. The infant should have a good follow-up within 24 hours. The infant can be given ceftriaxone 50 mg/kg IM and can then be placed on amoxicillin 40 mg/kg/day every 8 hours and can be discharged from the ED. Blood cultures should be drawn and checked at the follow-up examination within 24 hours.

    Children with sickle cell anemia need special care. Splenic infarctions will leave these children asplenic, thus making them susceptible to overwhelming infections. *S. pneumoniae* and *H. influenzae* are the major organisms that cause infection in the asplenic patient. A reticulocyte blood count should be drawn. The chance of infection is increased in a sickle cell patient when neutrophils on the peripheral WBC are greater than 1000/mm³. Lumbar puncture, stool cultures, and *Mycoplasma* titers should also be performed. Localized unrelieved pain should enter into the diagnosis of osteomyelitis in the patient with sickle cell disease. *Salmonella* osteomyelitis and *Salmonella* sepsis should be considered in any sickle cell patient presenting with a fever.

    The two best rules in pediatrics are, when in doubt admit the patient to the hospital and consult a pediatrician so that the child can be admitted as soon as possible. If a follow-up is questionable, admit the child to the hospital.

FEBRILE SEIZURE

Definition

Febrile seizures occur in 2 to 5% of all children. They involve a febrile illness in which a general seizure occurs lasting from 10 to 15 minutes. Meningitis occurs in children 2% of the time with fever and seizures. A diagnosis of meningitis must not be missed. The greatest risk of meningitis is in children younger than 18 months of age.

Epidemiology

Febrile seizures usually occur in children between the ages of 5 months and 5 years with the peak incidence between 8 and 20 months.

Pathology

The seizure is usually accompanied by an upper respiratory tract infection, otitis media, pharyngitis, pneumonia, a UTI, or gastroenteritis. Exanthema subitum (roseola) is accompanied with a high fever and is often present with a febrile seizure. *Shigella* infection also produces a high fever secondary to the neurotoxins. Seizures are often present with severe *Shigella* infections.

Clinical Presentation/Examination

Usually upon presentation to the ED the child usually looks well, especially if the seizure occurred less than 30 minutes ago. The average febrile seizure lasts from 10 to 15 minutes. Ask the parents if the seizure was generalized tonic-clonic or focal. Was it followed by a period of transient or persistent neurologic changes? Complex seizures last longer than 15 minutes. A child is usually postictal after a febrile seizure. The child usually returns to baseline in 30 minutes. If the child is not back to baseline in 30 minutes, question the diagnosis of a febrile seizure.

Diagnosis/Laboratory Findings

In the child with a new onset of seizure activity, the diagnosis of a febrile seizure is a diagnosis of exclusion. A lumbar puncture should be performed on any child younger than 1 year of age or less than 2 years of age with a temperature higher than 41° C, who, after aggressive antipyretic therapy, is not back to his or her baseline or who is still lethargic or irritable.

A CBC and blood culture, glucose test sticks, electrolytes, and BUN should also be evaluated. A sterile urine sample should be obtained for culture and sensitivity. Serum sodium should be evaluated, and a history of drinking pure tap water should be obtained. Increased intake of free water by children whose parents have attempted to treat vomiting and diarrhea with tap water will cause hypernatremia and mental status changes with seizures in young children. A chest x-ray should also be obtained as indicated by the physical examination. If a history of trauma is noted, a CT scan of the head should be performed. If trauma is suspected, a careful evaluation of extremities for fractures should be performed. An abdominal examination for internal injuries should also be performed. If child abuse is suspected, proper referral and consultation should be made and the child should be admitted to the hospital.

Treatment

The patient is usually not actively seizing upon arrival in the ED. If the patient is actively seizing:

1. Establish and maintain proper airway control with suction and manual maneuvers.
2. Administer oxygen.
3. Gain IV access.
4. Give dextrose 0.5 to 1 g/kg/dose, 2 to 4 ml D25W/kg/dose IV.
5. If the patient is actively seizing give:
    a. Diazepam (Valium) 0.2 to 0.3 mg/kg/dose IV over 2 to 3 minutes (not exceeding 1 mg/min), with a maximum dose of 10 mg. You can repeat the dose every 5 to 10 minutes, *or*
    b. Lorazepam (Ativan) 0.05 to 0.15 mg/kg/dose IV over 1 to 3 minutes, with a maximum adult dose of 5 mg, *or*
    c. Phenobarbital 15 to 20 mg/kg/dose IV, 25 to 50 mg/min, with a maintenance dose of 3 to 5 mg/kg/24 hr PO or IV, *or*
    d. Phenytoin (Dilantin) 10 to 20 mg/kg/dose IV (not exceeding 40 mg/min or 0.5 mg/kg/min) with a maximum loading dose of 1250 mg and a maintenance dose of 5 mg/kg/24 hr IV or PO.

All patients with a febrile seizure should be aggressively treated with antipyretic medications:

1. Acetaminophen 10 to 15 mg/kg/dose every 4 to 6 hours PO or per rectum
2. Ibuprofen 10 mg/kg/dose every 6 hours PO
3. Do not give aspirin, secondary to Reye's syndrome

Obtain a family history of febrile seizures. Determine if the seizure was generalized or focal. Did the seizure last longer than 15 minutes? (Complex seizures last longer than 15 minutes.) Was there any abnormal neurologic or developmental history before the seizure? When in doubt, work the child up to include a lumbar puncture, CBC, electrolytes, and chest x-ray.

Disposition

Children who have completely recovered, have a source of infection, are back to baseline and afebrile, and who had a simple febrile seizure can be discharged home with good follow-up and good patient education. Reassurance of the parents and the use of antipyretics are the key to discharge. Explain to the patients that this was probably not the onset of epilepsy and that control of fever is the key to childhood febrile seizure. Forty percent of children who have one febrile seizure will have recurrent febrile seizures within 6 months of the first seizure.

The child should have a follow-up examination within 48 hours of discharge from the ED and should return to the ED if another febrile seizure lasts longer than 15 minutes, if abnormal neurologic abnormalities occur, or if fever is unrelieved by antipyretics. When in doubt consult a specialist early and admit the patient to the hospital. Always consider meningitis as a possible diagnosis.

HIRSCHSPRUNG'S DISEASE OR CONGENITAL AGANGLIONIC MEGACOLON

Definition

Hirschsprung's disease is caused by a congenital aganglionosis of the distal colon and rectum.

Epidemiology

Hirschsprung's disease is the cause of 15 to 20% of all neonatal intestinal obstruction. It is the most common cause of partial intestinal obstruction in the neonate.

Pathology

The lack of parasympathetic ganglion cells 4 to 25 cm in the rectosigmoid or rectal area of the colon is the leading cause (90%) of Hirschsprung's disease. Only about 5% of patients present with involvement of the entire colon.

Clinical Presentation

Children with Hirschsprung's disease present with vomiting, reluctance to feed, and abdominal distention. The newborn can present in shock. The first clue to the possible diagnosis of Hirschsprung's disease is the failure of the newborn to pass meconium. The newborn can also present looking like a child who is failing to thrive. Peristaltic patterns can be seen. The vomiting may be bilious and later can have fecal material present. The stool can be ribbon-like. The onset of Hirschsprung's disease can present as late as 2 to 3 weeks after birth.

The stools may consist of diarrhea and may be infrequent. They may be explosive in nature. The child can have a fever. Bowel perforation (especially perforation of the cecum) is often present, and sepsis is common.

Necrotizing enterocolitis secondary to *Clostridium difficile* can occur. Malnutrition, urinary tract obstruction, and appendicitis can also occur.

Examination

On rectal examination, the rectal ampulla will be absent of stool. Gas and liquid stool will often be passed after the examiner's finger is removed, secondary to stimulation of the parasympathetic nerve ganglions that are still present.

Diagnosis

A diagnosis is made by histologic examination of the biopsied colon, which will show aganglionosis. The biopsy should be taken at 3, 4, and 5 cm into the rectum. Histochemical evidence of increased acetylcholinesterase activity also suggests Hirschsprung's disease.

Laboratory Findings

A CBC with electrolytes and stool and blood cultures should be performed on every child with suspected Hirschsprung's disease. The child can present with hypochromic anemia and hypoproteinemia. Abdominal films can show distended gas-filled proximal segments of bowel.

A barium enema is performed by inserting a small catheter with the tip barely past the anal sphincter. A narrowed segment of bowel will be noted on x-ray examination. A 12- to 24-hour postevacuation film will show retained barium secondary to the lack of peristalsis of the colon. This is especially diagnostic after the age of 6 weeks.

Treatment

The treatment in the ED is having a high index of suspicion for the diagnosis of Hirschsprung's disease and evaluating the child for sepsis and fluid and electrolyte abnormalities. Use D5W 0.9% NS at 20 ml/kg for the first hour; then replace any deficit and maintain IV fluids. Place an NG tube, and decompress the bowel. Administer appropriate antibiotics. Consult a surgeon and admit the child to the hospital. The goal of surgery is to place the normal ganglion-containing bowel within 1 cm of the anal opening.

Enterocolitis before or after surgery is associated with a 30% mortality rate; therefore, be aware of the postsurgical patient with Hirschsprung's disease who looks ill and has diarrhea.

KAWASAKI SYNDROME

Definition

Kawasaki syndrome also known as *mucocutaneous lymph node syndrome* is a disease that causes a vasculitis with a fever higher than

104° F for more than 5 days. It is usually a self-limiting syndrome, but if there is involvement of the coronary arteries, the mortality rate is high. The syndrome has three phases: the *acute* phase with a febrile illness lasting 7 to 10 days, the *subacute* phase lasting 10 to 14 days, which can last up to 25 days. The syndrome presents in the subacute phase with cardiovascular disease, desquamation, anorexia, with the highest mortality rate during this phase. The third phase, the *convalescence* phase, lasts for 6 to 8 weeks. There is still a high mortality rate during the convalescence phase. Coronary artery dilatation is the most common coronary disease finding.

Etiology

Its cause is believed to be related to a lymphotropic retrovirus. It has also been associated with rug shampoos, house mites, and house dust.

Epidemiology

Kawasaki syndrome is a syndrome that affects boys more than girls and is seen in the late winter and early spring. It is a multisystem disease that usually affects children younger than 5 years of age.

Clinical Presentation

There are six major criteria for the diagnosis of Kawasaki syndrome. The criteria,* signs, and symptoms of Kawasaki syndrome are:

1. Fever higher than 101.3° F (38.5° C) for at least 5 days
2. Bilateral nonexudative conjunctivitis
3. Oral inflammatory changes
   a. Erythema, fissuring, or crusting of the lips
   b. Oropharyngeal erythema
   c. Strawberry tongue
4. Skin changes on the extremities:
   a. Induration of the hands or feet (early finding)
   b. Erythema of the hands and feet (early finding)
   c. Desquamation of the skin on the tips of the fingers and toes (usually a late presentation, 2 to 3 weeks after the onset of the syndrome).
5. Erythematous, polymorphous skin rash, with fever, resolves in 5 to 7 days
6. Lymph node enlargement, involving the cervical lymph nodes, 1.5 cm in size

Cardiac involvement can cause congestive heart failure (CHF), pericardial effusion, summation gallop, and coronary artery aneurysm. Aseptic meningitis, obstructive jaundice, hydrops of the gallbladder, uveitis, urethritis, and diarrhea can occur.

---

*Five of the six aforementioned criteria should be present to make the diagnosis of Kawasaki disease.

Diagnosis

As mentioned, five of the six major criteria must be established for the diagnosis of Kawasaki syndrome. Twenty percent of the patients will develop coronary artery disease, arteritis, aneurysm, or thrombosis within 45 days of the onset of fever. Fifty percent of these abnormalities will resolve on their own. The extremes of age (<1 year or >5 years of age) are at the greatest risk of coronary disease. The mortality rate from coronary disease in Kawasaki syndrome is 1 to 2%. Seventy percent of the deaths will occur within 15 to 45 days of the onset of fever and usually occur during the subacute and convalescent stages. CHF can also occur.

Laboratory Findings

An elevated WBC count greater than 20,000/mm^3, with predominance of neutrophils and a reduced hematocrit will be present. The ESR rate will be elevated higher than 55 mm/hr. Platelets are often higher than 1 million/mm^3. A urinalysis will often show proteinuria with sterile pyuria. Serum alanine aminotransferase (ALT) will often be elevated. An ECG is often not helpful in making the diagnosis. Echocardiography is helpful at 7 to 12 days after the onset of illness.

Treatment

1. Fluid support is essential, with treatment of CHF if present.
2. Aspirin at a dose of 100 mg/kg/24 hr every 6 hours for 14 days, then 3 to 5 mg/kg/24 hr for 2 to 3 months through the convalescence phase is recommended. High doses of aspirin may be needed because of the poor absorption of aspirin. Aspirin inhibits platelet function and reduces the risk of thrombosis and coronary artery disease.
3. IV gamma globulin administered in high doses of 400 mg/kg/24 hr over a 2-hour period for 4 days will decrease the chance of coronary artery disease if given with aspirin within 10 days of the onset of the syndrome. An alternate dosing of 2 g/kg in a single dose over 10 to 12 hours has also been recommended.
4. In children with known coronary artery lesions and platelet counts more than 1 million/mm^3, dipyridamole 5 mg/kg/24 hr can be used.
5. Antibiotics and steroids should not be used in Kawasaki syndrome.
6. The child should be admitted to the hospital, and a pediatric cardiologist should be consulted.

MITRAL VALVE PROLAPSE

Definition

Mitral valve prolapse (MVP) is caused by redundant valve material or abnormal tissue comprising the mitral valve apparatus.

Epidemiology

MVP is the most common abnormal auscultatory finding in the pediatric population. It is found in 2 to 20% of the population and has the highest incidence in slender teenage females. MVP is usually found in female children who are older than 6 years of age and who have a slender habitus and bony thoracic abnormalities.

Pathology

The redundant valve tissue causes the mitral valve to move either posteriorly or superiorly into the left atrium during ventricular systole.

Clinical Presentation

Most patients with MVP are asymptomatic. Patients with MVP present with dizziness, palpitations, and chest pain. Some studies have shown that these symptoms are no more prevalent in people with MVP than in the normal population. Dysrhythmias and exercise intolerance are uncommon.

Examination

A midsystolic click is best heard with the patient standing or squatting and is diagnostic of MVP. A systolic click is heard as the valve moves and is the clinical hallmark of MVP. To diagnose MVP, the patient should be auscultated in several positions. Systolic murmurs with or without clicks are best heard in the standing or squatting positions. The click will be heard earlier in children than in adults, and the click will be more midsystolic than systolic.

Diagnosis

The diagnostic test of choice is the echocardiogram. If there is significant posterior systolic movement of the posterior mitral valve leaflet, this is considered diagnostic for MVP.

Laboratory Findings

Basic laboratory studies should be performed—CBC, electrolytes, and urinalysis (UA). An ECG will rarely show T wave inversion in precordial lead V_6.

Treatment

Most patients are asymptomatic and require no treatment. If chest pain is a major complaint of MVP, oral propranolol can be given. If mitral insufficiency is also present, prophylaxis is indicated for subacute infectious endocarditis.

OTITIS MEDIA

Definition

Acute otitis media is a suppurative effusion of the middle ear that often follows a eustachian tube dysfunction. This dysfunction is caused by abnormal patency or obstruction of the eustachian tube. Serous otitis media, mastoiditis (now rare), cholesteatoma (keratinized, stratified, and squamous epithelium causing a sack-like structure of accumulated desquamated epithelium in the middle ear), perforations, and persistent or recurrent otitis media and meningitis are all complications of acute otitis media.

Epidemiology

Eskimos, American Indians, and children with Down syndrome are at higher risk of otitis media infection.

Pathology

The most common pathogens are *H. influenzae, Branhamella catarrhalis,* and *S. pneumoniae.* Thirty percent of otitis media middle ear cultures show no bacteria. *Mycoplasma pneumoniae* has been associated with bullous myringitis. Several viruses have been isolated in otitis media: adenovirus, enterovirus, RSV, and parainfluenza. Rarely tuberculosis may be the cause of acute otitis media.

Clinical Presentation

Children can present with ear pain, irritability, and lethargy with accompanying upper respiratory infection symptoms. If the tympanic membrane is ruptured, drainage from the ear may be present. Hearing loss may be present. Foreign bodies in the ear, trauma, external otitis media, mastoiditis, dental abscess, sinusitis, parotitis, lymphadenitis, or peritonsillar abscess can all present as acute otitis media.

Diagnosis

A diagnosis is made by visualization of the tympanic membrane (TM). An infected ear will have increased erythema and vascularity of the TM. Landmarks will be obscured, and the TM can be bulging. The "gold standard" for the diagnosis of acute otitis media is the use of a pneumatic otoscope. If an effusion is present, there will be decreased mobility of the TM. Twenty-five percent of treated children will have a persistent or recurrent otitis media. There is controversy as to when or if a child should have a follow-up ear check. Recommendations range from 14 to 21 days after the start of antibiotics for a follow-up ear check. It is a good policy in the ED to refer all children back to their primary health care provider within 14 days for a follow-up evaluation.

Laboratory Findings

In uncomplicated otitis media in children older than 6 months and who look well and do not have a fever higher than 102° F, no laboratory examinations are needed. If the child is 3 to 6 months of age, a CBC, blood culture, urine culture, and lumbar puncture should be considered in the work-up, because of the high incidence of meningitis in association with otitis media in this age group. Children in this age group should be admitted to the hospital. Throat cultures are usually not very helpful in the diagnosis of acute otitis media.

Treatment

Children younger than 2 months of age should be admitted to the hospital. The antibiotics of choice for this age group are ampicillin and gentamicin or cefotaxime. From 2 months to 8 years amoxicillin (Augmentin), erythromycin, sulfisoxazole (Pediazole), trimethoprim-sulfamethoxazole (Septra, Bactrim), cefotaxime, or cefaclor (PO) can all be used as initial antibiotic therapy. In children over 9 years of age, because of the high incidence of *S. pneumoniae* and group A streptococci, penicillin V or erythromycin can be used. For recurrent or persistent otitis media, amoxicillin or trimethoprim-sulfamethoxazole can be used.

Perforations of the TM secondary to otitis media do not usually require therapy but a referral should be made to the patient's primary health care provider for a follow-up examination to determine if the acute otitis media has resolved.

Serous otitis media can occur in up to 42% of children with otitis media. Serous otitis media is a sterile effusion behind the TM that can cause a temporary hearing loss. If the serous otitis media effusion lasts longer than 2 months, the child should be referred for audiologic testing.

Tympanocentesis has been recommended for children younger than 8 weeks of age who are symptomatic or immunocompromised, for those with persistent acute otitis media (after two or three courses of therapy), and also for children with painful bullous myringitis. Tympanocentesis is carried out to relieve pain and to obtain fluid for a Gram's stain and culture of fluid. Tympanocentesis can be performed by using a slightly bent 3½ inch, 18-gauge spinal needle that is attached to a syringe. The needle is inserted in the posterior, inferior area of the TM under otoscopic visualization. Fluid contents are aspirated for a Gram's stain and culture. Decongestants and antihistamines are usually not effective in resolving acute otitis media. Acute ear pain can be treated with glycerin (Auralgan) drops. If the TM perforates, the pain is usually relieved. If otitis externa occurs secondary to the otitis media, polymyxin (Cortisporin) otic drops can be used as therapy.

Antipyretics should be used—acetaminophen 10 to 15 mg/kg/dose q4 to 6 hr PO or per rectum or ibuprofen 40 mg/kg/24 hr PO every 6 to 8 hours.

The parents should be told that any child who does not show signs of improvement in 36 hours, or who is becoming more ill, should be re-evaluated by the primary health care provider or should return to the ED for re-evaluation.

PEDIATRIC ANALGESIA AND SEDATION

Analgesia and sedation are probably underused in the pediatric population in the ED. The major reason is the lack of understanding of analgesia and sedation and how they can be used safely. A child's injury hurts as much as an adult's injury; thus their pain should be relieved or prevented before a painful procedure. The major risk factor in pediatric sedation is respiratory depression. Current literature shows that there is approximately a 15% failure rate with any sedative in children. Children tolerate sedation better than do adults in most cases. One complication of sedation in children is that a paradoxic excitement can occur instead of sedation.

When sedating a child, starting an IV, heparin lock, or infiltrating a wound, do not lie to the child. Tell the child that this is going to hurt. If you violate the child's trust, you will create a "white coat" mentality for the child and the parents.

Assess the child's pain. Treat the pain in relation to the procedure that needs to be performed. Use the correct medication in the appropriate dose for the kind of procedure that you are going to perform.

Local Analgesia

Lidocaine is the most commonly used local analgesia. The two most common mistakes when using lidocaine are running it into the wound too quickly and not buffering it with 8.4% sodium bicarbonate. By infiltrating slowly and buffering the lidocaine with sodium bicarbonate in a 1:10 mixture, the procedure is almost painless.

Lidocaine comes in 1 or 2% solutions, with or without epinephrine. Epinephrine is a vasoconstrictor and will reduce bleeding. Do not use lidocaine with epinephrine on the pinna of the ear, penis, nose, or a distal phalanx. The maximum dose of lidocaine with epinephrine is 7 mg/kg, and the maximum dose without epinephrine is 5 mg/kg.

Bupivacaine is a local analgesia that is four times more potent than is lidocaine. Bupivacaine is more acidic than is lidocaine, and bupivacaine should also be buffered with sodium bicarbonate. Bupivacaine comes in 0.25 and 0.5% solutions, with or without epinephrine. The maximum dose of bupivacaine is 2 to 3 mg/kg, with or without epinephrine.

Topical Analgesia

There are many topical analgesia preparations on the market for superficial wound repair. Tetracaine 0.5%, epinephrine 1:2000, and cocaine 11.8% (TAC) can be used as a topical preparation. Half-strength TAC is also as effective as full-strength TAC and is safer. TAC is only effective when applied to a highly vascular area. TAC contains epinephrine and should be used with caution on the distal phalanx secondary to vasoconstriction.

Hallucinations, seizures, disorientation, and death have been reported secondary to systemic absorption of cocaine and tetracaine. These problems have been associated with improper use of TAC, by repeatedly applying it to the eyes, nose, and mouth. Do not use TAC near mucous membranes or in children with a history of seizures or cardiac arrhythmias.

The maximum dose of TAC is believed to be 3 ml of one-half strength. After TAC has been applied, supplemental buffered lidocaine can be applied at a reduced pain level.

SYSTEMIC ANALGESIA AND SEDATION

There are numerous single or combinations of analgesia and sedation available for use in the ED. The American Academy of Pediatrics defines conscious sedation "as a minimally depressed level of consciousness that retains a patient's ability to maintain a patent airway . . . and responds appropriately to physician stimulation and/or verbal commands."

Morphine is the oldest analgesic drug and the basis for all other analgesic drugs to be measured. Morphine can cause respiratory depression, especially in children younger than 3 months of age when given via rapid IV push. Morphine can also cause hypotension; however, the effect can easily be reversed by giving naloxone at 5 to 10 μg/kg. The dose of morphine is 0.1 mg/kg IV. It cannot be given orally. The time of onset is 3 to 10 minutes, and the effect of morphine lasts for 3 to 4 hours. The patient's discharge time from the hospital will therefore be prolonged. An additional dose of morphine at 0.05 mg/kg can be given to titrate to effect.

Meperidine is a synthetic derivative of morphine that is one tenth of the potency of morphine. It is not very effective when given orally. Meperidine is better given for short procedures. Side effects include vomiting and respiratory depression. If meperidine is given with hydroxyzine 0.5 mg/kg PO or IM, the likelihood of vomiting will be reduced. The effects of meperidine can be reversed with naloxone 5 to 10 μg/kg. The dosage of meperidine is 1 mg/kg IV, IM, or 1 to 2 mg/kg PO. When given IV, the onset is rapid in 10 to 15 minutes. When given IM or PO, the onset of effect starts in 15 to 30 minutes. Its duration is 2 to 3 hours. A supplemental dose of meperidine at a dose of 0.5 mg/kg to a maximum of 100 mg IV, or IM, and 150 mg PO may be given.

Fentanyl is a synthetic narcotic that is 100 times more potent than is morphine. The effect of fentanyl lasts only for a short time (30 minutes) and the onset is immediate. Fentanyl will cause minimal respiratory depression if the drug is administered over 3 to 5 minutes.

Quick Reference for Sedation and Analgesia in Children

Topical Viscous Cocaine
Indications: Face, scalp, head, or neck
  1. May replace lidocaine injection in some cases
  2. Wait 10 to 15 minutes after application
  3. Poor results in distal extremities in older adults; may try proximal extremities in children

TAC Solution
  a. Indications: Face, scalp, head, or neck
    1. May replace lidocaine injection in some cases
    2. Wait 10 to 15 minutes after application
  b. Dosage: Tetracaine 2% 5 ml
         Epinephrine 1:1000 5 ml
         Cocaine 5 g
  c. Apply 1 ml/cm of wound

Sedation

Oral Midazolam (Versed)
  a. Dosage: 0.5 mg/kg PO to a maximum dose of 10 mg, usually not necessary to dilute (may mix with orange juice or cola, but not as effective). Use in children who weigh less than 30 kg.
  b. Onset: 10 minutes (be ready)
  c. If spat out by the child, repeat the same dose
  d. Not an analgesic, therefore lidocaine is necessary
  e. If child is younger than 12 months of age, consider intranasal midazolam at 0.4 mg/kg
  f. Can use injectable midazolam as oral or nasal sedation (works the same and has slower onset)
  g. Precautions:
    1. Monitoring as with conscious sedation*
    2. 10 to 20% of children will have hyperactivity in 1 to 2 hours after dosing

Rectal Thiopental
  a. Dosage: 25 to 45 mg/kg rectally. Use in children weighing less than 30 kg and older than 4 years of age
  b. Precautions: Monitoring as with any conscious sedation*

Chloral Hydrate (Noctec)
  a. Dosage: 50 to 80 mg/kg PO (use for CT)
  b. Precautions: Monitoring as with any conscious sedation*

Methohexital (Brevital)
  a. Dosage: 20 mg/kg rectally
  b. Precautions: Monitoring as with any conscious sedation*

Pentobarbital (Nembutal)
  a. Dosage: 4–5 mg/kg IV or IM
  b. Precautions: Monitoring as with any conscious sedation*

Diazepam (Valium)
  a. Dosage: 0.1 mg/kg IV
         0.2 mg/kg PO or rectally
  b. Precautions: Monitoring as with any conscious sedation*

Quick Reference for Sedation and Analgesia in Children
Continued

Analgesia

Fentanyl
   a. Dosage: 2 to 3 μg/kg IV
   b. Precautions: Monitoring as with any conscious sedation*

Ketamine
   a. Dosage: 0.1 mg/kg IV
              4 mg/kg IM

Morphine
   a. Dosage: 0.1 mg/kg IV
   b. Precautions: Monitoring as with any conscious sedation*

Meperidine (Demerol)
   a. Dosage: 1 mg/kg IV or IM
              1 to 2 mg/kg PO
   b. Precautions: Monitoring as with any conscious sedation*

Glycopyrrolate (Robinul) Ketamine/Midazolam (Versed)
   a. Dosage: Glycopyrrolate (Robinul) 0.01 mg/kg IM (decreases the secretions
              of ketamine)
              Ketamine 2 to 4 mg/kg IM
              Midazolam (Versed) 0.1 to 0.2 mg/kg IM
   b. Use as a single injection in children 3 to 5 years old. (Do not use
      glycopyrrolate in asthmatics.)
   c. Precautions: Monitoring as with any conscious sedation*

*Standard Precautions for any conscious sedation follow:
   1. The child should be placed on a cardiac monitor.
   2. The child should be placed on pulse oximetry.
   3. The child should have IV access or IV access equipment should be readily
      available.
   4. The child should be placed on oxygen.
   5. An airway chart with appropriate intubation equipment should be readily
      available.
   6. Naloxone (Narcan) 1 mg/kg should be readily available to reverse the effect of narcotics.
   7. Flumazenil (Romazicon) 0.1 to 0.2 mg should be available to reverse the effect
      of benzodiazepines.

There have been reported cases of chest wall rigidity if fentanyl is administered by too rapid an IV push. The dose is 2 to 3 μg/kg IV, over 2 minutes, and the dose lasts for 30 minutes. Fentanyl can be titrated to effect in increments of 0.5 μg/kg. Side effects are respiratory depression, bradycardia, and muscle rigidity. Naloxone in a dose of 5 to 10 μg/kg should be available to reverse the effects of respiratory depression.

Ketamine is a dissociative analgesic that has sedative properties. Ketamine can be given IV, IM, or PO. Side effects of ketamine are laryngospasm and hypersalivation. This drug can cause hallucinations in older children. Ketamine can raise intracranial pressure and blood pressure. It should be used with caution in head trauma. Ketamine used with atropine will reduce hypersalivation. Ketamine used with midazolam will reduce the likelihood of hallucinations.

Nitrous oxide is delivered as a 30 to 50% mixture with oxygen. Nitrous oxide is an effective analgesic, and it also induces a state of sedation and a feeling of euphoria and dissociation. A fail-safe delivery system must be available for proper delivery. The system should have a mouthpiece that allows, when the patient is oversedated, for the mask to fall off and the patient to breathe room air. The system should have an oxygen analyzer and a scavenger device. Pulse oximetry should be in place before sedation is attempted. The onset of nitrous oxide is 1 to 2 minutes. Side effects include altered mental status, eye injury, obstructed viscus, pneumothorax, and dyspnea. There is limited experience with nitrous oxide in young children, and nitrous oxide is contraindicated in children who have had another sedative in the preceding hours.

Midazolam is the drug of choice for sedation in many EDs. It can be given PO, IV, rectally, IM, subcutaneously (SQ), or intranasally. Midazolam's duration of action is 30 to 40 minutes. Children require higher doses of midazolam than do adults. Children usually remain awake but are disinhibited. It is used for CTs, placement or removal of sutures, and orthopedic procedures. The effect of midazolam can be reversed by giving flumazenil 0.1 to 0.2 mg IV. The dose of midazolam is 0.15 mg/kg IV or IM. Midazolam can also be given intranasally or rectally at 0.2 to 0.3 mg/kg. The oral dose of midazolam is 0.5 mg/kg. Complications of midazolam are respiratory depression, apnea, anterograde amnesia for 1 to 2 hours, and hypotension especially when midazolam is combined with fentanyl.

Diazepam has been used for many years and is an effective anxiolytic and amnestic. It is also used as an anticonvulsant agent. Diazepam can cause respiration depression, apnea, and amnesia. The pediatric dose of diazepam is 0.1 mg/kg IV, and the rectal dose is 0.2 mg/kg. The onset of action of diazepam in IV doses is rapid. With PO or rectal route of administration onset is 30 to 60 minutes. The duration of action is from 1 to 2 hours. The maximum IV dose is 0.6 mg/kg over 8 hours. The oral dose is 10 mg over 6 to 8 hours.

Chloral hydrate is one of the oldest sedative agents. It can be used both orally and rectally and is unlikely to cause respiratory depression. It has a wide success rate and is from 70 to 85% effective when used. Chloral hydrate has a slow onset of from 30 to 60 minutes, and it has a prolonged sedative effect up to several hours (3 to 4 hours). Side effects include mucosal and gastric irritation, cardiac arrhythmias, and hyperbilirubinemia in premature infants. The dose for PO or rectally administered chloral hydrate is 75 mg/kg with onset in 30 minutes or more. The maximum dose is 2 grams.

Phenobarbital is a long-acting barbiturate. It can be administered IV or IM. The IM or IV dose is 4 to 5 mg/kg. The onset of action when given IV is rapid. The onset of action when given IM is 15 minutes. The effect of phenobarbital when given IV lasts for 30 minutes, and the IM effect lasts for 2 hours. The maximum dose is 100 to 200 mg. Give phenobarbital slowly. Supplemental phenobarbital can be given at 1 mg/kg slowly.

Methohexital is a short-acting sedative. The onset of methohexital is in 15 minutes when administered rectally. Its duration is 20 minutes. Methohexital is dosed at 20 mg/kg rectally. The maximum rectal dose is 25 mg/kg. It has side effects similar to those of phenobarbital.

ASTHMA

Definition

Asthma results from bronchoconstriction, inflammation with increased secretion, and mucus plugging from intrinsic mechanisms related to automatic dysfunction from extrinsic sensitizing agents or substances in the lungs. It is a chronic disease defined as increased reactivity of the pulmonary airways. Remember that "all that wheezes is not asthma." Foreign bodies, CHF, and congenital heart disease can all cause wheezing. A precipitating or aggravating extrinsic factor usually causes an asthma attack. Cystic fibrosis, tracheoesophageal fistula or tracheal anomaly, hyperventilation, or metabolic acidosis can present as asthma. Neoplasms, mediastinal or pulmonary, can cause wheezing and shortness of breath that resemble asthma. Vocal cord dysfunction can mimic asthmatic wheezing. Pulmonary edema, pulmonary embolism, CHF, aspiration, bronchiolitis, and pneumonia can all mimic asthma.

Epidemiology

Asthma is a very common presentation to the ED. It is found in 6.7% of children in the United States. There is an increasing death rate from asthma in the United States, especially in the black population.

Pathology

Bronchodilatation is caused by an increase in intracellular cyclic adenosine $3',5'$ monophosphate (cAMP). This increase in cyclic AMP is caused by the promotion of biosynthesis (β-adrenergic agents) or by the inhibition of its degradation (e.g., theophylline). These pathways cause bronchodilatation. Cyclic AMP is also increased by activation of adenylate cyclase, causing an increased intracellular concentration of cyclic AMP. Protein kinase A is increasingly released, which inhibits phosphorylation of myosin and lowers intracellular ionic calcium concentrations. This process causes the relaxation of smooth muscles in the airways.

Cyclic guanosine monophosphate (cGMP) is produced when there is parasympathetic stimulation. The parasympathetic stimulation arises by activation of cholinergic receptor stimulation, thus causing bronchoconstriction. Early bronchoconstriction is thought to be due to the release of mast cell mediators in response to an allergen. Later in the exacerbation, alveolar macrophages and eosinophils assume a dominant role in the inflammatory process. Edema of the microvasculature causes epithelial shedding and thus produces an obstruction in the lumens of the small airways. This causes bronchial hyperresponsiveness by exposing sensory nerves to direct and specific stimuli, causing an axon reflex and thus increased bronchoconstriction.

Viral infections cause between 19 and 42% of asthma exacerbations. Other precipitating or aggravating factors include:

Smoke	Pollutants	Aerosols	Chemicals
Pollen	Molds	Animal dander	Chlorine
Ammonia	Exercise	Emotional stress	Food
Food additives	Aspirin	Bronchoconstrictors	
Nonsteroidals	β-Blockers		

Examination/Clinical Presentation

Asthma can present in numerous ways (e.g., coughing, wheezing, shortness of breath, chest tightness, rhinitis, atopic dermatitis, wheezing upon expiration, sinusitis, and respiratory arrest). Increased breathing rate, tachypnea, is the hallmark of asthma. A patient can present with a prolonged expiratory phase, expiratory wheezing, nasal flaring, accessory muscle use, and supraclavicular retractions. Upon initial examination of the lung fields, the patient may be so "tight" that no wheezing can be heard, but tachypnea will be present. Only after several nebulizer treatments does the child start to "wheeze." Remember that agitation, confusion, and headache can all be responses to hypoxia. If the child has been in respiratory distress for a long time, he or she will eventually become tired. Don't mistake this presentation for the child getting better. Wheezing can decrease because the inspirations are decreasing secondary to respiratory failure.

Cyanosis indicates hypoxia. The child should have serial examinations while in the ED. If possible, peak flow forced expiratory volume in 1 second (FEV_1) should be obtained before and after each nebulizer treatment. Ask the child to state his or her name. If the child cannot give his or her name or the name of his or her mother or father, this is a sign of respiratory distress. Can the older child speak a whole sentence? If the child is unable to do this, he or she is in respiratory distress.

Prior history of hospitalizations, intubations, steroid use, and home nebulizer use can help you estimate the extent of the disease. If the family has made more than three trips to the ED in the past 7 days, or two trips in the past 72 hours, this is a good indicator that the child probably needs to be admitted to the hospital for treatment. Remember that only 50% of asthma patients who leave the ED are completely "cleared" at time of discharge. The child's pulse rate should decrease with respiratory rate as the child improves. The child will interact more with the environment as he or she improves. The ABG is the "gold standard" for evaluating respiratory function.

This is often difficult to obtain in a small child. Respiratory failure is defined as a PaO_2 of less than 50 mm Hg and a $PaCO_2$ greater than 50 mm Hg on room air and at sea level. Pulse oximetry is an excellent alternative if the sensor is placed correctly on the finger or toe.

Pulsus paradoxus should be determined if possible. It can be present in pericardial tamponade, pneumothorax, and severe asthma. It is obtained by asking the patient to breathe quietly while the health care provider lowers the blood pressure cuff toward the systolic level. When the first sound is heard, it is noted. The cuff is further deflated and the systolic sound is listened for throughout the respiratory cycle. A difference of 10 mm Hg or greater is an indication of pulsus paradoxus.

Complications of asthma are:

1. Pneumothorax or pneumomediastinum
2. Pneumonia
3. Dehydration
4. Syndrome of inappropriate antidiuretic hormone
5. Death secondary to respiratory failure

Laboratory Findings

CBC, electrolytes, ABG, chest x-ray, blood culture, and urine cultures should be guided by the severity of the illness and by the likelihood of precipitating factors. If the child is taking theophylline, a serum theophylline level should be obtained. Normal values, depending on the laboratory, range from 5 to 15 μg/ml or 10 to 20 μg/ml. Prolonged use of albuterol can cause hypokalemia; therefore be sure to check the child's potassium level.

X-ray Findings

On chest x-ray, the classic pattern of hyperinflation will be seen with asthma. Also look for infiltrates and atelectasis. Signs of infiltrates on a chest x-ray will show a normal diaphragm, no mediastinal shift, and the presence of air bronchograms. Atelectasis on a chest x-ray will show an elevated diaphragm, a mediastinal shift toward the lesion, and variable air bronchograms.

Treatment

Oxygen is the mainstay of treatment of asthma and respiratory distress. Administration of oxygen via blow-by, nasal cannula, or facemask can all be used. Use your imagination to get oxygen to the child. Give preferably humidified oxygen at 3 to 6 l/min. Cardiac monitoring is essential when adrenergic agents or theophylline-containing medications are used.

Aerosols of β_2-agonists are used as initial therapy for an acute exacerbation of asthma.

1. Albuterol (0.5% solution or 5 mg/ml) (Proventil, Ventolin) 0.03 ml (0.15 mg)/kg/dose to a maximum dose of 1 ml (5 mg)/dose with 2 ml of NS can be administered every 20 minutes in the initial stabilization phase, then every 2 to 4 hours. In the severely ill child, continuous albuterol treatment can be used. The peak onset is from 30 to 60 minutes with a duration of 4 to 6 hours.
2. Terbutaline can be given as a 0.1% solution or 1 mg/ml parenterally or 0.03 mg (0.03 ml)/kg/dose, to a maximum dose of 0.5 ml/dose in 2 ml of 0.9% NS every 4 hours.

Parenteral agents have long been used. Inhaled agents have a greater efficacy than do parenteral agents. Parenteral agents can be used in the severely ill patient or when it is impractical for the child to inhale the nebulized solution.

1. Epinephrine (Adrenalin) (1:1000) at 0.01 ml (0.01 mg)/kg/dose, with a maximum dose of 0.35 ml is given subcutaneously (SQ) every 20 minutes for a total of three doses or a heart rate greater than 180 beats/min. The peak onset is in 20 minutes, with a duration of 2 hours.
2. SusPrine, a long-acting epinephrine (1:200) at 0.005 ml/kg/dose, with a maximum dose of 0.15 ml SQ.
3. Terbutaline (0.1% solution) (Brethine), 0.01 ml/kg/dose, with a maximum dose of 0.25 ml (0.25 mg) SQ is given every 20 minutes for a total of three doses.

Anticholinergic agents can be given:

1. Atropine 0.02 mg/kg/dose, to a maximum dose of 2 mg, with 2 ml of 0.9% NS can be given as a nebulizer treatment every 4 to 6 hours.
2. Ipratropium (Atrovent), which is a derivative of atropine, can be administered as an inhaled agent. The pediatric dose is not known.

Oral agents can also be utilized.

1. Albuterol (Proventil) Syrup, (2 mg/5 ml) 0.1 to 0.15 mg/kg/dose PO every 6 to 8 hours, with a maximum dose of 4 mg, can be used in children in whom home nebulizer treatments are impractical or the child refuses to inhale nebulized solutions. Two- and 4-mg tablets are also available.
2. Fenoterol (0.5% solution) can be used.
   a. Less than 2 years, 0.1 ml/dose
   b. From 2 to 9 years, 0.2 ml/dose
   c. Above 9 years, 0.3 ml/dose

Metered dose inhalers (MDI) are a mainstay of outpatient treatment. Albuterol, terbutaline, ipratropium, steroid, and cromolyn are all used to prevent asthma exacerbations. When used with a "spacer," they are much more effective than when used alone.

Cromolyn (Intal) bullets (20 mg) can be given to neonates, infants, and older children in 10 to 20 mg/dose three to four times a day.

Theophylline is a β-agonist that has long been used in the treatment of asthma. It has a narrow therapeutic range. It has not been shown that the administration of theophylline shortens the hospital stay or benefits patients in the hospital setting. Dosing is as follows:

- If the patient is already on theophylline therapy and is at a subtherapeutic level, give half of the loading dose.
- Parenteral administration of aminophylline (100 mg in 100 ml 0.9% NS) will give you 1 mg/ml of aminophylline or 0.85 mg/ml of theophylline.

Aminophylline doses are as follows:

a. 1 to 6 months, loading dose of 6 to 7 mg/kg, maintenance dose of 0.5 mg/kg/hr
b. 6 to 12 months, loading dose of 6 to 7 mg/kg, maintenance dose of 1 mg/kg/hr
c. 1 to 9 years, loading dose of 6 to 7 mg/kg, maintenance dose of 1.5 mg/kg/hr
d. 10 to 16 years, loading dose of 6 to 7 mg/kg, maintenance dose of 1.2 mg/kg/hr

Increased doses of theophylline must be adjusted for concurrent drug use, such as phenobarbital, rifampin, carbamazepine, and marijuana. Patients with cystic fibrosis or hyperthyroidism, smokers, and patients who are on a high-protein diets must also have increased doses of theophylline.

Decreased doses of theophylline must be used in children who are on cimetidine and erythromycin therapy. In older children who take oral contraceptives, the dose of theophylline should be decreased. Viral illness, CHF, abnormal renal function or renal disease will also cause the decreased metabolism of theophylline; thus the theophylline dose should be decreased. Infants younger than 3 months of age and pregnant women (especially during the third trimester) require less theophylline.

Conversion from IV aminophylline to oral sustained-release preparations can be achieved by calculating the total infusion rate of theophylline (1 mg/ml of aminophylline = 0.85 mg/ml of theophylline) over the last 24 hours.

1. Preterm infants up to 40 weeks after conception (postconception age = gestational age at birth + postnatal age) 1 mg/kg every 12 hours
2. Term infants at birth or 40 weeks after conception:
   a. Up to 4 weeks postnatally: 1 to 2 mg/kg every 12 hours
   b. 4 to 8 weeks: 1 to 2 mg/kg every 8 hours
   c. After 8 weeks: 1 to 3 mg/kg every 6 hours

Careful monitoring of theophylline levels must be ensured for an infant younger than 6 months of age.

A patient on long-term theophylline therapy can be maintained at a dose of 16 mg/kg/24 hr PO to maintain a serum level of 5 to 15 μg/ml.

Steroids are now a main form of treatment of asthma. Patients who have been admitted to the hospital in the last 12 months or who have been on steroids for the last 12 months should have steroids administered early, with the first nebulizer treatment.

1. Methylprednisolone (Solu-Medrol), 1 to 2 mg/kg/dose every 6 hours IV, can be used in children with moderate or severe asthma.
2. Oral prednisone, 1 to 2 mg/kg PO every 6 to 12 hours for 5 days, can be used effectively in the outpatient treatment of asthma.
3. Oral MDI of steroids, beclomethasone (Vanceril, Beclovent), 42 to 50 μg/puff with a "spacer," can be used in outpatient therapy every 6 to 8 hours.

Magnesium sulfate ($MgSO_4$) has been used in the treatment of adult asthmatic patients, who have shown signs of improvement. Further studies are needed in children.

Admission Criteria

Any child who presents to the ED three times in 7 days or twice in 72 hours should be admitted to the hospital. Any child who, after 3 to 10 nebulizer treatments with steroids and 6 hours in the ED, has not shown signs of improvement should be admitted to the hospital. Any child who cannot take PO liquids should be admitted to the hospital. A child with theophylline toxicity should be admitted to the hospital. Any child who is hypoxic, tachycardiac, or tachypneic after several treatments of steroids and several hours in the ED should be admitted to the hospital. Ask the parents if the child is back to baseline status. Has the child improved enough to go home? Is this exacerbation like the last exacerbation when the child was admitted to the hospital? When in doubt, admit the child to the hospital.

PEDIATRIC DIARRHEA

Definition

Diarrhea is defined as an acute increase in stool number and water content. Numerous viral, bacterial, and parasitic agents can cause diarrhea.

Epidemiology/Pathology

In children, 39% of diarrhea is caused by rotaviruses. Diarrhea usually occurs in the cooler months. Norwalk virus is common in summer camps and is more common in the adolescent and adult popula-

Predicted Average Peak Expiratory Flow for Normal Children and Adolescents (Males and Females)*

Height (inches)	Peak Expiratory Flow (l/min)
43	147
44	160
45	173
46	187
47	200
48	214
49	227
50	240
51	254
52	267
53	280
54	293
55	307
56	320
57	334
58	347
59	360
60	373
61	387
62	400
63	413
64	427
65	440
66	454
67	467

*From the National Asthma Education Program: Guidelines for the Diagnosis and Management of Asthma (Publication 91-3042/3042A). Bethesda, MD, National Institutes of Health, US Department of Health and Human Services, 1991.

tions. *Salmonella* usually affects children younger than 2 years of age; *Shigella* affects children younger than 5 years of age. *Campylobacter* is transmitted by contaminated food or by person-to-person contact. *Yersinia enterocolitica* occurs in the cooler months. Enterotoxigenic or invasive *E. coli* is seen in young children and infants.

Diarrhea can also be caused by food poisoning. *Staphylococcus, Clostridium botulinum*, and *C. perfringens* can all occur secondary to contact with contaminated food. *C. difficile* occurs secondary to administration of antibiotics.

Clinical Presentation

1. *Rotavirus*
   a. The virus can affect a child aged 6 to 18 months.
   b. Vomiting is an early and prominent symptom.
   c. More than five stools daily will be present.
   d. Blood or mucus rarely will be seen in the stool.

    e. Respiratory symptoms may be present.
    f. Symptoms usually last for 2 to 3 days.
  2. *Norwalk virus*
    a. Nausea and vomiting occur.
    b. Abdominal pain is present.
    c. Lethargy is present.
    d. Fever is present.
    e. The symptoms last for approximately 3 days.
  3. *Astrovirus*
    a. Winter is the peak time.
    b. This virus can present in infants up to 7 years of age.
    c. Transmission occurs from one person to another.
    d. Contaminated water or shellfish can also be sources of infection.
  4. *Adenovirus*
    a. The incubation period is 3 to 10 days.
    b. The virus lasts for 5 to 12 days.
    c. Symptoms include watery diarrhea, vomiting, and dehydration.
  5. *Salmonella*
    a. Children younger than 5 years of age can be affected.
    b. Fever, vomiting, and diarrhea occur with loose, slimy stools that have a foul odor.
    c. The incubation period is 24 to 48 hours after exposure.
    d. Abdominal pain will be severe and can be confused with acute appendicitis.
    e. Poultry, pet turtles, eggs, unpasteurized milk, and cantaloupes are vehicles for transmission.
    f. The WBC count is often elevated.
    g. Children with sickle cell disease or who are immunocompromised are at increased risk for septicemia from *Salmonella*. Meningitis, osteomyelitis, endocarditis, UTIs, and septic arthritis have all been reported.
    h. *Salmonella typhi* causes a severe form of diarrhea. The patient presents with malaise, headache, myalgias, hepatosplenomegaly, and rose spots.
  6. *Shigella*
    a. Children younger than 5 years of age are affected.
    b. Fever, cramping abdominal pain, and diarrhea occur.
    c. Stools are watery with blood and mucus with PMN leukocytes.
    d. Febrile convulsions are common and are often described as seizures by the parents.
    e. The WBC count is elevated and results of blood cultures are usually negative.
  7. *Y. enterocolitica*
    a. This species is prevalent in the cooler months.
    b. *Y. enterocolitica* can be found in contaminated food and water.
    c. The incubation period is 3 to 4 days after exposure.

    d. Fever and abdominal pain are present; abdominal pain can present as right lower quadrant pain mimicking acute appendicitis.

    e. The stool is watery and rarely contains blood or leukocytes.

8. *Campylobacter*

    a. The incubation period lasts from 2 to 7 days.

    b. Person-to-person contact takes place.

    c. Presents in children younger than 6 months of age during the winter.

    d. Diarrhea is profuse and watery with blood, mucus, and leukocytes.

    e. Vomiting with abdominal cramps, headache, fever, and myalgia occurs.

    f. The virus lasts for 2 to 5 days.

9. *E. coli*, either enterotoxigenic or invasive

    a. Organism is tissue invasive, producing an enterotoxin.

    b. Severe, profuse, watery diarrhea is present, with mucus, blood, and PMN leukocytes in the stool.

10. *C. perfringens*

    a. The onset is within 12 to 24 hours of contamination with food containing *Clostridium*.

    b. Fever, vomiting, and nausea are present.

    c. Abdominal pain is present.

    d. Symptoms resolve in 24 to 48 hours.

11. *C. botulinum*

    a. This species does *not* cause diarrhea.

    b. *C. botulinum* is contracted after contact with contaminated fruit, fish, or home-preserved vegetables. Honey has been implicated in children younger than 1 year of age.

    c. Physical signs include diplopia, dysphagia, dysarthria, dry mouth, nausea, and vomiting. Paresis of extraocular muscles, nystagmus, ptosis, and mydriasis can all be present.

12. *C. difficile*

    a. *C. difficile* is caused by the use of antibiotics; it is also called pseudomembranous colitis

    b. It occurs rarely in infants younger than 1 year of age

    c. Bloody stools with rare leukocytes are present.

13. *Giardia lamblia*

    a. The patient can be asymptomatic.

    b. The patient presents with watery diarrhea, right upper quadrant pain, flatulence, and bloating.

    c. Epigastric pain or cramping can be present.

    d. *G. lamblia* can be found in the immunocompromised patient or in patients who have multisystem disease.

Examination/Diagnosis

Look for signs of dehydration, poor skin turgor, sunken eyes, sunken fontanel, altered mental status (mother giving tap water causing hypernatremia), decreased urination by history. Look to see if the child cries and, if so, whether tears are present. Examine the oral mucosa to check if it is moist and if the lips are cracked. Is the child tachycardiac or tachypneic? Look for other sources of infection, otitis media, pneumonia, a UTI, and hemolytic uremic syndrome, acute tubular necrosis, lactose intolerance, meningitis, septic arthritis, or postinfectious malabsorption syndrome.

Laboratory Findings

Stool cultures should be performed on all children with blood or mucus in the stool or who have had diarrhea for more than 3 days. A methylene blue smear for fecal leukocytes is positive in 90% of the examinations for *Salmonella* and *Shigella*. Fecal leukocytes are also found in *E. coli, Y. enterocolitica, Campylobacter*, and *Vibrio parahaemolyticus*.

Mucus can be placed on a slide with two drops of methylene blue and examined on a high-power field. If five or more PMN leukocytes are present in the mucus, then the mucus sample is positive for fecal leukocytes.

A CBC for WBC should be performed. Look at the ratio of neutrophils (segmented + bands). If the ratio of band forms is over 0.10% in ratio of neutrophils, then suspect *Campylobacter, Shigella,* or *Salmonella*. Blood cultures should be drawn for the very young, the sickle cell patient, or the immunocompromised patient.

An enzyme-linked immunosorbent assay (ELISA) test is available for rotavirus testing. If parasites such as *Giardia* are suspected, stool cultures for ova and parasites and cysts should be performed.

Treatment

Rehydration is an essential part of the treatment of diarrhea. Clear liquids, Rehydrate, Ricelyte, Pedialyte, and Lytren are excellent choices of oral rehydration. Defizzed soda can be used in children older than 2 years of age. Avoid tap water secondary to hypernatremia. Gatorade is an excellent choice in older children. Soy formulas such as Isomil, ProSobee, or Soylac are excellent choices when lactose intolerance is suspected.

IV rehydration with 0.9% NS, D5W lactated Ringer's solution, or D5W 0.9% NS can be administered as a 20 ml/kg bolus then as a maintenance infusion. Antibiotics are reserved for specific organisms (see table).

Antidiarrheal agents are not recommended for treatment in the pediatric population. Both diphenoxylate and atropine (Lomotil) and loperamide (Imodium) decrease intestinal contraction, motility, and peristalsis. Diphenoxylate and atropine may have a detrimental effect in patients who are infected with *Shigella*. If used, the recommended doses are:

1. For children 13 to 20 kg: 1 mg three times a day (TID) for the first day, then 0.1 mg/kg/dose after each unformed stool

2. For children 20 to 30 kg: 2 mg BID for the first day, then 0.1 mg/kg/dose after each unformed stool
3. For children > 30 kg: 2 mg TID for the first day, then 0.1 mg/kg/dose after each unformed stool
4. For children > 2 years of age: a dose of 0.4 to 0.8 mg/kg/dose every 6 to 12 hours PO can be used. Bile acids such as aluminum hydroxide (Amphojel) 2.5 to 5 ml every 16 hours can be given to children with secretory diarrhea for 2 to 4 days during an episode of diarrhea. Cholestyramine (Questran) 1g/24 hr can be given to infants younger than 1 year of age for diarrhea. Cholestyramine absorbs and combines with bile acids, fatty acids, and bacterial enterotoxins to reduce diarrhea.

Bismuth subsalicylate, 2 tablets four times a day or 30 ml every 30 minutes for 3½ hours, can help to reduce "travelers diarrhea."

Organism	Drug of Choice	Dose
Campylobacter	Erythromycin	30 to 50 mg PO every 6 to 8 hours
Giardia	Furazolidone *or*	6 to 8 mg PO every 6 hours
	Metronidazole *or*	15 mg PO every 8 hours
	Quinacrine	6 mg PO every 8 hours
Salmonella	Ampicillin *and*	200 to 400 mg/kg IV every 4 to 6 hours
	Gentamicin	5 to 7.5 mg/kg IV every 8 hours
Shigella	Trimethoprim-sulfamethoxazole	8 to 18/40 to 58 mg PO every 12 hours
Y. enterocolitica	Trimethoprim-sulfamethoxazole	8 to 18/40 to 58 mg PO every 12 hours

PHARYNGOTONSILLITIS

Definition

Pharyngitis in association with tonsillitis is an acute bacterial or viral infection of the oral pharynx. It can involve the nasal mucosa in infants.

Epidemiology

Ten percent of children with a sore throat have group A streptococcal infection. If left untreated, group A streptococci can cause rheumatic fever or suppurative complications, such as peritonsillar abscess, cervical adenitis, otitis media, septicemia, or cellulitis. Glomerulonephritis is a late complication of untreated acute group A streptococcal infection.

Exudative pharyngitis in infants younger than 3 years of age is most commonly of a viral nature. In the age group older than 6 years, pharyngotonsillitis is commonly caused by group A streptococci.

Pathology

Viral pharyngotonsillitis can be caused by influenza, Epstein-Barr virus (mononucleosis), herpes simplex, or parainfluenza.

Bacterial infections are often caused by group A streptococci. Less common bacterial pathogens causing pharyngotonsillitis are other streptococcal pathogens, *Neisseria meningitidis, N. gonorrhoeae*, and *C. diphtheriae*.

Mycoplasma pneumoniae is a common cause of pharyngotonsillitis in school-aged children.

Clinical Presentation/Examination

Children at different ages will present with different symptoms. The infant with group A streptococcal infection will present with anorexia, rhinitis, and listlessness with adenitis, excoriated nares, and minimal fever.

School-aged children with group A streptococcal infection will present with sudden onset of sore throat, tonsillar erythema, tonsillar exudate, palatal petechiae, and a high fever. They can also present with a scarlatiniform rash. This age group can also present with abdominal pain, headache, and vomiting.

Children with viral pharyngotonsillitis will present with symptoms of gradual onset of sore throat, cough, rhinitis, and conjunctivitis. Hoarseness and loss of voice are common with viral pharyngotonsillitis. Nasal congestion is also common. Tonsils can be either exudative or nonexudative.

Epstein-Barr virus (mononucleosis) can present as exudative pharyngitis. Petechiae of the soft palate are found in both group A streptococci and Epstein-Barr virus infections. Vehicles or ulcers on the posterior tonsillar pillars are common in enterovirus. Herpesvirus infections are usually seen with anterior palate ulcers and adenopathy.

Diagnosis

The entire child should be examined.

Laboratory Findings

A throat culture is indicated in all children who have a sore throat. Infants should have their nasal passages cultured along with their throats. Cultures that have low colony counts are indicative of a carrier state of streptococci. Serum Streptozyme should be ordered to determine the titer status. If *C. diphtheriae* is considered, a special culture for *C. diphtheriae* should be taken.

Rapid strep screens are available, but these tests have high false-negative rates.

Treatment

In EDs, we often do not have rapid strep screens and do not have the luxury of follow-up on strep cultures; therefore, anyone who presents clinically with pharyngotonsillitis should be treated.

Choice of treatment includes:

1. Penicillin VK 25 to 50 mg (40,000 to 80,000 units)/kg/24 hr every 6 hours PO
2. Benzathine penicillin G IM dosing as (900,000:300,000 Bicillin C-R):

Benzathine penicillin G,	<30 lb	300,000 units
	31 to 60 lb	600,000 units
	61 to 90 lb	900,000 units
	>90 lb	1,200,000 units

3. Erythromycin, 30 to 50 mg/kg/24 hr every 6 to 8 hours PO for 10 days

PNEUMONIA

Definition

Pneumonia is an acute bacterial, mycoplasmal, or viral infection. It presents as an interstitial infection of the lung parenchyma involving either the alveoli or the alveolar walls. Bacterial pneumonia, *Mycoplasma* pneumonia, and viral pneumonia can be differentiated clinically by age, onset of symptoms, type of fever, presentation of cough, myalgia, and social habits.

Epidemiology/Pathology

S. pneumoniae, H. influenzae, S. aureus, and group A streptococci are the most common types of community acquired pneumonia in children. *M. pneumoniae* is more common in children older than 5 years of age.

Less common organisms causing pneumonia in children include pertussis, in the catarrhal stage, which is followed by a staccato cough or a paroxysmal cough. *Pseudomonas aeruginosa* must be considered in the immunocompromised patient and in those with cystic fibrosis. *P. carinii* must also be considered in the immunosuppressed or malnourished patient. *Klebsiella pneumoniae* will be seen in people at the extremes of age (the very young and the very old), alcoholics, and the immunocompromised.

Viral pneumonias, such as parainfluenza and RSV, will be the prominent viral infections in children under 2 years of age. After the age of 2, influenza A and B are the most common organisms causing viral pneumonia. Chickenpox, adenovirus, and measles can also cause viral pneumonia. *Chlamydia trachomatis* pneumonia usually presents from the second to the sixth week after birth.

M. tuberculosis should be considered if there is a history of exposure. Fungal infections can cause pneumonia. Histoplasmosis and coccidioidomycosis are the most common types. A rare form of pneumonia is caused by Q fever, a rickettsial organism. *E. coli* should be considered in children younger than 2 months of age with pneumonia.

Clinical Presentation

S. pneumoniae presents in children younger than 4 years of age with a rapid onset, poor feeding, cough, irritability, fever, and toxic appearance. Abdominal pain is the hallmark of *S. pneumoniae.* Effusion, empyema, and bacteremia are complications that occur with *S. pneumoniae.*

H. influenzae usually presents in children younger than 8 years of age, and its onset is gradual. The child presents with a fever, cough, and toxic appearance. Sometimes otitis media will complement the pneumonia. Meningitis, bacteremia, bronchiectasis, and lung abscess are all complications of *H. influenzae* pneumonia.

Group A streptococci presents in children older than 10 years of age. Its onset is gradual, with tachypnea, fever, pleuritic pain, chills, and hemoptysis. A complication of group A streptococci is empyema (serosanguineous).

S. aureus presents in infants younger than 1 year of age. Its onset is rapid with acute respiratory distress, nausea, and vomiting with an elevated fever. The patient often looks toxic. Pyopneumothorax, pneumothorax, empyema, and pneumatocele are common complications of *S. aureus.*

K. pneumoniae in children will present with gastroenteritis, neurologic signs, and explosive pulmonary symptoms. A child with *C. trachomatis* presents with conjunctivitis, tachypnea, and a staccato cough. *M. tuberculosis* pneumonia will present with anorexia, nocturnal cough, night sweats, and fever. *P. carinii* presents in the immunosuppressed patient as dyspnea, fever, tachycardia, cough, hypoxia, and cyanosis. A patient with Q fever can present with headache, fever, chills, chest pain, sore throat, and respiratory symptoms.

Examination

All children should be fully examined to rule out other sources of infection. Otitis media, sinus infections, gastroenteritis, meningitis, and bacteremia are all infections that can occur with pneumonia.

Remember that a patient with chest pathology, pneumonia, pericarditis, or pneumothorax can present with abdominal pain. Pneumonia is often misdiagnosed as an acute abdomen; therefore always get a chest x-ray as part of your work-up for an acute abdomen.

Diagnosis

A presumptive diagnosis of pneumonia is made by chest x-ray, the onset of symptoms, the patient's age, and the physical examination.

A definitive diagnosis is made after blood cultures, sputum cultures, purified protein derivative (PPD), or aspirations of sputum have been taken.

M. tuberculosis pneumonia is diagnosed by sputum culture or by gastric aspirate culture. A PPD skin test can be used as a screening test for family contacts.

P. carinii is diagnosed by lung aspirate or biopsy using methenamine silver nitrate stain. Coccidioidomycosis and histoplasmosis are diagnosed by complement fixation testing and skin tests. Q fever is diagnosed by complement fixation.

Laboratory Findings

A CBC with differential, blood cultures, and serum electrolytes (calcium, magnesium, and phosphorus) should be drawn. A urine culture should be performed if the child is younger than 2 years of age. An ABG should be taken if the child appears toxic, in respiratory distress, cyanotic, or has a history of apnea.

Sputum cultures should be obtained if possible, but they are usually contaminated by the normal oral flora. Tracheal suctioning via direct laryngoscopy is a reliable but difficult method to obtain cultures. Transtracheal aspiration is difficult to perform in children. The best method is direct aspiration by bronchoscopy with a brush border biopsy; however, this procedure is expensive and is dictated by the availability of equipment and experienced personnel to perform the procedure. In the critically ill immunocompromised child, direct needle lung aspiration should be considered. A patient with histoplasmosis will present with anemia on the CBC.

X-ray Findings

Group A streptococci will have a single or multiple infiltrates.

S. aureus on x-rays will show a segmental lobar infiltrate.

H. influenzae on a chest x-ray will show unilateral lobar consolidation.

S. pneumoniae will show lobar consolidation and patchy bronchopneumonia on a chest x-ray.

K. pneumoniae will have bulging fissures on x-ray.

C. trachomatis pneumonia will present with hyperexpansion on a chest x-ray.

M. tuberculosis pneumonia will have hilar adenopathy and apical findings on a chest x-ray.

P. carinii presents on x-ray as diffuse interstitial pneumonitis.

Coccidioidomycosis will show effusion, cavitations, and granulomas.

Histoplasmosis will show pulmonary calcification on a chest x-ray.

Treatment

Antibiotic therapy is usually based on the most likely organism suspected of causing the pneumonia for children in the patient's age group, x-ray findings, and positive blood or sputum cultures. The following children should be admitted to the hospital: any child younger than 3 months of age with pneumonia, any child who appears hypoxic or tachypneic, or any immunocompromised child with pneumonia.

Infants younger than 2 months of age with pneumonia (the major etiologies being *E. coli*, group B streptococci or *S. aureus*, or *C. trachomatis*) should be admitted to the hospital and started on ampicillin, 100 to 200 mg/kg/24 hr every 6 to 12 hours IV, and gentamicin, 5 to 7.5 mg/kg/24 hr every 8 to 12 hours IV.

Children 2 months to 8 years (the major etiologies being *S. aureus* [rare], *S. pneumoniae*, *H. influenzae*, or viral), who do not appear toxic and who have good follow-up care, can be placed on amoxicillin 30 to 50 mg/kg/24 hr every 8 hours PO; amoxicillin 50 mg/kg/24 hr every 8 hours PO; or cefaclor 40 mg/kg/24 hr every 6 hours PO. Some health care providers recommend ceftriaxone 50 mg/kg IM along with the PO amoxicillin before discharge. If the child is too ill to be discharged, ampicillin 100 to 200 mg/kg/24 hr every 4 hours IV or ceftriaxone 50 to 100 mg/kg/24 hr every 12 hours IV should be given. If there is a poor therapeutic response to the ampicillin or ceftriaxone, add nafcillin 100 mg/kg/24 hr every 4 hours.

For children older than 9 years of age (the major etiologies being viruses, *S. pneumoniae, Mycoplasma*, and rarely *H. influenzae*, group A streptococci, and *S. aureus*), give erythromycin 30 to 50 mg/kg/24 hr every 6 hours. Erythromycin/sulfisoxazole (Pediazole) 200 mg erythromycin/600 mg sulfisoxazole/5 ml, dose as 40 mg/kg of erythromycin and 120 mg of sulfisoxazole (per 24 hours given as a QID dose) PO can be used also. If the child is too ill to be discharged, admit the child and place the child on ampicillin 200 mg/kg/24 hr every 4 hours IV or ceftriaxone 50 to 100 mg/kg/24 hr every 12 hours IV. If there is a poor therapeutic response, add erythromycin PO or IV nafcillin. Q fever is usually self-limiting in 3 weeks and requires no antibiotic therapy.

Viral pneumonias do not require antibiotics, but if the patient is younger than 6 months of age or looks toxic, the patient should be admitted for fluid maintenance and fever control. Tuberculosis should be treated with appropriate medications for geographic region or current therapy for immunocompromised patients.

Children who are wheezing or are having reactive airway symptoms can be given nebulizer treatments with albuterol solution 0.5% at a dose of 0.03 ml/kg/dose with 2 ml NS every 20 minutes (given three times). If after three nebulizer treatments the child is still tachypneic or still has a low pulse oximetry reading (<92%), consider admitting the child to the hospital. Albuterol 2 mg/5 ml at 0.1 to 0.2 mg/kg/dose every 6 to 8 hours PO, with a maximum dose of 4 mg, can be given as outpatient therapy. Any child who appears to be tired of breathing should be admitted to the hospital. Intubation should be considered if on an ABG the patient's Po_2 reading is approximately 50% or the Pco_2 is almost 45%. Any child who has a pulse oximetry reading below 92% or is tachypneic should be placed on oxygen therapy.

Many children are dehydrated at the time of presentation to the ED due to pneumonia. A bolus of 20 ml/kg of NS and dextrose 5% can be given, and the child's response to fluid can be judged. If the patient is still tachycardiac after a fluid bolus, and not because of albuterol therapy, consider giving the child another fluid bolus and admitting the child to the hospital.

Patients or parents should be informed to return to their primary health care provider or the ED if the child is not afebrile or has not shown marked improvement in 48 hours. They should also be advised to return to the ED if a new onset of tachypnea, cyanosis, wheezing, costal retractions, high fever, difficulty breathing, trouble with taking medications, or apnea occurs.

PYLORIC STENOSIS

Definition

Pyloric stenosis is caused by hypertrophy and hyperplasia of the circular antral and pyloric musculature. This hypertrophic musculature causes a gastric outlet obstruction.

Epidemiology

Pyloric stenosis can occur from birth to 5 months and appears most commonly in males three to four times more often than in females. Pyloric stenosis occurs in 1 in 500 live births, and it has an increased occurrence in twins and in sons of fathers who had pyloric stenosis. Pyloric stenosis appears more often in first-born white males and most commonly occurs at the third or fourth week of life.

Clinical Presentation

Children will commonly present with gradual onset of vomiting at 3 to 4 weeks of life. The vomiting progresses to projectile vomiting, which is nonbilious emesis. Poor weight gain and weight loss will be present. The child will be hungry and will be easily re-fed. The child can be dehydrated. Constipation is common. Visible peristaltic waves may be noted and will travel from the left upper quadrant to the right upper quadrant. Twenty percent of the children will present with esophagogastritis and blood-tinged vomitus. Children can present with jaundice secondary to glucuronyl transferase deficiency.

Children can present with failure to thrive and neurologic sequelae. They can present with GI hemorrhage or perforation. Pyloric stenosis can mimic pylorospasm or antral webs. In pylorospasm, there will be no "string" sign on barium swallow. The elongated narrow pyloric canal is not present. No right upper quadrant "tumor" will be present.

In achalasia, the food is undigested when vomited. In annular pancreas, the vomitus contains bile.

Examination

On examination of the abdomen, a palpable olive-sized mass "tumor" can be felt in the right upper quadrant. It can be found just below the edge of the liver and lateral to the right rectus abdominis muscle. It is best located just after vomiting.

Laboratory Findings/Diagnosis

A CBC, electrolytes, LFTs, blood and urine cultures, and chest and abdominal x-rays should be performed. Hypochloremic alkalosis secondary to dehydration can be found. Elevated conjugated bilirubin can occur in 2 to 3% of patients presenting with pyloric stenosis. Hypokalemia is often present. The hemoglobin and hematocrit are often elevated secondary to the hemoconcentration.

Abdominal x-rays will show gastric dilatation. A barium swallow will show the classic "string" or "beak" sign. This sign is indicative of an elongated pyloric canal.

An abdominal ultrasound will show a hypoechoic ring in front of the right kidney and medial to the gallbladder.

Treatment

Treatment in the ED is based on a high index of suspicion. IV access should be obtained, and dehydration should be treated. Give D5W 0.9% NS 20 ml/kg during the first hour to treat the fluid deficit, and then maintenance fluid should be given. Check for hypernatremia or hypokalemia and treat the patient accordingly. Treat sepsis with antibiotics. Place a nasogastric (NG) tube, and decompress the stomach and bowel.

Consult a surgeon early on, and admit the child to the hospital. Pyloromyotomy is the procedure of choice for pyloric stenosis. There is usually an excellent outcome after surgery.

REYE'S SYNDROME

Definition

Reye's syndrome is an acute life-threatening illness that causes noninflammatory encephalopathy, hepatic dysfunction, altered level of consciousness, cerebral edema, with fatty metamorphosis of the viscera. It occurs in two phases. The first phase is the infectious phase, followed by the encephalopathic phase. Reye's syndrome was first described in 1963 and is poorly understood. There is a 10% mortality rate.

Epidemiology

Black urban infants and white suburban children are at the greatest risk for Reye's syndrome. Only 101 cases were reported in 1986. Reye's syndrome has been decreasing since 1981. It has occurred in epidemic proportions and sporadically. Reye's syndrome occurs in all ages, seasons, and geographical locations, but it usually affects young children. The average age is 7 years. It often follows a viral infection, chickenpox, or influenza illness. The use of aspirin or salicylates has been implicated as a precipitating factor in Reye's syndrome.

A Reye-like syndrome has also been suggested when there are defects in urea and fatty acid metabolism. It is suggested that a Reye-like syndrome is caused by toxicologic injury with impaired gluconeogenesis. Reye's syndrome has been described as a five-stage disease by the National Institutes of Health in 1981.* With regard to the diagnosis of Reye's syndrome, the Centers for Disease Control and Prevention (CDC) have stated that "there must be no more reasonable" explanation for the hepatic and cerebral dysfunction.

Pathology

Viruses, toxins, metabolic disorders, genetic predisposition, and interactions between toxins and viruses have all been proposed as causes of Reye's syndrome. No matter what the cause, there are pathologic changes in the liver. There is mitochondrial damage throughout the body. The liver will have a diffuse microvesicular accumulation of lipids without inflammation or necrosis. There can also be an accumulation of lipids in the skeletal muscle, kidneys, and myocardium. The brain will have ultrastructural abnormalities and cerebral edema. As the liver fails, hepatic encephalopathy occurs despite normal or falling ammonia levels.

Clinical Presentation/Examination

The child will present with a history of respiratory or GI symptoms for 2 to 3 days. Within 24 to 48 hours, vomiting will occur. This is the infectious phase. Soon after vomiting starts, the encephalopathic phase occurs. Behavioral changes, delirium, combativeness, disorientation, and hallucinations will occur. The more change in mental status, the greater will be the increase in cerebral edema and intracranial pressure. Finally, coma will ensue. The five stages that occur are:

Stage 0: Alert and awake

Stage I: Lethargic, with normal posture, brisk pupillary light

---

*From the National Institutes of Health Consensus Conference: Diagnosis and treatment of Reye's syndrome. JAMA 246:2441, 1981.

reflex, normal oculocephalic reflex, and the patient will follow verbal commands.

Stage II: The patient will progress to combativeness and inappropriate verbalization. The patient will have normal posturing but will be stuporous, with a purposeful or nonpurposeful response to pain, sluggish pupillary reaction, and conjugate deviation on doll's eyes maneuver.

Stage III: The patient will progress to decorticate posturing, decorticate response to pain, sluggish pupillary reaction, conjugate deviation on doll's eyes maneuver, and will be comatose.

Stage IV: The patient will be comatose in stage IV. Decerebrate posturing and decerebrate response to pain, sluggish pupillary reaction, and inconsistent or absent oculocephalic reflexes occur.

Stage V: The patient will proceed to flaccid paralysis. The patient will be comatose and will have no response to pain, no pupillary response, and no oculocephalic reflex.

Pancreatitis and hepatomegaly may also be present in any stage of Reye's syndrome. Children can progress to respiratory failure, herniation secondary to cerebral edema, and can die of cardiac dysrhythmias.

A Reye-like syndrome can also present with many of the same symptoms as Reye's syndrome. These symptoms are nonspecific in presentation and diagnosis.

Diagnosis

All other possibilities should be ruled out before the diagnosis of Reye's syndrome is made. The possibility of hypoglycemia, electrolyte abnormalities, infections, and trauma should be addressed. A liver biopsy is recommended to demonstrate characteristic changes; however, these changes are not pathognomonic of Reye's syndrome.

Laboratory Findings

An ABG should be obtained. It will often show metabolic acidosis and respiratory alkalosis. BUN and creatinine should be followed to manage fluid volume status and renal status. A CBC will not be very helpful. A serum amylase and lipase should be obtained to detect possible pancreatitis. Serum and urine ketones should be drawn. Salicylate and acetaminophen levels should be drawn acutely if Reye's syndrome is suspected and ingestion of salicylates is suspected.

The ammonia level is usually three times the normal level. The ALT and aspartate aminotransferase (AST) are universally elevated. The PT is usually prolonged. Bilirubin can be normal or elevated. A lumbar puncture is recommended to rule out other possibilities of altered mental status and infection. To meet the diagnosis of Reye's syndrome, the CSF must have less than 9 WBC mm³. Increased opening pressures are present. A small needle should be used, and only the smallest amount of CSF should be withdrawn secondary to the possibility of increased pressure and the risk of herniation. A CT scan is recommended to rule out other possibilities of altered mental status.

Treatment

The treatment of Reye's syndrome is generally supportive, and particular attention should be paid to electrolyte and fluid support. Serum glucose should be kept between 125 and 175 mg/dl. Serum osmolality should be kept below 310 mOsm/kg of water. Recommended IV fluids are D10W or D20W. Arterial and venous pressures should be monitored. A urinary catheter should be placed to monitor urine output at 1 ml/kg/hr.

If seizures are present, a loading dose of phenytoin, 10 to 20 mg/kg/dose over 30 minutes, and a maintenance dose of 5 mg/kg/24 hr every 6 hours should be administered.

If the PT and PTT are prolonged and coagulation abnormalities are present, give:

1. Fresh frozen plasma 10 ml/kg/dose every 12 to 24 hours IV or as needed
2. Vitamin K, 1 to 10 mg/dose IV slowly
3. An exchange transfusion as indicated

Intracranial monitoring will be needed as the patient's mental status deteriorates and intracranial pressure increases. This treatment should be in consultation with a neurosurgeon. Intracranial pressure should be maintained below 15 to 18 mm Hg. If intracranial pressure is elevated above 20 mm Hg, mannitol should be given at 0.25 to 0.5 g/kg/dose IV over 20 minutes. Serum osmolality should be kept below 210 mOsm/kg of water. Hyperventilation should be used to decrease intracranial pressure by keeping the $PaCO_2$ below 25 mm Hg. Furosemide, 1 to 2 mg/kg/dose every 4 to 6 hours can also be used to decrease intracranial pressure.

The child should be intubated and placed in a barbiturate coma for 2 to 3 days while intracranial pressure is monitored using:

1. Pancuronium, 0.05 to 0.1 mg/kg/dose every 1 to 2 hours or PRN
2. Pentobarbital 3 to 20 mg/kg IV slowly. Keep the infusion rate at 1 to 2 mg/kg/hr for a maintenance level of 25 to 40 µg/dl.

ACUTE RHEUMATIC FEVER

Definition

Rheumatic fever is caused by a group A streptococcal infection. If left untreated it can cause carditis, valvulitis, or polyarthritis.

Epidemiology

Rheumatic fever is a disease in transition. It has declined significantly during the last 50 years secondary to penicillin therapy. It presents between the ages of 6 and 15 years of age in the United States. It is more prevalent in inner city blacks and is more common in girls than in boys. Approximately 0.3% of untreated children will acquire rheumatic fever. In North America, the attack rate is less than 1 in 10,000.

Pathology

Group A β-hemolytic streptococcal infection from the respiratory tract infection is the essential trigger that predisposes an individual to rheumatic fever. After colonization of the pharynx by group A streptococci, the B lymphocytes are sensitized by streptococcal antigens. There are formations of antistreptococcal antibodies. These formations cause immune complexes that cross-react with cardiac sarcolemma antigens, causing myocardial and valvular inflammation.

Clinical Presentation

Children can present in many ways. They can present looking fairly well or toxic in appearance. They can present with back, abdominal, or precordial pain. Vomiting, epistaxis, malaise, weight loss, or anemia can all be present. Erythema multiforme can be a presenting complaint. A prior sore throat in the past 3 weeks that was not treated is an important element of history to be obtained.

Examination

The entire child should be examined. Look for petechiae on the soft palate and exudates on the tonsils. Look for hepatosplenomegaly or enlarged lymph nodes.

Diagnosis

Rheumatic fever is diagnosed by the Jones criteria. Two major criteria or one major criterion and two minor criteria must be met for the diagnosis of rheumatic fever to be made.

Major Criteria

1. Carditis: A valvulitis will be present that is diagnosed as a new murmur. Tachycardia out of proportion to fever will be present. Pericarditis or CHF can be present. The aortic or mitral valves are the most common valves involved.
2. Polyarthritis: Two or more joints must be involved. The knees, wrists, ankles, and elbows are the most commonly involved. They will present with redness, swelling, and severe pain and

will be hot to touch. The arthritis can last for 4 weeks but responds dramatically to salicylates.
3. Sydenham's chorea: Emotional lability with involuntary motor movements can last for several months or can be self-limiting.
4. Erythema marginatum: This ringed eruption spreads rapidly, forming serpiginous or wavy lines over the trunk and extremities. This rash does not blanch and is not pruritic or indurated.
5. Subcutaneous nodules: These nodes will be hard and painless and will vary in size. They will most often be seen in patients with carditis. They will most often be seen over the spine, scalp, and overlying joints.

Minor Criteria

1. Arthralgia, pain in one or more joints without evidence of inflammation.
2. Fever above 39.4° to 40° C (103° to 104° F)
3. ECG changes; prolongation of the PR interval.
4. Elevated acute-phase reactants (ESR or C-reactive protein) in a patient with polyarthritis or acute carditis.
5. Supportive evidence of group A streptococcal infection; antistreptolysin O (ASO) titer, Todd of at least 240 units in adults or 320 units in children.

Laboratory Findings

A CBC, blood culture, urine culture, ESR, and C-reactive protein tests should be obtained. ASO, antihyaluronidase (AH), antistreptokinase (ASK), and antinicotinamide-adenine dinucleotidase (ANA-Dase) should be obtained. A throat culture should be obtained. An ECG and a chest x-ray should also be obtained.

Treatment

1. To treat an acute episode of rheumatic fever, give benzathine and procaine penicillin or PO penicillin V. Penicillin V 25,000 to 50,000 units/kg/24 hr every 6 hours PO for 10 days or benzathine penicillin G as follows:

<30 lb	300,000	300,000:100,000
31 to 60 lb	600,000	600,000:200,000
61 to 90 lb	900,000	900,000:300,000
>90 lb	1,200,000	

2. If cardiac status is compromised, give digoxin and treat CHF with furosemide, 1 mg/kg/dose IV.
3. The best anti-inflammatory agent is aspirin in a dose of 30 to 60 mg/dose four times a day (QID). Aspirin often gives the patient dramatic relief from arthritis and fever. The salicylate level should be maintained between 20 and 30 mg/dl.

4. Corticosteroids are rarely indicated; however, if they are needed, use prednisone 2 mg/kg/day. Use corticosteroids for patients who have severe carditis and CHF. Give 2 mg/kg/day for the first week, then decrease the dose to 1 mg/kg/day during the second week. Start aspirin at 50 mg/kg/day, and taper the dose of prednisone over the next 2 weeks.
5. Treat chorea with haloperidol 0.01 to 0.03 mg/kg/24 hr every 6 hours in children PO, adults 2 to 5 mg/24 hr every 8 hours.
6. Strict bed rest is required for acute episodes followed by gradual ambulation.
7. Give prophylactic antibiotics oral penicillin VK 200,000 to 250,000 units every 12 hours for 3 to 4 weeks or benzathine penicillin 1,200,000 units every 3 weeks. Patients with cardiac involvement or initial chorea should receive penicillin indefinitely. Patients who have no cardiac involvement should receive prophylactic antibiotics for at least 5 years to prevent endocarditis.

SEIZURES AND STATUS EPILEPTICUS IN CHILDREN

Definition

A seizure or convulsion is an episodic, paroxysmal disturbance in motor activity, behavior, sensation, or psychic or autonomic function. A seizure is a physiologic abnormality that occurs suddenly with excessive electrical discharge of gray matter neurons and that propagates down the white matter neuronal processes and affects end organs. The International Classification of Epileptic Seizures is used to classify seizures types:

Partial seizures (seizures beginning locally)
1. Partial seizures with elementary symptomatology (generally without impairment of consciousness)
   a. With motor symptoms (includes jacksonian seizures)
   b. With special sensory or somatosensory symptoms
   c. With autonomic symptoms
   d. Compound forms
2. Partial seizures with complex symptomatology (generally with impairment of consciousness)
   a. With impairment of consciousness
   b. With cognitive symptomatology
   c. With affective symptomatology
   d. With "psychosensory" symptomatology
   e. With "psychomotor" symptomatology
3. Partial seizures secondarily generalized
Generalized seizures (bilaterally symmetric without local onset)
1. Absence (petit mal)
2. Bilateral massive epileptic myoclonus

3. Infantile spasms
4. Clonic seizures
5. Tonic seizures
6. Tonic-clonic seizures (grand mal)
7. Atonic seizures
8. Akinetic seizures

Unclassified epileptic seizures

Status epilepticus is seizure activity that lasts longer than 30 minutes and is repeated so often or is so prolonged that it creates a fixed and lasting epileptic condition. In a primary generalized grand-mal status epilepticus, the seizure can be of a tonic-clonic, myoclonic, or clonic-tonic status. In secondary generalized convulsive status epilepticus, the seizure can be either tonic or tonic-clonic status with partial onset. Both primary and secondary status epilepticus can be continuous or noncontinuous. Status epilepticus can also present as simple partial status, complex partial, or absence status seizures.

Many toxic substances can cause seizures. Aspirin, lead, cocaine withdrawal, theophylline, anticholinergics (e.g., phenothiazines) or tricyclic overdose, carbon monoxide, propoxyphene, alcohol, and withdrawal of seizure medication can all cause seizures.

In children, the most common neoplasm is a glioma. The supratentorial lesion is most likely to cause seizures. Vascular intracranial hematomas, cerebral, subarachnoid, or extradural, can all cause seizures. Embolism, hypertensive encephalopathy, and transient ischemic attacks can also cause seizures in children.

Degenerative and deficiency disorders such as Tay-Sachs disease, juvenile Huntington's chorea, pyridoxine deficiency, and metachromatic leukodystrophy can all present as seizures in children.

Epidemiology

Up to 73% of first seizures are idiopathic. Idiopathic seizures recurred in 17% of children within 20 months of the first seizure and 26% of the children will have another seizure within 36 months. There is an increased occurrence in siblings who have had seizures. There is also a higher incidence of a recurrence in children who have generalized spike waves on electroencephalograms (EEGs).

Pathology

Seizures can have many etiologies. From birth to 6 months, hyperglycemia, hypoglycemia, trauma at birth, hypoxia, drugs, infection, hypocalcemia, hyponatremia, hypernatremia, inborn error of metabolism, intracranial hemorrhage, pyridoxine deficiency, and illicit drug withdrawal secondary to use by the mother are the main causes of seizure activity. From 6 months to 3 years, febrile seizure, trauma, infection, toxic ingestion, metabolic disorders, cerebral degeneration disorders, and birth injury are the most common causes of seizure activity. In children older than 3 years of age, infection, trauma, cerebral degeneration disease, and idiopathic problems are the most common causes of seizure activity.

In a child with a fever, febrile seizure, meningitis, encephalitis, and intracranial abscess are the most common causes of seizures. Infectious diarrhea, such as with *Shigella*, or pertussis, tetanus, or DPT immunizations can also cause fever and thus seizure activity.

Endocrine causes such as phenylketonuria (PKU), uremia, and amino and organic acidemias can cause seizure activity. Hypoglycemia or hyperglycemia in any age group, DKA, or new onset of diabetes can cause seizure. Hyponatremia or hypernatremia caused by the parents giving tap water while trying to rehydrate a child who has vomiting and diarrhea can cause seizures and altered mental status.

Infantile spasms occur between 3 and 9 months of age. The onset is sudden. The child will have a very brief spasm of flexion or extension of the head and trunk that lasts for seconds. Spasms will come in bursts of 5 to 20 spasms. The child will present with a history of regressive development, and mental retardation can be as high as 85%. Spasms will occur after a sudden auditory or physical stimulation or upon awaking from sleep. Metabolic disorders, trauma, infection, and vitamin B_6 deficiency have all been related to infantile spasms. The EEG will be abnormal.

Clinical Presentation

Different kinds of seizures will present with different symptoms. The key to diagnosis is to take a good history from the parent or from someone who witnessed the seizure.

Absence (petit mal) seizures usually last only a few seconds. There are very brief lapses in awareness that are often associated with rhythmic eye blinking, head dropping, or just staring ahead. Absence seizures are often noted by the child's teacher while in the classroom.

Complex partial or psychomotor seizures are of two types: (1) temporal lobe seizures that impair consciousness, and (2) those that are generalized. In complex partial seizures, there is usually an "aura" before the onset of the seizure. Hallucinations or an alteration in perception can occur.

Patients who have partial seizure will have no loss of consciousness and can present in many ways. They can present with a jacksonian march presentation. They can present with somatosensory complaints, such as a different taste in the mouth or a severe headache. They can present with déjà vu or autonomic sweating, rhinorrhea, or flushing. Generalized seizures will present with specific movement patterns.

Juvenile myoclonic epilepsy presents with early morning neck, head, and arm myoclonus tonic-clonic or absence seizure activity. Benign rolandic epilepsy involves hemifacial seizures and a simple partial seizure. The onset is from 3 to 13 years. It usually resolves by the age of 16 years.

Examination

All children should be given a complete examination, including a complete neurologic examination. Particular attention should be made to ensure that no evidence of trauma is present. Vital signs, including attention to fever, should be taken. Look for asymmetry in your examination. Ask about premature birth history, complications at the time of birth, perinatal asphyxia, or if there is a family history or a history of siblings having seizures or febrile seizures.

Diagnosis

A diagnosis is made by history, physical examination, and ancillary data.

Laboratory Findings

Upon presentation to the ED, a blood glucose determination must be made. A CBC with differential, UA, and complete electrolytes with special attention to sodium and potassium levels should be obtained. If the child is febrile, a lumbar puncture should be performed for a Gram's stain and cultures. A blood culture should also be obtained. If there is an abnormal neurologic finding or a history of trauma, a CT scan of the head should be performed. Aspirin, acetaminophen, phenytoin, valproate, theophylline, lead, cocaine, and toxicologic levels should be drawn as indicated. A chest x-ray should be performed if indicated.

Treatment

If the child is actively seizing, oxygen, dextrose, and anticonvulsants should be administered. Metabolic abnormalities should be addressed as needed. Seizures after trauma require an immediate CT scan of the head and a neurosurgical consultation. If meningitis or infectious etiology is suspected, antibiotics should be administered.

If a child presents to the ED in status epilepticus, perform the following steps:

1. Establish an airway and administer oxygen.
2. Obtain an IV access.
3. Administer an IV bolus of 25% glucose, 2 ml/kg.
4. Obtain blood for a CBC, calcium, electrolytes, blood culture, BUN, and creatinine.
5. If the child is actively seizing give:
   a. Diazepam 0.2 mg/kg IV, with a maximum dose of 5 mg for infants up to 2 years of age, and 10 mg for infants over 2 years of age. The dose can be repeated three times. Give 1 mg/min and watch for respiratory depression. Doses of up to 2.6 mg/kg have been established as safe. Diazepam is the drug of choice in status grand mal seizures. Tonic-clonic generalized

seizures respond very well to diazepam. Noncontinuous clonic or tonic-clonic seizures are refractory to diazepam, *or*

b. Lorazepam, 0.05 mg/kg IV, with a maximum dose of 0.2 mg/kg, can be repeated twice. Give over 2 minutes. Lorazepam has a slower onset of action and has a longer duration than does diazepam.

6. If the child is still seizing after a trial of diazepam or lorazepam, give phenytoin 15 mg/kg at a rate of 25 mg/min.

7. If the child is still in status epilepticus, give phenobarbital 10 to 15 mg/kg IV slowly.

8. If the child is still in status after lorazepam, diazepam, phenytoin, and phenobarbital, give paraldehyde 0.3 ml/kg rectally mixed with mineral oil. Paraldehyde should only be administered using glass syringes and rubber tubing secondary to degradation into toxic formations by certain plastics.

9. If still in status epilepticus, give IV lidocaine 2 mg/kg.

10. Give clonazepam (Klonopin) via an NG tube, 0.2 to 0.6 mg/kg as a single dose.

11. If the child is still in status epilepticus, consult an anesthesiologist for general anesthesia.

The treatment for infantile spasms is early diagnosis and aggressive treatment with adrenocorticotropic hormone (ACTH). These children should be admitted to the hospital and should have a consultation with a pediatric neurologist.

Juvenile myoclonic epilepsy is treated with valproate with good results. Benign rolandic epilepsy is treated with phenytoin or carbamazepine. Absence seizures are treated with valproate or ethosuximide.

Side Effects of Seizure Medications

Phenytoin has a narrow serum level concentration. Toxicity occurs above 25 μg/ml. Nausea, diplopia, dysarthria, and impaired level of conciousness can occur. Ataxia and lethargy can occur. When phenytoin is given IV, there can be burning of the limb at the IV site. Chronic phenytoin use can cause folate deficiency, peripheral neuropathy, lupus-like syndrome, myasthenic weakness, and macrocytic anemia. Phenytoin levels are reduced when used with valproic acid.

Valproic acid (Depakene) can cause hepatic failure, vomiting, behavioral changes, and increased lethargy. GI side effects are common. Pancreatitis has also been reported.

The use of the antibiotic erythromycin with theophylline and carbamazepines can cause a toxic rise in the levels of these medications. Clonazepam and diazepam can cause bladder dysfunction. Choreic movements can occur after use of ethosuximide or carbamazepines. These movements can be relieved by the use of diphenhydramine (Benadryl), 12.5 to 25 mg IV.

If the child is already on anticonvulsive medications and the child has a "breakthrough seizure" secondary to noncompliance of medications, viral or bacterial infections, change in sleep habits, new job, emotional stress, or use of alcohol or illicit drugs assume that the anticonvulsant level is low. Give the patient a partial loading dose of the current medication. If the patient is compliant and this fact is verified by the parent, give the child his or her daily dose of phenobarbital or phenytoin. If the patient is noncompliant or blood levels are low, give a dose that is twice the normal daily dose. Give the normal daily dose if the child seizes, and repeat the second dose no matter what the serum level is.

Children are usually placed on anticonvulsant medication for 2 years. If after 2 years the child has been seizure free, an attempt is made to discontinue the medication.

SUDDEN INFANT DEATH SYNDROME

Definition

Sudden infant death syndrome (SIDS) is defined as a sudden unexpected death of an infant under the age of 1 year for which no postmortem examination or pathologic cause can explain the sudden death of the infant. There are more than 70 theories as to what causes SIDS.

Epidemiology

SIDS occurs in nearly 10,000 infants each year (2 per 1000 live births). It is the leading cause of death in children between the ages of 1 month and 1 year. The peak ages for SIDS is between 2½ months and 4 months. Thirty to 50% of children have an acute infection, usually an acute upper respiratory infection (URI). Respiratory syncytial virus, otitis media, and gastroenteritis have all been associated with SIDS. SIDS has a higher incidence in the winter. There is a higher incidence of male to female deaths if there is acute infection, and there is no sexual disparity if no infectious cause is found on autopsy. Native American infants have the highest death rate for SIDS (5.93 per 1000), and Asian American children have the lowest death rate (0.51 per 1000). Twins of a SIDS victim possibly have a 20-fold increased risk of SIDS. There are four groups of children who are at increased risk for a SIDS event:

1. Previous life-threatening episode of apnea (actual life-threatening event [ALTE])
2. Low birth rate or premature delivery
3. Family history of a brother or sister who has died of SIDS
4. Children whose mothers have abusive histories or have used illicit drugs

The diagnosis of SIDS is made on autopsy.

Pathology

Apnea is believed to be the central cause of SIDS. Apnea causes hypoxia, which leads to respiratory failure. Arrhythmias and cardiac arrest, secondary to hypoxia, are a terminal event in the SIDS process. Wolff-Parkinson-White syndrome is a rare arrhythmia in SIDS. On autopsy, brain stem gliosis is the only regularly reported finding. Smooth muscle thickening in the small pulmonary arteries, hematopoiesis in the liver, increased periadrenal brown fat, right ventricular hypertrophy, and abnormalities of the carotid bodies are all signs of chronic hypoxemia on autopsy.

The association of ALTE with SIDS is not clearly defined. Possible depressed ventilatory response to CO_2 breathing, prolonged sleep apnea, obstructive apnea, hypoventilation with chronic hypoxemia, mixed obstructive and central apnea, immaturity, lead injury, infections, primary failure of respiratory center control, abnormal response of peripheral chemoreceptors to hypercarbia and hypoxia, and dive reflex could all be contributing factors in SIDS.

Clinical Presentation

Children can present to the ED in complete cardiopulmonary arrest or looking completely well. The history of events prior to presentation is very important in the diagnosis of SIDS.

Seizures can present with what the parents describe as "stiffening" or "jerking," which are really signs of tonic or clonic movements. The complaint of "stopped breathing" could be associated with a postictal apnea event. With a seizure, an infant is usually awake before becoming apneic.

If a history of feeding just prior to the event is given, gastroesophageal reflux or aspiration should be considered to be the cause of the apneic event. Pertussis should be considered in the young infant if the history of a URI is given. Sepsis, infantile botulism (especially with a history of ingestion of honey is given), cardiomegaly, and hypoglycemia can all present with seizure or what can look like a postictal apneic event.

The history of CPR is important. If no resuscitation was performed, and the child looks well, this was probably not an ALTE or SIDS event. If mouth-to-mouth resuscitation was needed to revive the infant, re-evaluate the infant to ensure that the infant has been fully resuscitated. Signs of incomplete resuscitation include poor muscle tone, poor motor response to pain, bradycardia (bradycardia is usually a terminal event in infants), abnormal skin color, and shallow or slow breathing rate. The infant should be resuscitated vigorously and should be given high-flow oxygen. Remember that an infant usually has a young, very healthy heart and can be resuscitated after prolonged apnea.

Examination

The child should be fully examined. Care should be taken to note signs of physical abuse. Long bone fractures, bruising, trauma around the head and orbits on funduscopic examination (to look for hemorrhages secondary to shaken child syndrome signs), or poor hygiene should all be clues of physical abuse. Münchausen by proxy should be considered if a history is inconsistent or bizarre, or if injury is unexplainable by history.

Diagnosis

A diagnosis of SIDS is one of exclusion. All children with a suspected ALTE event should be admitted to the hospital and placed on apnea monitoring until all possible causes of the apneic event are ruled out. Polysomnography testing to measure air flow in the mouth and nose can detect obstructive apnea. Pneumograms can detect abnormalities related to periodic breathing and episodes of apnea.

Laboratory Findings

CBC, serum electrolytes, calcium, magnesium, phosphate, blood cultures, CSF, urine culture, ECG, and chest x-ray should all be performed. Stool samples for botulinum toxin testing and clostridial cultures should be taken. Lead levels should be considered if appropriate by examination or by history. X-rays of long bones should be taken if trauma is suspected. A CT scan or x-rays of the skull should be performed if a head injury is considered.

Treatment/Prevention

The use of home apnea monitoring is the cornerstone of treatment. There are three groups of infants in which the National Institutes of Health and Consensus Statement of 1986 believe that the use of home monitoring would decrease the incidence of death.

1. Group 1: term infants with unexplained apnea of infancy, usually manifested by a life-threatening episode or an abnormal pneumogram. A normal pneumogram does not preclude the use of a monitor.
2. Group 2: a preterm infant who has continued to manifest apnea beyond term (40 weeks after conception).
3. Group 3: subsequent siblings of two or more SIDS victims, but not of one SIDS victim.

Children with known respiratory disease such as bronchopulmonary dysplasia and infants who require a tracheostomy or who are oxygen-dependent at home are also candidates for monitoring.

Parents of a SIDS victim will have enormous grief about the loss of their child. They should be referred for counseling. The National Foundation for Sudden Infant Death Syndrome, 101 Broadway, New York, New York 10036 can provide information to the practitioner or family members about SIDS.

TETRALOGY OF FALLOT

Definition

Tetralogy of Fallot is caused by a severe obstruction to right ventricular outflow secondary to a ventricular septal defect. This intracardiac shunt is predominantly from right to left. The term tetralogy of Fallot is used to describe both right ventricular infundibular level obstruction and valvular level obstruction associated with right ventricular hypertrophy and an overriding aorta.

Epidemiology

Tetraology of Fallot is the most common type of cyanotic heart disease and accounts for 10 to 15% of cyanotic heart disease.

Pathology

The ventricular septal defect is usually located in the membranous portion of the septum and may be totally surrounded by muscular tissue. This obstruction may be at the right ventricular infundibular area (50 to 74%) or at the valvular level (rarely) or both places (25%). The aorta is often overriding secondary to the presence of a large septal defect causing a dilatation of the aorta. These three factors—right ventricular hypertrophy with overriding aorta with a large septal defect—cause tetralogy of Fallot.

The right-to-left shunt caused by these lesions causes cyanosis. The larger the shunt, the more the arterial blood will be desaturated. The larger the obstruction, the larger the ventricular septal defect, the lower the systemic vascular resistance will be and the greater the right-to-left shunt. The key to this lesion/disease (and thus the tetralogy) is the hemodynamics of the shunt. As long as the right ventricular pressure does not exceed the left ventricular pressure, oxygenated blood will be perfused. The left side of the heart is usually quite able to maintain this pressure without causing heart failure.

Clinical Presentation

Clinical symptoms of tetralogy of Fallot depend on the severity of the disease. A patient with mild disease will present with mild cyanotic or acyanotic events. A patient with minimal disease, previously undiagnosed, can present with CHF. Children with severe disease can present with cyanosis at birth. Most children will have cyanosis by 4 months of age. These children will present with failure to thrive (FTT) and growth retardation with dyspnea and tire easily. Older children who can walk can present with a parent's initial complaint of the child "squatting" when he plays hard.

Children will often present with sudden onset of cyanosis or worsening cyanosis, sudden onset of dyspnea, change in consciousness, from increased irritability to a true syncopal episode. The classic systolic murmur will decrease or completely disappear during a cyanotic episode.

Examination

The child should be given a complete examination. The oxygen level should be measured by a pulse oximetry device. Look for clubbing of the fingers and toes. The child will usually be thin, small, and pale or cyanotic. There will be a right ventricular lift, but no thrill will be present. There will be an ejection click at the apex of the heart. The first heart sound will be normal. The second heart sound will be heard best at the left lower sternal border at the third and fourth intercostal spaces. There will be a rough grade I to III/VI systolic ejection murmur heard best at the left sternal border at the third intercostal space. This murmur can radiate to the anterior and posterior lung fields.

Diagnosis

A diagnosis is made by echocardiography, cardiac catheterization, and angiocardiography. An echocardiogram will show thickening of the right ventricular wall and an overriding aorta with a membranous ventricular septal defect or obstruction at the infundibular area and pulmonary valves.

Cardiac catheterization and cineangiocardiography are the definitive tests. Usually pulmonary artery pressure is low at 5 to 10 mm Hg. Cineangiocardiography is diagnostic. The injection into the right ventricle will show a right ventricular outflow obstruction.

Laboratory/X-ray Findings

A CBC, electrolytes, ABG, ECG, and chest x-ray should be obtained. The hematocrit, hemoglobin, and red blood cell count are mildly elevated. The chest x-ray will usually show a normal heart size in most cases. The right ventricle sometimes will show hypertrophy and, on the posteroanterior x-ray, the apex will be "upturning" (boot-shaped). The pulmonary artery will usually be concave, and the aortic arch (25%) will arch to the right.

The ECG will show an axis to the right +90 to +180 degrees. There might be some right atrial hypertrophy shown by P wave changes.

Treatment

1. The initial treatment of tetralogy of Fallot is to place the child in the knee-chest "fetal" position and administer oxygen.
2. If acidosis is present, give IV sodium bicarbonate.
3. Give morphine 0.1 to 0.2 mg/kg IV.
4. Give propranolol 1 mg/kg PO every 4 hours.
5. Early surgical and pediatric consultation is indicated for surgical correction.

THE ABUSED CHILD

Definition

Child abuse or nonaccidental trauma (NAT) occurs in over 1 million children each year in the United States. Emergency health care providers are frequently the first persons to see the abused child. There are three kinds of abuse: (1) child neglect, (2) sexual abuse, and (3) physical abuse. Münchausen by proxy is another type of physical abuse in which the child is kept ill by the parent to draw attention or sympathy to the parent.

Child neglect is when the parent or guardian fails to provide basic physical and emotional needs for the child. It usually occurs in children younger than 3 years of age. If neglect is from birth, the child can present with FTT syndrome.

Environmentally neglected children over the age of 2 to 3 years are called psychosocial dwarfs. They will present with short stature and low weight. They manifest a triad of a disturbed home situation, short stature, and bizarre voracious appetite. Psychosocial dwarfs often have low to normal growth hormone.

Sexual abuse can present to the ED in many different ways. Fifteen percent of sexual abuse victims present to the ED with unrelated complaints. Presentations can include excessive masturbation, vaginal discharge, vaginal bleeding, genital fondling, encopresis, nightmares, UTI, regression, and provocative behavior.

It is the norm for the child to reveal the abuse after a significant time lapse from the event of abuse or the onset of abuse. More than 90% of sexual abuse is repetitive, and the assailant is known to the child and family.

Physical abuse encompasses a large spectrum of intentional trauma. One third of abused children are younger than 6 months of age, and two thirds of these children are under 3 years of age. Signs of physical abuse include a history of trauma that does not correlate with the type of injury or the mechanism of injury that the parent describes. A history that changes over time is suspect for abuse when the mechanism of injury is in question. The patient's delayed presentation to the ED after injury should bring into question abuse.

A knowledge of childhood developmental stages is necessary for evaluating child abuse. Children younger than 6 months of age cannot ingest drugs in significant quantities by themselves to cause poisoning. The milestones of rolling over, sitting up, standing, and walking must be taken into consideration when evaluating the mechanism of injury and the age of the child.

It is important to take into consideration who is the primary child care provider, who brought the child to the ED, and the concern of the parent over the injury. Is the parent intoxicated or does the parent appear to be abusing drugs? Always ask the child, if appropriate for age, what happened and enter the child's explanation into the medical record.

Epidemiology

It is estimated that six infants per 1000 live births are abused during their childhood. An estimated 500 per 1 million children are abused annually in the United States. One fourth of all girls and one sixth of all boys are sexually abused during their childhood. Ten percent of all injured children seen in the ED have injuries sustained secondary to child abuse. Five percent of children will die of future child abuse who visit the ED, and 35% will suffer serious injury in the future.

Clinical Presentation

Neglected and malnourished children will present with protruding ribs and very little subcutaneous tissue, and the skin will hang loosely from the buttocks. Muscle tone will also be increased, particularly in the lower extremities, and infants may present with scissoring positioning. The child will present to the ED with physical signs of long-standing malnutrition. Hygiene will be poor, skin rashes may be present, and diaper dermatitis can also be present.

Children who present with FTT will be wide-eyed and will turn away with close eye contact. FTT children will be hard to console and will refuse cuddling. These children prefer to be left alone and will keep their hands in their mouths. They will lie in the "straphanger's position," i.e., with their arms flexed at the elbows and extended over their shoulders. They prefer inanimate objects.

In sexually abused children the physical examination can be quite difficult. The genitalia and perianal areas should be inspected. A speculum examination is usually not required unless vaginal trauma is suspected. The frog-leg position is the best position for examining the genitalia and perianal area in children. Look for bruising, abrasions, and lacerations. Toluidine blue dye applied to the genitalia can increase the likelihood of detecting subtle injuries.

The knowledge of the normal anatomy for the particular age group for a female patient is of the utmost importance. The female genitalia normally change with age. Prepubescent females have a thin, small labia minora and a full labia majora. The hymen is reddish-orange and thin-edged and covers the vagina. The hymen will change as the child grows older. During infancy, the hymen is thick. From infancy to puberty, it is thin, smooth-edged, and annular or crescent shaped. The hymen should be examined for trauma or notches. An indentation at the 6 o'clock position is suggestive of penetration trauma. White areas or swirling vascularity are signs of scarring. Redness can be a sign of inflammation, irritation, or chronic manipulation and is not necessarily a sign of abuse. Signs of venereal disease, vaginal discharge, and condylomata lata or acuminata should be noted. Anal penetration is often easier than vaginal penetration in the young female; therefore do not focus on the vagina alone.

The sexual abuse examination on males is even more difficult than on females. Rarely are there bite marks on the male genitalia. The perianal area should be examined for fissures, lacerations, loose sphincter tone, abrasions, hematomas, skin tags, or discharge. Look for changes in the anal rugae, thickening, or thinning.

Don't forget to examine the oropharyngeal area. Consider orogenital contact in all suspected sexually abused children. Look for exudate, trauma, lip lacerations, and bruising in and around the mouth.

If venereal disease is considered, culture the oropharnyx, anus, and penis or cervix/vagina.

The examination of the physically abused child is based on the knowledge of childhood milestones. Children who are learning to walk will have numerous bruises on the shins, forehead, and bony prominences. If bruising is found over multiple areas of the body in different stages of bruising, physical abuse must be considered. Linear bruising from light cords, belts, or buckles should be suspected. Bruising can be aged. Knowledge of the color of aging of bruising can verify the age of the injury. Within 1 to 2 days, a bruise will have a reddish-blue color. In 5 to 7 days, the bruise will turn green. At 7 to 10 days, the bruise will turn yellow, and between 10 and 14 days the bruise will turn brown.

Children who live in one-parent families, or in families where a live-in boyfriend is present, or a household where known alcohol or drug abuse is present are at increased risk for abuse. Children who are in the toilet-training age group are at increased risk for "punishment" after accidents.

Often abuse will take the form of forced feeding the infant. Look in the mouth for lacerations of the frenulum or lacerations of the oral mucosa. If present, consider trauma secondary to forced feeding if the presenting complaint includes poor feeding and "the baby cries all the time."

If head injury or "shaken child syndrome" is suspected, do a good funduscopic examination and check for retinal hemorrhages, lens dislocation, hyphema, or retinal detachment.

Examine the skin for burns. If circular burns to the hands, feet, or buttocks are present, suspect that the child's hands have been placed on the stove burner as punishment. If the burns are in the stocking-glove presentation, suspect that the child's hand or leg has been placed in hot water and held there. If the child is made to sit in hot water, the lower extremities will be drawn up into the fetal position. The genitalia will be burned, and horizontal burn marks will be present on the thighs. The knees will be spared, and the feet will be burned.

Laboratory Findings

Laboratory tests are guided by the suspected trauma and physical examination. A CBC, PT, PTT, liver function tests, amylase, and lipase should be drawn in the case of suspected abdominal trauma. An SMA-7, calcium, magnesium, and phosphorus test should also be included in the laboratory work-up. A urinalysis should be performed to rule out kidney contusion or trauma. If "shaken child syndrome" is suspected or if head injury is considered, a CT scan or MRI should be included in the tests.

Plain film x-rays of long bones should be performed as indicated. Remember that spiral fractures are caused by a twisting motion. If the history is not consistent with a twisting injury and a spiral fracture is noted, suspect physical abuse. Metaphyseal chip fractures in children younger than 6 months of age are indicative of inflicted injury. If physical abuse is considered, a trauma series of x-rays should be performed. Look for multiple periosteal elevation, indicating several healing fractures in different stages of healing. An abdominal series of x-rays should be included if abdominal trauma is suspected. Look for the "double-bubble" sign that is indicative of duodenal hematoma.

Interaction with Parent or Guardian

The interaction between the child and parent or guardian and the health care provider can give numerous clues in suspected child abuse cases. Be suspicious of a parent who hesitates to share the mechanism of injury with the health care provider; a parent who refuses x-rays or tests; or a parent who is not supportive of the child or the health care provider. Suspicion should also be raised in the case of a parent who ignores major injuries and addresses minor complaints or if a parent or guardian expresses the feeling of "losing control" of the child or is overwhelmed by the child's behavior. These statements should be regarded as very serious "cries for help."

Treatment

Physical injuries should be addressed first. If child abuse is suspected, do not be judgmental. Know your state laws regarding the reportability of child abuse, because you could be held accountable for future injuries if suspected abuse is not reported. In most states, physical and sexual abuse along with neglect must be reported to the police and social work services. When in doubt report suspected abuse, consult a pediatrician, and have the child admitted to the hospital for a "cooling off period." This will ensure the child's safety and allow the police and social work service to perform the necessary investigation. Always place the child's safety above all other concerns.

THE CHILD WITH DIABETES MELLITUS AND DIABETIC KETOACIDOSIS

Definition

There are two types of diabetes. The onset of type I, insulin-dependent diabetes mellitus (IDDM) or juvenile diabetes is at a young age, and the onset of type 2 or noninsulin-dependent diabetes is usually in adulthood.

DKA in the diabetic child can be caused by a viral or bacterial infection, emotional or environmental stresses, drugs, change in diet, trauma, or surgery.

Epidemiology

The onset of diabetes before the age of 20 reduces life expectancy by one third. The incidence of IDDM affects 1 in 300 children. The mean onset is at 12½ years of age for males and at 11 years of age for females. Males and females are equally affected and present more commonly in the summer and winter. DKA accounts for approximately 14 to 31% of hospital admissions (160,000 per year) for diabetes. The mortality rate is approximately 15%.

Pathology

Epstein-Barr virus, rubella, CMV, mumps, and coxsackievirus have all been implicated in the cause of type I diabetes. Type I diabetes is believed to be an autoimmune disease. It is believed that circulating islet-cell antibodies and autoreactive T lymphocytes cause an autoimmune reaction that causes the destruction of pancreatic insulin-secreting beta cells. HLA-DR3 and HLA-DR4 are present in 90% of patients with diabetes. HLA-B7 and HLA-DR2 seem to have protective properties from diabetes.

DKA is caused by a relative lack of insulin secondary to an increased activity of the counterregulatory hormone glucagon. Glucose rises, glucagon is mobilized, and muscle breakdown with proteolysis occurs. Free fatty acids increase, and amino acid levels increase. Acetoacetate and beta-hydroxybutyrate and ketone bodies increase secondary to muscle breakdown, causing metabolic acidosis and ketosis. Hyperglycemia causes an increase in serum osmolality and thus osmotic diuresis and dehydration. This diuresis causes an increased loss in sodium, phosphate, and potassium. The liver produces acetoacetate and beta-hydroxybutyrate (both of which are organic acids), thus causing ketoacidosis. This acidosis causes respiratory alkalosis and, therefore, a compensatory increased respiratory rate or Kussmaul respirations. Cardiac depression or collapse can occur secondary to volume depletion or arrhythmias secondary to metabolic acidosis.

Clinical Presentation

The classic triad of polyuria, polydipsia, and hunger should alert the health care provider to the possible diagnosis of diabetes. The diagnosis of DKA should be suspected in any patient who presents with hyperventilation, acetone-smelling breath, polydipsia, polyuria, lethargy, abdominal pain, and vomiting. In children younger than 2 years of age, sepsis can mimic DKA.

Children can present with cerebral edema with 8 to 12 hours

of onset of DKA. Seizures can be a presenting complaint. Visual disturbances, weight loss, weakness, anorexia, altered mental status, ileus, muscle cramps, and arrhythmias can also be presenting complaints.

Laboratory Findings

Hyponatremia secondary to urinary loss can be present. Sodium can be artificially depressed secondary to hyperglycemia or hyperlipidemia. True serum sodium can be estimated by:

Corrected serum Na$^+$ (mEq/l) = measured serum Na$^+$ (mEq/l)
+ (plasma glucose [mg/dl] − 100) × 0.016.

There is usually a total body potassium deficit, and the serum potassium may be normal. The serum potassium will increase 0.5 mEq/l for each decrease of 0.1 in pH. The BUN is usually elevated.

Glucose is elevated above 300 mg/dl with glucosuria. If serum glucose is above 100 mg/dl, serum osmolarity should be evaluated. The measurement of serum ketones is not of very much clinical value in DKA. Serum ketones measure serum acetoacetate not beta-hydroxybutyrate. Beta-hydroxybutyrate is in a ratio of 3:1 to acetoacetate.

There is a renal threshold of 180 mg/dl of glucose. Any glucose level above 180 mg/dl will produce glucosuria.

The WBC count and amylase will usually be elevated. A blood culture should be taken to rule out sepsis, and a throat culture and urine culture should also be obtained. Glycosylated hemoglobin can be used as a measurement of the degree of long-term control.

Treatment

1. In children with DKA, fluid replacement is of the utmost importance. Fluid deficit is usually from 100 to 150 ml/kg. Give 20 ml/kg over the first hour. If the patient is in shock, give a repeated bolus of fluid at 20 ml/kg until shock is corrected. Use 0.45% NaCl as a bolus solution and maintenance fluid until the serum glucose is less than 250 mg/dl, then change to D5W, 0.45% NaCl. Do not correct the fluid deficit too quickly or cerebral edema will occur. The total water deficit should be corrected, as follows, over a 24-hour period: a 20 ml/kg bolus of fluid over the first hour; then, one half of the deficit fluids plus one third of the maintenance fluids from the 1st to 9th hours of fluid replacement; and one half of the fluid deficit plus two thirds of the maintenance fluid over the last 9 to 24 hours.
   a. If pH is below 7.0 or HCO$_3$ is below 10 mEq/l, sodium bicarbonate 1 to 2 mEq/kg can be added over 30 minutes to 0.45% CaCl as an IV fluid.
   b. Potassium should be added to the infusion solution secondary to total body deficit. If the pH is less than 7.10, replacement should begin immediately. Hypokalemia exacerbates as the pH

improves. If the potassium level is greater than 6.0, do not give potassium until iatrogenic hypercalcemia is ruled out. Potassium phosphate 20 mg/l or potassium chloride 20 mEq/l can be utilized. Forty milliequivalents of KCl can be added to each liter of fluid.

2. Laboratory data, including a CBC, electrolytes, calcium, phosphorus, magnesium, BUN, creatinine, blood culture, UA with culture, throat culture if indicated, chest x-ray if indicated, and serum ketones, should be drawn if an IV is started. A lumbar puncture should be performed if indicated.

3. Insulin should be given IV. Regular insulin, 50 units, should be mixed with 250 ml of 0.9% NS (0.2 units/ml), and an infusion rate of 0.1 to 0.2 units/kg/hr should be started. A 50-ml flush should be performed through the tubing before the infusion is started. There is controversy as to whether a bolus should be administered. If a bolus of insulin is given, give the bolus at 0.1 units/kg IV. Insulin can also be given IM at a dose of 0.1 to 0.2 units/kg/hr. Glucose should fall between 50 and 100 mg/dl/hr. The insulin infusion should be continued until the serum glucose reaches 250 mg/dl or the pH is above 7.30. The IV solution should be changed to D5W 0.45% CaCl when the serum glucose falls below 250 mg/dl. When glucose is below 250 mg/dl and the pH is above 7.30, short-acting SQ NPH insulin can be started 1 hour before IV insulin is stopped. SQ insulin at a dose of 0.25 to 0.5 units/kg every 4 to 6 hours should be administered for the change from IV to SQ insulin.

4. If cerebral edema occurs, death ensues in 90% of the cases. The patient should be intubated and hyperventilated, and mannitol, 1 to 2 g/kg, should be administered. A fluid restriction should be instituted. A slow correction of metabolic derangements and fluid deficits should be undertaken.

UPPER RESPIRATORY EMERGENCIES IN PEDIATRICS

Definition

Stridor is the physical sign of upper airway obstruction. It can be inspiratory, biphasic, or expiratory. Stridor is a type of wheezing that is a continuous sound originating from the airway. Wheezing is usually referred to as isolated expiratory stridor, and stridor proper is referred as inspiratory noises.

Inspiratory stridor is caused by an obstruction *above* the larynx. Expiratory stridor is caused by an obstruction *below* the carina. Biphasic stridor is heard in both the inspiratory and expiration phases of breathing and is a sign of obstruction *in* the trachea. The common URI infection is the main cause of stridor in the pediatric population.

Pathology/Epidemiology

Causes of stridor can be divided into those that cause stridor in children younger than 6 months of age and those that cause stridor in children older than 6 months of age. Congenital causes such as congenital vocal cord paralysis, vascular rings, laryngomalacia, laryngeal or tracheal webs, cysts or tumors, or ectopic thyroid or thyroglossal duct cysts are the major causes of stridor in children younger than 6 months of age.

Viral croup, epiglottitis, and aspiration of a foreign body are the major causes of stridor in the age group older than 6 months of age. Retropharyngeal abscesses, diphtheria, tetanus, esophageal foreign bodies, tetany, trauma, tumors, and gastroesophageal reflux can all cause stridor.

Epiglottitis is usually caused by *H. influenzae* and affects children in the 2- to 7-year age group. Gram-positive cocci are also a common cause of epiglottitis.

Viral croup is usually caused by a parainfluenza virus. Severe croup is usually more common in boys than in girls. Bacterial tracheitis is a severe form of croup caused by *S. aureus.* Spasmodic or allergic croup is caused by allergies.

Foreign bodies will present clinically with an acute upper airway obstruction. Bronchial foreign bodies will produce a less acute course than do laryngotracheal foreign bodies. Nuts, seeds, grapes, hard candy, raisins, or sausage-shaped meats like hot dogs or carrots can be easily aspirated by children. Objects that are 32 mm or less are more likely to be aspirated and completely obstruct the airway. Children from birth to 48 months are at the highest risk of aspiration, and children from 1 to 2 years of age are at the peak age group for aspiration. Bronchial foreign bodies will present in four ways:

1. A bypass valve, which produces a partial obstruction to both inflow and outflow with decreased aeration on the affected side.
2. A check valve, in which air is inhaled, but not expelled, causes emphysema.
3. A ball valve, in which the foreign body is dislodged during expiration and is resealed against the bronchi during inspiration, causes atelectasis.
4. A stop valve allows no air to be inhaled, thus resulting in distal atelectasis.

Examination/Clinical Presentation

The child's pulse, respiration rate, blood pressure, temperature, and pulse oximetry should be measured. Normal respiratory rates for children are:

Newborns, 40 to 50 breaths/min
At 1 year, 30 to 35 breaths/min
At 4 years, 20 to 25 breaths/min
At 8 to 10 years, 12 to 15 breaths/min

The skin should be evaluated for cyanosis. The nail beds should be evaluated for capillary refill. A capillary refill time of less than 2 seconds is a sign of hypoxia. Cyanosis is determined by the hemoglobin concentration and the peripheral circulation of the child. Cyanosis in a black infant may be difficult to determine; use the capillary refill test and look at the mucous membranes for cyanosis. Cyanosis is always a late finding. Tachypnea, nasal flaring, intercostal retractions, ancillary muscle use, and subdiaphragmatic and supraclavicular retractions are all signs of respiratory distress and are probably better indicators of respiratory distress than the respiratory rate alone. Tachypnea is also seen in cardiac disease, diabetic ketoacidosis, and salicylate intoxication.

Determine if the child has been coughing or grunting or has (or had) stridor. Children under the age of 6 months do not cough. In a child with a cough, *Chlamydia* pneumonia, pertussis, or cystic fibrosis should be included in the differential diagnosis. If the child is grunting, the respiratory disease is usually located in the lower respiratory tract. Grunting is caused by a delay in the closure of the glottis during expiration. It is the child's attempt to cause positive end-expiratory pressure secondary to lower respiratory tract disease. Grunting is specific for lower respiratory tract disease and correlates with the severity of the disease.

Stridor correlates with an upper respiratory tract obstruction. Stridor occurs early in the disease process and correlates with the severity of the disease. Children with asthma, pneumonia, or bronchiolitis do not usually have stridor unless there is another cause of the stridor.

Take a history of the onset and duration of stridor. Did the onset of stridor occur rapidly or slowly over weeks or months? The slower the onset, the more likely that the stridor is of a congenital nature, especially if the child is younger than 6 months of age. Laryngomalacia is the most common cause of stridor in children younger than 6 months of age. It is caused by the collapse of a weak larynx during inspiration. This condition usually resolves in 6 to 12 months without treatment.

The rapid onset of stridor in children older than 6 months of age is caused by epiglottitis, viral croup, foreign body aspiration, or retropharyngeal abscesses.

In epiglottitis, there is an abrupt onset of stridor over several hours. There will usually be a high fever, sore throat, the classic sign of drooling, and inability to swallow oral secretions. Stridor is of late onset. The child will sit very still in the parent's lap, will appear toxic, ashen-gray, anxious looking, and very apprehensive. The child will sit in the parent's lap with the neck extended, chin up, and in the classic "sniffing" position. There is usually no history of a cough. Viral croup will present with a cough. Children with epiglottitis will present without cough. True epiglottitis is a medical emergency.

Viral croup with URI symptoms will usually occur over a 2- to 3-day period. The cough worsens over 2 to 3 days and is worse at night. The cough sounds like the "barking of a seal." Dyspnea, stridor, and anxiety can occur. Croup can be differentiated from epiglottitis by the slow onset over days of symptoms: a barking cough that is worse at night and the absence of apprehension and drooling. Chest and lateral neck x-rays are usually not necessary to make the diagnosis of croup. In severe croup and when a PA chest x-ray is taken, the tracheal air column will be in the form of a "steeple" instead of the "square shoulder" appearance of the tracheal air column on a normal chest x-ray.

Children with foreign body airway obstruction will present with an acute obstruction. They can have cyanosis, apnea, stridor, wheezing, dysphonia, cough, or facial petechiae secondary to increased intrathoracic pressure. At least one component of the triad of wheezing, coughing, and decreased breath sounds is not present in 61% of acute airway obstructions. Dysrhythmias are a late result of foreign body obstruction and are secondary to hypoxia.

Chest x-rays can help to determine not only the type of object that was aspirated but also its location. Flat, round objects (e.g., coins) will lie in the frontal plane on an PA x-ray, if they are in the esophagus. Flat, round objects will lie in the sagittal plane and will appear end-on-end if they are in the trachea, due to the cartilaginous rings of the trachea. They will appear flat on the lateral view if they are in the trachea. Inspiratory and expiratory chest x-rays should also be taken. If there is a bronchial obstruction, where a "check valve" obstruction is present, upon expiration the obstructed lung will not deflate. If there is a "stop valve" obstruction upon inspiration, no air will go into the obstructed lung. In a "ball valve" obstruction, the lung fields will be equal on expiration and unequal on inspiration. A "bypass valve" obstruction will have both decreased inflow and outflow signs on an x-ray.

Laboratory Findings

In epiglottitis or bacterial tracheitis, a CBC, electrolytes, ABG, blood cultures, UA, and chest x-ray should be performed.

Treatment

In epiglottitis, the child should be taken to the operating room after consultation with an anesthetist and an eye, ear, nose, and throat (EENT) specialist. After administration of anesthesia, the patient's airway is examined with a laryngoscope, and the patient is intubated if epiglottitis is diagnosed. If an examination in the operating room by laryngoscope cannot be performed, a portable lateral neck x-ray can be performed to diagnose an enlarged epiglottis. The x-ray should be taken on inspiration, because the retropharyngeal space normally opens during expiration.

Four areas of the lateral x-ray should be examined. The epiglottis is located at C2–C3 in children rather than at C5–C6 in adults.

1. The epiglottis is normally tall and thin, projecting up into the hypopharynx. In epiglottitis, the epiglottis will appear as a thumb print, squat and flat at the base of the hypopharynx.
2. The retropharyngeal or prevertebral space is usually 3 to 4 mm wide. Any tissue swelling more than 3 to 4 mm is suspect for epiglottitis.
3. The tracheal air column should be the same size in its entire length. If there are densities in the air column, suspect foreign bodies or epiglottitis.
4. The normal hypopharynx will distend proximal to the point of an obstruction. This distention is indicative of an upper respiratory tract obstruction.

There is controversy in regard to an attempt at direct visualization of the epiglottis in the ED. If direct visualization is attempted in the ED, experienced intubation personnel should be readily available with anesthesia and an ENT consultation.

High-flow oxygen should be given without causing increased anxiety; usually high-flow "blow-by" oxygen will increase oxygenation. The child will usually not tolerate a mask over the face. The airway cart should be readily available for rapid intubation. The child *must not be left alone* until the diagnosis of epiglottitis is ruled out. If the airway is obstructed and the child becomes apneic, the child can be bagged effectively. Emergency surgical airway should not be performed unless absolutely necessary. There is a higher morbidity rate in patients in whom a tracheostomy is performed. A good bagging technique can effectively ventilate almost any child with epiglottitis.

Cefotaxime 50 to 150 mg/kg/24 hr every 6 to 8 hours IV or ceftriaxone 50 to 75 mg/kg/24 hr every 12 hours IV or cefuroxime 100 to 150 mg/kg/24 hr every 6 to 8 hours IV are the drugs of choice due to the resistance of *H. influenzae* to ampicillin. Steroids are not indicated in epiglottitis.

Viral croup is treated by cool mist and PO or IV rehydration. Oxygen is usually not necessary in the treatment of viral croup. A child who has stridor at rest should be hospitalized. Racemic epinephrine can be used in the management of croup patients. Racemic epinephrine as a diluted 2.25% solution can be used in the following doses:

- \>20 kg, 0.25 ml in 2.5 ml NS as nebulizer treatment every 2 hours
- 20 to 40 kg, 0.5 ml NS as nebulizer treatment every 2 hours
- Above 40 kg, 0.75 ml NS as nebulizer treatment every 2 hours

Racemic epinephrine will last for 4 hours. It is also a bronchodilator and can cause a "rebound" stridor. Antibiotics are not needed because of the viral etiology of croup. Steroids usually shorten the course of croup, but controversy still exists regarding their use. Dexamethasone (Decadron) 0.6 mg/kg/dose IV, IM, or PO can be given every 6 to 12 hours for one to four doses. If, after treatment in the ED with racemic epinephrine and dexamethasone, the child is asymptomatic for 4 to 8 hours and the child has a good follow-up examination, the child can be discharged from the ED.

The patient with bacterial tracheitis will have more respiratory distress and will have purulent secretions. That patient will need to be admitted to the hospital and will require intubation and antibiotics.

Spasmodic or allergic croup is treated with racemic epinephrine as mentioned earlier. Spasmodic croup has a rapid onset and is rapidly resolved with treatments of racemic epinephrine. Children with spasmodic or allergic croup usually need further nebulizer treatments of racemic epinephrine and will require hospitalization for further treatment with humidified air and hydration.

Treatment of foreign body airway obstruction should be based on the patient's oxygen saturation level and on the clinical presentation of the patient. Shock, respiratory or cardiac arrest, or hypoxia should be treated appropriately. Remember that the primary cause of anxiety, altered mental status, and apprehension is hypoxia! If you suspect that your patient has a foreign body obstruction and is getting apprehensive, check the patient's pulse oximetry for the blood oxygen concentration. The guidelines of the American Heart Association for clearing the airway blocked by a foreign object should be utilized. Back blows and manual abdominal thrusts appropriate for age should be utilized. In infants younger than 12 months of age, five back blows are used to attempt to dislodge the foreign body. If five back blows are not successful, then five chest thrusts should be performed. Repeat this sequence as necessary. In older children, the Heimlich maneuver can be utilized.

Blind probing for foreign bodies can cause the object to be pushed further into the trachea; therefore this procedure is discouraged. If the foreign body can be seen, Magill forceps or Kelly clamps may be utilized to remove the object. The use of a laryngoscope with a pair of Magill forceps or Kelly clamps can be used to remove distal foreign objects in the trachea.

Bronchoscopy should be performed on all patients who present with symptomatic airway obstruction. If bronchoscopy is not immediately available and the patient is in severe respiratory distress, a cricothyroidotomy should be performed.

Any patient with a foreign body with significant hypoxia or other complications should be admitted to the hospital until definitive bronchoscopy is performed.

URINARY TRACT INFECTIONS IN CHILDREN

Definition

UTIs in children can indicate an infection or can be a warning sign of significant pathophysiologic disease. Pyelonephritis is an associated infection of the kidneys.

Epidemiology

There can occur significant morbidity, including renal insufficiency and hypertension in later years related to poorly or untreated UTIs in children. Most damage occurs before 5 years of age. Children younger than 3 months have a 1% rate of bacteriuria. If the child is febrile (>38.1° C), the incidence of UTI increases tenfold, from 7 to 17%. In this age group, males are three times more likely to have a UTI than are girls. The incidence of a male with a UTI is 80 to 90% more likely in uncircumcised males. In children younger than 3 months, the incidence of sepsis with a UTI is 10 to 35%.

After the age of 3 months, female children have a higher rate of UTIs than do males. The chance of a UTI in females after 3 months of age is 3 to 5%.

Untreated UTIs can lead to sepsis, bacteremia, renal failure secondary to recurrent pyelonephritis, perinephric abscess, and urolithiasis.

The risk of recurrence after the first infection is 30%. After three infections, the recurrence rate rises to 75%.

Pathology

The normal flora of the GI tract and rectal and perineal areas are the major causes of UTIs in children. *E. coli* (90%), *Klebsiella, S. aureus, S. epidermidis,* and enteric streptococci are the major organisms that cause UTIs. Recurrent infections in children present with enterococci, *Pseudomonas,* and *Proteus* organisms as their cause.

Clinical Presentation

The clinical presentation of children with a UTI is often confusing and nonspecific. A high index of suspicion is required when evaluating children for a UTI. Children will present with different complaints at different ages. Children can present asymptomatic, with fever, vomiting, irritability, diarrhea, FTT, feeding problems, incontinence (dribbling), enuresis, dysuria, frequency constipation, fussiness, crying, abdominal pain, back pain, flank pain, and vulvovaginitis.

Sexual activity should be documented. If sexual or physical abuse is questionable, address the issue appropriately. Males with UTIs have a higher risk of anatomic abnormalities. Neonates can present with hypothermia or fever, cyanosis, jaundice, or feeding poorly. Vomiting, fever, diarrhea, and poor feeding are often presenting complaints for infants. Older children present with adult-presenting complaints, e.g., dysuria, urgency, frequency, lower abdominal pain, vomiting, and enuresis.

Any patient who presents with chills, high fever, and costovertebral angle tenderness or pain should be considered to have pyelonephritis. Obtain a prior history of UTIs and surgical anatomic abnormality corrections.

Examination

The child should be totally examined secondary to the vague and often confusing presenting complaints. Sepsis, bacteremia, acute appendicitis, surgical abdomen, and meningitis should rank high on the differential diagnosis when evaluating a child with a UTI.

The evaluation of a child after his or her first UTI is somewhat controversial. A radiologic evaluation of the urinary tract should be performed 4 to 6 weeks after infection in the following cases. Every male should be evaluated after his first UTI secondary to the higher risk of a physical anomaly. Females should be evaluated after their second UTI. Any child who presents with pyelonephritis or clinical or laboratory signs of renal disease or elevated BUN or creatinine should have further evaluation. The type of evaluation is also controversial. The most recommended evaluation is the voiding cystourethrogram (VCUG), which detects reflux in males. In females, the nuclear cystogram is also used. If these tests are negative, often a renal ultrasound is used to evaluate renal size, the possibility of obstruction pathology, and the vesicoureteral junction for deformity or obstruction. No further studies are required if these studies are normal. If an obstruction is still considered, an IVP can be ordered. If the VCUG shows abnormalities, both a renal ultrasound and an IVP should be ordered.

Diagnosis

Urine culture is the gold standard for diagnosis of UTIs and antibiotic treatment choices. *N. gonorrhoeae, C. trachomatis, Trichomonas,* pinworms, chemical vaginitis, and viral, mycobacterial, and fungal agents can all cause pyuria. Sterile pyuria in adolescent boys is highly suggestive of sexually transmitted urethritis, and the urethra should be cultured for *N. gonorrhoeae* and *C. trachomatis.* If sexual abuse is considered, remember to also culture the oral pharynx and the rectum for the aforementioned organisms and consult a pediatrician, social work services, and the police.

Laboratory Findings

The urine culture is the gold standard for UTIs. It can be obtained via a suprapubic tap, catheterization, clean catch midstream into a cup, or bag catch. Catheterization is the most desirable way to obtain urine, because there is less contamination of the urine. All urine should be cultured in 30 minutes or refrigerated. Pyuria is present if more than 5 WBC/hpf are present on a UA. Numerous causes of pyuria include pelvic infections, dehydration, renal tuberculosis, trauma, appendicitis, gastroenteritis, bubble bath, masturbation, irritation, and oral polio vaccine. Positive nitrate in the urine is pathognomonic for a UTI. Leukocyte esterase, when WBCs are present, correlates with a UTI.

If the child appears ill, febrile, and younger than 6 months of age, a CBC, electrolytes, BUN, and creatinine should be ordered. If the child appears septic or younger than 6 months of age or if pyelonephritis is considered, a blood culture should be obtained.

1. A midstream clean catch is positive if there are 10^5 colonies of a single organism per milliliter of urine. Colonies between 10^4 and 10^5 are uninterpretable.
2. In a catheterized urine or a suprapubic specimen, the presence of 10^3 colonies per milliliter of catheterized urine is positive for infection.

Treatment

All children with a suspected UTI should have a urine culture obtained before treatment. Any child with suspected pyelonephritis, bacteremia, sepsis, or urolithiasis should be admitted to the hospital. Any child who cannot keep fluid down or is immunocompromised or dehydrated or has had previous renal disease should be admitted to the hospital. Any child under 3 months of age with a UTI should be admitted to the hospital. A simple uncomplicated UTI, with or without fever, which is treated on an outpatient basis, must have a follow-up in 48 hours to access the results of the urine culture.

Uncomplicated lower UTIs can be treated with:

1. Amoxicillin 40 to 50 mg/kg/24 hr every 8 hours PO for 5 to 7 days
2. Sulfisoxazole (Gantrisin) 120 to 150 mg/kg/24 hr every 6 hours PO for 5 to 7 days
3. Trimethoprim and sulfamethoxazole (Septra) 8 mg trimethoprim and 40 mg sulfamethoxazole/kg/24 hr every 12 hours (1 tsp for every 10 kg BID) PO
4. Cephalexin (Keflex) 25 to 50 mg/kg/24 hr every 6 hours PO

If the child is diagnosed with pyelonephritis give amoxicillin, sulfamethoxazole, or sulfisoxazole along with gentamicin or tobramycin 5 to 7.5 mg/kg/24 hr every 8 to 12 hours IM or IV.

If urgency, dysuria, or frequency is present, you can give phenazopyridine (Pyridium) 12 mg/kg/24 hr every 8 hours for 1 to 3 days, with a maximum dose of 200 mg/dose.

All children should return in 14 days for a follow-up UA and culture.

BIBLIOGRAPHY

Avery ME, First LR (eds): Pediatric Medicine, 2nd ed. Baltimore, Williams & Wilkins, 1994
Brandenburg RO, Fuster V, Giuliani ER, et al (eds): Cardiology Fundamentals and Practice. Chicago, Year Book Medical Publishers, 1987
Hamilton GC, Sanders AB, Strange GR, et al (eds): Emergency Medicine: An Approach to Clinical Problem-Solving. Philadelphia, WB Saunders, 1991

Hathaway WE, Groothuis JR, Hay WW (eds): Current Pediatric Diagnosis and Treatment, 10th ed. Norwalk, CT, Appleton & Lange, 1991

Kravis TC, Warner CG, Jacobs LM (eds): Emergency Medicine: A Comprehensive Review, 3rd ed. New York, Raven Press, 1993

May HL, Aghababian RV, Fleisher GR (eds): Emergency Medicine, 2nd ed. Boston, Little, Brown, 1992

Oski FA, DeAngelis IM, Feigin RD (eds): Principles and Practice of Pediatrics. Philadelphia, JB Lippincott, 1990

Schwartz GR, Cayton CG, Manglesen MA, et al (eds): Principles and Practice of Emergency Medicine, 3rd ed. Philadelphia, Lea & Febiger, 1992

Tierney LM, McPhee SJ, Papadakis MA (eds): Current Medical Diagnosis and Treatment, 33rd ed. Norwalk, CT, Appleton & Lange, 1994

Chapter **14**

Psychiatric Emergencies

ANXIETY DISORDERS AND PANIC ATTACKS

Definition

A patient presenting to the emergency department (ED) with an anxiety or panic attack is very common. Panic disorders are a subcategory of anxiety disorder. Anxiety disorders can include agoraphobia, which involves a fear of places or situations from which escape or assistance is believed to be difficult or embarrassing. Many medical conditions can mimic anxiety disorders. The primary cause of anxiety in the ED is hypoxia. Never assume that anyone who is anxious is just suffering from an anxiety attack.

The *Diagnostic and Statistical Manual of Mental Disorders-Revised (DSM-IV-R)* divides anxiety into eight different categories:

1. Panic disorder with avoidance (agoraphobia)
2. Panic disorder without agoraphobia
3. Agoraphobia without a prior history of panic disorder
4. Simple phobia
5. Obsessive-compulsive neurosis
6. Post-traumatic stress syndrome
7. Generalized anxiety disorder
8. Anxiety disorder not otherwise specified

Epidemiology

Anxiety disorders affect as many as 13 million persons in the United States. Generalized anxiety disorders affect 2.5/100 persons; phobic disorders affect 1.4/100 persons; panic disorders affect 0.4/100 persons. There is a high failure to diagnose anxiety disorders, and thus as many as 75% are untreated.

Clinical Presentation

Several behavioral and social factors produce or exacerbate the anxiety disorder. A patient with an anxiety disorder usually presents before 45 years of age, and there is a high incidence of first-degree relatives with anxiety disorders.

Generalized anxiety disorders result in excessive anxiety secondary to two or more life circumstances in at least 6 months. The patient presents with motor tension, autonomic hyperactivity or vigilance, and scanning. There is often associated mild depression. There is usually only mild occupational or social impairment.

True panic disorders present in the early phase with brief intermittent episodes of panic lasting for less than 10 minutes. Patients present with symptoms of numbness, dizziness, difficulty breathing, and heart palpitations with somatic complaints of tachypnea, tachycardia, and chest tightness.

Agoraphobia is believed to occur after repeated panic attacks due to associated situations. It is believed that patients with panic disorders suffer from noradrenergic and serotonergic system abnormalities.

Social phobia is a fear of social situations in which an individual is humiliated by the scrutiny of others. If the fear is great, it can affect the person's occupational and social interaction. When the person is exposed to phobic stimuli, severe anxiety develops. Social phobia is more common in males than in females and usually presents in late childhood.

Simple phobia is a persistent fear of a single stimulus. Common fears involve dogs, cats, spiders, or snakes. As long as the phobic stimulus is avoided, there is no anxiety.

Obsessive-compulsive neurosis is manifested by persistent, repetitive thoughts, ideas, impulses, or obsessions that cause distress to an individual, consume a person's time, or interfere with a person's normal daily function. This disorder is chronic and develops in early childhood in both sexes. Often there is an associated major depressive disorder that complicates the disorder.

Post-traumatic stress disorder is a result of a severe traumatic stress, secondary to a stress that is out of the range of normal human experience. The patient will avoid any stimulus that represents the initial trauma, which would cause the patient to relive the experience. The patient will often complain of "flashbacks," recurrent nightmares, headaches, decreased responsiveness to others, difficulty sleeping, impulsive behavior, and emotional lability. There is also a degree of substance abuse associated with post-traumatic stress disorder.

Treatment

Treatment of any anxiety disorder begins with taking a good history. Signs of organic disease must be interpreted correctly and addressed. The ED health care provider must assume that there is an organic basis for the panic attack. Respiratory, cardiovascular, dietary, neurologic, drug-related, hematologic, and immunologic causes and secreting tumors can all cause anxiety.

Management of the patient who has an acute panic attack includes treatment of the patient's hyperventilation by reassuring the patient that hyperventilation is not life threatening. Encourage the patient to control his or her breathing. If this does not work, the drugs of choice are the benzodiazepines: alprazolam (Xanax), chlordiazepoxide (Librium), clorazepate (Tranxene), diazepam (Valium), lorazepam (Ativan), flurazepam (Dalmane), oxazepam (Serax), midazolam (Versed), temazepam (Restoril), or triazolam (Halcion). These drugs can all be used to treat anxiety disorders. No patient should be given refills or a supply of any benzodiazepine medication for more than a few days, secondary to the risk of suicidal gestures or attempts, the high rate of dependency, and the need for continuity of care with the primary care physician. All patients with an anxiety disorder should be referred for follow-up psychiatric care.

CONVERSION REACTIONS

Definition

Conversion reactions are common in the young adult. For the diagnosis of a conversion reaction to be made, five criteria must be met:

1. There must be a loss of physical function, suggesting a physical disorder.
2. The patient has undergone a recent psychological stressor or conflict.
3. The patient unconsciously produces the symptoms.
4. The symptoms cannot be explained by a known organic etiology.
5. The symptoms are not limited to pain or to sexual dysfunction.

Pathology

Conversion reactions are secondary to a psychically unacceptable urge to avoid a required action. The symptoms persist until the patient allows expression of the urge without consciously confronting the feeling that led to the wish. The symptom often has a symbolic relationship to the conflict, but this is not always present. Conversion reactions are nonverbal responses to stress in an attempt to control the patient's environment.

Two mechanisms are responsible for the occurrence of the symptoms. "Primary gain" allows the patient to avoid confronting uncomfortable feelings, and "secondary gain" involves avoidance of uncomfortable situations. Support is given by others that might not usually be given for the patient's situation.

Clinical Presentation

Conversion reactions are quite rare but usually occur with neurologic or orthopedic complaints. Conversion reactions are often seen in military conflicts, industrial accidents, and in victims of violence. These reactions occur most commonly in early adulthood and adolescence and are more common in the less educated, rural, and lower socioeconomic populations. Up to 21% of those with a conversion reaction have a dependent personality. Often there is an associated schizophrenia, borderline personality disorder, depressed state, and passive aggressive personality disorder.

Patients with conversion reactions present with symptoms of paralysis, aphonia, seizures, akinesia, coordination disturbances, dyskinesia, tunnel vision or blindness, anesthesia, anosmia, or paresthesia.

Pseudoseizures present as an associated diagnosis in 10 to 20% of the cases. Often the patient is indifferent to his or her condition.

Examination

The physical examination includes the motor drop test, the Bowlus and Cirrier test, the yes-no test, the stretch reflex test, the thigh adduction test, the Hoover test, and the sternomastoid test to help rule in or rule out a conversion reaction. In an awake patient, the corneal reflex will remain intact. In a patient in a true coma, the eyes will remain in the neutral position when the head is moved and the eyelids, when opened, will close rapidly. In patients who are awake, the eyelids will stay open, snap shut, or flutter.

If the patient presents with a true seizure, the corneal reflex will usually be absent. In a pseudoseizure, the corneal reflex will be intact. There will also be an absence of contractions of certain muscle groups during a pseudoseizure.

If the patient presents with blindness, alternating black and white striped pieces of tape with alternating black and white sections pulled laterally in front of the patient's open eyes will produce nystagmus in a patient with intact vision.

Diagnosis

Before the diagnosis of conversion reaction is made, all organic causes must be ruled out. Conversion reaction should not be the first diagnosis. It is a diagnosis of exclusion only after all organic causes have been ruled out. A diagnosis is made by the clinical history of the single sudden onset of a symptom related to a severely stressful event. The patient, family, or friends will often separately need to be interviewed to obtain the whole history of the event. The most diagnostic criterion for conversion reaction is the presence of a somatization disorder, which is found in one third of the cases, or a previous history of a conversion reaction.

Treatment

The treatment of a conversion reaction is based on eliminating the stressor that caused the reaction. Confronting the patient that there is no organic or "real" cause of the symptoms is usually of no help. The patient requires reassurance that he or she has no serious medical problems. All patients who have a conversion reaction require a psychiatric referral.

PERSONALITY DISORDERS

Definition

The main components of a person with a personality disorder are that the person's personality traits are inflexible, rigid, and maladaptive.

Personality traits are a combination of genetic factors and environmental influences in early life. The core personality traits develop into a person's temperament, distinctive character, and individuality.

Social factors play an important factor in what is defined as maladaptive behavior. What is considered maladaptive in one society might not be considered maladaptive in another society. The personality disorder usually does not cause discomfort to the individual with the disorder but can cause frustration in regard to that person's function in society.

Epidemiology

Five to 10% of the adult population of the United States has some type of personality disorder. Personality disorders occur more commonly than does schizophrenia or a mood disorder.

Most studies have found that there is a genetic link to personality disorders. Family dysfunction is often present and acts as an environmental multiplier in the presentation of the disease. Signs of antisocial behavior often begin in the person's youth, especially in children whose parents are antisocial (e.g., due to alcoholism, drug use, early crime, and association with other antisocial persons).

A person with a borderline personality disorder is an individual who over time becomes more impulsive and dependent. The person can escalate to *acting-out* behavior or suicidal behavior, frequently in a competitive manner, while rejecting the borderline personality parent. Borderline personality disorders are more common in females than in males and are thought to be present in 15 to 20% of the adult population.

Antisocial behavior is six times more common in males than in females, but these persons are more likely to marry other antisocial individuals. There is a 4% rate of personality disorders in males who are 25 to 44 years of age. The rate declines to 0.45% by the age of 65 years. There is a strong genetic predisposition for antisocial behavior.

Clinical Presentation

Patients with a personality disorder present to the ED usually in one of two ways: with *externalization* or *acting-out* behavior. Those who are externalizing project outside themselves the discomfort and frustration experienced in their lives. They often blame others for their failures and are impulsively dissatisfied. They have major conflicts with authority figures and often change jobs secondary to their conflict with authority figures. They have major resentment toward school rules, work rules, living arrangements, or community settings. Those who are acting out provoke conflicts or invite assaults, altercations, or arguments.

Individual personality disorders present in five disorder types:

1. Narcissistic personality disorder
2. Borderline personality disorder

3. Antisocial or sociopathic personality disorder
4. Paranoid personality disorder
5. Histrionic personality disorder

A patient with a *narcissistic personality disorder* presents with a sense of elevated accomplishments, talents, and self-importance, and the person strives for and requires constant attention and admiration. The person exploits relationships and often his or her relationships are unstable and fragile.

A person with a narcissistic personality disorder is preoccupied with fame, beauty, power, and success. The more the person demands, the worse that person's disease becomes. The individual demands special attention in the ED. This patient will have to be admitted to the hospital if he or she presents with self-destructive behavior, dangerous impulses, or a threat to himself or herself or to others.

A person with a *borderline personality disorder* presents with extraordinary instability of mood, affect, self-image, and interpersonal relationships. The person often has stormy relationships and is unstable, overanxious, prone to anger, destructive to self and to others, and very impulsive.

A patient with a borderline personality disorder has an increased risk of suicidal threats, gestures, and attempts. The patient is prone to self-mutilating behavior and is often very reflective of the psychologically painful nature of his or her life.

A patient with borderline personality disorder often presents to the ED in crisis with anxiety or depression. It is very common for individuals presenting to the ED to fake illness or provoke self-injury to ensure immediate and complete attention from the staff.

On examination, these patients exhibit a very immature emotional state despite their age. It is believed that their emotional development arrested somewhere in their youth. These patients never developed an emotional self-sufficiency (autonomy). They did not complete the two phases of separation and individualism of childhood. There is usually a parent (often the mother) who also suffers from borderline personality disorder and who frustrates the child's attempt to separate and obtain self-sufficiency. The parent often has an axis I or axis II disorder that prevents him or her from providing the necessary parental support and encouragement that the child needs to become self-sufficient.

The parent often requires a self-serving dependent child as part of his or her disease. There is usually a complex pattern of withholding support and encouragement, clinging to prevent separation, and discouraging growth and independence by the parent toward the child.

In early childhood, borderline personality disorder is manifested by learning problems in school, temper tantrums, school phobias, juvenile delinquency, and truancy. As the child grows into adolescence and adulthood, these symptoms manifest as drug abuse and alcoholism. Females often marry early, become pregnant in their teens, become prostitutes, and are victims of poor marriages and relationships. The patient's relationships are based on fear, dependency, rage, anger, and hostility.

When a patient with a borderline personality disorder presents to the ED, this is a true cry for help. This presentation can be a prelude to a suicidal gesture or escalation of violent behavior. A patient with a borderline personality disorder is emotionally immature and has very few social survival skills. Often a visit to the ED is a temporary safe haven from the world, family, and the patient's psychiatrist or psychologist who is demanding that the patient "grow up." This is manifested by the patient making grandiose demands on the ED staff to remove his or her anxiety. The patient may at one time be very thankful for your help, and the next minute, when the patient discovers that his or her expectations are not going to be satisfied, the health care provider is met with anger, violence, and threats of suicide.

In the patient with borderline personality disorder there are no prolonged psychotic episodes, thought disorders, or the classic schizophrenic signs. Fifty percent of all patients with borderline personality disorder will meet the criteria for histrionic, antisocial, or schizoid disorders.

Patients with borderline personality disorder are difficult to treat. The main job of the emergency health care provider is to recognize that these patients are at an increased risk of violence and suicidal attempts and gestures, all of which must be taken seriously. No medications are available for the treatment of persons with borderline personality disorder unless an axis I disorder is present.

Antisocial or *sociopathic personality disorder* is seen in patients with very violent or aggressive behavior. Studies have found that the antisocial behavior begins in early childhood and is manifested by inappropriate childhood aggression. Violent children grow up to be violent adults. Seventy-five percent of these patients are educationally retarded and have a short attention span and reading disorders.

These children are bound for academic failure and are frequently truant. They have a long history of suspension and expulsion from school. As they approach adulthood, they start stealing and lying and have a history of early marriage, divorce, infidelity, separation, and promiscuous heterosexual and homosexual behavior. They have trouble keeping a job and find themselves in the lower socioeconomic classes.

Treatment of antisocial or sociopathic personality disorder is very difficult. Do not confront the patient about his or her antisocial behavior, because it will cause more antisocial behavior. This behavior is normal to the patient. The ED health care provider must evaluate the patient's potential for violence, suicide, and organic disease. The patient should be referred for psychiatric help, and if the patient poses a threat to himself or herself or to others, the patient should be admitted to the hospital.

Patients with a *paranoid personality disorder* insist that nothing is wrong with them. Patients will resist questioning and will appear normal upon presentation, often believably so. These patients will resist psychological questioning or consultation, and they are usually not violent, suicidal, or dangerous to others. They require a psychological referral.

A patient with a *histrionic personality disorder* desires attention, exaggerates his or her thoughts and feelings, has dramatic presentations, and is extremely extroverted. The person is flamboyant and pays great attention to his or her physical attractiveness. The person is usually very creative and imaginative but lacks good analytical thought processes.

A patient with a histrionic personality disorder has poor relationships based on control and is very superficial. Women present with this disorder more often than do men. Women are very good at drawing others into their desire for admiration in order to counter their anxiety. A real threat exists to their self-esteem when they are faced with illness or injury.

These patients often present to the ED with dramatic suicidal attempts or gestures. They will dramatize minor complaints or manifest conversion symptoms and somatization. The ED health care provider must take all threats of suicide seriously, and these patients should be admitted to the hospital secondary to their high level of acting-out impulsive behavior.

The rule for treating any borderline personality disorder is that when in doubt, consult with a psychiatric specialist early and admit the patient to hospital. All suicidal threats must be taken seriously. Complete diagnostic criteria for all types of personality disorders can be found in the DSM-IV-R.

SUICIDE

Definition

Unfortunately, the concept of suicide has existed since the beginning of recorded history. It is recorded in the Bible and in ancient Egyptian writings. The definition of suicide is an intentional taking of one's life. Suicides are defined as attempted or complete suicides.

Epidemiology

There is a 20% chance that a person who attempts suicide will do so again within 1 year. One in 20 of those persons will be successful in their second suicide attempt. Adolescents who attempt suicide have a 400% greater mortality rate than have those who do not attempt suicide.

Suicide is probably under-reported secondary to the social stigma associated with it. The suicide rate in the United States is approximately 11 to 12/100,000 people. The suicide rate for young men has been increasing, especially between the ages of 15 and 24. The suicide rate has risen 50% between 1970 and 1980 in young males.

There is also an increase in the use of firearms as a vehicle for suicide in the United States. Forty-seven percent of suicides in the United States were completed by people who used firearms in 1974; by 1980, 57% of all suicides were completed by firearms.

Pathology

Many different theories are given as to why a person attempts suicide; however, there is no good scientific explanation. The reasons are as individual as the person and involve depression, psychiatric illness, antisocial behavior, and social norms.

Depression is a major component of suicide. Of those who die of suicide, 15% have the diagnosis of endogenous depression. Depressed persons have a stronger desire to actually kill themselves and are at a higher risk of suicidal behavior. There is a strong association between the diagnosis of panic disorder and suicide. Patients with panic disorder have a greater rate of suicidal ideation and suicide attempts than any other psychiatric disorder.

There is also a higher rate of suicide among alcoholics and those who are intoxicated by alcohol at the time of their suicide attempt. Alcohol lowers the patient's inhibitions and can draw the person to attempt suicide. There is a 25% alcohol association rate in the United States for those who attempt suicide.

Schizophrenic patients also have a higher rate of suicide attempts, and 10% of schizophrenic patients will die of suicide. Fifty percent of all schizophrenic patients will attempt suicide at least once in their lives. Schizophrenic patients attempt suicide at a younger age than their peer population age group. Hallucinatory or persecutory delusions are frequently a factor in the schizophrenic patient's suicide attempt. Often voices tell the patient to kill himself or herself.

Clinical Presentation

Usually we do not see the successful suicide patient in the ED. We see the patient who attempts suicide. Bancroft and Marsack categorize patients who attempt suicide into three groups. The first group consists of the chronic habitual repeaters. They have self-destructive behavior. Their chronic suicidal behavior is secondary to their attempt to deal with stress. The second group of patients consists of individuals who make a burst of attempts surrounding a particular life stress. The last group consists of patients who make occasional attempts throughout their lives when confronted with overwhelming stresses.

Examination/Evaluation

The goal of the ED health care provider is to prevent the person from harming himself or herself and to evaluate the patient for admission to the hospital. An appropriate referral should be obtained. To do this, you must understand the type of person who is at risk for suicide. Men have higher rates of successful suicide than do women. Women attempt suicide at a greater rate than men do (a rate of 1.4 to 3.0:1). Completed suicide rates increase with age, whereas suicide attempts are higher in the younger population. Patients with chronic illness and a family history of suicide are at a greater risk than are the rest of the population.

Marital status also has a positive predictive value in the likelihood of suicide. Seventy-two percent of patients attempting suicide were single, separated, widowed, or divorced. Married persons have the lowest suicide rate. Men with children also have the lowest suicide rate of all.

Rosenbaum and Richman found five consistent characteristics in families of those who commit suicide by overdose. They also found that 89% of overdoses were at home or in the presence of family members, and in 40% of the cases they found that the patient had actually obtained the medication from a family member. The five consistent characteristics are:

1. An expectation by the family that the person will take an overdose.
2. Imitation and identification by the patient of others in the family who had attempted suicide by the same method.
3. Oral preoccupation and fixation by both the patient and the family.
4. A high rate of general trauma in the family (e.g., divorce, death).
5. Frequent direct participation by other family members in the suicidal act.

Diagnosis

Patterson and associates developed the SAD PERSONS mnemonic in 1983 to help persons who are not psychiatrists to evaluate the potentially suicidal patient and to help determine the need for the patient's hospitalization.

A patient with a score of 5 or less can safely be sent home. Patients with a score of 6 to 9 require psychiatric evaluation in the ED, and those with a score greater than 9 will require admission to the hospital. Also any patient who is intoxicated and is threatening or has attempted suicide should be admitted to the hospital.

The patient should be asked specifically about suicidal or homicidal ideations and if the patient has a plan—if so, who, where, how, and when can give you a clue to the patient's intent.

Treatment

Any patient who presents to the ED with a suicide attempt should be placed on suicide precautions. There should be a standard policy for

Mnemonic	Characteristic	Score
S—Sex	Male	1
A—Age	<19 or >45 years	1
D—Depression or hope-lessness	Admits to depression or decreased concentration, appetite, sleep, or libido	2
P—Previous attempts or psychiatric care	Previous inpatient or outpatient care	1
E—Excessive alcohol or drug use	Stigmata of chronic addiction or recent frequent use	1
R—Rational thinking loss	Organic brain syndrome or psychosis	2
S—Separated, widowed, or divorced		1
O—Organized or serious attempt	Well thought out plan or "life threatening" presentation	2
N—No social supports	No close family, friends, job, or active religious affiliation	1
S—Stated future intent	Determined to repeat attempt or ambivalent	2

the department with regard to what is done when a person who has made a suicide attempt presents to the ED. The patient should be searched for dangerous objects or medications. If the patient is physically violent to himself or herself or to others, the patient should be physically restrained and pulses and neurologic checks should be maintained at least every 15 minutes. Physical restraint protocols should be part of every ED.

For the most part, all patients who attempt suicide should be admitted to the hospital. This will give the patient support and a cooling off period. You will need to know the individual state's law regarding involuntary commitment for suicidal patients or for those who threaten others.

BIBLIOGRAPHY

Brandenburg RO, Fuster V, Giuliani ER, et al (eds): Cardiology Fundamentals and Practice. Chicago, Year Book Medical Publishers, 1987

Braunwald E, Isselbacher KJ, Petersdorf RG, et al (eds): Harrison's Principles of Internal Medicine, 11th ed. New York, McGraw-Hill, 1987

Diagnostic and Statistical Manual of Mental Disorders (DSM-IV-R). Washington, DC, American Psychiatric Association, 1994

Hamilton GC, Sanders AB, Strange GR, et al (eds): Emergency Medicine: An Approach to Clinical Problem-Solving. Philadelphia, WB Saunders, 1991

Hockberg RS, Roth RJ: Assessment of the suicide potential by nonpsychiatrists using the SAD PERSONS score. J Emerg Med 99:6, 1988

Kolb LC, Brodie HKH (eds): Modern Clinical Psychiatry, 10th ed. Philadelphia, WB
    Saunders, 1982
Kravis TC, Warner CG, Jacobs LM (eds): Emergency Medicine: A Comprehensive
    Review, 3rd ed. New York, Raven Press, 1993
May HL, Aghababian RV, Fleisher GR (eds): Emergency Medicine, 2nd ed. Boston,
    Little, Brown, 1992
Patterson WM: Evaluation of suicidal patients: The SAD PERSONS scale.
    Psychosomatics 343:24, 1983
Rosen P, Barkin RM (eds): Emergency Medicine: Concepts and Clinical Practice, 3rd ed.
    St Louis, Mosby-Year Book, 1992
Schwartz GR, Cayton CG, Manglesen MA, et al (eds): Principles and Practice of
    Emergency Medicine, 3rd ed. Philadelphia, Lea & Febiger, 1992
Tintinalli JE, Krone RL, Ruiz E (eds): Emergency Medicine: A Comprehensive Study
    Guide, 4th ed. New York, McGraw-Hill, 1996
Wolberg LR: The Technique of Psychotherapy. Philadelphia, Grune & Stratton, 1988
Yodofsky SC, Hales RE (eds): Textbook of Neuropsychiatry, 2nd ed. Washington, DC,
    American Psychiatric Press, 1992

Chapter 15

Pulmonary Emergencies

ADULT BACTERIAL PNEUMONIA

Definition

Pneumonia is defined as an infection of the pulmonary parenchyma. Pneumonia is caused by aspiration of an oropharyngeal organism, hematogenous spread from another site, or direct introduction of the organism into the pulmonary parenchyma or by an iatrogenic process. Pneumonias are classified as atypical, hospital-acquired, or community-acquired.

Epidemiology

Pneumonia is the sixth leading cause of death in the adult patient in the United States. There are more than 500,000 hospital admissions annually for pneumonia in the United States, accounting for 10% of all hospital admissions. There is an increased risk of a recurrence of pneumonia in patients who have had a previous admission to the hospital for pneumonia. Institutional living also increases the risk of a recurrence of pneumonia.

Smokers, patients with chronic obstructive pulmonary disease (COPD), congestive heart failure (CHF), cancer (leukemia, lymphoma), diabetes, hypogammaglobulinemia, and sickle cell disease are at increased risk for pneumonia. The very old or very young are at increased risk for pneumonia. Patients with chest wall trauma, patients who are intubated, and patients with acute stroke are also at higher risk for pneumonia. Patients who are alcoholics or who have chest wall myopathies and neuropathies are also at increased risk for pneumonia.

Viral pneumonia occurs in epidemics in small groups. School-aged children, debilitated older persons, persons living in nursing homes, and army trainees are at a higher risk for acquiring viral pneumonias.

Pathology

The majority of cases of adult bacterial pneumonia in the United States are caused by *Pneumococcus* (90%), with *Escherichia coli, Pseudomonas aeruginosa, Klebsiella pneumoniae, Staphylococcus aureus, Haemophilus influenzae,* and group B streptococci making up the other 10% of pneumonias in the adult population.

The majority of viral pneumonias in the United States are caused by the parainfluenza and influenza viruses. Parainfluenza virus causes a severe upper respiratory virus in children. The influenza virus causes significant mortality and morbidity secondary to bacterial superinfections. These viruses belong to the orthomyxovirus group.

Other viruses that cause pneumonia in humans include Coxsackie A and B viruses, echoviruses, adenoviruses, rhinovirus, herpesviruses, lymphocytic virus, measles, and varicella-zoster in the adult or child.

Atypical pneumonias include:

Viral pneumonias	*Chlamydia* pneumonia
Mycoplasma pneumoniae	*Legionella* pneumonia
Rickettsial pneumonia	

Bacterial pneumonias include:

Streptococcus pneumoniae	Gram-positive encapsulated diplococci
Pseudomonas	Gram-negative cocci-bacilli
H. influenzae	Gram-negative, encapsulated cocci-bacilli
E. coli	Gram-negative cocci-bacilli
Group A streptococci	Gram-positive cocci in chains or pairs
K. pneumoniae	Gram-negative, encapsulated paired cocci-bacilli
S. aureus	Gram-positive cocci in pairs and clumps

The major hospital-acquired (nosocomial) pneumonias (>50%) are gram-negative bacilli in origin. They include:

Klebsiella

E. coli

P. aeruginosa

Nosocomial infections caused by Enterobacteriaceae organisms include:

S. aureus

S. pneumoniae

Legionella

Moraxella catarrhalis

Anaerobic oral flora

L. pneumophila is found in natural or synthetic water systems and has been cultured from mud. *L. pneumophila* is the causative organism in 6 to 30% of all pneumonias. It causes both hospital-acquired pneumonia and community-acquired pneumonia. It occurs in outbreaks and epidemics and appears more commonly in the summer and early fall. It is assumed that it is transmitted by airborne droplets. The exact mode of transmission is still controversial. The incubation period is from 2 to 10 days. Direct person-to-person contact is unlikely as a mode of transmission. Middle-aged men with a 2.6:1 ratio to women is most common. Risk factors include patients who are diabetic, smoke, use alcohol in excess, have chronic lung disease, renal disorders, neoplastic disorders, or kidney transplants, and also patients who are immunocompromised or who live or work near construction sites.

Pneumocystis carinii pneumonia (PCP) must be considered in the human immunodeficiency virus (HIV)/acquired immunodeficiency syndrome (AIDS) population. Of all patients with AIDS, 80% will have at least one episode of PCP. It is often found in asymptomatic persons and does not cause illness in nonimmunosuppressed patients. The organism is a trophozoite that develops into a cystic structure containing sporozoites. It is seen in patients with AIDS, lymphomas, leukemias, organ transplants, and collagen vascular diseases and also in patients with malignant tumors. Respiratory failure occurs in 5 to 30% of hospitalized patients. Failure of response to therapy after 4 to 5 days necessitates a search for another cause of the acute illness. The mortality rate for *P. carinii* is 18%. When other organisms are present in a mixed flora, the mortality rate approaches 92%.

Chlamydia pneumoniae and *M. catarrhalis* are two atypical pneumonias that are on the rise. *Mycoplasma* and viral pneumonia are common in young adults and in older children. Alcoholic and diabetic patients are at increased risk of infection by gram-negative bacteria and *P. aeruginosa.*

Clinical Presentation/Examination

Pulse oximetry should be used on any patient with a respiratory complaint, and the readings should be noted on the patient's chart. The organism and presentation will be different for community-acquired versus hospital-acquired pneumonia. The age of the patient, the underlying illness, and the immunosuppression status must all be taken into consideration in your diagnosis of the type of pneumonia that the patient is infected with. Seasonal variation of the pneumonias must be considered.

The setting in which the patient lives is very important with regard to how and what kind of pneumonia is acquired. Recent travel or current hobbies should be considered. Patients from the Ohio and Mississippi River valleys can present with *Histoplasma capsulatum.* Patients who live in the southwestern part of the United States can present with *Coccidioides immitis. Coxiella burnetii,* or Q fever, is found in cows and is found especially in California. Patients who handle birds such as parakeets, turkeys, or parrots can be infected by *C. psittaci*. Tularemia is caused by fleas or ticks from dead animal carcasses.

Patients with any kind of pneumonia generally present with cough, sputum production, fever, pleuritic chest pain, and chills or any combination of the aforementioned symptoms.

Patients with viral pneumonia present with fever, cough, dyspnea, especially in flu season with accompanying chest pain. Presenting complaints are often mild and can vary greatly. On examination, viral pneumonia will present with fine rales and sometimes wheezing.

Patients with *S. pneumoniae* will present with acute shaking chills, tachypnea, and tachycardia. They will often give the history of a single episode of "rigors" lasting for several minutes. If more than one rigor occurs, the pneumonia is probably not caused by *S. pneumoniae*. Patients will present 70% of the time with sharp chest pain on the side of the infection. Patients can present with anorexia, general malaise, flank pain, abdominal pain with vomiting, back pain, and myalgias. Patients will present on examination with signs of consolidation, bronchial breath sounds, and increased tactile or vocal fremitus. They can present with cyanosis and jaundice. Make sure that you examine the abdomen. The patient may have abdominal distention or paralytic ileus.

H. influenzae has six capsular forms of the organism. *H. influenzae* is a gram-negative pleomorphic rod. Type b (a-f) is a capsular form of the organism that causes 95% of all *H. influenzae* infections. The uncapsulated form can also cause pneumonia. *H. influenzae* usually presents in the early spring and is more common in the extremes of age and in the immunocompromised or debilitated patient. On examination, the patient will have rales. The patient will present with fever, shortness of breath, and pleuritic chest pain.

Klebsiella is the pneumonia of patients with underlying diseases of COPD, alcoholism, and diabetes. It is seen most frequently in the right upper lobe and is a necrotizing lobar pneumonia. Empyema occurs within 2 to 48 hours with intrapulmonary abscess formation in 4 to 5 days. The patient with *Klebsiella* pneumonia will present with malaise, shortness of breath, sudden onset of rigors, and cough. Eighty percent of the patients with *Klebsiella* will have pleuritic chest pain. A physical examination will show cyanosis and consolidation.

Staphylococcal pneumonia only causes 1% of all bacterial pneumonias. It is seen in intravenous (IV) drug users, hospitalized patients, and the debilitated patient population. Patients with staphylococcal pneumonia usually present after an acute viral illness with an abrupt onset of multiple chills, fever, pleurisy, and a productive cough. On examination, there will be fine coarse rales or rhonchi. No signs of consolidation are usually present. It is a gram-positive organism.

Streptococcal pneumonia (group A) is a rare cause of pneumonia. It rapidly progresses to pneumonitis. The patient presents with a productive cough, sudden onset of fever, and chills. On lung examination, the patient presents with fine rales without signs of consolidation.

Chlamydial pneumonia is an atypical pneumonia. *C. psittaci* is acquired by coming in contact with birds who are infected. *C. trachomatis* and the new TWAR strain cause infection in humans also. Patients present with upper respiratory infection (URI) symptoms, cough, and chest pain, with a history of mucoid-to-green sputum production.

Mycoplasmal pneumonia is the most common community-acquired pneumonia behind viral pneumonias. This type of pneumonia presents with a mild URI, high fever, chills, dyspnea, and chest pain. The cough is usually nonproductive. The patient can complain of a headache. Mycoplasmal pneumonia is seasonal and epidemic in presentation. *Mycoplasma* can present as laryngitis, tracheobronchitis, pharyngitis, and bronchitis. The illness can last for 4 to 6 weeks if not treated. The illness usually lasts for 10 days. Bullous myringitis can occur with a mycoplasmal pneumonia infection. *Mycoplasma* has a cell wall that is resistant to most common antibiotics that act on cell walls. It causes 25% of all community-acquired pneumonias. It can also cause hepatitis, pericarditis, and encephalitis.

Complications of *Mycoplasma* include Guillain-Barré syndrome, meningitis, encephalitis, pneumothorax, pleural effusion, mediastinal adenopathy, atelectasis, and increased respiratory response in patients with COPD or asthma. Rarely renal failure can occur secondary to hemolysis. Disseminated intravascular coagulation (DIC) and thromboembolism have been reported. Pericarditis and myocarditis have also been reported.

L. pneumophila presents with acute onset and is rapidly fatal. The patient presents with malaise, cough, shaking chills, anorexia, and watery diarrhea. Weakness is often the only complaint. Fever starts out low-grade and rises to 103.1° to 104° F. The patient will complain of a headache and drenching sweats with nausea. Pleuritic chest pain, dyspnea, and hemoptysis are seen in one third of the patients. The patient's cough will be nonproductive but will become bloody or watery over time. On lung examination, fine inspiratory rales will be present in many lung fields. The patient will look acutely ill to toxic with sepsis. One third of the patients will present with confusion and disorientation. Coma will occur in 15 to 20% of patients with *L. pneumophila*. The mortality rate is as high as 75% in patients who are not treated or undertreated.

The onset of *P. carinii* in the immunocompromised patient is slow and insidious, and the symptoms are mild upon first presentation. The three symptoms of *P. carinii* are: (1) HIV positive, (2) nonproductive cough, and (3) dyspnea. The dyspnea is exertional 30 to 95% of the time. The patient will present with fatigue, tachypnea, night sweats, weight loss, and chest pain. Fever is almost universal.

When the patient's lungs are auscultated, no rales, wheezing, or rhonchi are noted.

Diagnosis

The diagnosis is made in the emergency department (ED) by history, physical examination, and x-ray. The patient is treated with the antibiotic that is most likely to cause the pneumonia for the age group that the patient is in, underlying disease, and previous living condition. Note if the pneumonia is community-acquired or hospital-acquired or if the patient is immunosuppressed or if the pneumonia is an aspiration pneumonia.

Older children usually have *Mycoplasma* or viral pneumonia. Older adults are most likely to have pneumonia caused by gram-negative bacillary organisms like *H. influenzae* and *K. pneumoniae.* Pneumonococcal pneumonia, *Legionella, Moraxella,* and *M. tuberculosis* are also common in the elderly.

Laboratory Findings

The laboratory examination should be directed by the severity of the patient's presentation, the knowledge of underlying disease, the patient's age, and the likelihood that a certain organism may be causing the illness. If a patient has underlying diseases such as diabetes, COPD, anemia, sickle cell disease, or HIV/AIDS or is a transplant patient, then the likelihood of a secondary infection, bacteremia, or sepsis should be considered. The likelihood of a severe illness developing should direct your laboratory tests. A complete blood count (CBC), electrolytes, sputum cultures, blood culture, urinalysis (UA) with urine culture, and chest x-ray should be performed on any patient suspected of having pneumonia.

The sputum should be examined under a low-power (100×) field. If there are more than 10 squamous epithelial cells on low power, then the sputum specimen is contaminated and should not be used for culture. An adequate specimen will have 25 or more polymorphonuclear leukocytes and less than 10 squamous epithelial cells.

The sputum from a patient who has group A streptococcal pneumonia will be purulent and bloody. Bloody or rusty looking sputum is indicative of pneumococcal pneumonia. Thick "currant jelly" sputum is produced by *K. pneumoniae,* and type 3 pneumococcus. *P. aeruginosa, S. pneumoniae* and *H. influenzae* organisms produce green sputum. Foul-smelling sputum is produced by anaerobes.

Immunofluorescent staining can be used to isolate the offending virus. Leukocytosis of 10,000 to 15,000 is often common.

S. pneumoniae will present a white blood cell (WBC) count from 12,000 to 25,000. Decreased WBCs suggest overwhelming infection caused by *S. pneumoniae.* A patient with *H. influenzae* will have a WBC count greater than or equal to 30,000. *Klebsiella* pneumonia will have an elevated WBC count in 75% of the presenting cases. Patients with staphylococcal pneumonia will present with a CBC higher than 15,000. *M. pneumoniae* will have a WBC count greater than 10,000, but rarely increases to 25,000. There can can a false-positive Venereal Disease Research Laboratory (VDRL) test and a negative tuberculin skin test in the presence of *Mycoplasma*. A complement-fixing serology test for antibody titers can be diagnostic if there is a fourfold increase in the titers. If the initial titer is higher than 1 in 64, it is highly suggestive of infection. Immunoglobulin M (IgM) rises around the 10th day and peaks between 4 and 6 weeks. Nonspecific cold agglutinins can also be used to diagnose *Mycoplasma* pneumonia. On an x-ray, chlamydial pneumonia will show the normal signs of atypical pneumonia.

L. pneumophilia will present with a WBC count from 10,000 to 20,000 with a left shift. The erythrocyte sedimentation rate, serum glutamic-oxaloacetic transaminase (SGOT), lactate dehydrogenase (LDH), bilirubin, and alkaline phosphatase levels will often be elevated. On urine examination, microscopic hematuria can be present in 10% of patients. The patient can present with electrolyte abnormalities. Hyponatremia and hypophosphatemia are the two most common electrolyte abnormalities. Immunofluorescence assays are highly specific but have low sensitivity for *L. pneumophila*. The problem with immunofluorescence testing is that the antigens of *L. pneumophila* are excreted for long periods of time and can represent a prior infection rather than a current infection. For titers to be positive, they must be at least 1:128 for a serologic diagnosis of *L. pneumophila*.

Respiratory failure is very common, and ventilator support is usually needed. Shock occurs in 10% of patients who ate diagnosed with *L. pneumophila.* The outcome is predicted to be poor.

X-rays of *P. carinii* will almost always be abnormal. When radiographic findings are present, alveolar infiltrates or diffuse bilateral interstitial infiltrates are usually present. The classic "bat-wing" appearance in the perihilar area is the most common x-ray presentation. In long-standing infections or as the disease progresses, the x-rays will reveal consolidations in all lung fields or asymmetric infiltrates, infiltrates near the periphery, or unilateral infiltrates.

X-ray Findings

On x-ray presentation viral pneumonia may show as patchy infiltrates or interstitial involvement. *S. pneumoniae* usually has one single lobar or segmental pattern on an x-ray. Elderly patients and infants can have patchy involvement on x-ray examination. The infiltrate usually presents in the right or left lower lobes or in the right middle lobe. Pleural effusions can be present in 10% of patients with *S. pneumoniae.*

An x-ray of *M. pneumoniae* will show patchy densities to dense consolidation involving the whole lobe. An abscess, cavity, pleural effusion, pneumatocele, and mediastinal adenopathy can all be noted on an x-ray.

H. influenzae will present with patchy infiltrates usually without effusion. Abscess formation is rare, but lobar consolidation does occur.

On an x-ray, *Klebsiella* will show as right upper lung necrotizing lobar pneumonia. Thirty-five percent of patients will have a bulging minor fissure. Perihilar and patchy infiltrates can also be seen on x-ray.

An x-ray of *staphylococcal pneumonia* will present with a patchy infiltrate that will progress to lobar consolidation and abscess formation. Empyema is common. X-rays of *streptococcal pneumonia* will present with multilobar bronchopneumonia and large pleural effusions.

X-rays of *L. pneumophila* will show small unilateral alveolar infiltrates in 70% of the patients. These infiltrates will often progress to multiple bilateral patchy or nonsegmental pulmonary infiltrates in two thirds of the patients. By the 10th day of the illness, the x-ray will show pulmonary consolidation. Pleural effusions and cavitary lesions are also common in the later processes of the disease. The patient should have serial x-rays to document the process of the disease. Infiltrates can still be seen on x-rays from 6 to 12 months after resolution of the illness.

When examining x-rays on a patient with *P. carinii,* keep in mind that *P. carinii* can simulate tuberculosis. Therefore, any patient with tuberculosis should be considered to be HIV positive, and any HIV-positive patient should be considered to have tuberculosis.

Treatment

Viral pneumonias are treated supportively. Bed rest, antihistamines, expectorants, analgesics, and increased fluids are the norm. If the patient is wheezing or having bronchial spasms, bronchodilators or aerosolized β_2-agonists should be used. If the patient becomes more severely ill, consider a secondary bacterial infection and treat the patient accordingly. The World Health Organization has recommended the influenza vaccine for influenza types A and B for high-risk patients. The following people are at high risk for infection with influenza types A and B: the elderly, patients with COPD, nursing home residents, patients with diabetes, renal failure, immunosuppression, asthma, anemia, cystic fibrosis, or medical personnel. *S. pneumoniae* usually resolves without treatment in 7 to 10 days. It often takes 14 to 21 days for all physical signs to resolve. The patient is treated with one of the following drugs:

1. Phenoxymethyl penicillin 500 mg by mouth (PO) four times a day (QID) for 10 days
2. Erythromycin 500 mg PO QID for 10 days
3. Aqueous penicillin 20 million units/day q4 to 6 hours
4. Procaine penicillin G 1.2 million units intramuscularly (IM) followed by phenoxymethyl penicillin 500 mg PO QID for 10 days
5. Vancomycin 1 g every 12 hours IV

H. influenzae is treated with one of the following drugs:

1. Ampicillin 500 mg PO QID for 10 days
2. Tetracycline 500 mg PO QID for 10 days
3. Cefuroxime 0.75 to 1.5 g IV every 8 hours for 10 days
4. Cefamandole 6 to 12 g/day IV every 4 to 6 hours
5. Chloramphenicol 50 to 100 mg/kg/day IV QID
6. Cefaclor (Ceclor) 250 to 500 mg PO QID

Klebsiella is treated with:
1. Cefazolin (Ancet, Kefzol) 0.25 to 1 g every 8 hours IV, *or*
2. An aminoglycoside
   a. Gentamicin 1 mg/kg every 8 hours

Staphylococcal pneumonia is treated with:

1. Cefazolin 1 to 2 g IV every 6 hours
2. Penicillinase-resistant penicillins:
   a. Cloxacillin (Novocloxin) 250 to 500 mg PO QID *or*
   b. Nafcillin (Nafcil) 1 g IV every 8 hours

Streptococcal pneumonia is treated with one of the following drugs:

1. Erythromycin 250 to 500 mg PO QID
2. Penicillin V 500 mg PO QID
3. Amoxicillin 500 mg PO QID
4. Cephalexin 500 mg PO QID
5. Cefazolin 1 to 2 g IV every 6 hours

Chlamydial pneumonia is treated with:

1. Erythromycin 250 to 500 mg PO QID for 10 days *or*
2. Tetracycline 500 mg PO QID for 10 days

Mycoplasmal pneumonia is treated with:

1. Erythromycin 250 to 500 mg PO QID for 1 to 14 days

L. pneumophila is treated with:

1. Erythromycin 750 to 1000 mg IV every 6 hours for 10 days, *and*
2. Erythromycin 500 mg PO QID for 3 more weeks
3. Rifampin is an alternative choice but is not as good as erythromycin

P. carinii is treated with:

1. Trimethoprim-sulfamethoxazole (TMP-SMX): 15 to 20 mg/kg/day of TMP and 75 to 100 mg/kg/day of SMX IV every 6 hours for 21 days, *or*
2. Pentamidine isethionate, 4 mg/kg IV over 1 to 3 hours daily for 14 to 21 days, can cause hypotension; therefore, give this drug slowly.
3. Patients with severe respiratory disease, PO_2 less than 70 mm Hg

or $P(A\text{-}a)O_2$ gradient greater than 35 mm Hg should be given corticosteroids. Oral prednisone 40 mg PO BID for days 1 to 5, 40 mg PO daily for days 6 to 10, and 20 mg PO daily for days 11 to 21 has been shown to be very beneficial in patients with *P. carinii*. Methylprednisolone can be given IV in place of PO prednisone.

4. Prophylaxis treatment with TMP-SMX in patients with CD4 counts below 200 cells/ml should be the norm.

ADULT RESPIRATORY DISTRESS SYNDROME

Definition

Adult respiratory distress syndrome (ARDS) is a syndrome secondary to an acute lung insult. It is a syndrome of intrapulmonary shunting, hypoxemia, reduced lung compliance, and parenchymal lung damage.

Epidemiology

ARDS can occur in a neutropenic patient, a patient with a cardiac event, or a traumatized patient. The permeability edema can be secondary to direct bacterial endotoxins and endothelial exposure to complement. Patients who are on high-dose oxygen are at increased risk of oxygen toxicity and thus damage to the pulmonary endothelium that can lead to ARDS. There is a 50% mortality rate for patients with ARDS.

Pathology

ARDS is caused by acute lung permeability edema. The classic pathway involves the release of immune complexes, plasmin, and a cascade of C1 to C9 complexes. The alternative pathway is caused by the activation of aggregated immunoglobulin E (IgE) and complex polysaccharides to a cascade of C3 to C9 complexes, both leading to membrane damage.

Permeability edema is unlike cardiac, high-pressure, or hemodynamic pulmonary edema. In ARDS, the microvascular membrane is no longer a barrier to protein; thus there is an increased leakage of fluid into the lungs without the usual Frank-Starling fluid movement of hydrostatic and oncotic forces. With an increase in the normal hydrostatic pressure, there is greater hemodynamic edema. This leakage causes an inflammatory response in the lungs, and an enzyme cascade response will be noted. This enzyme cascade can trigger an antibody response of endotoxins and exposure to the surface cells of bacteria or fungal organisms or complex polysaccharides. The production of C3a and C5a leads to neutrophil aggregation and the release of protease and superoxide radicals, which can cause damage to the pulmonary vascular endothelium and thus increased leakage. There is also the formation of arachidonic acid, which will cause the formation of leukotrienes and prostaglandins. This in turn will increase endothelial and alveolar injury.

When collagen is exposed to subendothelial basement membranes, the Hageman factor (factor XII) causes an enzymatic cascade of the fibrinolytic and kinin systems to activate. This action results in an additional mediator release and an increase in endothelial damage. As the mechanical properties of the lung decrease, surfactant is inactivated and the lungs become stiffer and require greater pressure to inflate; thus, a cycle of endothelium destruction and lung stiffness occurs as the continued interaction of enzymatic and biochemical cascades ensues. This is a three-tiered response of classic or alternative pathways, collagen exposure to basement membrane, and the formation of arachidonic acid.

Clinical Presentation

ARDS develops in the severely ill or traumatized patient usually in the surgical intensive care unit (SICU) or medical intensive care unit (MICU). It usually occurs in 12 to 72 hours after the initial medical or surgical insult. The patient will develop tachypnea, labored breathing, and arterial PO_2 will be less than 50 mm Hg with an FIO_2 of more than 0.5. Pulmonary compliance will be reduced, and there will be an increased need for ventilation pressures to maintain oxygenation. Serial chest x-rays will show progressive bilateral alveolar infiltrates. Airways pressures will steadily increase until complete respiratory failure occurs.

Diagnosis/Laboratory Findings

A sample of lung fluid should be taken if the patient is believed to have ARDS. In high-pressure edema, the colloid osmotic pressure is less than 60%. In permeability edema (ARDS), the edema:plasma ratio or colloid pressure ratio is greater than 60%. In the lung fluid of a patient with ARDS, there will be an increase in angiotensin-converting enzyme, collagenase, and elastinase.

Treatment

If a patient develops ARDS, the primary concern is to treat the underlying cause of ARDS. Mechanical ventilation is the main treatment for ARDS. Positive end-expiratory pressure (PEEP) is the mainstay of mechanical ventilation for ARDS. Cardiac output, arterial and mixed venous oxygen tensions, and pulmonary artery pressures should be monitored. The pulmonary artery wedge pressure (PAWP) should be maintained as low as possible. All patients with ARDS should be admitted to a MICU or a SICU.

ASPIRATION PNEUMONIA

Definition

Aspiration pneumonia is defined as an inflammation of the lung parenchyma secondary to the entrance of a foreign substance into the tracheobronchial tree. A lung abscess is a cavitation of the pulmonary parenchyma. Empyema is a collection of purulent material in the pleural space between the lung fissures.

Epidemiology

A patient who has a decreased gag reflex secondary to altered normal physiologic handling of secretions or gastric contents or has structural alterations in the normal protective mechanisms of swallowing is predisposed to aspiration. When the pH of aspirated particles or fluid is below 1.8 and 2.5, the mortality rate is between 40 and 70%. In patients who aspirate fluid from a bowel obstruction or fluid that is grossly contaminated, the mortality rate is approximately 100%.

Pathology

When a foreign substance is introduced into the lungs, ensuing damage is based on the pH of the material, the size of the material, and the form of the material. Large particles can cause acute upper airway obstruction. The lower the pH, the more significant will be the pleural damage. Severe injury occurs when the pH is below 2.5. The resultant foreign substances cause reflex airway closure, interstitial edema, and collapse or expansion of individual alveoli.

There are six basic types of foreign material that are aspirated: lipids, gastric juices, nontoxic liquids, dissolved food, pyogenic material, and particulate matter.

Aspiration causes an inflammatory process that results in a hemorrhagic pneumonitis within 6 hours of aspiration. This inflammation causes a chronic granulomatous reaction that can be seen on x-ray.

Particulate matter is usually neutral, and the response is based on the size and composition of the particulate matter aspirated. The aspirated particle will travel down the bronchial tree until it becomes lodged somewhere. If the particle is very large and blocks large bronchials, an obstruction occurs, and the patient will die. Peanuts, pinto beans, and talc powder are common causes of aspiration. Aspiration of talc powder will have a lag time of 4 to 6 hours, then an acute onset of tachypnea, cyanosis, wheezing, and rhonchi with prolonged expiration will take place. Atelectasis and pulmonary edema will ensue, and the patient will die if respiratory support is not ensured.

Vomitus from the stomach in a patient with altered mental status secondary to drug or alcohol intoxication is the main cause of aspiration pneumonia. The particles are usually very small and travel deep into the lung, causing an inflammatory response. The pH is very low and can cause symptoms similar to an acid aspiration. Hemorrhage pneumonitis with erythrocytes, granulocytes, and macrophage and giant cell invasion of the bronchial tree and alveoli occur. After 48 hours, there is massive giant cell invasion and a granulomatous reaction. Within 72 hours, the alveoli walls become thickened and the reaction becomes mononuclear with the presence of granulomas and obstructive bronchitis. By the fifth day, the macrophage infiltration declines.

Fluid aspiration is of two types: toxic and nontoxic. All fluid aspiration, regardless of whether it is toxic or nontoxic, causes a reflex constriction or dilatation of the alveoli. This dilatation or construction of alveoli causes a ventilation-perfusion (V/Q) mismatch and hypoxemia. There is increased fluid leakage from the capillaries and an increase in the interstitial spaces. *Toxic fluid* aspiration pneumonia is usually secondary to gastric fluids. After the fluids enter the lung, a rapid onset of pneumonitis occurs. Initially patchy atelectasis takes place, followed by pulmonary edema. Intra-alveolar hemorrhage with marked interstitial and peribronchial edema are present. Within the first 24 hours, bronchiolitis and necrotizing bronchitis occur with frank necrosis of the lung parenchyma. The ensuing pneumonitis causes an increase in fibrin, which causes atelectasis and emphysema. In the next 48 hours, atelectasis and pneumonitis occur with hyaline membrane formation. After 72 hours, the process begins to resolve. It can take up to 3 weeks for healing to take place. Parenchyma scarring can be seen on an x-ray.

Nontoxic fluids (usually saline or water) cause little damage to the lung parenchyma. This usually takes place in drowning or near-drowning victims. When water enters the lungs, there is a separation of endothelial cells from the basement membrane, diapedesis of erythrocytes, pulmonary edema, and bronchial neutrophilic infiltration. There is very little cellular necrosis in nontoxic fluid aspiration. When water enters the lungs, there is a marked rapid reduction in lung compliance. The airways close, and microatelectasis ensues.

Pyogenic aspiration occurs when infected material is aspirated. This material is usually infected gastric contents or normal flora of the oropharynx. This infected material can cause lung abscess, empyema, or necrotizing pneumonia. Hospitalized patients who aspirate and develop aspiration pneumonia have an increased risk of developing pneumonia from:

Gram-negative rods

E. coli	*Pseudomonas*
Proteus	Anaerobes

A *lung abscess* is a cavitation of the pulmonary parenchyma that develops as a continuation of an aspiration pneumonia. The abscess is secondary to the necrosis of the lung parenchyma. Cavitation and lung abscess occur 1 to 2 weeks after aspiration.

Organisms that cause lung abscesses include:

Anaerobic organisms

Fusobacterium	*Bacteroides*
Anaerobic streptococci	Microaerophilic streptococci

Aerobic organisms

Pseudomonas	*S. aureus*
S. pneumoniae	*Proteus*
E. coli	*K. pneumoniae*
Alpha streptococci	

Other organisms that can cause lung abscesses

Lung fluke	*Entamoeba*
Coccidioides	

Empyema usually occurs secondary to lymphatic or hematogenous spread from pneumonia. It can also occur secondary to a lung abscess rupture into the pleural space. Esophageal perforation, rupture of a mediastinal lymph node, mediastinitis, or retropharyngeal or subdiaphragmatic abscess can all cause empyema. Surgical complications such as thoracostomy tubes, needle aspirations, or thoracotomy can also cause empyema.

Clinical Presentation/Examination

Aspiration can occur at any time. A patient can present with hypoxemia, tachycardia, tachypnea, wheezing, fever, rales, rhonchi, and large amounts of frothy or bloody sputum. A patient can present with hypotension and shock. Many patients present with signs and symptoms of CHF or pulmonary edema.

With a lung abscess, the onset is insidious and often occurs after the patient leaves the hospital. The patient presents with a productive cough, bloody or foul-smelling sputum, chest pain, fever, weight loss, shortness of breath, and weakness.

A patient with empyema will present with weight loss, fever, chills, pleuritic chest pain, shortness of breath, clubbing of fingers, dullness to percussion, decreased breath sounds, and diminished excursion of the affected hemothorax.

Complications of empyema are bronchopleural fistulas, permanent loss of parenchyma, or empyema necessitatis. Empyema necessitatis occurs when the encapsulated empyema dissects into the subcutaneous tissues through the chest wall.

X-ray Findings

The chest x-ray for a patient with aspiration pneumonia will show a diffuse alveolar and interstitial infiltrate or a lobar or segmental infiltrate. A patient who has chronic aspirations will have chronic right lower lobe or axillary segment of the right upper lobe involvement on serial chest x-rays.

The x-ray for a patient with a lung abscess will usually show an air-fluid level. The abscess is usually located in the posterior segment of the right upper lobe and the superior segment of the right and left lower lobes. To diagnose a lung abscess versus empyema, look for the following:

1. Air-fluid levels that extend to the lateral chest wall
2. A cavity with an air-fluid level that tapers at the pleural border
3. An air-fluid level that crosses a fissure

Diagnosis

A diagnosis is made by clinical history, physical examination, and x-rays. Often bronchoscopy will be necessary to obtain sputum cultures or a parenchymal sample. The diagnosis of empyema is made by thoracentesis and by the aspiration of purulent material.

Laboratory Findings

All patients with suspected aspiration pneumonia, empyema, or lung abscess should have a CBC, arterial blood gas, electrolytes, blood and urine cultures, sputum cultures, cardiac enzymes, liver function tests (LFTs), prothrombin time (PT), and partial thromboplastin time (PTT) drawn.

Treatment

The goal of treatment is early removal of foreign aspirate, reduction of hypoxia, and prevention or correction of hypovolemia if present.

1. Good airway control is very important. All patients should receive high-flow oxygen. Any patient suspected or known to have aspirated should be placed in the left lateral decubitus position, and vigorous tracheal and mouth suction should be performed prior to intubation.
2. An arterial blood gas should be drawn, and a chest x-ray should be taken. The patient should be intubated, and intermittent positive-pressure ventilation (IPPV) should be started.
3. Two large-gauge IV lines should be started.
4. A central line should be started to monitor central venous pressure (CVP) or PAWP secondary to the extravasation of fluid across the pulmonary capillary membranes. These pressures should be used to guide fluid management in a patient who has aspirated. Fluid management should be guided by the CVP or PAWP and by serial measurements of plasma and edema colloid osmotic pressures.
5. The pulmonary edema is noncardiac pulmonary edema; thus digitalis or diuretics are not indicated.
6. Steroids should probably not be given prophylactically in aspiration pneumonia.
7. Antibiotics should not be given prophylactically. Antibiotics are indicated when:

    a. New or expanding infiltrate appears more than 36 hours after aspiration

    b. A new or higher fever exists in a patient who already has a fever

    c. Cultures of sputum grow pathogenic bacteria

    d. Positive Gram's stain

    e. Leukocytosis

    f. Unexplained deterioration of the patient

    g. Purulent sputum

       1. When antibiotics are needed, they should be specific to the organism based on sputum cultures or blood cultures.

       2. If antibiotics can be given specific for the organism, then:

          a. Penicillin G 6 to 12 million units/day until clinical improvement takes place. Then give 500 mg PO QID for 6 weeks.

          b. Clindamycin 600 mg IV every 6 hours for a patient with an allergy to penicillin, *or*

          c. Chloramphenicol 500 mg IV every 4 hours, *or*

          d. Cefoxitin 1 to 2 g IV every 4 hours

8. Bronchoscopy can be used to remove large foreign particles, biopsy, facilitate drainage, or culture lung contents.

9. If there is a life-threatening hemoptysis, the patient should be placed in the Trendelenburg position with the bleeding side down, and vigorous suction should be performed. A pulmonologist should be consulted immediately so that a double-lumen endobronchial tube (Robert Shaw, Carlens, or White) can be placed.

10. Empyema requires appropriate antibiotics and tube thoracostomy for drainage of purulent infectious material.

ADULT ASTHMA

Definition

Asthma is defined by the American Thoracic Society as "a clinical syndrome characterized by increased responsiveness of the tracheobronchial tree to a variety of stimuli." This hyperresponse causes the classic symptoms of dyspnea, wheezing, and cough with variable airway response. Asthma is a chronic disease. Asthma has been defined as *extrinsic* or allergic and *intrinsic* when no obvious extrinsic causes are found.

Today it is understood that asthma is triggered by many combinations of stimuli or by a single stimulus.

Epidemiology

Asthma is on the increase in the United States, especially in the black population. It is suggested that approximately 10% (15 million persons) of the United States' population has asthma and that 2 to 5 million children are affected by asthma. Asthma is more prevalent in males than in females.

Pathology

Asthma is a reversible air flow obstructive disease. It is associated with increased responsiveness of the tracheobronchial tree to many different stimuli. It is a condition of bronchial hyperactivity.

The autonomic nervous system influences the smooth muscles of the airways. When the vagus nerve is stimulated there is a release of acetylcholine, which causes constriction of the airways to 1 to 5 mm. Stimulation of the larynx and lower airways can cause vagus stimulation and bronchial constriction. These reactions are secondary to an exaggerated parasympathetic reflex action. Any stimulation of the α-adrenergic receptors will cause bronchial constriction.

The sympathetic nervous system plays a small role in bronchial constriction by constricting the smaller airways.

Some of the triggers that can provoke an acute asthmatic attack are:

1. Dusts, molds, fumes, and chemicals of occupational exposure
2. Viral respiratory infections
3. Exercise
4. Gastroesophageal reflux
5. Odors including chemicals and perfumes
6. Sinus infections
7. Deep or forceful inspiration or expiration
8. Aspirin
9. Nonsteroidal anti-inflammatory drugs
10. β-Adrenergic blocking agents
11. Yellow dye number 5
12. Immunologic reactions to an antigen-mediated release

Possible mechanisms of bronchial hyperactivity in asthma are:

1. There is a decrease in bronchial caliber.
2. Bronchial smooth muscle becomes hypertrophied and hyperplasic.
3. There is an increase in mast cell release.
4. There is then an increase in the synthesis of mediators.
5. This lowers the receptor threshold.
6. The damaged epithelial cells cause a greater exposure to subepithelial irritant receptors.
7. There is an imbalance in the regulation of the autonomic nervous system causing an increase in parasympathetic activity, a decrease in β-adrenergic responsiveness, an increase in α-adrenergic responsiveness, and a decrease in the nonadrenergic inhibitory system.

The extrinsic asthma is an IgE–related response, thus causing the release of mast cells. When the mast cells degenerate, this causes bronchial constriction. This process is implicated in exercise-induced asthma. Mast cells also release mediators, including platelet activation factor, causing bronchial constriction, vasodilatation, and the release of neutrophils and eosinophil chemotaxis. This causes the release of allergen-mediated histamine release from mast cells.

There is an early and late response to a stimulus in asthma. The early response is bronchial constriction, which usually occurs within 10 minutes of exposure, peaks in 30 minutes, and resolves in 3 to 4 hours. The late response occurs if the early response lasts longer than 3 to 4 hours. The early response is thought to be mast cell mediated. The late response continues with increased airway constriction and mucous plugging. Within the mucous plugging, eosinophils and sloughed mucosal epithelial cells are found. Charcot-Leyden crystals (crystalline structures representing coalescence of free eosinophilic granules), Creola bodies (large compact clusters of sloughed mucosal epithelial cells), and Curschmann's spirals (bronchiolar casts of sputum) components will be found in the sputum.

When airway obstruction occurs there is increased airway resistance, decreased maximum expiratory flow, air trapping, increased airway pressure, hypoxemia, hypercarbia with the presence of pulsus paradoxus, and respiratory fatigue and failure.

Clinical Presentation

Asthma has variable presentations, even in the same person. The most common presenting complaints are progressive dyspnea, chest tightness, cough, and wheezing. The biggest mistake in the diagnosis of asthma is the failure to recognize a cough as an asthma attack. Attacks that last for several days, in phase two of asthma, will have significant mucous plugging and edema. Remember that "all that wheezes is not asthma." Conditions that can mimic asthma include:

1. New onset of CHF
2. Aspiration of a foreign bodies or gastric contents
3. Upper airway obstruction
4. Endobronchial obstruction secondary to bronchogenic carcinoma
5. Lymphangitic metastasis of metastatic carcinoma
6. Multiple pulmonary emboli
7. Vocal cord dysfunction
8. Endobronchial obstruction secondary to sarcoidosis

Examination

Look at the whole patient. Are there costal retractions or use of accessory muscles (prominent neck muscles)? If the patient is using accessory muscles with inspiration, the neck muscles are prominent with inspiration, and the upper abdomen moves inward with inspiration, this connotes diaphragmatic fatigue and impending respiratory failure.

Ask the patient to speak a whole sentence or say his or her name.

If the patient can't speak a whole sentence or at least his or her name, the patient is in severe respiratory distress. Look at the patient's skin color. Is the person cyanotic or blue? Look at the patient's eyes. If the patient can't speak his or her name and the patient has the look of fear in his or her eyes, be ready to intubate.

Sometimes you will be able to hear wheezing without a stethoscope. At other times an asthmatic will be so "tight" that you will not be able to here wheezing until the patient has had one or two nebulizer treatment. There will be hyperresonance to percussion on examination. Prolonged expiration is the hallmark of asthma. Remember that wheezing does not correlate with the severity of the asthma attack. A pulsus paradoxus above 20 mm Hg is indicative of a severe asthma attack.

Look for exhaustion or lethargy. Remember that the first sign of hypoxia is agitation or confusion. A confused asthmatic is hypoxic.

Perform pulmonary function tests on every patient before and after every nebulizer treatment. This will help you to objectively gauge how the patient is doing. The peak expiratory flow rate (PEFR) is a simple test with a hand-held flow meter. Ideally you want to check forced expiratory volume (in 1 second) vital capacity (FEV_1/VC) and the forced expiratory volume in 1 second (FEV_1). Nebulizer treatments should continue until the PEFR reaches 300 l/min or is greater than 60% of the patient's predicted performance.

Diagnosis

A diagnosis is made by the history and presentation of the patient. Most patients with asthma know that they are having an asthma attack. If the patient is a known asthmatic, ask the patient if this is a mild, normal, or severe asthma attack for him or her. Most asthmatics know when they are getting into trouble. Ask the duration of this attack. Ask if the patient knows the precipitating factor of this attack or if the patient has known this attack has been coming on for a short or long period of time. Ask about what medications the patient is taking currently or in the past (e.g., prednisone, the number and kind of inhalers). Does the patient have a home nebulizer, and has the patient used it in the past 24 hours? Has the patient ever been hospitalized because of asthma? Has the patient ever been intubated for asthma; if so, when was the last time that he or she was intubated and how many times? The most important question that you can ask an asthmatic is whether he or she is getting tired of breathing? If the patient states that he or she is becoming tired of breathing, be ready to intubate this patient.

Laboratory Findings

If the patient has a temperature, a CBC should be performed; however, a CBC does not routinely need to be performed for an acute asthma attack without fever. Eosinophilia is common in asthmatics who do not take steroids. Electrolytes should be performed if the patient looks extremely dehydrated or is on a diuretic.

If sputum analysis is performed, eosinophilia is characteristic. The sputum usually looks yellow or green. If a wet mount and a Wright stain are performed, eosinophilias will be seen. Less than 10 epithelial cells should be present, and Charcot-Leyden crystals, Curschmann's spirals, or Creola bodies can be noted on sputum examination under low power.

The arterial blood gas is not routinely performed, unless the pulse oximetry is below 90% or the patient is in severe respiratory distress.

The electrocardiogram (ECG) will show a right ventricular strain, a right axis deviation or a right bundle branch block, abnormal P waves, or nonspecific ST-T wave abnormalities.

A chest x-ray is not normally required unless the patient has a fever or there is suspicion of an underlying pneumonia or pneumothorax. If an x-ray is performed, there will be a marked increase in lung volume and hyperinflation. The anteroposterior (AP) diameter will be increased, and the diaphragm will be flattened. A chest x-ray should be performed on any patient who presents with asthma for the first time to rule out foreign body, aspiration, or new lung pathology.

Treatment

There are two main components to asthma: bronchial constriction and inflammation. Treat both components. The biggest mistake in the ED is not to treat both components of asthma. If you treat the asthmatic with just a β-adrenergic medication, the patient may get better in the ED but may return to the ED in 4 to 6 hours. Remember that asthmatic attacks take hours, if not days, to come on. Treatment follows for the asthmatic who presents to the ED:

1. Examine the patient as described earlier. Place the patient on pulse oximetry, and note the patient's oxygen saturation level. Obtain a PEFR or FEV_1. Place the patient on oxygen by nasal cannula at 2 to 4 l/min.
2. Most asthmatics are dehydrated; therefore, remember to rehydrate the patient either with IV or PO fluids. Start an IV line of normal saline 0.9% if the patient is dehydrated or in respiratory distress or if the patient needs steroids.
3. Aerosol β-adrenergic agonists are the mainstay of treatment of an acute asthmatic attack in the ED. Give a treatment every 15 minutes. If the patient is in severe respiratory distress, continuous nebulizer treatments can be given; however, take into consideration any underlying heart disease. Some common β-agonists used in the ED are:
   Albuterol sulfate 0.5% solution, 0.5 ml (2.5 mg) diluted with 2 to 3 ml of normal saline
   Metaproterenol sulfate 5% solution, 0.3 ml diluted with 2 to 3 ml of normal saline

4. If no response after one to two nebulizer treatments, give corticosteroids. Some suggested doses for corticosteroids are:
   Methylprednisolone 125 mg IV slowly, then 15 to 20 mg every 6 hours until the patient has improved. The patient can be switched to oral corticosteroids (e.g., prednisone). A common dose is 60 mg/day of prednisone for 5 days if the patient has not been on steroids in the past year. If the atient has been on steroids in the past year, the dose   should be tapered over a 3-week period.
5. Sometimes if the patient is extremely "tight" and cannot effectively utilize a nebulizer treatment, subcutaneous (SQ) β-adrenergic bronchodilators can be used. Common SQ β-adrenergic bronchodilators are:
   Epinephrine 0.3 mg SQ every 20 minutes for three doses
   Terbutaline sulfate 0.25 mg every 20 minutes for three doses
6. Magnesium sulfate is a bronchodilator and can be used in mild or severe asthma attacks. Give magnesium sulfate 2 to 3 mg intravenous piggyback (IVPB) slowly.
7. Theophylline was at one time the first-line drug of choice for asthma; however, when combined with nebulized β-adrenergic drugs, there is an increased risk of toxicity from theophylline. In theory, if a patient has a severe asthma attack, theophylline will sustain the bronchodilator effect. The new range for theophylline levels is 10 to 15 μg/ml. Cimetidine, erythromycin, allopurinol, and oral contraceptives will increase serum theophylline levels. Cigarette smoking, phenytoin, phenobarbital, or consumption of charcoal-broiled beef will all decrease serum theophylline levels. Theophylline is dosed as:
   Loading dose, with no previous doses of theophylline, at 5 mg/kg IVPB
   If the patient is taking short-acting theophylline for less than 12 hours, or long-acting theophylline for less than 24 hours, and serum levels are therapeutic, no loading dose is required.
   If the theophylline level is subtherapeutic, 3 mg/kg or half (desired level − observed level) mg/kg
   Maintenance doses:
     If the patient is taking oral theophylline and the serum level is subtherapeutic, increase the dose by 25%
     Smoker, 0.8 mg/kg/hr
     Nonsmoker, seriously ill, 0.5 mg/kg/hr
     CHF or liver disease, 0.2 mg/kg/hr
8. If the patient requires theophylline or does not respond to nebulizer treatments and corticosteroids or does not surpass 60% of the predicted values or 300 PEFR, the patient should be admitted to the hospital.
9. If the patient is in acute respiratory failure, the patient should be intubated and mechanical ventilation should be performed

with aggressive maximal bronchodilator therapy. Barotrauma and hypotension are complications of mechanical ventilation.
10. Pregnant patients should be treated somewhat differently from nonpregnant patients. Corticosteroids are safe in pregnancy. Epinephrine should be avoided secondary to the possibility of congenital malformations. Aerosolized β_2-adrenergics should be the mainstay of treatment in the pregnant patient. Theophylline should be avoided secondary to its ability to cross the placenta.
11. Any patient who returns for the third time in 5 days or for the second time in 24 hours should be considered for admission to the hospital.
12. All patients who are discharged should go home with the following instructions:
    a. I tell all asthmatics that I would prefer to see them too early than too late. If the patient takes four metered dose inhaler (MDI) puffs 10 to 15 minutes apart and there is no objective or subjective improvement, the patient should return to the ED.
    b. All patients should leave the ED with prescriptions for a steroid inhaler and a β-agonist inhaler, with or without a 5- to 21-day course of corticosteroids. All children need spacer devices, and most adults can benefit from spacer devices also. It does no good to give an asthmatic medication if the person does not know how to use the MDI properly.
    c. All asthma patients must have a follow-up examination within 72 hours before they leave the ED.

CHRONIC OBSTRUCTIVE PULMONARY DISEASE

Definition

Chronic obstructive pulmonary disease (COPD) is defined by the American Thoracic Society as two distinct types of disease.

1. *Pulmonary emphysema* (defined pathologically) is a condition of the lung characterized by abnormal, permanent enlargement of the air spaces distal to the terminal bronchiole, accompanied by destruction of their walls.
2. *Chronic bronchitis* (defined clinically) is a condition of excess mucus secretion in the bronchial tree, occurring on most days for at least 3 months a year for at least 2 consecutive years.

The patients who have these conditions are often referred to as "blue bloaters" and "pink puffers." They usually have a mixture of asthma, bronchitis, and emphysema.

Pathology

The primary cause of COPD is cigarette smoking. Environmental and industrial air pollution and passive cigarette smoke have all been implicated in COPD. This is a disease of chronic air flow obstruction, primarily expiratory air flow. The pathophysiology of COPD can be defined in stages:

Stage A: A patient has no respiratory symptoms, even on exertion, and minimal if any hypoxemia.

Stage B: The patient has mild or minimal symptoms and has little disability. There is detectable lung damage and dyspnea only on exertion, with slight hypoxemia.

Stage C: This stage marks the onset of ventilatory insufficiency and dyspnea at rest. There is erosion of normal lung function with hypocarbia and hypoxemia.

Stage D: The physiologic reserve of the lung is exhausted, followed by erosion of the baseline lung function. There is chronic ventilatory failure with the onset of cor pulmonale.

Stage E: At this final stage of lung disease, the patient will die without oxygen and ventilatory assistance.

Most COPD bronchitis is caused by the following organisms:

H. influenzae
Diplococcus pneumoniae
B. catarrhalis
Mycoplasma
Chlamydia
Bordetella pertussis

Clinical Presentation

The patient will present in one of two ways: A "blue bloater" is short and obese and a "pink puffer" is thin in stature. A patient with COPD will be tachypneic and will be using accessory respiratory muscles and will also be pursing his or her lips upon exhalation. Wheezing can be present on exhalation, or coarse crackles can be present, or both can be heard on examination. In long-term chronic disease the thorax will be hyperexpanded with increased anteroposterior (AP) diameter. Poor dietary intake and weight loss are common in end-stage disease. Confusion secondary to hypercarbia, plethora secondary to polycythemia, and cyanosis can all be present.

Chest X-ray Findings

The chest x-ray is a poor examination for determining the severity of COPD. Bronchitis pathology will be shown poorly on the chest x-ray. Emphysematous disease will show signs of hyperaeration with increased AP diameter, flattened diaphragm, increased parenchymal lucency, and attenuation of pulmonary arterial vascular shadows.

Examination

The most valuable examination or test to determine the severity of the COPD is the pulmonary function test. FEV_1 and forced vital capacity (FVC) are the two best measurements of lung disease. A reduction in FVC, in the absence of restrictive ventilatory disease, when bronchodilators are given, is a sign of emphysema. If FVC improves with bronchodilators, the underlying disease is probably more the bronchitis form of COPD.

Laboratory Findings

The arterial blood gas can be normal or exaggerated. The alveolar-arterial (A-a) gradient is almost elevated. Usually there is an increase in this gradient of more than 30. The normal $Paco_2$ is 35 to 45 mm Hg, less than 35 mm Hg representing excessive carbon dioxide elimination or hypoventilation. Remember that for every 10 mm Hg increase in $Paco_2$ over 40 mm Hg, the pH will decrease by 0.08 units, and for every 10 mm Hg decrease below 40 mm Hg, the pH will increase by 0.08 units. Also for every change in bicarbonate of 10, the pH should change by 0.15 units.

A sputum examination in the COPD patient in the ED is very helpful. Sputum with tiny dark specks that are 1 or 2 mm in diameter is characteristic of inspissated mucous plugs as seen in asthmatics and COPD patients. If the sputum contains only eosinophils, there is probably no infection. If the sputum contains polymorphonuclear cells, an infection is probably present. Gram's stain is helpful if infection is present.

An ECG will usually show right ventricular hypertrophy, which suggests cor pulmonale. The finding of "P pulmonale," peaked Ps in leads II, III, and avF suggests COPD. The classic triad of a low QRS voltage, poor R wave progression, and clockwise rotation is indicative of COPD on an ECG, but it is nonspecific and insensitive to COPD.

Treatment

Treatment must be directed toward both acute exacerbations and long-term therapy. The most important factor in preventing exacerbations is for the patient to stop smoking, if he or she is still smoking, and the cessation of exposure to secondary smoke if someone else is smoking in the home. Patients should receive antibiotics for bronchitis exacerbations. Bronchodilators are a main form of treatment for the asthma component of COPD. Corticosteroids are needed in short bursts or chronically to treat the inflammatory process of COPD. Oxygen is needed for acute exacerbations in the ED, and home oxygen is required for treatment of end-stage disease. All patients with COPD should receive the polyvalent (23) pneumococcal and the annual trivalent influenza vaccines to prevent viral infections and thus COPD exacerbations.

There is controversy as to whether theophylline therapy has a place in the treatment of patients with COPD. In theory, oral theophylline helps to keep the large and small airways open.

If the patient's resting room air oxygen saturation is less than 90%, home oxygen is indicated at 1 to 2 l/min.

Commonly used antibiotics for bronchitis include TMP-SMX (Septra), ciprofloxacin, first-generation cephalosporins, erythromycin (be careful if given with theophylline), ampicillin, and amoxicillin.

Most patients with COPD also have left-sided heart failure and are dehydrated at the time of presentation to the ED. Patients with end-stage COPD will have secondary pulmonary hypertension and cor pulmonale. There is a delicate balance in treating these patients. Bronchodilators increase heart rate and thus increase stress on the heart, which can cause the heart to fail. The patient with CHF can have heart failure due to rapid IV fluid administration in a dehydrated patient or to an attempt made to move the mucous plugs. It is recommended that the patient's lungs be listened to after every 250 ml of fluid administration.

All patients with COPD should have an ECG, especially those on theophylline therapy. Patients with COPD can present in atrial fibrillation (AF) or multifocal atrial tachycardia (MAT). Those patients who also have CHF are sometimes on digoxin therapy and should have an ECG and their digoxin levels drawn.

Many patients are also on diuretics and have the potential for hypokalemia. Hypokalemia can also promote dysrhythmias. Patients with COPD can have metabolic abnormalities. All patients with COPD should have a complete set of electrolytes drawn along with theophylline and digoxin levels if the patient is taking these medications. If there is a history or a suspicion of CHF or a prior myocardial infarction, cardiac enzymes should be drawn.

Expectorants are sometimes used; however, there is no objective evidence that they improve the expectoration of mucus or improve the quality of life.

Treatment of the Patient with COPD in the ED

1. The patient should be placed on a cardiac monitor, and pulse oximetry readings and vital signs should be monitored closely every 10 minutes.
2. The patient is placed on a nasal cannula at 1 to 2 l/min.
3. Give bronchodilators every 10 to 15 minutes, and monitor the patient's vital signs and response to treatment.
4. Give cortiocosteroids: methylprednisolone 125 mg IV.
5. Perform ECG, chest x-ray, CBC, electrolytes, cardiac enzymes as needed, and PEFR between treatments.
6. If the patient shows signs of pneumonia, give antibodies IV. If the patient is dehydrated, give IV fluids very slowly.

7. If the patient shows no improvement or has oxygen desaturation while on room air, admit the patient to hospital.

PNEUMOTHORAX

Definition

A pneumothorax is a collection of air in the potential pleural spaces. There are iatrogenic, spontaneous, tension, and traumatic pneumo-thoraces.

Epidemiology

A spontaneous pneumothorax usually occurs in tall, thin males 20 to 40 years of age. A spontaneous pneumothorax in a person younger than 40 years of age is usually secondary to a rupture of a subpleural bleb. An iatrogenic pneumothorax is usually secondary to pulmonary barotrauma, which is secondary to increased airway pressures from ventilatory assistance or a medical procedure or complication, such as percutaneous lung biopsy, cannulation of the subclavian vein, intercostal nerve block, thoracentesis, or ventilation of the lungs at high pressures (bag-valve-mask).

Pathology

When a bleb ruptures, there is a leakage of air from the alveoli into the pleural space and thus an increase in intrapleural pressure caus-ing a spontaneous pneumothorax. A spontaneous pneumothorax can occur in conjunction with Marfan's syndrome, Ehlers-Danlos syn-drome, asthma, COPD, emphysema, "honeycomb" lung or lung carci-noma, sarcoidosis, histiocytosis X, or tuberous sclerosis. A spontane-ous pneumothorax has also been reported in conjunction with diaphragmatic, pelvic, or pleural endometriosis. A spontaneous pneumothorax can occur more than once in any patient who has previously had a pneumothorax.

Clinical Presentation

A patient with spontaneous pneumothorax can present with a history of Valsalva maneuvers, coughing, or screaming. The patient usually presents with a sudden onset of sharp chest pain on the side of the pneumothorax. The pain is anterior and can radiate to the neck. The severity of symptoms will be related to the size of the pneumothorax and the patient's underlying disease. The patient will be tachycar-diac, tachypneic, and dyspneic. The patient will often be cyanotic and will have hypotension. There can be deviation of the trachea and mediastinal structures. This deviation of mediastinal structures can cause kinking of the inferior vena cava with a secondary decrease of venous return causing hypotension.

Examination

With an acute pneumothorax, the patient will be in acute respiratory distress. The breath sounds will be decreased on the side of the pneumothorax. There will be hyperresonance to percussion on the side of the pneumothorax and decreased tactile fremitus. Patients with COPD or emphysema who present with a pneumothorax can present with very mild or no symptoms. Even a small pneumothorax can lead to direct pulmonary failure in the patient with underlying lung disease or COPD.

Diagnosis

The diagnosis of a tension pneumothorax is a clinical diagnosis not a radiographic diagnosis. If the signs and symptoms are present for a tension pneumothorax, then the patient should be treated as if he or she has a pneumothorax with immediate lung decompression with a 14-gauge needle being placed in the second intercostal space, mid-clavicular line.

The diagnosis of a pneumothorax is made by x-ray examination. An inspiratory x-ray should be taken. On the x-ray, there will be a lack of lung marking on the peripheral edges or hyperlucency of the lung field on the side of the pneumothorax.

Treatment

All patients with a suspected pneumothorax should be placed on 100% oxygen with a nonrebreathing mask. An IV line of normal saline 0.9% should be started, and a portable chest x-ray should be ordered. A pulse oximetry reading should be obtained along with an arterial blood gas at room air.

The treatment of an acute pneumothorax is based on the size of the pneumothorax, the oxygen saturation, the patient's underlying disease, oxygen reserve, and life habits (e.g., a smoker). If the pneumothorax is larger than 20%, then a tube thoracostomy should be performed with a waterseal or vacuum drainage system. If the pneumothorax is under 20%, and no underlying lung disease is present, the pneumothorax can be watched. If the patient has severe underlying lung disease, a tube thoracostomy should be performed and a consultation should be made with a pulmonologist and a general surgeon.

PULMONARY EMBOLISM

A pulmonary embolism (PE) is caused by the classic triad of venostasis, hypercoagulability, and vessel wall inflammation. Most PEs arise from the deep vein system of the lower extremities. Popliteal thrombosis causes 50% of PEs. With femoral vein involvement, morbidity reaches 70%. The cause of PEs is seldom calf vein involvement. PEs are the third most common cause of death in the United States. A PE occurs when a fragment of a thrombus breaks off and is carried via the vena cava to the right side of the heart and then becomes lodged in the pulmonary artery tree, causing either complete or partial obstruction to the distal pulmonary tree. Seventy percent of proven PEs will have a clot in the pelvis or lower extremity. The PE causes a V/Q mismatch. Major causes of PE are:

1. Amniotic fluid PE in abortion or in the postpartum period at the end of the first stage of labor
2. Pelvic or leg thrombus
3. Right heart thrombus
4. IV drug use
5. Cardiac vegetations
6. Fat embolism in trauma patients
7. Fracture of the large long bones, tibia, and femur
8. Orogenital sex

Signs and symptoms of PE include:

1. Chest pain is the most common presenting complaint, often noted 3 to 4 days before presenting to the ED; 90% of patients will present with chest pain.
2. Dyspnea will occur sometime during the course of the presentation (in 80% of cases).
3. Hypoxia will produce anxiety and apprehension (in 60% of cases).
4. The patient may present with a history of syncopal episodes.
5. Tachypnea and respirations greater than 16 may occur in 90% of presenting patients.
6. The patient may present with rales, wheezing, friction rubs, or rhonchi.

Risk factors are:

1. Burns
2. Obesity
3. Deep vein thrombosis
4. Trauma
5. Heart disease, CHF, atrial fibrillation
6. Postoperative period
7. Prolonged immobilization

Three classic types of presentations are:

1. Pulmonary infarction or hemorrhage:
   a. Presents with pleuritic chest pain
   b. Resembles pleuritis or infectious pneumonitis
2. Submassive embolism without infarction:
   a. Presents with unexplained dyspnea on exertion or rest
   b. Will look like infection, CHF, asthma, hyperventilation
3. Massive embolism:
   a. Presents with acute cor pulmonale (enlarged right ventricle secondary to malfunction of the lungs)

b. Will look like an acute myocardial infarction (AMI), hypovolemia, or septic shock

The prognosis is:

1. Ten percent will die in 1 hour.
2. When the diagnosis is made, survivors have an 8% mortality rate.
3. Death occurs in chronically ill patients after 24 hours.
4. The incidence of recurrence will be high.

The arterial blood gas interpretation is:

1. The A-a gradient (room air at sea level) = 150 − (measured $PaO_2 + PaCO_2/0.8$) or A-a = 140 − ($PO_2 + PCO_2$)
2. Normal is less than 10 mm Hg in youth and 20 mm Hg in adults (The useful rule is that the A-a gradient should never be greater than 10 plus one tenth of the patient's age)
3. A patient with a decreased PaO_2 and an increased A-a gradient, in the setting of a suspected PE, is highly likely to be having a PE

ECG changes are:

1. Right-heart strain and tall, peaked P waves
2. Right axis deviation
3. New right bundle branch block
4. S1-Q3-T3 pattern, large S wave in lead I, large Q wave in lead III, ST depression in lead II, with T wave inversion in lead III
5. T wave inversion in V_1 to V_4
6. Tachycardia
7. Nonspecific ST-T wave changes
8. Atrial fibrillation

Chest x-ray findings are:

1. Nonspecific and insensitive
2. Hampton's hump, a triangular, pleural-based infiltrate that is frequently located at the costophrenic junction with the apex toward the hilum
3. Westermark's sign, dilated pulmonary vessels to the embolism, along with the collapse of those distal, with a sharp cut-off
4. Thirty percent will have a normal chest x-ray.
5. One half will have an elevated hemidiaphragm.
6. One third will develop transient parenchymal infiltrates.

The V/Q scan results are based on Bayes theorem, 4 V/Q scan interpretation:

1. Normal scan with no perfusion defects
   a. Sensitivity of 2% (2% of patients with this pattern will have a PE)
   b. Positive predictive value of 4% (4% do have a PE)
   c. 96% with this pattern do not have a PE

2. Low probability, small perfusion defects
   a. Sensitivity of 16% (16% of patients with a PE will have this pattern)
   b. Positive predictive value of 14% (14% have a PE)
   c. 86% with this pattern do not have a PE
3. Intermediate probability, any V/Q scan not classified as "high" or "low":
   a. Sensitivity of 41% (41% of patients with a PE will have this pattern)
   b. Positive predictive value of 30% (30% have a PE)
   c. 70% with this pattern do not have a PE
4. High probability, two or more segmental or larger defects
   a. Sensitivity of 41% (41% of patients with a PE will have this pattern)
   b. Positive predictive value of 87% (87% will have a PE)
   c. 13% with this pattern will not have a PE

Pulmonary angiography is the "gold standard" of PE diagnosis.
Treatment of a PE:

1. High dose of oxygen
2. Treat hypotension if present with IV crystalloids if the CVP is low; give dopamine 5 to 10 μg/kg/min if the CVP is normal or high.
3. Laboratory values: CBC, PT, PTT, sodium, potassium, chloride, CO_2, BUN, creatinine, glucose, creatine phosphokinase (CPK), CPK-MB, lactate dehydrogenase (LDH), aspartate aminotransferase (AST), alanine aminotransferase (ALT)
4. Arterial blood gas
5. Two 14- to 16-gauge IV lines of crystalloids
6. Placement of a Swan-Ganz catheter
7. Heparin: Start at 5,000 to 10,000 unit bolus, then 25 units/kg/hr, PTT to 1½ to 2 times control values (in case of abnormal bleeding caused by heparin, use protamine sulfate). (Each milligram of protamine sulfate neutralizes approximately 100 units of heparin activity.)
8. Thrombolytic therapy in PE
   a. Criteria:
      1. A hemodynamically compromised patient who has not responded to stabilization procedures
      2. Pulmonary angiography has documented a massive PE
      3. Consultation with a pulmonary specialist
9. A pulmonary embolectomy can be done in consultation with a thoracic surgeon.

TUBERCULOSIS

Definition

Tuberculosis is an acute or chronic illness caused by *Mycobacterium,* which forms tubercles. Tuberculosis can infect humans or animals (cattle). It has been known as white plague, phthisis, and consumption and was the primary infectious disease killer in the United States in 1900.

Epidemiology

Tuberculosis is transmitted from one person to another by aerosol contamination through droplets. Household members, fellow workers, and persons who live in tightly packed environments (e.g., jails and institutions) are at high risk for infection. With the increase in HIV and AIDS, new rapid-onset *Mycobacterium* are infecting the AIDS population. In the AIDS population, tuberculosis causes a massive systemic infection. Tuberculosis is most prevalent in the homeless, drug addict population, alcoholics, the elderly population, and the nursing home population. It is also prevalent in the immigrant population.

Pathology

Tuberculosis is a *Mycobacterium* organism of many types. They are all acid-fast staining. They are non–spore-forming, aerobic, and non-motile bacilli. They will cause a granulomatous reaction or infection. Types of tuberculosis include:

M. tuberculosis
Bacillus Calmette-Guérin
M. kansasii
M. fortuitum
M. bovis
M. avium
M. gordonae

Large numbers of the organism must be transmitted to cause the initial infection. It usually takes 2 to 3 weeks for the organisms to multiply before a patient is symptomatic, if at all. The organism is spread during this inflammatory response period, 2 to 3 weeks after initial infection, by the lymphatics and hematogenously. This spreading period usually takes the organisms to the upper lobes of the lungs secondary to the organisms' high oxygen requirement and the high oxygen tension of the upper lung. The organism usually starts in the superior segments of the lower lobes and the apical and posterior segments of the upper lobes. These sites are usually the initial site of infection.

Tuberculosis also likes to infect the vertebral column, renal cortex, the meninges, epiphysis of the long bones, and the pericardium. As the organism grows and spreads, granulomatous formations occur. Macrophages, giant cells, and histiocytes are then surrounded by the granulomatous tubercle. The granuloma begins to scar, and this scarring kills many of the organisms, thus stopping further spread of the infection.

Clinical Presentation

The usual presenting complaint is a mild upper respiratory or inflammatory response. The majority of infected patients do not develop significant sequelae. After the aforementioned pathologic process occurs, if the host organism is not immunocompromised, there is host immunity to further infections. The remains from the initial infection become a calcified focus in the lung or a calcified regional lymph node (Ghon's complex).

Primary tuberculosis occurs after the initial infection. Ninety percent of the time, there is no clinical illness. The purified protein derivative (PPD) skin test will be positive, and there will be hilar lymph node involvement. A subpleural lesion will be the primary lesion. The consolidation process that takes place will be one much like pneumonia.

Reactivation of tuberculosis is the classification of tuberculosis that is most commonly seen with a true clinical presentation. The patient presents with fever, weight loss, symptoms of a chronic illness, malaise, and a productive cough with occasional hemoptysis. The PPD will be positive in 80% of the cases, and the chest x-ray will show apical or posterior lobe involvement of the upper lobes.

Tuberculosis with a pleural effusion is a complication of primary tuberculosis. A fibrocaseous tuberculosis is seen in the bronchopleural fistula. Ninety percent of these patients will have a positive PPD. These patients present with pleuritic chest pain. There will be minimal sputum production, with a mild cough and a low-grade fever. The chest x-ray will show a pleural fluid. Fluid from the effusion should be analyzed. The fluid will show an elevated LDH and a low glucose with a decrease in fluid pH. Acute effusion fluid will show polymorphonuclear leukocytosis while chronic effusions will show lymphocytic leukocytosis.

Extrapulmonary tuberculosis is secondary to a disseminated infection. Pericarditis, skeletal tuberculosis, meningitis, and peritonitis can all be caused by extrapulmonary tuberculosis.

Miliary tuberculosis is an acute form of hematogenous tuberculosis. It presents with multisystem involvement. Splenomegaly, hepatomegaly, arthritis, pericarditis, peritonitis, and meningitis can all be presenting complaints of miliary tuberculosis.

Tuberculosis in the patient with AIDS has been on the rise since 1986. Ten percent of all patients with AIDS in the United States have tuberculosis. Haitians with AIDS have a 60% rate of tuberculosis. AIDS patients, being immunocompromised, are more susceptible to the initial infection and to rapid reactivation. Their decreased T-cell level sets up an environment for widespread dissemination, leading to an increased rate of extrapulmonary and miliary forms of tuberculosis.

Diagnosis

A diagnosis is made by a positive PPD, positive sputum cultures, bronchial washings, or biopsy of lung tissue. A chest x-ray is also helpful in the diagnosis of tuberculosis.

Laboratory Findings

Cultures of the patient's sputum are necessary for diagnosis. Specimens of gastric fluid, bronchoalveolar lavage, bronchial washing, and bronchial or lung biopsy are sometimes necessary to make a definitive diagnosis.

Treatment

Currently a 9-month regimen of isoniazid and rifampin is recommended in nonimmunocompromised patients. It should be supplemented with ethambutol, streptomycin, or pyrazinamide as needed.

Infants and children should be treated with isoniazid and rifampin. A 6-month regimen is acceptable if four drugs are used: isoniazid, pyrazinamide, rifampin, and streptomycin or ethambutol.

Immunosuppressed patients should receive 9 to 12 months of a four-drug therapy. Extrapulmonary tuberculosis should be treated with a four-drug therapy.

Persons who have come in close contact with a positive tuberculosis patient should be treated as if they have tuberculosis. Those persons include household members and other close contacts, newly infected persons, within 2 years of infection, and persons with a positive PPD or abnormal chest x-ray. The following people should also be treated as if they have tuberculosis: any person with a positive PPD who has diabetes mellitus; end-stage renal disease, corticosteroid therapy for COPD, silicosis, AIDS, or is positive for HIV, but does not have AIDS, hematologic or reticuloendothelial malignancies, chronic or rapid weight loss, and those younger than 35 years of age with a positive tuberculin skin test.

Doses of Tuberculosis Treatment Drugs	
Isoniazid	5 to 10 mg/kg/day, up to 300 mg PO or IM
Ethambutol	15 to 25 mg/kg/day PO
Rifampin	10 to 20 mg/kg/day, up to 600 mg/day PO
Streptomycin	15 to 20 mg/kg/day, up to 1 g/day IM
Pyrazinamide	15 to 30 mg/kg/day, up to 2 g/day PO

BIBLIOGRAPHY

Hamilton GC, Sanders AB, Strange GR, et al (eds): Emergency Medicine: An Approach to Clinical Problem-Solving. Philadelphia, WB Saunders, 1991

Kravis TC, Warner CG, Jacobs LM (eds): Emergency Medicine: A Comprehensive Review, 3rd ed. New York, Raven Press, 1993

May HL, Aghababian RV, Fleisher GR (eds): Emergency Medicine, 2nd ed. Boston, Little, Brown, 1992

Pearson RD, Guerrant RL, Isselbacher KJ, et al (eds): Harrison's Principles of Internal Medicine, 11th ed. New York, McGraw-Hill, 1987

Rosen P, Barkin RM (eds): Emergency Medicine: Concepts and Clinical Practice, 3rd ed. St. Louis, Mosby-Year Book, 1992

Schwartz GR, Cayten CG, Mangelsen MA, et al (eds): Principles and Practice of Emergency Medicine. Philadelphia, Lea & Febiger, 1992

Tierney LM, McPhee SJ, Papadakis MA (eds): Current Medical Diagnosis and Treatment, 33rd ed. Norwalk, CT, Appleton & Lange, 1994

Tintinalli JE, Krone RL, Ruiz E (eds): Emergency Medicine: A Comprehensive Study Guide, 4th ed. New York, McGraw-Hill, 1996

Chapter 16

Acute Resuscitation Emergencies

AIRWAY MANAGEMENT

Definition

Emergency airway management is a common problem encountered in the emergency department (ED) daily. It is the "A" in ABCs. Airway obstruction can be as simple as a tongue obstructing the airway or as complicated as a foreign body, or a tumor or angioedema. Airway obstruction causes hypoxia and hypercapnia with death to the brain within 5 to 6 minutes without oxygen. Cyanosis occurs when the hemoglobin has desaturated to 5 g/100 ml. (For pediatric airway management, see the pediatric airway management section.)

Clinical Presentation

Aphonia indicates a complete airway obstruction. Hoarseness is specifically localized to the larynx and is associated with edema and unilateral vocal cord dysfunction. Stridor is a high-pitched squeaking or crowing noise that is indicative of a partial airway obstruction of the larynx or trachea. For stridor to occur, the diameter of the airway must be less than 4 mm at rest and 4 to 6 mm on exertion. Patients with pharyngeal obstruction will present with "snoring" sounds. If an expiratory wheezing is present, it is indicative of an obstruction at the bronchial level. Coughing can be secondary to a mechanical, chemical, or thermal stimulus. A croupy barking cough is secondary to subglottic pathology such as croup. A "brassy" cough is usually secondary to tracheobronchial disease.

Treatment

Rescue breathing can be accomplished by mouth-to-mouth or bag-to-mouth breathing in the ED. Always remember to ask how the patient became unconscious, and always protect the patient's cervical spine if there is a possibility of injury or fracture. The patient should be given 100% oxygen at a rate of 12 to 20 breaths/min for a tidal volume of 1000 to 2000 mL in an adult by mask until intubation is accomplished. I do not recommend the use of the esophageal obturator airway (EOA). Good airway control with a well-fitting mask is superior to an EOA tube. Endotracheal or nasotracheal intubation is the recommended type of intubation. Indication for endotracheal intubation is airway obstruction, hypoxia, hypercarbia, and an emergent investigation without motion artifact.

The indication for nasotracheal intubation is: difficult or impossible direct laryngoscope intubation, possible cervical spine injury, or long-term ventilation. The contraindications of nasotracheal intubation include apnea, upper airway foreign body, tumor or abscess, central facial fractures, nasal obstruction, basal skull fracture, coagulopathy, acute epiglottitis, or cardiac or other prostheses. Nasotracheal intubation can cause epistaxis, bacteremia, turbinate mucosal avulsion, necrosis of the nares, sinusitis, otitis media, and retropharyngeal or piriform sinus perforation.

Rapid Sequence Induction

Preoxygenate the patient with 100% bag-to-face mask for 3 minutes with cricoid pressure

Pretreatment Options

- Atropine 0.02 mg/kg intravenously (IV), routine if older than 10 years of age
- Lidocaine 1.5 mg/kg IV (routine)

  OR

- Vecuronium 0.01 mg/kg IV (optional, not routine)

  OR

- Fentanyl 3 μg/kg IV (optional, not routine)

WAIT FOR 1 TO 3 MINUTES

Induction and Muscle Relaxation

Pick *One* Induction Agent:

- Thiopental 3 to 5 mg/kg for hemodynamically (HD) stable patients, 0.5 to 1 mg/kg for unstable patients

  OR

- Etomidate 0.3 to 0.4 mg/kg IV for HD stable patients, 0.1 to 0.2 mg/kg IV for unstable patients

  OR

- Methohexital (Brevital) 1 to 2 mg/kg IV for HD stable patients

Pick *One* Paralytic Agent:

- Succinylcholine 1.5 mg/kg IV

  OR
- Vecuronium 0.1 to 0.3 mg/kg IV

Rapid Sequence Induction in an Asthmatic Patient or Patient with COPD

Preoxygenate with 100% oxygen by facemask for 3 minutes with cricoid pressure

Pretreatment Options

- Atropine 0.02 mg/kg IV routine if younger than 10 years of age
- Lidocaine 1.5 mg/kg IV (routine)

Induction agent:

- Ketamine 0.5 to 1 mg/kg IV

Paralytic agent:

- Succinylcholine 1.5 mg/kg IV

There are two types of blades: the Miller (straight blade) and the MacIntosh (curved). Only by use and practice can you determine which blade is best for you. Fiberoptic intubation is an invaluable technique in difficult intubations in the ED. It can negate the necessity of a cricothyrotomy in many cases. Retrograde tracheal and

Rapid Sequence Induction in a Patient with a Head Injury

Preoxygenate with 100% oxygen by facemask for 3 minutes with cricoid pressure

Pretreatment Options

- Fentanyl 3 μg/kg IV

Induction agent:

- Thiopental 3 to 5 mg/kg IV for HD stable patients, 0.5 to 1 mg/kg for HD unstable patients

Paralytic agent:

- Succinylcholine 1.5 mg/kg IV

tactile endotracheal intubation both require special equipment and practice but should be known by anyone working in the ED.

Once patients are paralyzed, they can be kept paralyzed and sedated with vecuronium 1 to 2 mg IV and midazolam (Versed) in 1 to 2 mg IV every hour.

SHOCK

Definition

Shock is the acute reduction of blood flow secondary to diminished cardiac output and maldistribution of output with potential for reversal. Shock causes impairment of the brain, heart, lungs, kidneys, mesentery, muscles, and skin.

Patients present in three generalized types of shock: hypovolemic (traumatic or nontraumatic), cardiogenic (traumatic or nontraumatic), and vasogenic (septic, anaphylactic, neurogenic, pharmacologic).

Pathology

As the fluid loss progresses, the venous capacitance is decreased by about 10 to 20% before a patient is symptomatic, with an interstitial to intravascular compartment shift of fluid and arteriolar constriction. The central venous pressure (CVP) is decreased, even though there is compensation stroke volume and urine output decreases. There is decreased skin perfusion and decreased temperature regulation. The central nervous system (CNS) also has decreased perfusion, which causes altered mental status. There is a decrease in microvascular perfusion and cardiovascular dysfunction. As the process ensues, there is anaerobic metabolism and release of proteolytic enzymes and vasoactive substances. Platelet aggregation and myocardial function is depressed.

Clinical Presentation

Nontraumatic *hypovolemic* shock occurs secondary to dehydration or hemorrhage, secondary to decreased fluid volume. Patients with hemorrhage present with bloody stools, hematemesis, hemoptysis, signs of a ruptured aortic aneurysm, or severe epistaxis. An acute ectopic pregnancy should be considered in any female of childbearing years who is hypotensive.

Patients with hypovolemia due to dehydration appear very pale and have moist skin secondary to adrenergic stimulation. Patients with traumatic hypovolemic shock present with hypotension or tachycardia that responds to IV fluids and blood.

Other causes of hypovolemic shock are sedatives, anorexia, bulemia, gastrointestinal obstruction, CNS abnormalities, overdiuresis, diabetes, diabetic ketoacidosis, and adrenal insufficiency. Pancreatitis, peritonitis, and ascites can cause sequestration of fluids and hypovolemia.

Cardiogenic shock is most often seen in patients who have had a myocardial infarction (MI), papillary muscle rupture, or ventricular septal defect (VSD). VSD and papillary rupture can be detected by a loud systolic murmur that is louder than the first heart sound (S_1). Pericardial tamponade, air embolus, tension pneumothorax, and pulmonary embolus can all cause cardiogenic shock. Dilated, nondilated, restrictive, and hypertropic cardiomyopathies can also cause cardiogenic shock secondary to decreased stroke volume and decreased ejection fraction.

Symptoms of cardiogenic shock are the same as those for hypovolemia, including anxiety and obtundation. Tachypnea and tachycardia are often present, unless a heart block is also present, secondary to a new MI. The patient is usually hypotensive. There is elevated jugular venous distention (JVD) and an S_3 secondary to an increased left ventricular end-diastolic pressure. If a right-sided MI is suspected, perform a right-sided electrocardiogram (ECG). Remember that right-sided MIs are fluid dependent.

Traumatic cardiogenic shock is secondary to cardiac tamponade, tension pneumothorax, or myocardial contusion, all of which decrease cardiac output secondary to poor venous return to the heart.

Pericardial tamponade can be secondary to penetrating trauma to the chest or abdomen. It can be secondary to a gunshot wound or a stab wound. It only takes 200 ml of blood to create a hemodynamic compromise. Beck's triad is the presence of distended neck veins, decreased arterial pressure, and muffled heart sounds secondary to a cardiac tamponade.

A patient with a tension pneumothorax presents with agitation, dyspnea, cyanosis, hypotension, and tachycardia. Always look for a tracheal shift toward the good lung and away from the pneumothorax.

Cardiac contusion rarely causes cardiogenic shock, but if blunt trauma is a factor in the history, consider myocardial contusion. Usually the right atrium and ventricle are affected more than the left atrium and ventricle secondary to their posterior location to the sternum.

Vasogenic shock is secondary to arteriolar and venous dilatation. Vasogenic shock includes septic, pharmacologic, anaphylactic, and neurogenic shock.

Septic shock is secondary to infection, usually in the compromised patient with underlying disease. The patient can present with chills, hyperthermia, hypothermia, nausea, vomiting, or mental status changes.

Pharmacologic shock is a drug-induced shock secondary to sedative hypnotics, narcotics, nitrates, antidepressants, antihypertensives, and cholinergics.

Anaphylactic shock occurs secondary to immunoglobulin E (IgE) or immunoglobulin M (IgM)–mediated hypersensitivity of the immune system. The patient presents with hypotension, bronchial spasm, dyspnea, pruritus, increased vascular permeability, and arteriolar dilatation.

Neurogenic shock is secondary to a spinal cord injury. The patient presents with hypotension and bradycardia secondary to a loss of sympathetic tone to the distal level of the spinal cord injury.

Laboratory Findings

A complete blood count (CBC), hematocrit and hemoglobin, prothrombin time (PT), partial thromboplastin time (PTT), and electrolytes should be drawn in any shock patient. If shock is secondary to bleeding, type and crossmatched blood (6 to 8 units) should be ordered. Type-specific blood is the choice of blood for transfusion. It usually only takes 5 minutes more to determine a blood crossmatch from a type and screen. Blood, urine, and sputum cultures should be obtained if septic shock is considered. Cardiac enzymes should be obtained if an MI or injury is suspected. An arterial blood gas should be obtained to determine the acid-base status of the patient.

Treatment

The mainstay of treating any kind of shock is to treat or remove the underlying cause of the shock. Treatment goals are to maximize oxygenation, correct underlying metabolic abnormalities, and improve hemodynamic dysfunction.

To monitor the fluid status of the patient is to monitor the CVP. The CVP is the filling pressure of the right atrium, which is dependent on the right ventricle function, venous tone, intrathoracic pressure, and intravascular volume. The normal values for CVP lie between 50 and 120 mm H_2O. CVP is elevated in pericardial tamponade, pulmonary embolism, right ventricular failure, and vasogenic causes secondary to left ventricular failure. In nonvasogenic causes, venous tone is low and CVP will be low. CVP will be low in hypovolemic shock and increased in cardiogenic shock.

Hypovolemic shock is treated with crystalloid infusions of lactated Ringer's solution or normal saline 0.9%. Fluid should be given in boluses, and then the patient's vital signs should be rechecked with CVP monitoring. Hemorrhagic shock should be treated with blood. Usually 2 units of fresh frozen plasma should be given for every 10 units of blood. Platelets should be given as needed to keep the platelet count above 100,000 platelets/mm³.

Cardiogenic shock treatment is a delicate balancing act. Fluid levels should be monitored by a Swan-Ganz catheter. If the cardiac index is below 2.2 l/min/m², fluids should be given to obtain a wedge pressure of 15 to 18 mm Hg. Dysrhythmias should be treated aggressively. Oxygen, nitrates, and narcotics are used to relieve the pain of an acute MI.

If cardiogenic shock persists or if the patient is severely hypotensive, dopamine is the first drug of choice. It has alpha and beta effects at a renal dose of 5 μg/kg/min and at doses of 5 to 15 μg/kg/min.

This dose will cause increased cardiac output and peripheral vascular resistance. It has alpha effects at doses higher than 15 to 20 $\mu g/kg/min$. At this dose, a generalized vasoconstriction occurs with a greatly increased systemic vascular resistance and the likelihood of ischemia. Dopamine also raises the wedge pressure.

Dobutamine is the drug of second choice. It is primarily a β_1 receptor agonist and is a positive inotrope, which increases or maintains cardiac output. Dobutamine also lowers the wedge pressure.

If the cardiogenic shock is secondary to penetrating trauma to the chest and the patient loses his or her pulse within 2 minutes of arrival in the ED, a left anterior thoracotomy should be performed. This procedure increases afterload and decreases arterial bleeding inferiorly when the aorta is cross-clamped and the pericardium is opened, thus relieving pericardial tamponade. If cardiac tamponade is believed to be the cause of the hypotension, then a pericardiocentesis should be performed.

Vasogenic shock or septic shock is managed by treating the underlying infection. Blood, sputum, and urine cultures should be obtained, and the patient should be given broad-spectrum antibiotics. Antibiotics should include gram-negative coverage with a third-generation cephalosporin or an aminoglycoside. Penicillin or vancomycin should be added to cover staphylococcal infections. If the patient is neutropenic, antibiotic coverage for *Pseudomonas* should be included.

Pharmacologic shock secondary to narcotics should be treated with naloxone, fluid, and vasopressors if necessary. Neurogenic shock is treated with fluid and dopamine or ephedrine. If bradycardia is present, treat the patient with atropine or pacing if required. Neurogenic shock usually resolves in 3 to 8 days.

Anaphylactic shock is treated with epinephrine and fluids. If the patient's blood pressure is not responding to subcutaneous or IV epinephrine, then an epinephrine drip of 2 to 4 $\mu g/min$ should be started and titrated until a clinical response is achieved. The patient should also be given diphenhydramine 50 mg IV, aerosolized albuterol 0.5 ml in 3 ml of saline, methylprednisolone 125 mg IV, and cimetidine 300 mg IV.

Any patient in shock should be admitted to an intensive care unit.

BIBLIOGRAPHY

Brandenburg RO, Fuster V, Giuliani ER, et al (eds): Cardiology Fundamentals and Practice. Chicago, Year Book Medical Publishers, 1987

Braunwald E, Isselbacher KJ, Petersdorf RG, et al (eds): Harrison's Principles of Internal Medicine, 11th ed. New York, McGraw-Hill, 1987

Eagle KA, Harber E, DeSanctis A, Austen WG (eds): The Practice of Cardiology, 2nd ed. Boston, Little, Brown, 1989

Hamilton GC, Sanders AB, Strange GR, et al (eds): Emergency Medicine: An Approach to Clinical Problem-Solving. Philadelphia, WB Saunders, 1991

Hurst JW, Logue RB, Rackley CE (eds): The Heart, 6th ed. New York, McGraw-Hill, 1994
Kravis TC, Warner CG, Jacobs LM (eds): Emergency Medicine: A Comprehensive
Review, 3rd ed. New York, Raven Press, 1993
May HL, Aghababian RV, Fleisher GR (eds): Emergency Medicine, 2nd ed. Boston,
Little, Brown, 1992
Rosen P, Barkin RM (eds): Emergency Medicine: Concepts and Clinical Practice, 3rd ed.
St. Louis, Mosby-Year Book, 1992
Schwartz GR, Cayton CG, Manglesen MA, et al (eds): Principles and Practice of
Emergency Medicine, 3rd ed. Philadelphia, Lea & Febiger, 1992
Tintinalli JE, Krone RL, Ruiz E (eds): Emergency Medicine: A Comprehensive Study
Guide, 4th ed. New York, McGraw-Hill, 1996

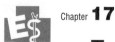

Chapter 17

Toxicology Emergencies

GENERAL PRINCIPLES OF THE POISONED PATIENT

Definition

Numerous words are used to describe the poisoned patient. Inebriation is used to describe the symptoms of alcohol ingestion. Intolerance is used to describe a low sensitivity to a nontoxic substance. Hypersensitivity is used to describe an altered immunologic response, independent of the metabolism of the compound. Intoxication is used interchangeably with inebriation, but intoxication can be from any substance that can cause alcohol-like effects. Idiosyncrasy is used to describe an aberration in the host's biochemistry that can lead to a disease peculiar to the metabolism or genetic composition of the host. Poisoning is used to describe a dose-dependent reaction that is usually harmful to the organism.

Epidemiology

There are over 1.5 million poisonings each year in the United States as reported by the American Association of Poison Centers. Actual poisonings may be twice this number secondary to the lack of reporting to poison centers. Fifty percent of all poisoning in the United States occurs in children between the ages of 1 and 5 years. These poisonings are usually always accidental. Approximately 10% of all hospitalizations are from acute poisonings.

Most adult poisonings are intentional. Eighty to 90% of all adult poisonings require admission to a medical intensive care unit (ICU) or a psychiatric unit. These intentional poisonings are from suicidal attempts, suicidal gestures, recreational drug abuse overdose, and occupational exposure. Poisoning accounts for approximately 7% of all ED visits. Ninety-two percent of all poisonings are in the home and take place between the hours of 5:00 PM and 9:00 PM. Most poisonings that occur in infants younger than 5 years of age are therefore accidental, and most adult poisonings are intentional or the adult has an underlying psychiatric illness. Forty-one percent of all accidental ingestions occur in the kitchen, and 21% occur in the bathroom.

Toxicokinetics and Pharmacokinetics

With every poisoning, several important questions must be answered about the toxin before appropriate treatment can be given. Important pharmacokinetic questions to be answered are:

1. What is the absorption rate of the toxin?
2. Where is the toxin stored in the body?

3. What is the volume of distribution of the drug in the body?
4. How is the drug excreted from the body?
5. How is the drug metabolized in the body?
6. Is the toxin protein bound?

The volume of distribution is the measurement of the amount of drug that is located in a certain part of the body (i.e., blood, fat, or organ tissues). The larger the volume of distribution of the toxin, the more of the toxin will be in the tissues. The smaller the volume of distribution of the toxin, the larger the amount of toxin that will be in the blood. The volume of distribution is required to determine the usefulness of dialysis, hemoperfusion, or exchange transfusions in therapy.

The way in which a toxin is excreted or eliminated is very important. Often excretion or elimination can be affected by therapy. Most toxins are eliminated by the liver, kidney, and lungs as bile, urine, sweat, or breathing.

Elimination is described as zero-order, first-order, or Michaelis-Menten order. Zero-order kinetics, or enzyme kinetics, means that a drug is metabolized only to a certain point, usually in the liver. Once the liver reaches this fixed point of metabolism, serum levels of the toxin rise dramatically. In zero-order kinetics, a constant amount of the toxin is eliminated over a certain period of time.

In first-order kinetics, renal elimination means that the higher the plasma concentration, the greater will be the amount of toxin eliminated by the kidneys. In first-order kinetics, a constant fraction of a toxin is eliminated over a certain period of time.

Michaelis-Menten elimination is a combination of both zero-order and first-order kinetics. Often after the enzymes in the liver are saturated, elimination is switched to zero-order kinetics.

Elimination can be increased by dialysis, diuresis, hemoperfusion, diuresis with ion trapping, and multiple doses of activated charcoal.

Approach to the Poisoned Patient

Always approach the poisoned patient in a cool and calm manner. Never be judgmental in your questioning or approach. Intentional ingestions are cries for help. Parents usually feel very bad that their child was poisoned in their own home. Always ensure appropriate psychiatric intervention.

Safety Net

Always establish a safety net on any patient who has been poisoned. With many acute drug ingestions, patients can have normal vital signs one minute and be dead the next. Always place the patient on a cardiac monitor and place at least one large-gauge IV line of normal saline or lactated Ringer's solution. Place the patient on pulse oximetry, and also place the patient on 2 liters of oxygen via nasal cannula.

Vital signs must be taken every 4 to 5 minutes until you have established the nature of poisoning. Vital signs include blood pressure, pulse, respiration, temperature, and pulse oximetry. Baseline vital signs are always necessary in the evaluation of any poisoned patient. They will guide how aggressive medical treatment will be.

History

A complete history of the event is always required. Often histories are difficult to obtain. In the pediatric population, the event is usually unwitnessed and the child is always a poor historian. A patient with intentional ingestion or a suicidal attempt usually does not want to give a history, and drug abusers are reluctant to give a history secondary to fear of prosecution.

A specific overdose history includes how much drug was taken, when was it taken, why was it taken, what else was taken, and whether the person took the medication before. Remember that many intentional overdoses are polyoverdoses.

Always obtain the past medical history to include a psychiatric history or a history of overdoses or prior suicide attempts. A social history should include IV drugs, alcohol, tobacco, and caffeine use. Recent divorce, marriage, death of a loved one, loss of job, start of a new job, new child in the home, or birth of a child are all important social histories to obtain. A family history should include a psychiatric history. A surgical history should include chronic pain or chronic pain medications. Information on a current or past medication use should be obtained. A record should be made of prior hospitalizations.

Clinical Presentation

Most poisoned patients present in one of six classic toxidrome classes: cholinergic, anticholinergic, opiate, sedative-hypnotic, sympathomimetic, and psychedelic poisoning.

Cholinergic poisoning patients present with the symptoms of SLUDGE—*s*alivation, *l*acrimation, *u*rination, *d*efecation, *G*I upset, and *e*mesis. These symptoms are due to the stimulation of the cholinergic receptors by cholinergic drugs that result in somatic and autonomic nervous system imbalances. This imbalance causes an increase in acetylcholine circulation. The increase in acetylcholine causes a cholinergic crisis that affects the parasympathomimetic nervous system, which causes the hypersecretory state of SLUDGE.

A patient will present with miosis and ciliary dysfunction, confusion, seizures, fasciculations to flaccid paralysis, pulmonary edema, or cardiac dysrhythmias. Atropine is the drug of choice for treatment of a cholinergic crisis.

Anticholinergic poisoning results from antagonism of acetylcholine by numerous medications or plant metabolites. A patient will present with the symptoms of the *Alice in Wonderland* paraphrase, "mad as a hatter, blind as a bat, red as a beet, hot as a hare, and dry as a bone." On physical examination, the patient will have dry eyes, skin and mouth, fever, urinary retention, hypoactive bowel sounds, decreased visual acuity, mydriasis, and photophobia. This patient is often psychotic or delirious.

Opiates are naturally occurring alkaloids and synthetic congeners. Patients with opiate overdose present with respiratory depression, coma, and miosis. Meperidine (Demerol) has some anticholinergic properties. Opiate poisoning is treated with naloxone and an opiate antagonist.

Sedative-hypnotics are a group of man-made compounds that are also found naturally. These compounds affect the CNS. They cause CNS depression much like the barbiturates, and they mimic ethanol intoxication. A patient with sedative-hypnotic poisoning presents with impaired judgment, lability of mood, dysarthria, ataxia, and often nystagmus. In an acute severe poisoning, flaccid paralysis, areflexia, and coma can occur. A patient in a barbiturate coma often presents with miosis, but some sedative-hypnotics can cause mydriasis. Treatment is usually supportive.

Sympathomimetics are amphetamine-like stimulants. People use sympathomimetics to cause anorexia for weight loss, decrease fatigue, create insomnia to stay awake at night, and be more alert. They can cause hyperkinesis, irritability, and anxiety. Paranoid schizophrenia can occur in high doses, along with stereotyped, semipurposeful movements, repetitive gestures, and bruxism. The treatment is mainly supportive.

The *psychedelics* are synthetic compounds derived from plant metabolites. They cause hallucinations and nonspecific behavioral changes. A patient will present with a diminished sense of personal and physical boundaries and philosophical introversion. On physical examination, the patient can present with tachycardia, mydriasis, hypertension, tremor, hyperthermia, hyperreflexia, and piloerection.

Examination

Every patient who presents to the ED with a suspected overdose should have a complete physical examination, including an examination of the skin, fingernails, toenails, and a complete cardiac, pulmonary, neurologic, rectal, and mental examination.

Treatment

Always evaluate the patient's basic life support when he or she arrives in the ED. Treatment is divided into supportive care, decontamination of the patient, antidotes, and elimination of poison and definitive care phases.

If exposure is dermal, the contaminated clothing should be removed and the patient cleaned with copious amounts of soap and water. Eye irrigations should take place for a minimum of 15 to 30 minutes in each eye. If ingestion took place, then GI decontamination should be the first priority after establishment of basic life support. Gastric decontamination can be achieved by syrup of ipecac or gastric lavage and activated charcoal. Currently, gastric lavage and activated charcoal are the recommended choices of gastric decontamination. Syrup of ipecac has fallen out of favor secondary to its risk of airway compromise when vomiting occurs and its ability to reduce absorption by only 30%.

Gastric lavage is performed with a No. 36 to 40 French orogastric hose with infusion of 250 to 300 ml of water or normal saline until the fluid return is clear. The patient's airway must be maintained at all times. After gastric lavage is performed, activated charcoal in a dose of 1 g/kg should be given to all patients. Not all ingestants bind to charcoal, but always give charcoal secondary to the large number of poisoned patients with co-ingestions. Approximately 50% of ingestants are absorbed by activated charcoal. Multiple doses of activated charcoal are often recommended in this chapter. Multiple doses of charcoal will often reduce gastric absorption by 50% each time a dose is given.

Cathartics decrease the transit time through the bowel of the poison and charcoal. Sorbitol, magnesium sulfate, and magnesium citrate all speed up GI motility, causing less exposure time of the poison in the gut.

Supportive care involves taking care of a compromised airway caused by vomiting, stridor, or diminished gag reflex. Bronchospasm should be treated with a β-antagonist, oxygen, positive end-expiratory pressure (PEEP) ventilation if the patient is intubated, and admission to the ICU. Hypotension is treated with fluid and vasopressors. Cardiac arrhythmias are treated as usual. Antidote treatment is agent specific.

Agents that cause concretions are remembered by the mnemonic BIG MESS:

B = Barbiturates
I = Iron
G = Glutethimide
M = Meprobamate
E = Extended-release theophylline
SS = Salicylates

Drugs that cause seizures are remembered by the mnemonic WITH LA COPS:

W = Withdrawal
I = Isoniazid
T = Theophylline and tricyclics
H = Hypoglycemia, hypoxia
L = Lead, local anesthetics, and lithium
A = Anticholinergics
C = Cholinergics, camphor, CO, and CN
O = Organophosphates
P = Phenothiazines, PCP, and propoxyphene
S = Sympathomimetics, salicylates, and strychnine

Drugs that cause nystagmus are remembered by the mnemonic SALEM TIP:

S = Sedative-hypnotics and solvents
A = Alcohol
L = Lithium
E = Ethylene glycol and ethanol
M = Methanol
T = Tegretol and thiamine depletion
I = Isopropanol
P = Phenytoin, PCP

Drugs that cause an altered level of consciousness are remembered by the mnemonic DONT:

D = Dextrose
O = Oxygen
N = Naloxone
T = Thiamine

Radiopaque substances are remembered by the mnemonic BETA A CHIP:

B = Barium
E = Enteric-coated tablets
T = Tricyclics
A = Antihistamines
C = Condoms, calcium, and chloral hydrate
H = Heavy metals
I = Iodine
P = Potassium and phenothiazines

Hydrocarbon additives are remembered by the mnemonic CHAMP:

C = Camphor
H = Halogenated hydrocarbons
A = Aromatics
M = Metals
P = Pesticides

Osmolol gaps are remembered by the mnemonic MAD GAS:

M = Mannitol
A = Alcohol
D = DMSO
G = Glycerol
A = Acetone
S = Sorbitol

AChE inhibitors are remembered by the mnemonic SLUG BAM:

S = Secretions, sweating, and salivation
L = Lacrimation
U = Urination

G = GI upset
B = Bronchoconstriction and bradycardia
A = Abdominal cramps
M = Miosis

Nicotinic effects of AChE inhibitors are remembered by the mnemonic M-T-W-tH-F:

M = Muscle twitching and mydriasis
T = Tachycardia
W = Weakness
tH = Hyperglycemia and hypertension
F = Fasciculations

ACETAMINOPHEN

Definition

Acetaminophen (*N*-acetyl-*p*-amino-phenol or APAP) is used as an antipyretic and analgesic. It has been used for more than 80 years in hundreds of prescription and nonprescription cough, cold, and pain relief medications. It is also used in muscle relaxants, antihistamines, barbiturates, caffeine, narcotics, phenothiazines, and anticholinergic and sympathomimetic medications. APAP is available in caplet, liquid, suppository, or pill form. In children, the therapeutic dose is 15 mg/kg every 4 to 6 hours. The maximum daily dose for children is 80 mg/kg. In adults, the therapeutic dose is 325 to 1000 mg every 4 hours. The maximum daily dose for adults is 4 g.

Epidemiology

The mortality rate from an overdose of APAP is relatively low secondary to the straightforward treatment of an APAP overdose. The mortality rate in the United States for APAP is approximately 0.4% of all poisonings. Of this 0.4% mortality rate, 50% of the death rate is secondary to respiratory depression from co-ingestion of propoxyphene or other opiates. Only 15% of all overdoses have a toxic serum level of APAP. Sixty percent of patients with toxic levels of APAP will have liver damage.

Pathology

Large overdoses of APAP can cause potentially fatal hepatic necrosis. The antipyretic action of APAP is caused by the inhibition of the hypothalamic prostaglandin synthetase. APAP is also an effective cutaneous vasodilator and inhibits the CNS and the peripheral prostaglandin system, which may cause the analgesic activity of APAP.

APAP is rapidly absorbed by the gut, and the peak serum level is obtained in 30 minutes to 2 hours. The volume of distribution of

APAP is 0.9 to 1 l/kg. APAP is rapidly taken up by liver hepatocytes. Protein binding is low with APAP. It is primarily metabolized by the liver, but small amounts are metabolized by the kidneys and then absorbed by the GI tract. Ninety percent of APAP is inactivated by glucuronide and sulfate conjugates and then excreted. In infants, the primary metabolization is by the APAP-sulfate route. In adults, the APAP-glucuronide route is the primary route of metabolization. The plasma half-life in adults is approximately 2 hours.

Large doses of APAP deplete hepatic glutathione stores. This causes toxic metabolites to combine covalently and irreversibly with nucleophilic proteins of the hepatocyte membranes, thus causing hepatocyte destruction.

Large doses of ethanol have an effect on the P450-MFO enzymes and may competitively inhibit the metabolism of APAP. Ethanol may lessen the likelihood that APAP will induce hepatotoxicity.

Clinical Presentation/Examination

A patient may present in one of four stages of APAP overdose. In stage I, the patient presents with nausea and vomiting. In children, these symptoms are more pronounced. Adults can present with mild symptoms or be asymptomatic. If respiratory depression, cardiac symptoms, or CNS symptoms are present, look for co-ingestion of opiates or other drugs.

In stage II, the patient will present with laboratory evidence of hepatic toxicity. The hallmark of stage II is a transient clinical improvement of symptoms (GI symptoms resolve). The serum transaminase levels begin to rise, and the patient develops right upper quadrant pain with hepatomegaly and liver tenderness. Dehydration and oliguria occur. An acute onset of pancreatitis is sometimes present.

In stage III, the liver function abnormalities peak. The aspartate aminotransferase (AST), alanine aminotransferase (ALT), gamma glutamyltransferase (GGT), and bilirubin levels will be elevated. Urinalysis will be abnormal, and the prothrombin time (PT) can be prolonged. In stage IV, the patient either recovers or dies of fulminant hepatic failure.

In the alcoholic patient, a syndrome of combined renal toxicity and hepatic failure is seen in patients who ingest even a normal dose of APAP. Acute tubular necrosis is seen in 50% of these patients.

Diagnosis

The toxic dose of APAP is 140 mg/kg in children and 7.5 g in adults. Children seem less susceptible than do adults to hepatotoxicity. Many drugs such as phenytoin, antihistamines, barbiturates, and other sedatives can cause a stimulation of the P450-MFO system and enhance APAP toxicity. Cimetidine may inhibit this system and thus reduce toxic effects.

Hepatotoxicity is defined as an AST or ALT level greater than 1000 international units (IU)/l. The best predictor of hepatotoxicity is an elevated APAP serum level between 4 and 24 hours after ingestion. The Rumack-Matthew nomogram can depict the risk of toxicity. A toxic dose is one with a level of 300 μg/ml at 4 hours and a level of 9.4 μg/ml at 24 hours.

An early elevation of ALT, AST, or GGT, is a good predictor for hepatotoxicity.

Laboratory Findings

A complete blood count (CBC), PT, partial thromboplastin time (PTT), electrolytes, blood urea nitrogen (BUN), creatinine, amylase, lipase, liver function tests (LFTs), AST, ALT, GGT, alkaline phosphatase, and total bilirubin, should all be drawn. A urinalysis and an arterial blood gas (ABG) should be drawn. The serum bilirubin, the indirect fraction, is usually increased and the PT is usually prolonged. There can be an increase in the creatinine and BUN. On urinalysis, protein-uria, glycosuria, hematuria, pyuria, and granular casts can be noted. An increased anion gap metabolic acidosis with a high serum lactate level is rare but can be seen in massive overdoses. Serum transami-nase levels will be elevated in stage II.

Treatment

The treatment for an acute APAP poisoning is early GI decontamina-tion with gastric lavage and placement of activated charcoal. APAP is 75 to 85% absorbed by activated charcoal. Sodium sulfate is the cathartic of choice for elimination of APAP and activated charcoal.

Patients who have ingested more than 7.5 g or 140 mg/kg of APAP in a 24-hour period should have N-acetylcysteine (NAC) given. The loading dose for NAC is 140 mg/kg followed by 17 more doses of 70 mg/kg every 4 hours. NAC is commercially available in a 20% (20 g/100 ml or 200 mg/ml) or a 10% (10 g/100 ml or 100 mg/ml) solution (Mucomyst). NAC has a very foul taste and smell. It can be mixed with fruit juices or soft drinks. If the patient drinks the solution through a straw, this sometimes helps to prevent nausea from the smell. Metoclopramide (Reglan) 0.1 to 1 mg/kg intravenously (IV) can be given to prevent vomiting. If signs and symptoms of hepatic encephalopathy develop, discontinue NAC therapy. IV NAC is avail-able in Europe and Canada and is currently under investigation for IV use in the United States.

If a patient has a toxic level of APAP between 4 and 24 hours of ingestion or is on two separate serum levels and the APAP is not decreasing, the patient should be admitted to the ICU.

AMPHETAMINES

Definition

Amphetamines were first synthesized in 1887. The term amphet-amine is a term used to describe the specific drug β-phenylisopropylamine. It is also used loosely to describe many substances that are similar to amphetamines that cause amphetamine-like catecholamine effects.

Epidemiology

Amphetamines were first used during World War II to combat battle fatigue. After World War II, amphetamines were used as therapeutic treatment for obesity. After the amphetamine abuse of the 1960s and 1970s, amphetamines are now listed as schedule II drugs.

In the 1980s and 1990s, drugs that closely resemble amphetamines were produced in "bootleg" laboratories. These "bootleg" amphetamines were called "designer" drugs, particularly 3,4-methylenedioxymethamphetamine (ecstasy or MDMA) or 3,4-methylenedioxyethamphetamine (eve or MDEA). These drugs are now listed as schedule I drugs. MDEA and MDMA are usually sold in pill form. The powder form is sold as crystal-meth and is usually inhaled intranasally, injected, or smoked.

Pathology

Amphetamines are metabolized primarily in the liver. They may be absorbed through the oral, nasal, or IV routes. The majority of the drug is excreted in the urine unchanged. Excretion of amphetamines in the urine is based on the pH of the urine. The lower the urine pH (acid), the more amphetamine is excreted. Excretion is also increased by increased volume of urine excreted.

Amphetamines are structurally similar to epinephrine and norepinephrine but have different effects on the CNS. CNS effects cause hyperactivity, restlessness, anorexia, sleep reduction, and repetitive or stereotyped behaviors. Convulsions and psychosis can occur in very large doses.

Stimulation of the α and β receptors can cause peripheral vasoconstriction, increased metabolism, pupillary dilatation, tachycardia, and bronchodilatation.

Clinical Presentation/Examination

A patient can present with dilated pupils (mydriasis), diaphoresis, piloerection, bizarre behavior, extreme restlessness, psychosis, coma, choreoathetosis, cerebrovascular accidents (CVAs), and cerebral vasculitis. Cardiac effects include facial flushing, tachycardia, arrhythmias, acute myocardial infarction, hypotension, polyarteritis nodosa, and hypertension. GI symptoms include diarrhea, nausea, and vomiting. Rhabdomyolysis, hyperpyrexia, and acute pulmonary edema have been reported.

Diagnosis

A diagnosis is made by a history of amphetamine ingestion, physical presentation, and physical examination.

Laboratory Findings

A CBC, PT, PTT, electrolytes, AST, ALT, GGT, creatinine phosphokinase (CPK), CPK-MB, BUN, creatinine, serum or urine toxicology
screen, urinalysis, and an amphetamine specific drug test should be
drawn. Leukocytosis and elevated T4 levels have been reported.

Treatment

Amphetamine intoxication is usually self-limiting, but the chronic
adult user can suffer an acute life-threatening withdrawal syndrome
with abrupt cessation. Any patient with a suspected amphetamine
overdose should be placed on a cardiac monitor, and one or two large-
gauge IV lines of normal saline should be placed. Oxygen should be
given via nasal cannula at 2 liters, and pulse oximetry should be
performed. An electrocardiogram (ECG) and a chest x-ray should be
performed along with the aforementioned laboratory examinations.

Emesis with syrup of ipecac should be avoided secondary to the
potential for seizures due to the CNS effects of amphetamines. Gastric
lavage should be performed with the placement of activated charcoal.

If the patient is extremely hyperactive, place the patient in a dark
room to decrease the sensory input. In extreme cases of hyperactivity,
give diazepam or haloperidol. Treat seizures with diazepam, phenytoin, or phenobarbital. In an uncontrollable seizure, paralyze the
patient with pancuronium.

If the patient is hyperthermic, aggressive cooling is a necessity
with cooling blankets, ice, and cold water. If hypertension is present,
treat the patient with a nitroprusside drip. Do not use β-blockers
secondary to the unopposed α effects that can cause hypertension.
Acidification of the urine and increased urination are theoretically
effective in increasing the excretion of amphetamines.

Any symptomatic patient who is highly agitated, mentally unstable,
or going through withdrawal symptoms should be admitted to the
hospital.

ANTICHOLINERGICS

Definition

Anticholinergics are a large family of plants and pharmaceuticals that
encompass the Solanaceae family of plants, belladonna alkaloids,
atropine, hyoscyamine, scopolamine, and hyocine drugs. Atropine
comes from the *Atropa belladonna* family of plants. Jimsonweed
(*Datura stramonium*) is an alkaloid that can cause major CNS effects.
The mushroom *Amanita muscaria* contains belladonna alkaloids that
can cause anticholinergic poisoning.

Epidemiology

Numerous overdoses or reactions to anticholinergic-containing drugs occur in the United States each year from antihistamine overdoses to therapeutic dosing of antiparkinsonian drugs.

Pathology

Anticholinergic agents are used as mydriatics, cardiac drugs, antiparkinsonian drugs, antihistamines, antipsychotic, antispasmodics, cyclic antidepressants, ophthalmic products, skeletal muscle relaxants, and belladonna alkaloid medications. They are absorbed by oral ingestion, smoking, or IV routes.

Anticholinergics work primarily by blocking the central and peripheral cholinergic receptors. The muscarinic and nicotinic receptors can both be blocked depending on the drug given. Peripheral effects of anticholinergic toxicity are decreased bronchial secretions, decreased GI motility, arrhythmias, decreased salivation, decreased sweating, hyperthermia, hypotension or hypertension, vasodilatation, and urinary retention. CNS effects cause agitation, amnesia, ataxia, coma, anxiety, delirium, confusion, dysarthria, disorientation, hyperactivity, hallucinations, somnolence, seizures, lethargy, mydriasis, and respiratory and cardiac failure.

Clinical Presentation

The classic patient presentation is described as:

Hot as Hades
Blind as a bat
Dry as a bone
Red as a beet
Mad as a hatter

A patient can present with seizures or a coma. Pulmonary edema can be present secondary to cardiac depression resulting from hypotension.

Examination

On physical examination, the patient will have absent bowel sounds, tachycardia, unreactive mydriasis, hypotension or hypertension, flushed skin, urinary retention, hyperthermia, very dry oral mucosa, dry skin, and visual and auditory hallucinations.

ECG

On an ECG, the QRS complex can be prolonged, a new bundle branch block can be present, and atrioventricular (AV) dissociation or atrial or ventricular tachycardia can be present. The most common rhythm is sinus tachycardia.

Diagnosis

The diagnosis of anticholinergic toxicity is made by clinical presentation, history of ingestion of anticholinergic-containing medications, physical examination, cardiac depression, and the classic signs of anticholinergic toxicity.

Laboratory Findings

A CBC, electrolytes, BUN, creatinine, urinalysis, toxic drug screen, and an ABG should be performed.

Treatment

A large-gauge IV should be started, and the patient should be placed on a cardiac monitor. An ECG and a chest x-ray should be performed. The aforementioned laboratory examinations should be performed.

The mainstay of treatment is supportive care. The patient's airway, breathing, and circulation should be monitored. If urinary retention is present, a Foley catheter should be placed for relief. If oral ingestion is known or suspected, perform gastric lavage followed by activated charcoal 1 g/kg. A cathartic should be given. Remember that one of the side effects of an anticholinergic overdose is decreased gastric emptying; therefore, gastric lavage, activated charcoal, and administration of a cathartic are very important in the decontamination of the patient's bowel.

Seizures should be treated with benzodiazepines or barbiturates. Hyperthermia should be treated with a cooling blanket. Arrhythmias should be treated as usual (i.e., per ACLS protocols), but class Ia agents should be avoided secondary to a quinidine-like effect. If the patient is agitated, give benzodiazepines; do not give phenothiazines.

Controversy lies in the use of physostigmine, a tertiary ammonium compound that can reverse the acetylcholinesterase inhibitor effect caused by anticholinergic toxicity. Physostigmine crosses the blood-brain barrier and reverses both peripheral and central actions of anticholinergics. Physostigmine is known to exacerbate seizures and aggravate arrhythmias; therefore, it must be used with extreme caution. Physostigmine is also used in the treatment of an overdose of cyclic antidepressants. Physostigmine should only be used as a last resort after all other therapies have failed. The initial dose is 0.5 to 2 mg IV every 5 minutes. Do not give physostigmine to patients with bronchospasm, cardiac vascular disease, intestinal obstruction, heart block, bladder obstruction, or peripheral vascular disease. If physostigmine is working, lacrimation, salivation, defecation, and urination will occur.

Any patient with severe anticholinergic symptoms or who requires physostigmine therapy should be admitted to the ICU.

ARSENIC

Definition

Arsenic is an odorless, tasteless metal that is found in a variety of industrial compounds. In gaseous form, it can be made into inorganic and organic compounds. Arsine is the gaseous form of arsenic.

Epidemiology

Arsenic is used in homicides and suicides and comes in various industrial forms. It is the second leading cause of chronic heavy metal poisoning. It is the most common cause of acute heavy metal poisoning.

Pathology

Arsenic can be absorbed through the skin, GI tract, and lungs. It is highly water soluble. Arsenic localizes in the leukocytes and erythrocytes, and within 24 hours it is distributed to the lungs, kidneys, GI tract, spleen, hair, nails, bone, muscle, and nervous tissue. Arsenic is 50% excreted by the kidneys within 30 hours of ingestion.

Arsenic blocks oxidative phosphorylation by binding with sulfhydryl groups and enzymes. Arsenic prevents the conversion of pyruvate to acetylcoenzyme A (acetyl-CoA) to α-ketoglutarate to succinyl-CoA in the Krebs cycle. This blocks the conversion of dihydrolipoate to lipoate. The substitution of arsenic for phosphate causes the loss of stable phosphoryl compounds, thus losing their high-energy phosphate bonds.

Clinical Presentation/Examination

The patient with acute arsenic poisoning presents with severe nausea, vomiting, and cholera-like diarrhea. This often leads to hypotension and tachycardia. Acute symptoms will occur within 30 minutes of ingestion. Arsenite (trivalent) is more toxic than the arsenate (pentavalent) form of arsenic. These gastric symptoms may last for days or weeks before a diagnosis is made. The patient will often complain of a metallic taste in the mouth or a garlicky breath odor.

A patient with arsenic poisoning can present with seizures, delirium, coma, pulmonary edema, acute renal failure, and rhabdomyolysis. Malaise, weakness, skin rashes, and peripheral neuropathy with a stocking glove distribution, which is initially sensory then becomes motor, are late signs. Ascending paralysis mimicking Guillain-Barré syndrome has been reported.

Hyperpigmentation and hyperkeratosis of the palms and soles, morbilliform rash, and epidermoid cancer have also been reported. The fingernails can develop Mees' lines, which occur 4 to 6 weeks after an acute ingestion. Mees' lines are 1- to 2-mm wide transverse white lines on the nails. Patients with chronic exposure can develop hepatatic angiosarcoma, leukemia, squamous cell cancer, basal cell skin cancer, and lung cancer.

Arsine gas is a colorless, nonirritating gas that is used in the semiconductor industry, ore-smelting industry, and refining industry. Many insecticides are mixed within arsine. Arsine can produce hemolytic anemia, jaundice, abdominal pain, acute renal failure, and hemoglobinuria-induced renal failure.

ECG

On ECG examination, nonspecific ST and T wave abnormalities with a prolonged QT are common with chronic ingestion. Torsades de pointes and ventricular tachycardia have been reported in cases of acute and chronic ingestion.

Diagnosis

A diagnosis is based on a high index of suspicion, occupational history, and physical presentation. Any patient who presents with hypotension of unknown etiology and severe gastroenteritis, in recurrent bouts, with peripheral neuropathy and typical skin manifestations should be considered to have arsenic poisoning. A definitive diagnosis is made by the finding of elevated arsenic levels in a 24-hour urine test. The normal urinary arsenic level is less than 0.05 mg/l. If this test is nondiagnostic and arsenic poisoning is still suspected, then perform the D-pencillamine mobilization test. Give 25 mg/kg of D-penicillamine, and then perform a 24-hour urine test.

Laboratory Findings

A CBC, reticulocyte count, electrolytes, BUN, creatinine, amylase, lipase, liver and cardiac enzymes, magnesium, calcium, phosphorus, and a 24-hour urine and a urinalysis should be performed. Arsenic levels in the blood are unreliable. Anemia can be present as either megaloblastic or normochromic anemia. The white blood cell (WBC) count can be elevated with a relative eosinophilia. Basophilic stippling of the red blood cells (RBCs) is often noted but is nonspecific. Often the reticulocyte count is elevated, and thrombocytopenia is present.

Treatment

A patient with acute or chronic arsenic poisoning should be placed on a cardiac monitor, and at least one large-gauge IV line of normal saline should be placed. The aforementioned laboratory tests, including a 24-hour urine test, should be performed. Gastric lavage should be performed, and activated charcoal 1 g/kg should be given. Arsenic is poorly absorbed by charcoal but is effective if other co-ingestants are taken.

X-rays of the chest and abdomen should be taken to check for radiopaque materials. Arsenic is radiopaque, and if radiopaque materials are present, whole bowel irrigation should be performed.

Hypotension should be treated with IV fluids, dopamine, or norepinephrine. Do not overhydrate the patient, because this can cause pulmonary or cerebral edema. Ventricular tachycardia or ventricular fibrillation should be treated with lidocaine, bretyllium, or defibrillation. If torsades de pointes is present, treat the patient with isoproterenol, magnesium, or overdrive pacing. Avoid class Ia agents, because they can prolong the QT.

If seizures occur, treat the patient with benzodiazepine, phenobarbital, phenytoin, or general anesthesia.

If severe toxicity is present give British antilewisite (BAL) 3 to 5 mg/kg IM every 4 hours for 2 days followed by 3 to 5 mg/kg every 6 to 12 hours until the patient improves. D-Penicillamine 100 mg/kg/day with a maximum dose of 2 g for adults and 1 g for children can be given in four divided doses for 5 days as an alternative drug to BAL. DMSA is under an investigational trial for arsenic poisoning. If the patient is in acute renal failure, consider hemodialysis.

Acute arsine gas poisoning is treated with an exchange blood transfusion to remove nondialyzable arsine and hemodialysis when acute renal failure is present.

Hospitalize all patients who have acute or chronic arsenic poisoning.

BARBITURATES

Definition

Barbiturates were first introduced in 1903 as sedative-hypnotics. The first barbiturate was barbital (diethylbarbituric acid). Barbiturates are now used in anesthesia, seizure disorders, and management of increased intracranial pressure. The early barbiturates have mostly been replaced by the benzodiazepines.

Barbiturates relieve anxiety and insomnia and possess euphoric properties similar to those of alcohol. Thirty percent of narcotic addicts are also addicted to barbiturates.

Epidemiology

Barbiturates have the highest mortality rate of all sedative-hypnotics. Most barbiturate overdoses are related to suicide or attempts at suicide. However, this suicidal association has been on the decline for the last 15 years. Cyclic antidepressants are now the primary cause of death by overdose. Whites overdose on barbiturates more than do blacks or Hispanics. Most overdoses occur in patients between the ages of 20 and 40, and the male:female ratio is 50:50. Abusers or long-term users develop a tolerance to barbiturates; thus the longer the use, the larger the dose that is needed to produce the desired effect.

Pathology

Barbiturates all have the same basic structure with no CNS activity. There are four categories of barbiturates based on their duration of activity, ranging from 18 minutes to 6 to 12 hours. The duration of action is based on the barbiturate's lipid solubility, which is determined by the side chain structure at the C-2 and pH gradients. The greater the lipid solubility, the faster the barbiturate diffuses into the body tissues. Barbiturates are mainly metabolized by the liver. The half-life of barbiturates is again based on the lipid solubility. Ultra-short-acting barbiturates have a half-life of 3 hours. The half-life of intermediate-acting barbiturates is up to 37 hours.

Long-acting barbiturates are 80% absorbed by oral dosing. The volume distribution is 0.8 l/kg. Fifty percent of barbiturates are bound by proteins. Barbiturates are metabolized by the liver, but 25% is excreted in the urine unchanged. The elimination half-life varies from 48 to 200 hours, and in children the elimination half-life is one half more than that found in adults and two to five times greater in infants than in adults.

Barbiturates, especially phenobarbital, can cause increased metabolism of anticoagulants, quinidine, phenytoin, digoxin, corticosteroids, tricyclic antidepressants, phenothiazines, and tetracycline.

Barbiturates depress nerve and muscle tissue at the synapse where they cause an inhibitory effect on the neurotransmission across the neuronal and neuroeffector junctions. Gamma-aminobutyric acid (GABA) receptors are single protein complexes located in the post-synaptic membrane, which is in association with a chloride ion channel, a benzodiazepine receptor, and a barbiturate receptor. GABA mediates the synaptic inhibition by binding to the principal GABA receptor and opening the chloride ion channel that causes excitatory depolarization to become more difficult. Barbiturates cause the GABA receptor's effect on the operation of chloride channels, in low doses, to open slightly, and it opens the chloride channel completely in high-dose contractions. Barbiturates are also believed to affect the presynaptic pathway by inhibiting the calcium-mediated neurotransmitter release.

This process affects the reticular activating system (RAS) in the brain stem, the cerebrum, and cerebellum. The action of barbiturates on the RAS is what causes their sedative-hypnotic effect. Barbiturates cause respiratory depression; they stop seizures; and they also affect the heart. They decrease GI and urinary bladder motility and ureter contraction, and they stimulate secretion of antidiuretic hormone.

Clinical Presentation

A patient with chronic use presents with withdrawal symptoms. Mild to moderate barbiturate intoxication produces the symptoms of alcohol intoxication, including emotional lability, lethargy, impaired thinking processes, slurred speech, incoordination, and nystagmus. In severe acute toxicity, coma and respiratory depression or arrest can be the presenting complaint. Hypotension, vasodilatation, hypothermia, flaccid muscle tone, loss of deep tendon reflexes, and shock can occur. Pupillary size can be either dilated or constricted. An electroencephalogram (EEG) can show a flat line.

Diagnosis

A diagnosis is based on the history of serum barbiturate levels and on physical examination. A rule of thumb for severe barbiturate overdose is 10 times the hypnotic dose capable of producing severe toxicity.

Laboratory Findings

A CBC, electrolytes, BUN, creatinine, LFTs, ABG, urinalysis, urine or blood toxicologic screen and, if known, type specific barbiturate level should be drawn. Specific barbiturate serum levels can be obtained, but they are unreliable in regard to actual barbiturate levels in the brain. Blood levels are poor predictors of toxicity.

Treatment

All patients with a suspected barbiturate overdose should be placed on a cardiac monitor and should have two large-gauge IV lines of normal saline placed. The aforementioned laboratory values should be drawn. An ECG should be performed. A chest x-ray should be performed if there is a question of aspiration. All patients should be monitored closely for respiratory depression, altered mental status, loss of gag reflex, cardiac arrhythmia, or acute hypotension or shock. If hypotension occurs, a fluid challenge is the first treatment of choice; however, if no response occurs, dopamine may be used.

Early gastric lavage with activated charcoal is the mainstay of treatment. Thirty grams per dose every six hours for a total of six doses should be used, especially in long-acting preparations.

Forced diuresis and alkalinization of urine are useful in the excretion of long-acting barbiturates. Sodium bicarbonate 1 to 2 mEq/kg every 4 to 6 hours can be used to maintain the urine pH at 7.5. Alkalinization of the urine can have a 5- to 10-fold increase in the excretion rate of phenobarbital.

Hemodialysis can remove large amounts of phenobarbital from the blood and is six to nine times more effective than are forced diuresis and alkalinization.

If the patient presents with chronic use of barbiturates, abrupt discontinuation of the barbiturate should not occur. These patients have both mental and physical dependence. Withdrawal symptoms usually occur 24 hours after the last dose. These physical symptoms include anxiety, restlessness, depression, insomnia, nausea, vomiting, sweating, abdominal cramping, and tremors. Severe withdrawal symptoms can also occur with abrupt discontinuation, including grand mal seizures, increased muscular tone and jerking, auditory hallucinations, delirium, cardiovascular collapse, hyperpyrexia, and death. Seizures should be treated with diazepam therapy. Physical withdrawal symptoms usually subside in 3 to 7 days.

Early deaths from barbiturate overdose are usually secondary to cardiovascular-related complications, such as shock or cardiac arrest. Most deaths occur secondary to pulmonary complications secondary to aspiration pneumonitis or pulmonary edema. Rarely, deaths are attributed to cerebral edema or renal failure.

Flumazenil (Romazicon) is a benzodiazepine receptor antagonist that can be used to reverse the effects of barbiturates. Flumazenil can precipitate seizures, secondary to its rapid withdrawal effect from the barbiturates and can cause a barbiturate withdrawal syndrome. Flumazenil should be given with caution. The recommended dose is 0.2 mg (2 ml) over 30 seconds. If the desired level of consciousness is not obtained in 30 seconds, a further dose of 0.3 to 0.5 mg can be administered every 30 seconds, up to a maximum dose of 3 mg. Another recommended therapy for flumazenil in chronic use overdose patients is a dose of 5 mg administered as 0.5 mg/min IV. If circumstances permit, you may dose as 0.2 mg/min over 10 minutes, which will help to reduce the signs and symptoms of sudden withdrawal. In patients who have a tolerance to benzodiazepines, flumazenil probably should not be used unless an acute life-threatening event is taking place.

β-BLOCKER OVERDOSE

Definition

β-Blockers are used to treat ischemic heart disease, hypertension, cardiac arrhythmias, obstructive heart disease, control of glaucoma, thyrotoxicosis, and prevention of migraine headaches.

Epidemiology

β-Blocker toxicity is usually secondary to underlying disease, such as chronic obstructive pulmonary disease (COPD), asthma, congestive heart failure, sinus node dysfunction, AV node conduction defects, or concomitant use with calcium channel blockers. In most cases, fatal toxicity is secondary to accidental or intentional acute overdose.

Pathology

There are two types of β receptors, β_1 and β_2. β-Blockers are often described as selective or nonselective. Nonselective β-blockers will stimulate both β_1 and β_2 receptors. Stimulation of β_1 receptors will cause an increase in myocardial contraction, AV node conduction velocity, and an increase in renin secretion and will cause bronchial constriction. β_2 stimulation causes a relaxation of smooth muscles in the blood vessels, the GI tract, the genitourinary tract, and the bronchial tree.

After ingestion β-blockers are rapidly absorbed by the gastric mucosa, and symptoms of overdose can occur in as little as 20 minutes. Long-acting β-blockers will have varying degrees of absorption. β-Blockers have variable half-lives.

β_2 stimulation will also promote glycogenolysis and gluconeogenesis in the liver, glycogenolysis in the skeletal muscle, and β_1 and β_2 receptors will act as competitive antagonists to catecholamines at all β-receptor sites.

Metoprolol, atenolol, esmolol, and acebutolol are selective β_1-blockers. Labetalol blocks both α_1 and β_1 and β_2. Acebutolol and pindolol have β-agonist properties that can stimulate catecholamine levels to increase when catecholamine levels are low. Pindolol, propranolol, and labetalol have membrane-stabilizing activity (quinidine-like effects) in high doses. Nadolol and atenolol are highly lipid soluble and have a greater degree of CNS effect and are better removed by hemodialysis.

Clinical Presentation/Examination

A patient with an acute overdose of β-blockers will present with bradycardia, new AV blocks, and hypotension. Cardiac output falls, causing negative inotropic effects, decreased myocardial perfusion, and death. The patient presents with dizziness and mental status changes, secondary to hypoperfusion, delirium, and coma. Grand mal seizures have been reported with β-blocker overdose. Respiratory arrest secondary to pulmonary edema in the presence of congestive heart failure, bronchospasm secondary to β stimulation, and hypoglycemia in unstable diabetic patients are often complications of β-blocker overdose.

ECG

On ECG examination, the ECG can show first-degree AV block, sinus bradycardia, ST changes, widening of QRS complexes, and peaked T waves. Practolol, sotalol, and pindolol have caused tachycardia in some patients who have taken overdoses.

Diagnosis

A diagnosis is made by a history of acute ingestion of β-blockers, use of timolol ophthalmic drops, physical examination, clinical presentation, bradycardia, hypoperfusion, and ECG changes.

Laboratory Findings

A CBC, electrolytes, BUN, creatinine, LFTs, urinalysis, and cardiac enzymes, including CPK and CPK-MB, should be drawn. Quantitative and qualitative β-blocker levels can be obtained but are usually not available in most hospitals.

Treatment

Any patient with a suspected acute β-blocker overdose should have at least two large-gauge IV lines and should be placed on a cardiac monitor. The patient should have an ECG performed and should be placed on oxygen therapy. Meticulous airway support with pulse oximetry should be performed, and the aforementioned laboratory tests should be drawn. Treatment is based on the principles of good supportive care with careful monitoring. Acute ingestions should be treated with gastric lavage and activated charcoal (1 mg/kg). Hypotension should be treated acutely with IV fluids.

Seizures should be treated with IV diazepam. Bronchospasms should be treated with oral nebulizer β-agonists. Hypoglycemia should be treated with IV glucose. Symptomatic bradycardia should be treated with 0.5 to 2 mg of atropine in adults and 0.01 to 0.03 mg of atropine in children until the desired heart rate is reached. Often dopamine, epinephrine, or isoproterenol in very large doses is needed to reach the desired heart rate and blood pressure. Trancutaneous or transvenous pacing should be considered in severe refractory bradycardia to drug therapy.

The mainstay of severe β-blocker poisoning is high-dose glucagon. Glucagon in a dose of 3 to 5 mg IV bolus should be given every 5 minutes until the desired response is achieved to a maximum dose of 10 to 15 mg. In children, 50 to 150 μg/kg should be given. Glucagon should be diluted in 5% dextrose. Glucagon stimulates glucagon receptors, which cause an increase in inotropic and chronotropic action by bypassing β receptors. The effects of glucagon should be seen in approximately 20 minutes. Glucagon should be given in complete cardiac arrest or in the presence of prolonged hypotension. Patients have recovered completely after prolonged cardiopulmonary resuscitation (CPR) when glucagon was given. Nadolol, atenolol, and acebutolol are responsive to charcoal hemoperfusion secondary to their small volume of distribution and low protein binding.

Any patient with an acute symptomatic β-blocker overdose should be admitted to the ICU for treatment and monitoring.

CALCIUM CHANNEL BLOCKERS

Definition

Calcium channel blockers are used in the United States to treat hypertension, angina, and tachydysrhythmias. They are divided into four groups: (1) the dihydropyridines: nifedipine (Procardia, Adalat), nicardipine, and nimodipine; (2) the phenylalkylamines: verapamil (Isoptin, Calan), and gallopamil; (3) the phenylpiperazines: cinnarizine and flunarizine; and (4) the benzothiazepines: diltiazem (Cardizem).

Epidemiology

Most overdoses of calcium channel blockers are secondary to suicidal or accidental verapamil overdoses. The sustained-release formulations of verapamil cause more accidental overdoses. Nifedipine and diltiazem rarely cause overdoses.

Pathology

Calcium channel blockers are highly protein bound and lipid soluble and have a large volume of distribution. Their serum half-life is 4 to 6 hours. They are metabolized mainly in the liver. If cirrhosis is present, their half-life will be greatly increased. Calcium channel blockers have a rapid onset of absorption after ingestion and a rapid onset of action within 1 hour after ingestion. Long-acting preparations can have up to a 5-hour lag-time between the time of ingestion and the onset of symptoms.

Calcium channel blockers inhibit the transportation of calcium through the "slow channel" during inward excitation-contraction phase, causing intravascular smooth muscle to relax and dilate. This slow-channel blockade of conduction causes the slowing of the sinoatrial (SA) node and the AV node, which impairs myocardial contraction and excitation.

Calcium channel blockers rarely affect the heart rate in the therapeutic ranges. If the patient suffers from sick sinus syndrome, verapamil and diltiazem can cause significant bradycardia. Verapamil can cause profound bradycardia and high-degree AV blocks, which can lead to life-threatening decreases in myocardial contractions and vasodilatation. Verapamil in high doses can also cause a class Ia antidysrhythmic effect, a "local anesthetic" effect, resulting in a decreased upslope in phase O of the action potential, causing a widened QRS complex.

Clinical Presentation/Examination

The patient presents with severe hypotension, dizziness, weakness, syncope, and sustained loss of consciousness. Nausea and vomiting are often presenting complaints. Palpitations from reflux tachycardia from nifedipine therapy can occur. If hypoperfusion is severe, chest pain, angina, and shortness of breath can occur. Seizures and focal neurologic symptoms are uncommon but have been reported. The onset of symptoms usually occurs within 1 to 2 hours of ingestion, but long-acting formulations can take up to 24 hours before symptoms occur.

Patients can often present with toxic symptoms after IV verapamil is given to terminate supraventricular tachyarrhythmias. Pretreatment with calcium will often block the verapamil-induced peripheral vaso-dilatation, but pretreatment with calcium will not affect the AV node conduction.

ECG

On ECG examination, in calcium channel blocker overdose, bradycardia, and high-degree AV blocks can be seen. The following can be present: a widened QRS complex, inverted P waves, low-voltage T waves, QT prolongation, nonspecific ST and T wave changes, and U waves.

Diagnosis

The diagnosis of calcium channel blocker overdose is based on a history of ingestion, physical presentation, laboratory studies, ECG, and the presence of hypotension.

Laboratory Findings

Hyperglycemia and metabolic acidosis can be present. Serum calcium channel blocker levels can be obtained but are not available in all hospitals and are not protective of severity or toxicity.

Treatment

Any patient with a suspected calcium channel blocker overdose should have at least one IV line of normal saline placed with a large-gauge needle and should be placed on a cardiac monitor. The patient should be given oxygen, and meticulous airway management should be adhered to. GI decontamination should be performed by gastric lavage, and then activated charcoal 1 g/kg should be given in the case of adults.

The mainstay of severe calcium channel blocker overdose is calcium gluconate or calcium chloride. Give 10 to 20 ml of 10% calcium chloride in adults (10 to 30 mg/kg in children) or calcium gluconate 10% as a dose of 0.2 to 0.5 ml/kg per dose, up to 10 ml per dose. IV calcium should be given slowly over a few minutes. Nifedipine-induced severe vasodilatation should be treated with dopamine. Fluids should be given with caution secondary to calcium channel blocker–induced myocardial depression. Norepinephrine, isoproterenol, and epinephrine can also be used for pressure support. Be careful when giving isoproterenol to patients with known coronary disease or idiopathic hypertrophic subaortic stenosis. Use atropine in symptomatic bradyarrhythmias. Transvenous or external pacing may be necessary to treat bradycardia.

If a patient with Wolff-Parkinson-White syndrome or Lown-Ganong-Levine syndrome receives verapamil for treatment of supra-ventricular tachycardia and a sustained ventricular acceleration occurs, treat the patient with cardioversion and procainamide or lidocaine.

Any patient with a calcium channel overdose, especially with a long-acting preparation, should be admitted to the ICU for treatment and observation.

CAUSTIC INGESTIONS

Definition

Caustic ingestions that damage GI mucosa are primarily from acids and alkali substances. These injuries can cause burns, perforations, and scarring of the gastric mucosa.

Epidemiology

The largest group that is affected by alkali and acid ingestion consists of children younger than 5 years of age. Five percent of all ingestions involve acid or alkali ingestions. Most caustic substances are found in the bathroom, kitchen, and garage in the home. Often these caustic substances are placed in old drinking containers (e.g., plastic soda bottles). The child believes that he or she is drinking a soft drink and accidentally ingests the caustic substance.

Common alkali substances found in the home include:

Dishwashing or soap powders
Button batteries
Toilet bowl cleaners
Automatic dishwasher detergents
Ammonia-metal cleaning product
Jewelry cleaners
Sodium hypochlorite (Chlorox) bleach

Clinitest tablets
Paint removers
Potassium permanganate
Sodium carbonate (Purex) bleach
Hair dyes and tints
Antirust products
Nonphosphate detergents

Common acid substances found in the home include:

Sulfuric acid in: battery acid, toilet bowl cleaners (sodium bisulfate)
Hydrochloric acid in: toilet bowl cleaners and swimming pool cleaners
Hydrofluoric acid
Oxalic acid
Slate cleaners
Bleach disinfectants
Carbolic (phenol) acid
Aqua regia (a mixture of hydrochloric and nitric acids)
Soldering fluxes

Pathology

Lye is the most commonly ingested caustic substance. It can burn the oral mucosa, esophagus, and stomach. When ingested it causes liquefaction necrosis, thus causing very deep and penetrating burns to exposed mucosa in seconds after exposure. Heat is produced immediately after contact. Saponification of fat occurs after lye ingestion but not from thermal injury.

Ingestion of acids causes superficial necrosis of exposed tissue of the esophagus. Excessive heat generation and dehydration are the main complications of acid ingestion. The stomach is more frequently injured with acid ingestion, whereas lye ingestion causes more damage to the esophagus than to the stomach.

Clinical Presentation/Examination

Presenting complaints will be determined by the duration of time since the substance was ingested. Immediate complications are usually secondary to the hyperthermic injury to the esophagus and stomach. These acute burns can cause hemorrhage, soft tissue edema, and airway compromise. Perforation of the esophagus or stomach is an acute concern in the first 48 to 72 hours.

After the first 72 hours, delayed complications of alkali and acid ingestions include strictures of the esophagus and the pylorus. Esophageal strictures occur usually after the ingestion of lye, and pyloric strictures occur after acid ingestions.

Diagnosis

A diagnosis of ingestion is determined by a history of ingestion, volume, concentration of the substance ingested, contact time with the GI mucosa, and the absence or presence of stomach contents at the time of ingestion. The tonicity of the pyloric sphincter is also very important in determining injury.

The patient should be given a complete examination with particular attention to the oral mucosa. The absence of oral lesions or burns does not rule out esophageal or stomach injury.

Laboratory Findings

A CBC, PT, PTT, electrolytes, BUN, creatinine, amylase, lipase, LFTs, urinalysis, ABG, and type and screen of 4 to 6 units of blood should be performed.

Treatment

Any patient with an acute ingestion of acid or lye should have two large-gauge IV lines of normal saline placed. The patient should be placed on a cardiac monitor and given oxygen by nasal cannula. Chest and abdominal x-rays should be performed. Meticulous attention to airway management is a necessity. If the patient is in acute respiratory distress and endotracheal intubation cannot be performed without additional trauma to the pharynx, a cricothyrotomy should be performed. Do not blindly intubate the patient. Do not intubate nasotracheally, secondary to possible injury to the hypopharynx. The acute risk of injury to the posterior pharynx is soft tissue swelling and hypoxia.

If the patient is in extreme pain, give morphine or meperidine IV. The patient should be placed on nothing by mouth (NPO) restriction. Diluents are of no value in lye ingestion secondary to their rapid tissue injury effect (often in seconds). There is controversy in regard to the use of diluents in the treatment in acid burns. The administration of water as a diluent has the risk of causing vomiting, thus re-injuring the esophagus, larynx, and oral cavity. The current recommendation is that no diluents be used in acid or alkali ingestion.

Likewise, gastric lavage and emesis are not recommended in alkali ingestions. There is an increased risk of perforation and new injury to burned tissue, aspiration of lye or acid ingestants, and re-exposure of the esophagus to acid or alkali ingestants. Also, activated charcoal and cathartics are not recommended in acid or alkali ingestions. Alkali substances are not absorbed by activated charcoal, and the injury occurs in seconds rather than minutes. The activated charcoal also limits the endoscopist's view of the esophagus and the stomach.

There is also a controversy with regard to the use of steroids. In some studies, it is shown that steroids reduce injury in alkali ingestions. Methylprednisolone 20 mg IV every 8 hours for patients under 2 years of age, 40 mg IV for patients older than 2 years of age has been recommended. Steroids should not be used in patients with an active bleeding ulcer, a gastric or esophageal perforation, or if more than 48 hours have passed since the substance was ingested.

There is also controversy with regard to the prophylactic use of antibiotics in alkali ingestions. There are no clinical studies that support the use of antibiotics in acid or alkali ingestions.

All patients with acid or alkali ingestion should be admitted to the ICU and a consultation should be made with a gastroenterologist who can perform an endoscopic examination of the patient. Immediate consultation with a surgeon is necessitated if esophageal perforation is suspected or determined by physical examination.

CLONIDINE

Definition

Clonidine hydrochloride is a synthetic imidazoline derivative that has a potent blood pressure–lowering effect. Clonidine is used as an antihypertensive agent and is used to decrease the symptoms of withdrawal from alcohol, nicotine, and opiates. Clonidine is available in 0.1-, 0.2-, and 0.3-mg tablets (Catapres). When clonidine is combined with chlorthalidone, it is called Combipres. Catapres patches are also available in 0.1 (2.5 mg total), 0.2 (5 mg total), and 0.3 mg (7.5 mg total)/day patches for a 7-day dose.

Epidemiology

There has only been one reported fatality from an overdose of clonidine. Toxic effects are mostly symptomatic.

Pathology

The primary site of action of clonidine is in the medulla oblongata, where it works as a presynaptic α_2-adrenergic agonist, which causes a decreased sympathetic outflow from the CNS. This decrease in sympathetic outflow causes a decreased cardiac output, heart rate, and peripheral vascular resistance. Clonidine can also depress the CNS and decrease the levels of norepinephrine and metabolites in the cerebrospinal fluid. In very high doses, clonidine can act as a peripheral α-adrenoreceptor agonist at vascular smooth-muscle sites and thus causes vasoconstriction.

The serum half-life of clonidine is approximately 12 hours (6 to 24 hours). Clonidine is lipid-soluble and is 20 to 40% protein bound with a volume distribution of 3 to 6 l/kg. Fifty percent of clonidine is excreted unchanged in the urine, and the other 50% is metabolized by the liver. Clonidine does not appear to be teratogenic.

Clinical Presentation/Examination

A patient with a clonidine overdose presents with symptoms of both central and peripheral effects. The onset of symptoms occurs usually 2 hours after ingestion and can last for up to 72 hours.

Symptoms are divided into two categories: cardiovascular and CNS complaints. CNS symptoms include hypotonia, apnea, miosis, respiratory depression, seizures, extensor plantar reflex, diarrhea, hyporeflexia, lethargy, or coma. Cardiovascular symptoms include hypotension; hypertension; first-, second-, third-degree AV blocks; and sinus bradycardia. Other complaints include hypothermia and pallor.

Often a patient with an overdose of clonidine will present much like he or she has a narcotic overdose. The symptoms are: respiratory depression, miosis, and coma.

Diagnosis

The amount of the substance ingested does not correlate with the severity of the symptoms. A diagnosis is based on the history, physical examination, and presentation of the patient.

Laboratory Findings

Laboratory tests are nonspecific and are of little help. Clonidine can be measured by high-pressure liquid chromatography. A CBC, PT,

PTT, electrolytes, BUN, creatinine, urine or blood toxicologic screen, LFTs, and ABG should be performed as needed.

Treatment

All patients with a suspected overdose of clonidine should have two large-gauge IV lines placed. The patient should be placed on pulse oximetry and also on oxygen and a cardiac monitor. An ECG should be performed. Any comatose patient should receive 100 mg of thiamine, IM or IV, 1 ampule of glucose 50%, and naloxone 0.4 to 2 mg IV. If respiratory complaints or findings are present, a chest x-ray should be performed. Remember that even though there has only been one reported fatality from clonidine, respiratory arrest and hypotension are possible. Always remember that co-ingestion must always be considered in any patient who has overdosed. If symptoms of respiratory depression are present, adequate airway and ventilation must be maintained. Treat hypotension with IV fluids.

All overdose patients should have a gastric lavage performed along with the administration of activated charcoal. Always protect the patient's airway when performing a gastric lavage.

The mainstay of clonidine overdose is supportive care. There is no proven antidote for clonidine. Any symptomatic patient should be admitted to the hospital for at least 12 hours. If the patient is asymptomatic after 4 hours of ingestion, it is highly unlikely that he or she has ingested a significant toxic dose.

A patient who has been on long-term therapy with clonidine and has had clonidine therapy abruptly withdrawn can experience an acute clonidine withdrawal syndrome. The patient will present with anxiety, headache, nausea, abdominal pain, diaphoresis, tachycardia, and hypertension. Hypertensive encephalopathy and ventricular arrhythmias have been reported with abrupt clonidine withdrawal. Clonidine therapy should always be tapered over 3 to 5 days. Treat severe hypertension with nitroprusside or β-blockers.

COCAINE

Definition

Cocaine (benzoylmethylecgonine) is a naturally occurring plant alkaloid found in the *Erythroxylon coca* plant. Cocaine can be abused by IV injection, smoking, oral ingestion, or nasal inhalation. It is also used medically as a topical anesthetic.

Epidemiology

Cocaine has had a long history of abuse. In 1990, it was estimated that more than 4 million persons in the United States were psychologically dependent on cocaine.

Pathology

Cocaine is extracted from the *Erythroxylon coca* plant by crushing the coca leaves and then placing the coca leaves in a hydrocarbon solvent where the extraction of the alkaloid takes place with sulfuric acid. The cocaine is then further purified until it is in the form of a water-soluble cocaine hydrochloride salt: The powder form is the one most commonly used. This hydrochloride salt can then be used intranasally or IV.

When cocaine is in the alkaloid form, it is heat stable and is commonly called "crack" cocaine and can be smoked. Street cocaine is usually "cut" with another substance such as lactose, mannitol, caffeine, ephedrine, phenylpropanolamine, amphetamine, procaine, lidocaine, tetracaine, or PCP. Stimulants and hallucinogens are commonly added to street cocaine also.

Cocaine is metabolized in the liver by liver esterases and plasma cholinesterase. Less than 20% of the cocaine is excreted in the urine. The serum half-life of cocaine is 40 to 90 minutes. Cocaine is eliminated by first-order kinetics.

Cocaine stimulates the adrenergic nervous system, which causes a potentiation of the response of the sympathetically innervated organs. This increased response causes a blockage of the re-uptake of catecholamines and serotonin at the adrenergic nerve endings. The blockage of the re-uptake of serotonin and catecholamines alters the metabolism of epinephrine, norepinephrine, and dopamine.

Clinical Presentation/Examination

A patient with chronic cocaine use can present with euphoric or withdrawal symptoms. Classically, the patient presents with adrenergic nervous system symptoms of hyperthermia, tachycardia, hypertension, increased rate of respiration, diaphoresis, and agitation. An acute myocardial infarction is a common presenting cardiac complaint. The patient will present with an anginal type of chest pain with a normal or nondiagnostic ECG. The acute myocardial infarction is probably secondary to the stimulation of the sympathetic nervous system, causing an increase in blood pressure, heart rate, and myocardial contractility. These changes increase myocardial oxygen demand; thus, if the patient has a fixed coronary lesion, these changes can induce an acute myocardial infarction. Cocaine is also a vasoconstrictor and can cause coronary vasospasm. Patients have presented with atrial and ventricular arrhythmias, aortic rupture, congestive heart failure, and myocarditis. Arrhythmias are probably secondary to an increased circulating level of catecholamines. On ECG, the QT interval is prolonged and the QRS interval is often widened.

Pulmonary complaints include spontaneous pneumothorax and pneumomediastinum. A patient can present with "crack lung," which is secondary to bronchospasm for an immunoglobulin E (IgE)-mediated entity. The chest x-ray will present with diffuse pulmonary infiltrates or pulmonary edema.

Hemorrhagic and ischemic cerebrovascular accidents have been reported. Hemorrhagic accidents can be intraparenchymal, subarachnoid, or intraventricular.

Muscle breakdown secondary to hyperthermia, seizures, and agitation of cocaine toxicity can lead to myoglobinuria, rhabdomyolysis, and myoglobinuric renal failure. Renal failure can also be secondary to hypotension, volume depletion, and hypotension secondary to cocaine toxicity.

Patients who inject cocaine are at risk for human immunodeficiency virus (HIV), acquired immunodeficiency syndrome (AIDS), hepatitis, osteomyelitis, thrombophlebitis, pneumonia, endocarditis, and abscess formation. The pregnant cocaine abuser is placing the maternal fetus at risk for spontaneous abortion, abruptio placentae, and congenital anomalies.

Persons who smuggle cocaine into the United States often do so by placing the cocaine in cellophane, condoms, foil, balloons, or latex gloves and then they swallow the package to keep the drug from being detected. These people are called "mules" or "body packers." If one of these packages ruptures and the cocaine is emptied into the GI tract, the patient can have a very large amount of cocaine rapidly absorbed, often resulting in death.

Topical cocaine is often used to anesthetize wounds in the form of TAC solution. TAC is *t*etracaine 0.5%, *a*drenaline 0.05%, and *c*ocaine 11.8%. A patient can become toxic from systemic absorption, especially if the substance is placed on the mucous membranes.

Diagnosis

A diagnosis of cocaine toxicity is made by history of ingestion of cocaine, physical examination, positive drug screen for cocaine, and presenting complaints.

Laboratory Findings

A CBC, PT, PTT, electrolytes, BUN, creatinine, amylase, lipase, LFTs, urinalysis, urine or serum drug screen, cardiac enzymes CPK, CPK-MB, LDH, AST, ALT, and GTT should be drawn.

Treatment

Most patients who die of cocaine poisoning die from cardiovascular and respiratory collapse. They will present with hyperthermia, metabolic acidosis, ventricular dysrhythmias, or status epilepticus.

Any patient who presents with possible cocaine poisoning should have two large-gauge IV lines placed. The patient should be placed on oxygen and on a cardiac monitor. The aforementioned laboratory tests should be drawn. If the patient is in acute distress, an ABG should be drawn to rule out metabolic acidosis. A chest x-ray and an abdominal series should be performed if a "body packer" is suspected or if rales or wheezing is heard on physical examination.

If the patient is acutely agitated, use haloperidol or lorazepam to treat the agitation. Remember, however, that the single most common cause of agitation is hypoxia. Always consider an intracranial bleed in any patient with altered mental status. Perform a computed tomography (CT) scan of the head if an intracranial hemorrhage or a history of head trauma is present.

Perform an ECG and a chest x-ray to rule out pulmonary edema, congestive heart failure, or acute myocardial infarction. Aggressive treatment of hyperthermia with cooling blankets is a necessity. Perform a glucose fingerstick to ensure that hypoglycemia is not present. If present, treat the patient with 1 ampule of D50W bolus.

If an opioid or heroin is suggested as a co-toxin in a comatose patient, give naloxone therapy. Treat seizures with diazepam or lorazepam therapy. Load the patient with phenytoin or phenobarbital. Prolonged seizures can cause rhabdomyolysis. Monitor the patient's urine output and correct metabolic acidosis with sodium bicarbonate. If rhabdomyolysis is present, treat the patient with IV fluids and mannitol-induced alkaline diuresis until myoglobinuria is cleared.

If severe hypertension is present, treat the patient with labetalol, nifedipine, sodium nitroprusside, or phentolamine. Anginal chest pain can be treated with a calcium channel antagonist, nitrates, or phentolamine. If hypotension occurs, treat the patient with norepinephrine.

If a body packer is suspected or if packages are seen on x-ray, give the patient an electrolyte bowel preparation solution (GoLYTELY). Do not attempt to remove the packages by colonoscopy or gastroscopy secondary to the potential to tear the packages. If a bowel obstruction is present, the bags should be removed by laparotomy.

Any patient with signs or symptoms of acute or chronic withdrawal should be admitted to the ICU for observation.

CYANIDE

Definition

Cyanide is one of the oldest known poisons. Cyanide can be found in cherry laurels and bitter almonds. The ancient Greeks and Romans used extracts of peach pits, cherry pits, and apricot pits to perform executions. Cyanide gas was first synthesized in 1786. Cyanide is a simple compound made of nitrogen and carbon. Tobacco smoke, certain fruit pits, nuts, fungi, bacteria, and plants contain cyanide.

Epidemiology

Acute accidental cyanide poisoning occurs in the United States secondary to accidental occupational poisoning, ingestion of plants, nuts, or fruits that contain cyanide, in persons working with metal polishes or acetonitrile-containing solvents, and iatrogenic-induced toxicity secondary to prolonged IV dosing of sodium nitroprusside. Hydrogen cyanide (HCN) is made by combining ammonia (NH_3) and methane (CH_4). Sodium cyanide (NaCN) and potassium cyanide (KCN) are synthesized from hydrogen gas. These cyanide compounds are used in the production of solvents, enamels, plastics, pesticides, herbicides, fertilizers, and wrinkle-resistant fabrics.

Cyanide has a very high affinity to metals, which is very helpful in extraction of ores, in electroplating metal, or in metal polishing. The leather industry uses cyanide products to strip hair from hides.

Poisoning can take place from exposure to the agent by inhalation or contact with the skin. One of the most common means of lethal exposure to cyanide gas occurs in an enclosed space in house fires. The burning of plastic-based products, polyurethane, vinyl, synthetic nitrogen-containing polymers, carpet, plastic furniture, drapes, and so forth, can release large amounts of cyanide.

In the Third World, the cassava plant is used for a source of carbohydrate. The active ingredient in the cassava plant is linamarin, which is a cyanogenic glycoside. It can cause ataxia and goiter with chronic exposure.

Pathology

Cyanide exposure causes a disruption in the metabolism by inhibiting the function of metal-containing enzymes. Ferric iron has the greatest affinity for cyanide. The mitochondria–oxidative phosphorylation is disrupted through the cytochrome A3 or cytochrome oxidase pathway with cyanide exposure. Cytochrome A3 catalyzes the final step in electron transport. At this step, oxygen is reduced to water. When cytochrome A3 enzyme is interfered with, the body tissues cannot utilize oxygen and only anaerobic metabolism occurs. Cyanide is bound rapidly and is labile and can be readily reversed. As cyanide poisoning increases, the inability of oxygen to be extracted from the blood increases; therefore, there is a direct increase in the oxygen content of venous blood.

Clinical Presentation

A patient will present with severe hypoxia but is not cyanotic. Only small amounts of cyanide bind to the ferrous iron on the hemoglobin molecule. Cyanide in small amounts does not interfere with the binding of oxygen to hemoglobin. If large amounts of cyanide are ingested, more binding will take place and cyanosis will occur as a terminal event. The blockage of the mitochondria to utilize oxygen produces a state of severe hypoxia in the presence of oxygen. Cyanide affects the brain first, then the heart; thus, mental status changes occur first, then cardiac symptoms occur. With acute cyanide poisoning, the classic "inspiratory gasp" followed by a hyperventilation history is often given by onlookers. The patient will be very anxious and breathless. A patient who is acutely subjected to a large dose of cyanide will present with altered mental status, unconsciousness, or coma. Acutely, the patient will present with tachycardia, atrial arrhythmia, and premature ventricular contractions. As exposure continues, bradycardia, apnea, and ventricular fibrillation will ensue.

Examination

The entire patient should be examined. Always check the patient's skin. Cyanide salts are caustic to the skin and can cause burns. On funduscopic examination, bright-red retinal vessels will be noted. Always smell the patient's breath. Often cyanide will have the smell of bitter almonds, but a large percentage of the population cannot smell the bitter almond odor.

A differential diagnosis in the unconscious acidotic patient includes exposure to carbon monoxide, hydrogen sulfide, natural gas, methanol, ethylene glycol, iron poisoning, and salicylate poisoning. In the occupational setting, often a history of smelling "rotten eggs" will be given just prior to the incident and will give a clue to hydrogen sulfide or natural gas exposure. Cocaine and isoniazid poisoning can also cause acidosis and seizures, which can mimic cyanide poisoning.

Diagnosis

A diagnosis is made by a history of occupational exposure (e.g., metal polishers, jewelry makers, laboratory technicians), herbal or nontraditional cancer therapy exposure, ingestion of laetrile or cyanogen-containing preparations, or exposure to burning plastic (e.g., in a house fire) or a suicidal ingestion of cyanide. The clinical presentation of hypoxia without cyanosis and bright-red retinal vessels with the odor of bitter almonds present are all clues to cyanide poisoning.

Laboratory Findings

A CBC, electrolytes, BUN, creatinine, calcium, magnesium, phosphorus, amylase, lipase, cardiac and liver enzymes, urinalysis, and an ABG should be performed on every patient with suspected cyanide or carbon monoxide poisoning. A carboxyhemoglobin (COHb) test should be performed also with each ABG. Cyanide levels can be obtained but are not readily available. A patient will present with a severe acidosis on ABG. Hypoglycemia occurs when poisoning is slow and is secondary to disruption of glycogen and lipid metabolism.

Treatment

If the patient has been contaminated topically, ensure adequate decontamination of the patient and proper protection for yourself and your staff. All patients with suspected cyanide or carbon monoxide poisoning should be placed on 100% oxygen by facemask or intubated and then given 100% oxygen, placed on a cardiac monitor, and have two large-gauge IV lines of normal saline placed. The aforementioned laboratory tests should be drawn with serial blood gases. If cyanide is ingested, gastric lavage and activated charcoal should be given; however, this should not be in place of or should not stop or slow down IV therapy with nitrates. The goal of therapy is to restore cellular respiration by providing an alternative source of ferric iron, thus freeing the cytochrome oxidase system. This is performed by the generation of MetHb by giving the *Lilly Cyanide Antidote Kit.* If the patient is unconscious, continue CPR and maintain airway control and oxygen therapy. The antidote kit contains sodium nitrate and sodium thiosulfate for IV administration and an ampule of amyl nitrate for inhalation. The adult dose of sodium nitrate is 300 mg, followed by 12.5 g of sodium thiosulfate. The pediatric dose is 0.33 ml/kg of a 10% sodium nitrate solution and 1.65 ml/kg of a 25% sodium thiosulfate. The goal of therapy is to form 25% methemoglobin.

Rapid reversal of cyanide poisoning and hypoxia has been well documented with just a small amount of methemoglobin formation. Therefore, even if CPR has been prolonged and the patient has no signs of life, give at least two doses of sodium nitrate and sodium thiosulfate. Watch the patient's blood pressure after administration of nitrates, because nitrates can cause vasodilatation and hypotension.

Special consideration for cyanide treatment occurs when a patient has been in a burning building and arrives at the ED unconscious. It is often impossible to determine acutely if the hypoxic and unconscious states are caused by carbon monoxide poisoning or cyanide poisoning. Nitrates will cause elevated levels of carboxyhemoglobin, which will decrease the oxygen-carrying capacity even more in patients who have inhaled carbon monoxide. Nitrates should not be given empirically to these patients. It will not be possible to distinguish immediately if the patient is suffering from an acute cyanide poisoning or carbon monoxide poisoning. If there is a high index of suspicion of cyanide poisoning by history and physical examination (hypoxia in the absence of cyanosis), give 100% oxygen and sodium thiosulfate *not* sodium nitrate. If on an ABG the carboxyhemoglobin level is not elevated and cyanide poisoning is suspected in a comatose acidotic patient, then sodium nitrite can be given. If carboxyhemoglobolin is elevated, then the treatment is 100% oxygen and hyperbaric chamber therapy.

Remember always to give dextrose, naloxone, and 100% oxygen to any unconscious patient.

Dicobalt edetate (Kelocyanor) is used in the United Kingdom to treat cyanide poisoning. 4-Dimethylaminophenol (DMAP) is used in Germany with some success in treating cyanide poisoning. It has less hypotensive effects than do the nitrates. Hyperbaric oxygen is also used in severe cases in which nitrate therapy has been only partially successful.

Any patient with suspected cyanide poisoning or carbon monoxide poisoning should be admitted to the ICU.

CYCLIC ANTIDEPRESSANT OVERDOSE

Definition

Cyclic antidepressants have been in use since the 1960s. The tricyclic antidepressants are the most popular therapy for depression in the United States. Cyclic antidepressants are also prescribed for insomnia, enuresis, chronic pain, and GI disease. More than 25 million prescriptions are written for cyclic antidepressants in the United States annually. There is often a lag time of 3 to 6 weeks before the cyclic depressants start to take effect.

Pathology

Cyclic antidepressants work by blocking the uptake of norepinephrine and at the synapse, they block the reuptake of serotonin. They also block the sodium channels in cell membranes. The different cyclic compounds have different degrees of anticholinergic and amine pump–blocking properties, all of which are related to the phenothiazines. The original agents consist of a basic three-ring structure, hence the name tricyclic antidepressants. Newer agents are now unicyclic, bicyclic, and tetracyclic. The treatment of older and newer cyclic drugs is the same. There are two exceptions to this rule of treatment. Amoxapine (Asendin) has a high incidence of seizures with overdose and death. Maprotiline (Ludiomil) also has a high incidence of seizures but not as high a mortality rate as amoxapine.

In overdoses, the cyclics are absorbed slowly from the stomach secondary to their ionization in the stomach acid. Cyclics can remain in the stomach for 12 hours or more. Once the cyclics are absorbed, they are 85 to 98% plasma protein bound. They then enter the mitochondria and endoplasmic reticulum. The cyclics are lipid soluble, and their ionic dissociation varies at various pH levels, which affects tissue entry. They will enter tissues at a higher rate if the pH of the tissue and plasma is higher. The volume distribution is higher in some tissues than in others, notably the heart, and is usually greater in tissues than in plasma.

The liver is the primary site of metabolism through glucuronidization, demethylation, and hydroxylation. Barbiturates, alcohol, and tobacco all enhance the metabolism of the cyclics. The half-life of cyclics of the β stage is measured in days, and a rebound effect can occur as the drug is redistributed from tissue compartments into the plasma.

The blocking of norepinephrine reuptake in the nervous system is the pathophysiologic reason for the reverse of depression. However, in the cardiovascular system, this leads to adrenergic blockade. The fast sodium channels are blocked, thus causing a decreased response in depolarization of conductive tissue of the heart. This also slows repolarization, causing a prolonged QT interval and depression of automaticity. There are also some α-adrenergic blocking effects present with cyclic overdoses.

Clinical Presentation/Examination

Any patient with any amount of cyclic ingestion can present with totally normal vital signs and can be awake and alert one minute and be in cardiac arrest the next. Seventeen percent of deaths due to overdose are from patients who presented to the ED with normal vital signs and are awake and alert. Forty-five percent have a normal sinus rhythm upon presentation to the ED. The signs of cyclic overdose are signs of CNS depression, depression of cardiac conduction and contractility, and anticholinergic toxicity. Patients present early with slurred speech, tachycardia, and lethargy.

CNS signs include coma, disorientation, myoclonus, clonus, and seizures. Cardiac effects include dysrhythmias, including new bundle branch blocks, aberrant conductions, ventricular arrhythmias, AV conduction blocks, idioventricular rhythms, and electromechanical dissociation (EMD). The QT and QRS intervals can be prolonged, and ST and T wave changes are common.

Diagnosis

The diagnosis is based on a history of ingestion and the clinical appearance of the patient. Always suspect a cyclic overdose in any patient who presents with decreased mental status, tachycardia, and mydriasis. An ECG with a rightward terminal QRS vector or a prolonged QRS of 100 msec or more in an obtunded patient is always suspect of a cyclic overdose. Do not rely on the alleged ingested dose. It is a poor predictor of outcome. One published guideline is that ingestion of less than 20 mg/kg is probably not fatal. A dose of 35 mg/kg is very serious, and 50 mg/kg or greater is probably fatal. However, these are only guidelines. Do not discharge a patient from the ED based on an ingested amount that is secondary to the cyclic drug's long half-life and protein binding in the tissues.

A patient with a Glasgow coma score of 8 or less upon presentation can be predictive of other serious complications with a sensitivity of 86% and a specificity of 89%.

Laboratory Findings

There are no specific laboratory tests for cyclic overdose. A CBC, electrolytes, calcium, magnesium, phosphorus, AST, ALT, total bilirubin, GGT, and cardiac enzymes CPK and CPK-MB should be drawn along with a drug screen. An ABG should be drawn to monitor acid-base balance.

Treatment

Any patient suspected of a tricyclic antidepressant overdose should be immediately placed on a cardiac monitor and have two large-gauge IV lines started. The patient should be given oxygen by nasal cannula and should be under constant observation. The aforementioned laboratory tests should be drawn, and an ABG should be performed. A gastric lavage should be performed if the patient has an intact gag reflex. Be prepared to intubate the patient before lavage is started. If the patient becomes unconscious, intubate and perform gastric lavage. This action could be lifesaving. If the patient has an intact gag reflex and has no altered mental status, activated charcoal should be given in multiple doses every 2 hours after gastric lavage. Peritoneal dialysis and forced diuresis are not effective in the removal of cyclics secondary to their high protein bonding. Hemoperfusion with activated charcoal can efficiently remove cyclics from the blood, but remember that most of the drug is bound to the tissues; therefore, this procedure has little effect on the overall removal of cyclic drugs from the body. Multiple charcoal doses shorten the half-life of cyclics from 36 hours to 4 hours. Magnesium sulfate can also be given to speed up the removal of cyclic-binded charcoal.

Monitor acid-base status with serial ABGs. Remember that there is less absorption in an alkaline environment. The arterial pH should be maintained above 7.50. Maintain a high normal PaO_2. Perform an ECG. If the QRS interval is greater than 100 msec, the sensitivity for major complications is 59%. Alkalinization of the blood to a pH above 7.5 is the best treatment to prevent cardiovascular toxicity. Alkalinization can be achieved by hyperventilation and by administration of IV sodium bicarbonate 1 to 5 mEq/kg. Titrate to a pH above 7.5. Sodium bicarbonate reverses the cyclic-induced blockage of cell membrane sodium channels. Isotonic saline should be used as a resuscitative fluid.

If life-threatening hypotension is present, use vasoconstrictors such as epinephrine, norepinephrine, and phenylephrine. Do not use isoproterenol or dobutamine secondary to their β-adrenergic effects. Dopamine at high doses is probably useful but would have β-adrenergic effects at low doses. Currently, the use of physostigmine is controversial. Physostigmine is a very short-acting cholinergic drug that reverses the anticholinergic effects of the tricyclics. It can cause seizures, worsen conduction blocks and hypotension, and produce cardiac arrest and asystole. Physostigmine should probably be avoided, except in a last-ditch effort. The dose of physostigmine is 2 mg IV over 2 minutes and then IV every 20 to 30 minutes or 2 mg IM every 2 hours.

Seizures have a 10% mortality rate in the 10% of tricyclic overdose patients who have seizures. The average seizure lasts less than 2 minutes; thus antiseizure medication is usually not required. Diazepam 5 to 10 mg IV can be used to stop a prolonged seizure; however, diazepam should be avoided because it slows hepatic clearance of tricyclic drugs. Diazepam also causes respiratory and CNS depression. Phenytoin and phenobarbital can both be used as treatment for prolonged seizures.

Any patient with an alleged cyclic overdose should be monitored for a minimum of 6 hours. If any signs of toxicity occur, the patient should be admitted to the ICU for treatment and observation. If after 6 hours the patient has had no tachycardia and has active bowel sounds, and the patient's clinical condition is improving, the patient can be discharged with psychiatric consultation and follow-up treatment.

DIGITALIS GLYCOSIDES

Definition

Digitalis is commonly used as a treatment for congestive heart failure and supraventricular tachyarrhythmias. Digitalis is a derivative of the foxglove plant *(Digitalis purpurea)*.

Epidemiology

Digitalis has been used in medical preparations since 1785. It has a very narrow therapeutic to toxic dose range. It can be given orally or IV. Toxicity is usually secondary to chronic use and rarely to intentional overdose.

Pathology

Digoxin's mechanism of action is related to the direct and indirect cardiac inotropic effect on the heart. Digitalis binds to and inactivates membrane-bound sodium, potassium, adenosine triphosphatase (ATP; Na^+, K^+-ATPase), which maintains the normal intracellular-to-extracellular concentration gradient of Na^+, Ca^+, and K^+. These actions cause an increase in intracellular Na^+ and Ca^+ and a decrease in intracellular potassium. The increased intracellular levels of calcium cause increased contractions of the heart. The volume of distribution is 7 to 10 l/kg. Digitalis preparations have a half-life of 36 to 48 hours. Digitalis in low doses does not affect the SA or AV node but does increase the vagal impulses and decrease sympathetic tone. In therapeutic doses, digitalis slows the AV node conduction and variably decreases the sinus rate of the heart.

Clinical Presentation/Examination

The GI symptoms of nausea and vomiting are usually first to appear. Patients with toxic levels of digoxin present with AV blocks, significant bradycardia, and sinus arrest. Always suspect digitalis toxicity in patients who are on digitalis and who present with new AV block or an AV block with junctional escape rhythms with a tachyarrhythmia. Bidirectional ventricular tachycardia and a narrow complex tachycardia with a new right bundle branch block are specific for digitalis toxicity. A patient can present with severe life-threatening hypokalemia with digoxin toxicity.

A patient on digoxin can be predisposed to toxicity secondary to chronic illnesses such as renal failure, heart disease, hepatic disease, COPD, and hypothyroidism. Drugs that interact with digoxin and that cause cardiac effects are calcium channel blockers and quinidine. A patient with severe digitalis toxicity will often present with the complaint of seeing yellow-green halos. Often symptoms are nonspecific, including anorexia, nausea, vomiting, headache, weakness, malaise, blurred vision, confusion, delirium, and hallucinations. A patient who presents with palpitations, near-syncope, syncope, and dizziness is probably experiencing cardiac toxicity. A patient who is on diuretics is at increased risk for toxicity.

ECG

A patient with digoxin toxicity on ECG examination will often present with the classic "dig effect" of downward sloping of the ST segment (sometimes with a slight elevation of the initial portion), an inverted T wave, and a subtle shortening of the RT interval. Bradydysrhythmia, tachydysrhythmia, and conduction defects are often seen. Atrial flutter or fibrillation are usually not found in digoxin toxicity; however, if present, look for another source of atrial fibrillation or atrial flutter.

Diagnosis

The diagnosis of digitalis toxicity is made by the clinical presentation of the patient, physical examination, serum digoxin level, and a history of acute or chronic ingestion of digitalis preparations.

Laboratory Findings

A CBC, electrolytes, BUN, creatinine, calcium, phosphorus, magnesium, LFTs, urinalysis, and serum digoxin levels should be performed on all patients with suspected digoxin toxicity. Normal serum digoxin levels are 0.5 to 2 ng/ml. Serum digoxin levels should be interpreted in the context of the overall patient presentation. Severe poisoning can be present in acute exposure with normal serum levels. Therapeutic doses do not rule out toxicity. A markedly elevated serum potassium level will not always be noted in digitalis toxicity. Serum potassium levels (hyperkalemia) are probably a better predictor of true digitalis toxicity in an acutely poisoned patient than are acute serum digoxin levels. Hyperkalemia is rarely seen in the chronically poisoned patient. Serial potassium and digoxin levels should be obtained.

Treatment

Any patient with suspected digoxin toxicity should have at least one large-gauge IV line of normal saline in place. The patient should be attached to a cardiac monitor, and the aforementioned laboratory tests should be drawn. An ECG should be performed. The patient should also be placed on oxygen therapy. In acute poisoning, gastric lavage should be performed and 1 g/kg of activated charcoal should be given.

If severe symptomatic toxicity is present, treat the specific symptoms. Establish an airway and treat hypoglycemia, hypoxia, and hypovolemia. If the patient is bradycardiac, give atropine or consider cardiac pacing. If ventricular arrhythmias are present, use phenytoin. Phenytoin accelerates the conduction at the AV node and is the drug of choice for digitalis-induced ventricular arrhythmias. Lidocaine and phenytoin also depress ventricular automaticity and increase the fibrillation threshold. Do not give class IA antiarrhythmics (quinidine or procainamide) because these agents depress AV node conduction, which will enhance cardiac toxicity. If electrocardioversion is necessary, use low 10 to 25 WS, secondary to the possibility of inducing ventricular fibrillation.

Hyperkalemia is treated with sodium bicarbonate, dextrose, insulin, and potassium-binding resin. Do not give calcium chloride, because hypocalcemia, hyperkalemia, sodium shifts, and hypomagnesemia are secondary to intracellular and extracellular shifts of electrolytes.

Digoxin-specific Fab (Digibind) is an immunoglobulin G (IgG) fragment of sheep antidigoxin antibodies. Fab directly removes digitalis from binding sites. Fab should be used in patients with severe bradyarrhythmias, ventricular arrhythmia, cardiac arrest, and severe hyperkalemia greater than 5.5 mEq/l. The Fab dose is based on an estimation of the total body load of digoxin.

$$\text{Total body load} = \frac{\text{serum digoxin level} \times 5.6 \text{ l/kg of the patient's weight (kg)}}{1000}$$

$$= \text{milligrams ingested} \times 0.80 \text{ (bioavailability)}$$

One vial (40 mg) of Fab fragments will bind 0.6 mg of digoxin. Calculate the number of vials needed for a dose by dividing the total body burden by 0.6. When the ingested dose cannot be calculated, give 10 vitals. Fab fragments must be given IV through a 0.22-μm filter over 30 minutes; however, if the patient is in full cardiac arrest, give Fab as a bolus. Clinical improvement is often seen in 1 hour after dosing.

All patients with symptomatic toxicity, who are hypokalemic, or are given Fab fragments, should be admitted to the ICU. After Fab is administered, serial potassium, calcium, sodium, and serum digoxin levels must be followed. Free digoxin levels fall to zero within minutes after the administration of Fab. However, serum digoxin levels will increase 10- to 20-fold, secondary to the digoxin being bound to the Fab fragments. Severe hypokalemia can occur after the administration of Fab; therefore watch the calcium level carefully.

Fab is a derivative of sheep IgG antibodies, and a hypersensitivity reaction can occur. Skin testing is available, but Fab should not be withheld in place of skin testing. Fab fragments are often lifesaving. Fab is eliminated by renal excretion.

Treat hypomagnesemia with magnesium sulfate 2 to 4 mg IV.

ETHANOL

Definition

Ethanol is a CNS depressant and is an aliphatic alcohol. It is used as a social stimulant. It is associated with motor vehicle accidents, suicide, homicide, and spouse and child abuse and is the drug of choice for co-dependent polydrug abusers.

Epidemiology

Ethanol is probably the most abused drug in the United States. Forty percent of all fatal traffic accidents involve ethanol alcohol. Twenty-three percent of all suicide attempts involve alcohol. Sixty-one percent of all drownings involve alcohol. It is estimated that 100,000 deaths each year are attributed to alcohol abuse.

It is estimated that the abusive use of ethanol reduces life expectancy by 12 years. It is also estimated that there are 10 million or more alcoholics in the United States alone. Half of all alcoholics are college educated and are functional within society.

Pathology

Ethanol is rapidly absorbed from the stomach and small intestine. Peak blood levels of ethanol are achieved in 30 to 90 minutes after ingestion. Ethanol's volume of distribution is approximately that of total body water at 0.6 l/kg.

Ethanol is metabolized by three different pathways: the microsomol ethanol oxidizing system, catalase, and alcohol dehydrogenase. The most important pathway is the alcohol dehydrogenase pathway, with NAD^+ as an oxidizing agent that converts ethanol to acetaldehyde. Ninety-five percent of ethanol is processed in the liver by this pathway. Ethanol is metabolized by zero-order kinetics. In nontolerant persons, ethanol is metabolized at 15 to 20 mg/dl/hr; in tolerant persons, such as alcoholics, ethanol is metabolized at 30 mg/dl/hr.

The CNS depression is probably secondary to the alteration of membrane lipid fluidity or the effect that ethanol has on the benzodiazepine-GABA-chloride complex.

Clinical Presentation/Examination

A patient with acute alcohol ingestion presents with primary CNS symptoms. As the ethanol blood level increases, the CNS symptoms increase until a coma is reached. Nausea and vomiting, ataxia, drowsiness, slurred speech, stupor, nystagmus, tachycardia, hypoventilation, hypothermia, hypotension, and loss of normal social restraints can occur. A patient will often present with facial flushing and diaphoresis.

Any chronic alcohol abuser or alcoholic who presents with an altered mental status should be considered to have Wernicke's encephalopathy. Wernicke's encephalopathy is a life-threatening illness that presents with the triad of ataxia, ophthalmoplegia (sixth nerve palsy and nystagmus), and altered mental status. A patient with Wernicke's encephalopathy will also present with hypotension, hypothermia, and coma.

Korsakoff's psychosis is also caused by a thiamine deficiency and is usually seen in conjunction with Wernicke's encephalopathy. Korsakoff's psychosis presents as retrograde and anterograde amnesia.

A patient who is an alcoholic is sometimes put on disulfiram (Antabuse) therapy. This drug inhibits aldehyde dehydrogenase and keeps the patient from ingesting alcohol. If alcohol is ingested or sometimes even topically applied, the patient can have an acute reaction consisting of nausea, vomiting, headache, skin flushing, and severe hypotension. Griseofulvin, chlorpropamide, metronidazole, and some third-generation cephalosporins can also cause a disulfiram reaction. This reaction can occur up to 2 to 3 weeks after the last dose of disulfiram.

The patient will often present in alcohol withdrawal, which is potentially fatal. The withdrawal symptoms are called delirium tremens (DTs) or "rum" fits. It is believed that DTs are caused by the direct effect that ethanol has on the benzodiazepine-GABA-chloride receptor complex. When ethanol is withdrawn, there is a substantial decrease in the activity of GABA. There is also an increase in the norepinephrine plasma concentration levels and an increase in the sympathetic activity.

A patient with DTs will present with highly variable symptoms. Most patients with DTs present with seizures, hallucinations, and tremors. These symptoms can be mild, moderate, or severe. Early symptoms of withdrawal include insomnia, irritability, and tremors. If the patient does not ingest alcohol, he or she can progress to hypertension, tachycardia, and diaphoresis. The patient will often complain of hallucinations, including auditory, visual, or olfactory symptoms. Approximately 90% of patients will progress to a grand mal type of seizure within 7 to 48 hours after their last drink of alcohol. Status epilepticus is rare, and if it does occur, consider another co-pathology to cause the seizures, such as head trauma. If DTs are left untreated, they can cause death secondary to cardiovascular collapse.

Alcoholic polyneuropathy is a result of nutritional deficiencies and direct alcohol toxicity. A patient with alcoholic polyneuropathy will present with symmetric loss of reflexes and vibratory sense. Autonomic and cranial nerves are spared. Their presenting complaints are usually paresthesias, pain, and extremity numbness.

Atrial fibrillation is the most common presenting cardiac complaint in the alcoholic patient. Atrial flutter, premature atrial contractions with re-entrant supraventricular tachycardia, premature ventricular beats, and nonsustained ventricular tachycardia can all occur in the alcoholic patient. These dysrhythmias are usually not secondary to underlying heart disease, but rather occur from the effect of toxicity of the alcohol on the heart muscle itself. These dysrhythmias usually resolve in 24 hours without treatment.

Congestive heart failure is very common in the chronic ethanol abuser secondary to alcoholic cardiomyopathy. Alcoholic cardiomyopathy is commonly seen in the 30- to 50-year-old man with more than 10 years of alcohol abuse. Treat congestive heart failure in the alcoholic the same as in any other patient with congestive heart failure.

The alcoholic patient can present with an acute Mallory-Weiss tear, an acute tear of the esophagus, secondary to forceful vomiting, or acute Boerhaave's syndrome, an acute rupture of the esophagus. Alcoholics can present with hemorrhage secondary to bleeding esophageal varices secondary to chronic cirrhosis.

Alcoholics can present with pancreatitis or hepatitis. The classic presentation of alcoholic hepatitis is anorexia, vomiting, low-grade fever, jaundice, and abdominal pain. Alcoholic cirrhosis presents 10 to 15 years after chronic alcohol ingestion, which leads to portal hypertension, which will cause splenomegaly, hepatic encephalopathy, coagulopathy, esophageal varices, and ascites.

Alcoholics are susceptible to pneumonias secondary to aspiration, co-use of tobacco, and immunocompromised host factors. Commonly, alcoholics are infected with the *Klebsiella* organism.

Diagnosis

Alcoholic beverages are labeled by their "proof." Proof is the ethanol content of the beverage. Two proof is equal to 1% ethanol content (1 g of ethanol is equal to 1.25 ml). In most states a blood alcohol level greater than 100 mg/dl is considered to be a level of intoxication. Decreased motor function occurs at 20 to 50 mg/dl; decreased coordination and impaired judgment occurs at 50 to 100 mg/dl; balance and speech are affected at 100 to 150 mg/dl; lethargy occurs at 150 to 250 mg/dl; coma occurs at 300 mg/dl; respiratory depression occurs at 400 mg/dl; and potential for death occurs at more than 500 mg/dl.

DTs are diagnosed by a history of a chronic alcoholic user who abruptly stops his or her alcohol ingestion and also the physical presentation and laboratory findings.

Laboratory Findings

A CBC, PT, PTT, electrolytes, BUN, creatinine, amylase, lipase, AST, ALT, GGT, LDH, total bilirubin, hepatitis panel, drug screen, and ethanol level should be drawn. If alcoholic ketoacidosis (AKA) or diabetic ketoacidosis (DKA) is suspected, draw an ABG.

Ethanol can cause hypoglycemia and AKA. Ethanol oxidation will shift the intracellular redox potential by increasing the $NADH/NAD^+$ ratio, which can cause the formation of lactate and β-hydroxybutyrate. This causes an increase in fatty acid metabolism for energy consumption and thus the possibility of AKA. Hypoglycemia secondary to ethanol ingestion is caused by the depletion of the body's glycogen stores because of total body starvation and depletion of pyruvate, which are needed for gluconeogenesis.

Patients with alcoholic hepatitis will present with leukocytosis and elevated liver aminotransferase. The AST will be greater than ALT in alcoholic liver disease, and there will be hyperbilirubinemia. In acute alcohol ingestion, the GGT is usually elevated.

Anemia is seen 75% of the time in alcoholic patients. The anemia is usually megaloblastic anemia secondary to vitamin B_{12} deficiency, and a high mean corpuscular volume (MCV) on CBC will also be present. If the hematologic indices show an iron deficiency anemia, assume that there is a blood loss from an acute or chronic GI bleed. Thrombocytopenia is common in alcoholics secondary to decreased platelet production and platelet survival from splenic sequestration. Always check the PT and PTT levels in alcoholic patients secondary to the vitamin K deficiency found in many alcoholic patients. If there is hepatic disease, hepatitis, or cirrhosis, the PT or PTT level can be elevated by both the liver disease and vitamin K deficiency.

Treatment

Treatment is mostly supportive. All patients with suspected acute alcohol abuse or chronic alcohol abuse with the possibility of DTs should have at least one large-gauge IV line of normal saline. The patient should be placed on a cardiac monitor and on 2 liters of oxygen via nasal cannula. An ECG and a chest x-ray should be performed, and the aforementioned laboratory tests should be drawn. A quick blood glucose test should be performed, and if the patient is hypoglycemic, give 1 ampule of D50W IV. If altered mental status is present, give naloxone 0.4 to 4 mg IV. If AKA or DKA is suspected, an ABG should be drawn. If a head injury is suspected or if the history of head injury cannot be determined, then a CT scan of the head should be performed, especially if the patient presents with altered mental status. All patients should be evaluated for co-ingestion of sedative-hypnotics or long-acting benzodiazepines.

All alcoholics are probably deficient in thiamine; therefore give 100 mg of thiamine intramuscularly (IM) or IV. Thiamine is a co-factor of pyruvate dehydrogenase, α-ketoglutarate dehydrogenase, and transketolase. Wernicke's encephalopathy, peripheral neuropathy, cardiomyopathy, and metabolic acidosis are all secondary to a thiamine deficiency. Alcoholics are usually deficient in magnesium, potassium, niacin, folate, and vitamins.

A common treatment in the ED for chronic or acute alcohol ingestion is a "Rally" pack or a "Banana" bag. In a bag of D5 normal saline, place 100 mg of thiamine, 2 g of magnesium, 1 mg of folic acid, a dose of multivitamins, and 20 mEq of potassium. Give this solution IV over 2 hours.

Treat acute seizures with diazepam or lorazepam (Ativan). Give diazepam 5 to 10 mg every 10 to 15 minutes as needed. Phenobarbital is a long-acting barbiturate that can be given in place of diazepam.

β-Blockers have been suggested as a treatment for alcohol withdrawal symptoms. Propranolol 0.5 to 1 mg IV or 40 mg PO has been suggested to control alcohol withdrawal tremors. Atenolol, 50 to 100 mg, has also been used to control tremors. Clonidine, 0.2 to 0.6 mg PO daily, or a clonidine patch can be used to decrease the withdrawal symptoms.

Remember that alcohol-intoxicated patients can be intoxicated *and* have meningitis, pancreatitis, liver disease, GI bleeds, or acute myocardial infarctions, or they could have fallen and struck their heads. Remember the first rule with the intoxicated patient is that if the patient does not have a normal mental status or if the patient can't walk out the door, the patient can't leave the ED and must be admitted to the hospital. Never attribute a change in mental status to ethanol intoxication alone. Never let your feeling about an intoxicated alcoholic patient overrule your clinical or medical judgment. Remember that alcoholic patients are at a higher risk for meningitis, cranial bleeds, and GI bleeds.

A patient with a potential withdrawal syndrome, DTs, cirrhosis, hepatitis, or altered mental status needs to be admitted to the hospital for detoxification.

ETHYLENE GLYCOL

Definition

Ethylene glycol is a colorless, odorless, sweet-tasting form of alcohol. It is used in antifreeze, coolants, polishes, paints, de-icers, lacquers, detergents, and pharmaceuticals.

Epidemiology

Ethylene glycol ingestions are either intentional (e.g., in a suicide attempt or gesture) or accidental.

Pathology

The volume of distribution of ethylene glycol is 0.6 to 0.8 l/kg. Ethylene glycol is absorbed rapidly by all tissues of the body. It reaches peak blood levels in 1 to 4 hours. The half-life is 3 to 8.4 hours. The metabolites of ethylene glycol affect the brain, heart, kidneys, and lungs. Nonmetabolized ethylene glycol has the same effect on the body as does ethanol. It is the metabolites glycolate, glycoaldehyde, glyoxate, and oxalate that inhibit oxidative phosphorylation, protein synthesis, and the sulfhydryl-containing enzymes from their normal function. Glycolic acid is the byproduct of ethylene glycol metabolism, which causes the severe anion gap acidosis.

Clinical Presentation/Examination

A patient will present in three stages. In stage I (the CNS stage), the onset of symptoms occurs in 30 minutes to 12 hours. The patient will present as if intoxicated with ethanol with an odor of alcohol on the breath. Ataxia, slurred speech, stupor, convulsions, hallucinations, and coma are often presenting complaints. The patient's primary complaint is nausea or vomiting, and the patient will be tachycardiac and hypertensive.

In stage II, the patient will present with cardiopulmonary complaints. This stage occurs 12 to 24 hours after ingestion of ethylene glycol. The patient will present with muscle tenderness, myositis, hypertension, tachycardia, and acute congestive heart failure.

Stage III, the patient will present with flank pain and costophrenic tenderness 24 to 72 hours after ingestion of ethylene glycol. Calcium oxalate monohydrate and dihydrate crystalluria are common findings on urinalysis. Oliguria is common in the first 12 hours after ingestion of ethylene glycol. Anuria often occurs in stage III. A patient who reaches stage III can develop adult respiratory distress syndrome (ARDS).

Diagnosis

The lethal dose of ethylene glycol is 1 to 1.5 ml/kg of a 100% solution. Unlike methanol and ethanol, any dose of ethylene glycol should be considered toxic and lethal. A diagnosis is made by the history of ingestion of ethylene glycol, large anion gap metabolic acidosis, hypocalcemia, oxalate crystals in the urine, and renal dysfunction.

Often fluorescein is placed in antifreeze. Therefore, if an ingestion of antifreeze is suspected, fluorescein will be seen in the urine with a Wood lamp examination.

Laboratory Findings

A CBC, electrolytes, BUN, creatinine, amylase, lipase, calcium, AST, ALT, GGT, CPK, LDH, acetone, serum ketones, magnesium, salicylate, ethanol and ethylene glycol, urinalysis, and ABG should be performed. A serum or urine drug screen should also be performed. Ethylene glycol causes a severe anion gap metabolic acidosis secondary to the accumulation of oxalate, lactate, and glycolate. On urinalysis, calcium oxalate crystals, hematuria, proteinuria, and renal epithelial cells are often found. Hypocalcemia is noted on an electrolyte panel.

There will be an osmolal gap before the onset of an abnormal anion gap. There is often leukocytosis and an elevated CPK secondary to muscle injury.

Treatment

The treatment of ethylene glycol overdose is based on correction of metabolic acidosis, correction of electrolyte abnormalities, prevention of ethylene glycol metabolism, removal of the unmetabolized ethylene glycol, and removal of its metabolites.

All patients with suspected ethylene glycol ingestion should have two large-gauge IV lines of normal saline placed. The patient should be placed on a cardiac monitor and given oxygen therapy. The patient should have a chest x-ray and an ECG performed. The aforementioned laboratory tests should be drawn to include an ABG and serum osmolality. A gastric lavage should be performed if ingestion is within 2 hours of presentation or if co-ingestion is considered. Ethylene glycol is poorly absorbed by charcoal. A Foley catheter should be placed to evaluate for an adequate urine output.

The mainstay of treatment is correction of anion gap metabolic acidosis by the administration of sodium bicarbonate and the removal of ethylene glycol. The patient should be given thiamine 100 mg and pyridoxine 1 mg/kg IV. Thiamine and pyridoxine are both co-factors in the detoxification of ethylene glycol.

To remove ethylene glycol from the patient, ethanol is given. Ethanol has a greater affinity for dehydrogenase than does ethylene glycol. Ethanol levels should be maintained at a serum concentration of 100 to 150 mg/dl. If the ethylene glycol level is above 25 mg/dl, then hemodialysis should be considered. The ethanol infusion rate needs to be doubled if hemodialysis is performed, secondary to the increased ethanol clearance rate with hemodialysis. An ethanol infusion should be maintained until the ethanol glycol level is zero.

All patients with an ethylene glycol overdose should be admitted to the ICU and have an ophthalmology consult to follow current or future eye pathology.

HALLUCINOGENS

Definition

Hallucinogens are a generic term for a group of drugs that cause hallucinations. They include lysergic acid diethylamide (LSD), phencyclidine (PCP), mescaline from the peyote cactus (*Lophophora williamsii*), morning glory from the Convolvulaceae family of mind-altering alkaloids, two types of mushrooms, psilocybin- or ibotenic acid-containing mushrooms, marihuana, nutmeg, and jimsonweed (*Datura stramonium*).

Pathology/Clinical Presentation

LSD is the most potent psychoactive drug known. LSD was discovered in the 1930s by Albert Hoffman and was named LSD-25. The drug was used in the 1960s. There has been a decrease in use during the past 10 years, but there is now a rise in use in the United States. The exact mechanism of action of LSD is unknown. It is believed that LSD is both an agonist and antagonist on the central dopamine receptors, which can cause sympathomimetic effects. LSD is believed to cause its effects through inhibition of the serotoninergic neurotransmission system. The inhibition of serotoninergic neurotransmission causes a decrease in the inhibitory tone in higher cortical centers, which results in perceptual distortions or hallucinations.

LSD is toxic in very small amounts ranging from 25 to 500 μg. It can be injected, insufflated, or inhaled. The oral route is the most popular route of ingestion. After ingestion, symptoms occur in 30 minutes to 1½ hours. Symptoms include an increase in blood pressure, mydriasis, increase in heart rate, increase in respiratory rate, and mild elevation in temperature. Mild piloerection, salivation, and nausea can occur. Tremor, hyperreflexia, and neuromuscular weakness are common. In about 2 hours after ingestion of LSD, hallucinations occur. Thought content becomes disordered, and paranoia can occur. Symptoms can last from 4 to 12 hours after ingestion.

Rhabdomyolysis, life-threatening hyperpyrexia, seizures, CNS veno-occlusive disease, acute psychosis, and coagulopathy can occur. If the patient has an underlying psychiatric pathology and uses LSD, that patient can be subjected to a "flashback" phenomenon for weeks, months, or even years after the last dose of LSD.

Mescaline is ingested by eating dried or cooked peyote buttons. Peyote buttons have been used in religious ceremonies for 8000 years by Native Americans and Indians of Mexico. Peyote was legal for use in the United States by the Native American Church until April 7, 1990. Peyote has an extremely bitter taste, and the ingestion results in severe nausea and vomiting. It takes 6 to 12 buttons or about 270 to 540 mg of peyote to produce hallucinations. Nausea and vomiting usually occur within minutes of ingestion. The onset of hallucinations occurs approximately 2 hours after ingestion and lasts for 6 to 12 hours. The hallucinations can be olfactory, visual, tactile, auditory, or gustatory. Hypotension, tachycardia, respiratory depression, and bradycardia can all occur.

Psilocybin is found in mushrooms usually in Florida, Louisiana, and Texas (*Psilocybe cubensis* or gold caps). They are often called "magic mushrooms." In these states, these mushrooms are usually found growing in cow dung. In the Pacific Northwest, the *P. semilanceata* (liberty cap) is found growing in pastures and lawns. Psilocybin is resistant to oxidation and remains active when dried or cooked. There is often an onset of gastric upset within minutes of ingestion. Mild hypertension, tachycardia, and mydriasis are common symptoms. The onset of hallucinations is usually within 1 hour, and the symptoms last for 4 to 12 hours. Seizures, hyperthermia, and coma have all been reported.

A second type of mushrooms contains the toxin ibotenic acid and its metabolite muscimol. It is found in the *Amanita muscaria* and *A. pantherina* species of mushrooms. Ibotenic acid and muscimol are isoxazole compounds that can cause illusions and visual perceptions but not true hallucinations. Ibotenic acid causes a modification of gamma-aminobutyric acid (GABA), glutamate, and serotonin function. No anticholinergic symptoms are produced after ingestion of these mushrooms. After ingestion, symptoms of dizziness, headache, and ataxia occur 30 minutes to 1½ hours after ingestion. The illusions and distortion of visual perceptions occur 2 to 4 hours after ingestion. The duration of the effect lasts for 6 to 12 hours. Seizures and muscle twitching have occurred.

Marihuana is obtained from the dried leaves and flowers of the *Cannabis sativa* plant. Hashish is the dried resin of the plant. Both contain the toxin delta 9-tetrahydrocannabinol (THC). THC has been used in China for over 4000 years. Marihuana is usually smoked but can be placed in food, such as brownies, or other drugs can be placed in a marihuana cigarette to increase the effect or "high." THC blood level peaks 7 to 8 minutes after smoking. The "high" usually lasts for 2 to 6 hours after inhalation. This "high" consists of euphoria, an increased sense of well-being, perceptual alterations, mild stimulation, depersonalization, hallucinations, dysphoria, and paranoia.

The exact mechanism of THC is yet unknown. It is believed that there are specific THC receptor sites, along with nonspecific effects on cell membranes (like general anesthetics), and interactions with serotonergic, dopaminergic, noradrenergic, and GABA systems. The physical effects of marihuana are dry mouth, hunger, conjunctival irritation, mild tachycardia, and unsteady gait.

Morning glory seeds from the *Convolvulaceae* family of plants, contain mind-altering alkaloids (e.g., D-lysergic acid amide) much like the ergots. The *Ipomoea violacea* (*Ipomoea rubrocaerulea*) is the most common plant. Acute ingestion of morning glory will cause symptoms similar to those after ingestion of LSD and hallucinations. It takes more than 200 seeds to cause the same effect as 200 μg of LSD. Symptoms resolve in 8 to 10 hours after ingestion.

Diagnosis

A diagnosis of hallucinogen ingestion is made by a history of ingestion, physical examination, and presenting complaints.

Laboratory Findings

There are no specific laboratory tests to rule in or out the use of hallucinogens.

Treatment

A patient who is intoxicated with LSD is treated symptomatically with cooling blankets, sedation, and volume resuscitation. Usually, by keeping the sensory input to a minimum, hallucinations and agitation symptoms will be decreased.

The treatment of mescaline toxicity includes IV rehydration and sedation. GI decontamination is of little help secondary to the usual vomiting within minutes of ingestion. Use benzodiazepines for sedation. Do not use phenothiazines secondary to their increased risk of flashback phenomenon. A patient with acute mushroom poisoning is treated mainly with supportive care. If the patient is having a seizure, treat the patient with diazepam. A patient who presents or is brought to the ED with marihuana intoxication usually only needs supportive care.

HYDROCARBONS

Definition

Hydrocarbons are organic compounds that contain carbon and hydrogen ions. Hydrocarbons are divided into the aliphatic, halogenated, and aromatic hydrocarbon groups. The aliphatic hydrocarbons are the gasolines, kerosenes, paraffins, and olefins. Aliphatic hydrocarbons consist of the open-chain mixtures of hydrocarbons of different chain length. The aromatic hydrocarbons all contain a benzene ring and are the halogenated hydrocarbons that are widely used in industrial solvents.

Common aliphatic hydrocarbons are:

Gasoline and automobile fuel
Naphthalene and cigarette
  lighter fluid
Mineral seal oil and furniture
  polishes

Kerosene and camping store
  lamp and stove fuel
Diesel oil and lubricants
N-hexane, rubber, and plastic
  cement

Aromatic hydrocarbons include:

Xylene, degreasers, cleaning agents, and industrial solvents
Benzene and gasoline
Toluene, acrylic paints, plastic cements, and airplane glues

Halogenated hydrocarbons include:

Trichloroethylene (TCE) used in degreasers, spot removers, and typewriter correction fluid
Trichloroethane (TCA) used in degreasers, spot removers, and typewriter correction fluid
Carbon tetrachloride, aerosol propellants, solvents, and refrigerants
Tetrachloroethylene, degreasers, and dry cleaning agents
Chloroform, chemical intermediates, and solvents
Methylene chloride, aerosol paints, paint stripper, varnish remover, and degreasers

Epidemiology

Hydrocarbon ingestion of gasoline, kerosene, mineral oil, lighter fluid, and turpentine involves approximately 3 to 10% of all accidental childhood ingestions. In 1989 there were approximately 58,000 exposures to hydrocarbons, with 1600 moderate to severe toxicity cases and 31 deaths secondary to hydrocarbon ingestion.

Older children and teenagers sniff glue, paint, and solvents to get "high," all of which contain hydrocarbons. Adult workers are exposed to hydrocarbons in the workplace via fuels, plastics, solvents, and insecticides. Medical personnel are exposed to hydrocarbons in the operating suite, via halothane, and in the care of patients with diethylstilbestrol and gamma benzene hexachloride.

Pathology

In evaluating a patient who has been exposed to hydrocarbons, it must be determined what the volatility, viscosity, and surface tension of the hydrocarbon is. It must also be known if the hydrocarbon is aliphatic, aromatic, or halogenated. Knowledge of other toxic additives, such as heavy metals or pesticides, also needs to be determined. The route of exposure and the concentration of the hydrocarbon or other chemical content must also be determined.

Viscosity is the resistance to flow. Viscosity is measured in Saybolt seconds universal (SSU). The lower the viscosity, the greater will be the risk of aspiration.

Volatility denotes the hydrocarbon's ability to vaporize. The higher the volatility, the more readily the hydrocarbon is inhaled and thus the greater the systemic absorption and potential for systemic toxicity. Surface tension is the "creeping" ability or ability of the hydrocarbon to move.

Low-viscosity hydrocarbons have a tendency to be aspirated during ingestion and spread over the lung fields, causing patchy pulmonary edema, bronchospasm, atelectasis, hemorrhage, and necrosis of lung tissue. Volatile hydrocarbons have a greater tendency to be inhaled as a vapor and cause increased neurologic symptoms.

No matter how hydrocarbons are absorbed, their metabolites cause lipid peroxidation and metabolic acidosis. Lipid peroxidation causes oxidate deterioration of polyunsaturated lipids, which damages lipids and produces free radicals that cause damage to enzymes and anion acids.

The kidneys are the primary excretory mechanism of soluble metabolites. Volatile hydrocarbons are primarily excreted by the lungs, and small amounts are excreted by the biliary tract and small intestine.

Clinical Presentation/Examination

A patient will often present to the ED as if drunk with alcohol ingestion. The patient will present with complaints of vomiting and shortness of breath. Often the patient will complain of palpitations or chest pain.

A patient with pulmonary complaints will complain of aspiration-associated symptoms. This patient is usually a small child who accidentally aspirates a small amount of an aliphatic, low-viscosity hydrocarbon. This patient usually presents with choking, gasping for air, coughing, dyspnea, and burning of the oral mucosa and tracheobronchial tree with CNS symptoms. The severity of aspiration is not dependent on the volume ingestion. Very small amounts (0.2 ml) can cause a significant pneumonitis in children. The amount of hydrocarbon absorbed by the GI tract does not cause the CNS symptoms, but rather the CNS symptoms are caused by even the smallest amount of direct aspiration of a hydrocarbon.

Direct aspiration of hydrocarbons causes direct destruction of the pulmonary parenchyma. Hydrocarbons cause destruction of the alveolar and capillary membranes, which in turn causes an increase in vascular permeability and pulmonary edema along with an altered surfactant function. CNS symptoms are secondary to hypoxia caused by the acute pneumonitis, which is caused by the direct damage to the pulmonary parenchyma. Pneumothoraces, pneumomediastinum, and pneumatoceles are all associated with hydrocarbon aspiration.

On examination, a patient will present with tachypnea, tachycardia, retractions, grunting respirations, and cyanosis. Thirty percent of patients will have a fever. There is often an odor of hydrocarbons on the patient.

A patient who is severely toxic with hydrocarbon exposure will die within 24 hours from necrotizing pneumonitis and hemorrhagic pulmonary edema. The patient who survives for the first 24 hours usually resolves all of the symptoms in 2 to 5 days. If the patient develops a pneumatocele and lipoid pneumonia, the symptoms can last for weeks to months.

The solvent-containing aromatic hydrocarbons toluene (glue and acrylic paint) and trichloroethylene (typewriter correction fluid) cause the most CNS symptoms. They are abused mostly by teenagers, young adults, and Native Americans. Chronic abusers of these aromatic hydrocarbons are called "baggers" or "huffers." They place these hydrocarbons in a bag or on a rag and inhale the hydrocarbons. These agents, once in the body, act much like inhaled anesthetic agents. The patient will often be mistaken for being intoxicated with ethanol. The patient presents with dizziness, slurred speech, lethargy, ataxia, and coma.

The desired effect of the inhalation of these aromatic hydrocarbons is euphoria and exhilaration. Often what does occur are hallucinations, perceptual changes, confusion, and psychosis. If the patient is a chronic abuser of these hydrocarbons, a chronic syndrome of cerebellar ataxia, recurrent headaches, emotional lability, chronic encephalopathy with tremors, mental status changes, cognitive impairment, and psychomotor impairment can occur. These syndromes are thought to be associated with the chronic ingestion of tetraethyl lead and its toxic metabolites, which are often found in spray paint.

If a patient is chronically exposed to the six-carbon aliphatic hydrocarbons, a characteristic peripheral polyneuropathy secondary to demyelinization and retrograde axonal degeneration will occur. This peripheral polyneuropathy is secondary to chronic exposure to *N*-

hexane and methyl N-butyl ketone six-carbon aliphatic hydrocarbon groups. The demyelinization is secondary to the metabolite 2,5-hexanedione produced by the cytochrome P450-mediated biotransformation of the parent compounds.

These patients present with wrist and foot drops, numbness, and paresthesias for months or years after the initial exposure. A diagnosis can be made by electromyelogram, which will show decreased nerve conduction velocity.

A patient can present with life-threatening arrhythmias, ventricular tachycardia, and ventricular fibrillation after systemic absorption. Often sudden cardiac arrest, "sudden sniffing death," can occur after a sudden release of catecholamines secondary to an acute panic attack, exertion, or fright. Epinephrine should not be used in these patients except in cardiac resuscitation secondary to the increased catecholamine release.

GI complaints are secondary to direct intestinal irritation. Patients will present with vomiting, diarrhea, nausea, belching, acute abdominal pain, and mouth and throat burning.

Carbon tetrachloride and chloroform, both halogenated hydrocarbons, can be hepatotoxic after inhalation. The free radical metabolites of these two agents can cause lipid peroxidation and thus hepatocellular destruction. A patient will present with elevated LFTs 24 hours after ingestion and will develop liver tenderness and jaundice in 48 to 96 hours. If the patient is a chronic user, he or she can develop hepatomas and cirrhosis.

A patient who chronically "huffs" hydrocarbons can develop a "huffer's flush or rash" on the face and hands. Pruritus and a defatting dermatitis, which appears similar to eczematoid dermatitis, can occur. "Huffers" are prone to cellulitis and sterile abscesses. Severe full-thickness burns have been reported in patients who immerse body parts in hydrocarbons. Chronic benzene exposure can cause aplastic anemia, multiple myeloma, and myelogenous leukemia.

If toluene is abused, acute renal tubular acidosis can occur. A patient with acute renal tubular acidosis presents with a non-anion gap metabolic acidosis, hypophosphatemia, and hypokalemia. Serum potassium can be as low as 2 mEq/l with the presence of severe muscle weakness and quadriparesis. Rhabdomyolysis can also be a presenting complaint of this syndrome.

Diagnosis

A diagnosis is made by a history of hydrocarbon ingestion, aspiration, inhalation, physical examination, and patient presentation.

Laboratory Findings

A CBC, PT, PTT, electrolytes, calcium, magnesium, phosphorus, BUN, creatinine, AST, ALT, GGT, bilirubin, urinalysis, and an ABG should be performed on every patient in whom a suspected hydrocarbon ingestion has taken place. On an ABG, there will be a markedly widened alveolar-arterial (A-a) oxygen gradient. Metabolic acidosis is secondary to lipid peroxidation in the mitochondria.

If the patient has been using lead-based paint for huffing or sniffing, or exposure to lead is suspected, a lead level can be helpful in making the diagnosis, especially if peripheral neuropathy is present.

Treatment

A patient with a hydrocarbon ingestion should have at least one IV line of normal saline started and pulse oximetry performed. The patient should be placed on a cardiac monitor and on oxygen therapy. A chest x-ray and an ECG should be performed. Pulmonary changes on an x-ray can be seen in 4 to 6 hours after aspiration and are usually always evident within 18 to 24 hours. Infiltrates will be from streaking to flocculent to homogeneous in appearance and are almost always in the dependent lobes and multilobar.

The mnemonic CHAMP (*c*amphor, *h*alogenated hydrocarbons, *a*romatic hydrocarbons, *m*etals, and *p*esticides), can be used to recall which hydrocarbons require GI decontamination. Activated charcoal does not absorb most hydrocarbon compounds. In fact there is an increased risk of aspiration secondary to gastric distention by activated charcoal use. Activated charcoal has been used in benzene and toluene ingestion with some success. Gastric lavage is the recommended method of GI decontamination for wood distillate ingestions. Always protect the patient's airway, especially in a patient with an altered mental status. Do not use syrup of ipecac secondary to the increased risk of aspiration. Most other, non-CHAMP hydrocarbons require no GI decontamination secondary to their rapid gastric absorption.

A patient who presents with hypotension should be treated with fluids. Dopamine and epinephrine, which increase circulating catecholamines, can precipitate dysrhythmias, especially after ingestion of halogenated hydrocarbons.

The mainstays of treatment are oxygen therapy, IV fluids, and supportive care. Hemodialysis and hemoperfusion have been successful in the treatment of tetrachloride intoxication. Asymptomatic patients who have been observed for 6 hours and are still asymptomatic after 6 hours, can be discharged home with drug rehabilitation follow-up.

IRON

Definition

Iron is a naturally occurring element. Ten percent of ingested iron, mainly ferrous iron (Fe^{2+}), is absorbed from the small intestine. Unbound or free iron is very toxic to all organs of the body.

Epidemiology

Intentional and accidental ingestion of iron are important causes of mortality and morbidity, especially in children. There were approximately 20,000 exposures to iron in the United States in 1988 as reported by the American Association of Poison Control Centers. The current mortality rate for iron poisoning is approximately 1%. The most common patient group that ingests iron consists of children between the ages of 9 and 24 months who "eat" their mother's iron-containing vitamins or prenatal iron tablets.

Pathology

The toxicity of iron is caused by the direct caustic effect on the GI mucosa, prolonged bleeding times, and the effects that iron has on the body's hepatic, CNS, metabolic, and cardiovascular systems. Iron is absorbed via first-order kinetics. After ferrous iron is ingested, it is changed into ferric iron (Fe^{3+}) and is stored in the intestinal mucosa complexes as the protein ferritin. When iron is needed, it is transported to the spleen, bone marrow, and liver for use in heme molecules. During this transportation it is protein bound and is called transferrin. The total amount of iron that can be bound to transferrin is called the total iron-binding capacity (TIBC). The normal TIBC is 300 to 435 μg/dl. The total normal serum iron is 50 to 150 μg/dl.

Iron is a very caustic substance, especially to the gastric mucosa. It can cause hypovolemia secondary to hemorrhagic gastroenteritis. Iron in large doses can have damaging effects on the brain, lungs, kidneys, and heart. It accumulates primarily in the liver.

In toxic doses, iron accumulates in the mitochondria. This increased accumulation of iron levels disrupts oxidative phosphorylation and catalyzes the formation of oxygen free radicals, which lead to rapid peroxidation and cell death in the liver. Ferritin complexes also cause dilatation of venules and thus venous pooling. Iron also increases membrane permeability and thus third spacing of fluids.

Hypoperfusion, hypovolemia, and dehydration all cause shifts of cells from anaerobic metabolism. This shift causes the oxidative phosphorylation to be impaired, thus causing lactic acidosis. Coagulopathy is caused by the direct ability of iron to inhibit the serine proteases, like thrombin, and thus increase PT bleeding time.

Clinical Presentation/Examination

A patient may present in one of four stages of poisoning; however, a patient can die in any of the four stages, thus be prepared for the worst in any stage.

In stage I, the patient presents with symptoms of the direct corrosive effects of iron, i.e., abdominal pain, nausea, vomiting, and diarrhea. If large amounts are ingested, hematemesis may be present. Metabolic acidosis, hypovolemia, anemia secondary to GI bleeding, and tissue hypoperfusion can occur.

In stage II, toxic amounts of iron are absorbed by the body. If a large amount of iron was ingested, and the patient's condition is rapidly deteriorating, this stage may not be present. If present, the GI symptoms may resolve and the patient is often quiet and sleeping. This improvement of symptoms can give a false sense of reassurance to the patient and the health care provider.

In stage III, toxic amounts of iron have moved into the tissues; cellular metabolism is interrupted; and third spacing occurs. This venous pooling produces shock and metabolic acidosis. Hepatic dysfunction, heart failure, and renal failure can occur. If peak iron levels remain under 500 µg/dl, there is usually no hepatic injury.

In stage IV, the patient recovers over days or weeks. The danger of this stage is the long-term risk of gastric outlet syndrome or small bowel obstruction secondary to scarring from the acute corrosive injury of iron poisoning.

Often a patient has a normal serum iron level at the time of death secondary to peak levels 2 to 6 hours after ingestion. Remember that the iron goes from the blood into tissues and causes systemic toxicity often after the serum iron levels have normalized.

Diagnosis

A diagnosis is made by a history of ingestion of iron products, physical examination, serum iron level, and TIBC level and presentation of symptoms. To determine a toxic dose of iron, the amount of elemental iron must be determined. A 300-mg tablet of ferrous sulfate contains 20% elemental iron. A tablet containing ferrous gluconate contains only 12% elemental iron, and a tablet containing ferrous fumarate contains only 33% elemental iron.

Toxic doses of iron vary with each patient. As little as 20 mg/kg has been known to be toxic. Moderate poisoning is present if 40 mg/kg of elemental iron is ingested. More than 60 mg/kg of elemental iron ingestion is indicative of severe poisoning. An oral dose of greater than 200 to 250 mg/kg is considered to be lethal. Children with a WBC count greater than 15,000 mm^3 or a serum glucose level greater than 150 mg/dl will have a serum iron level greater than 300 µg/dl.

A quick test for ferrioxamine in the urine is to inject the patient with deferoxamine 50 mg/kg, up to 1 g, IM or 10 mg/kg IV over 1 hour, and if the urine becomes rose wine in color than ferrioxamine is present. If the deferoxamine challenge test is positive, aggressive management is indicated. This test is, however, a poor indicator of iron poisoning.

Laboratory Findings

A CBC, PT, PTT, electrolytes, BUN, creatinine, amylase, lipase, LFTs to include AST, ALT, GGT, and bilirubin, TIBC, and serum iron should be drawn. The initial serum iron and TIBC should be drawn 4 hours after ingestion (iron levels peak 3 to 5 hours after an acute ingestion). If the iron preparation is a sustained release or an enteric-coated preparation, iron levels should be drawn 6 to 8 hours after ingestion. A 4-hour serum level of greater than 300 µg/dl should cause concern. TIBC may not be of great value in the presence of an acute iron ingestion. It is neither sensitive nor specific for predicting systemic toxicity. Leukocytosis and hyperglycemia are often present in both children and adults.

Treatment

Any patient who presents to the ED with a history of ingesting more than 20 mg/kg of iron or greater should have two large-gauge IV lines of normal saline placed. The patient should be placed on a cardiac monitor, and the aforementioned laboratory examinations and an ABG should be drawn. An abdominal x-ray should be performed. Iron is radiopaque, and the presence of iron tablets correlates with the severity of the ingestion.

A gastric lavage should be performed. Activated charcoal does not bind to iron, but charcoal should be given if a co-ingestion is suspected. It has been recommended that gastric lavage with sodium bicarbonate or phosphate solutions be performed, but this is usually not recommended over saline or water gastric lavage. Cathartics are also not recommended in a case of an acute iron ingestion. This is secondary to the already present diarrhea in most patients who are suffering from iron ingestion and the increased risk of dehydration and metabolic acidosis.

Deferoxamine mesylate is a highly specific chelating agent that can remove iron from tissues and free iron from plasma. You should never wait for the results of serum iron or TIBC blood tests to start deferoxamine mesylate treatment. If the patient is symptomatic, give deferoxamine mesylate. One-hundred milligrams can remove 8.5 mg of elemental iron from the body. Deferoxamine can be given PO, IV, or IM. The recommended dose for IM deferoxamine mesylate is 90 mg/kg, up to 1 g, every 8 hours. The IV dose of deferoxamine mesylate is 15 mg/kg/hr. Much larger doses can be used if needed. Deferoxamine can cause hypotension in high doses above 45 mg/kg/hr.

Criteria for deferoxamine include:

1. Serum iron level greater than 350 µg/dl
2. Severely symptomatic patient, hypotension, lethargy, or severe gastroenteritis
3. Serum iron level greater than the TIBC

In severe cases of iron poisoning, dialysis and charcoal hemoperfusion can remove some ferrioxamine and will as deferoxamine. Deferoxamine therapy should be continued during dialysis.

Any patient with a serum iron level greater than 350 µg/dl or a history of ingestion of 20 mg/kg or greater of elemental iron should be admitted to the hospital for observation and treatment. A patient who is asymptomatic after 6 hours of ingestion and has a completely normal examination can be discharged from the ED without medical treatment.

ISOPROPANOL

Definition

Isopropanol alcohol is commonly found in "rubbing" alcohol. It is used in cosmetics, industrial solvents, cleaning agents, antifreeze, hair and facial products, and disinfectants. Isopropanol is less toxic than methanol and ethylene glycol but is more toxic than ethanol. Isopropanol is three to four times more potent than ethanol as a CNS depressant.

Epidemiology

Isopropanol is ingested most commonly by children in the home, suicidal patients, and alcoholics who cannot obtain ethanol. It is common for small children who are given the home remedy of "rubbing" alcohol sponge baths to lower fever to become toxic secondary to transdermal absorption. Death from isopropanol is uncommon. Isopropanol can be absorbed by the gut or skin or by inhalation.

Pathology

The volume of distribution of isopropanol is 0.6 to 0.7 l/kg. Metabolism is by first-order kinetics. The major metabolite of isopropanol alcohol is acetone, which is not associated with cardiac, renal, eye, or metabolic problems. Eighty percent of isopropanol is absorbed by the gut in 30 minutes after ingestion. Isopropanol is a CNS depressant. The kidney excretes 20 to 50% of isopropanol unchanged. The liver metabolizes the remaining 50 to 80% into acetone by alcohol dehydrogenase. Acetone is then excreted by the kidneys and expired by the lungs; thus, the odor of acetone is smelled on the patient's breath. Acetone can also cause CNS depression.

Clinical Presentation/Examination

Isopropanol metabolites can cause CNS depression, myocardial depression, hypotension, vasodilatation, and gastric irritation. The CNS depression can last up to 24 hours with an acute ingestion of isopropanol. Hypotension is a common side effect from isopropanol ingestion secondary to vasodilatation and direct myocardial depression. Hemorrhage from gastric bleeding can be severe and rapid in onset. A patient can present with rhabdomyolysis, hepatocellular toxicity, and acute tubular necrosis secondary to prolonged hypoperfusion and prolonged hypotension.

Diagnosis

A diagnosis is made by a history of ingestion of isopropanol, physical examination, and laboratory tests. A lethal dose of isopropanol is 240 ml (2 to 4 ml/kg) in adults.

Laboratory Findings

Patients will have a very high osmolal gap, acetonuria, or acetonemia with the absence of acidosis. Acetone is not a ketoacid; therefore isopropanol does not cause metabolic acidosis by itself. If acidosis is present, it is secondary to hypotension, hypoperfusion, or starvation. If severe acidosis is present, consider co-ingestion with ethylene glycol or methanol. Hypoglycemia is often present in the acute isopropanol ingestion. Hypoglycemia is secondary to starvation and an increased $NADH/NAD^+$ ratio. Acetone also interferes with the colorimetric assay of the creatinine test; thus the creatinine level is sometimes falsely elevated.

Treatment

A patient with any overdose should have two large-gauge IV lines of normal saline or lactated Ringer's solution and the aforementioned laboratory tests drawn. The patient should be placed on a cardiac monitor, and oxygen should be given. An ECG and a chest x-ray should be performed. A gastric lavage should be performed, and activated charcoal should be given. Isopropanol is poorly bound to charcoal, but if co-ingestion is considered, always perform a gastric lavage.

Treatment for isopropanol ingestion is mostly supportive. Hypotension is treated with fluids and vasopressors. Hemodialysis and peritoneal dialysis are effective in removing isopropanol and acetone from the blood. Hemodialysis should be considered if the isopropanol blood level exceeds 400 mg/dl. If the patient is symptomatic with hypotension, obtundation, headache, nausea, or vomiting he or she should be admitted to the hospital. If the patient is asymptomatic for 6 hours, the patient can be discharged.

LEAD

Definition

Lead is a common organic or inorganic compound found in paints, insecticides, herbicides, rodenticides, soldering material, batteries, smelters, jewelry manufacturing, taxidermy, contaminated seafood, and wood preservatives.

Epidemiology

Lead is a common environmental contaminant. From 1976 to 1980, the National Health and Nutrition Examination Survey II found that 1.9% of persons aged 6 months to 74 years had a lead blood level of equal to or greater than 30 μg/dl. Lead poisoning is more common in children and in the lower socioeconomic groups.

Pathology

There are two types of lead: inorganic and organic lead. Organic lead primarily affects the CNS. Although inorganic lead poisoning also affects the CNS, it also affects the peripheral nervous system, the kidneys, the GI tract, the liver, the heart, and the reproductive and hepatic systems. Lead is absorbed primarily by ingestion or by inhalation and, to some extent, by the skin.

Ninety percent of lead is stored in the bones. The half-life of lead is approximately 30 years. Lead combines with sulfhydryl groups and is protein bound and inhibits enzymatic activity. Anemia is caused by interference with porphyrin metabolism. Iron deficiency is caused by lead's interference with the enzymes deptal-aminolevulinic acid dehydratase and ferrochelatase, which catalyze the transfer of iron from ferritin to protoporphyrin to form hemoglobin. In children, microcytic anemia is common. If anemia is already present when toxicity occurs, a synergistic effect can occur that will increase the severity of the anemia.

Hemolytic anemia occurs secondary to the interference with pyrimidine 5'-nucleotidase, which is the enzyme that is responsible for clearing cellular ribonucleic acid (RNA) degeneration products from the cell. RBC basophilic stripping will be present on peripheral smear in both acute and chronic lead poisoning.

The peripheral nervous system will suffer segmental demyelination followed by a secondary axonal degeneration of the motor neurons. The CNS will suffer cytotoxicity and cerebral edema.

Lead will cause a Fanconi-like syndrome with acute renal tubular acidosis, glycosuria, aciduria, and phosphaturia. Interstitial nephritis and increased uric acid levels will also be noted. Often the presenting complaints will be gout, acute renal failure, or hypertension. A patient can present with hypothyroidism secondary to depressed levels of thyroxine secondary to chronic lead exposure.

Lead has the effect of fetal wasting on the unborn fetus in a pregnant female. In the male, abnormal sperm counts, a decreased sperm count, and sterility can be seen. The liver is damaged by acute or chronic lead poisoning, and this is reflected by elevated serum transaminase levels.

Clinical Presentation

A patient can present with vague symptoms or acute encephalopathy. Clinical effects of inorganic lead poisoning are divided into chronic and acute symptoms. Acute symptoms include confusion, coma, papilledema, vomiting, optic neuritis, and ataxia with generalized or focal seizures. Peripheral nervous system symptoms include paresthesias. Acute gastric symptoms of abdominal pain, often colicky in nature, nausea, and vomiting will be present. On blood smear, basophilic stripping can be present along with hemolytic anemia on CBC examination. An acute Fanconi-like syndrome can be present. Bone pain is often a common presenting complaint.

Signs and symptoms of chronic ingestion of lead include chronic headaches, depression, fatigue, irritability, behavioral changes, sleep disturbances, memory deficit, and apathy. Peripheral nervous system symptoms are: a motor weakness, including the classic "wrist drop" of chronic lead poisoning. Often absent or reduced deep tendon reflexes (DTRs) are present with normal sensory function. GI complaints of constipation or diarrhea can be present. Arthralgias, weakness, and weight loss are common complaints. Interstitial nephritis is a symptom of chronic lead poisoning.

Men will present with decreased libido, impotence, decreased sperm count, and sterility. Women will present with chronic abortions and premature births.

Examination

The entire patient should be examined. The mouth should have special attention. Often a bluish gingiva will be present in lead poisoning. Always ask the patient what food tastes like. They will often complain of a metallic taste in the mouth.

X-ray Findings

In children on radiographic examination, the classic "lead bands" are often found. "Lead bands" are horizontal lesions at the metaphyseal plate, which are attempts of the bone to remodel itself after deposits of lead, in the long bones, have occurred, especially seen at the knees on x-rays. This is often seen in chronic exposure.

Diagnosis

A diagnosis is made by a history of exposure, neurologic presentation, hemolytic anemia, and a toxic lead level. A definitive diagnosis is made by the finding of elevated lead levels (PbB) and a positive result on a chelation provocation test. The PbB level is the best diagnostic tool for a diagnosis of lead toxicity. It may be misleading if the exposure is in the remote past. Also calcium disodium versenate ($CaNa_2$-EDTA) provocation tests may be necessary for the diagnosis of remote lead poisoning. The erythrocyte protoporphyrin (EP) test is also helpful in diagnosing chronic lead exposure. EP levels are diagnostic for end-organ damage. Iron deficiency will also cause elevations in EP levels.

The Centers for Disease Control and Prevention (CDC) has established that lead toxicity in children is defined as a PbB level of equal to or more than 25 μg/dl and an elevated EP level equal to or greater than 35 μg/dl. In adults, a PbB less than 40 μg/dl is accepted as normal, levels between 40 and 50 μg/dl require increased surveillance, and levels higher than 50 μg/dl require removal of the persons from their job until PbB levels fall to less than 40 μg/dl.

Gasoline sniffing of tetraethyl lead (TEL), which is found in leaded gasoline, can be metabolized into inorganic lead and triethyl lead. These patients can present with behavioral changes, insomnia, irritability, nausea and vomiting, tremor, chorea, convulsions, restlessness, mania, muscle and renal and hepatic damage.

Laboratory Findings

A CBC, reticulocyte count, PT, PTT, electrolytes, BUN, creatinine, AST, ALT, GGT, LDH, bilirubin, alkaline phosphatase, magnesium, phosphorus, urinalysis, and serum lead levels (PbB) should be obtained. Erythrocyte protoporphyrin levels should be obtained. Anemia, if present, can be normocytic or microcytic. An elevated reticulocyte count is often present. The transaminase levels will be elevated, and the bilirubin and alkaline phosphatase levels will be normal. On examination of a peripheral smear, basophilic stripping can be noted but is nonspecific for lead poisoning.

Treatment

The mainstay of treatment of lead poisoning is the elevation of the PbB levels and the removal of lead from the body. A patient rarely presents with encephalopathy, but when the patient does, it is often fatal. Seizures are treated with benzodiazepines, phenobarbital, phenytoin, and general anesthesia.

X-rays of the abdomen and chest should be performed. In acute ingestion, often radiopaque flecks will be noted. If flecks are noted, then whole bowel irrigation should be performed with polyethylene glycol electrolyte solution (GoLYTELY, Colyte). This infusion should be continuous until all flecks have disappeared. The continuous rate for adults should be 2000 ml/hr, and for children the rate should be 500 ml/hr. Be careful with fluid administration, because cerebral edema has been reported with overhydration.

The mainstay of treatment is chelation therapy. Dimercaprol (British antilewisite or BAL) should be used. Dimercaprol at 75 mg/m^2 should be given IM every 4 hours, followed by CaNa$_2$-EDTA 1500 mg/m^2 every 24 hours in a continuous infusion. Children are treated with dimercaprol 50 mg/m^2 and CaNa$_2$-EDTA 100 mg/m^2 every 24 hours. Dimercaprol can also be given as a continuous infusion if very high PbB levels are present. Dimercaprol is excreted in the bile and chelates both intracellular and extracellular lead. When CaNa$_2$ is given, there is a danger of renal toxicity; thus urine output must be monitored carefully. Other chelating agents include D-penicillamine and DMSA.

In asymptomatic children, chelation therapy is not required until the PbB level is higher than 56 μg/dl or the PbB level is 25 to 55 μg/dl, and the CaNa$_2$-EDTA provocation test is positive. In asymptomatic adults, no chelation is required unless they are symptomatic, but removal from exposure in the environment is necessitated and close follow-up of PbB levels are required.

All patients who are symptomatic, children with PbB equal to or higher than 56 μg/dl and adults with CNS symptoms, should be hospitalized.

LITHIUM

Definition

Lithium has been used for bipolar (manic-depressive) disorders since the 1970s in the United States. Lithium has a very narrow therapeutic range. Acute lithium toxicity occurs when there is an ingestion greater than 40 mg/kg. Toxicity can occur with a deliberate ingestion or a change in the kinetics of the drug with chronic therapy.

Lithium is usually given in a 900- to 1200-mg daily dose. Lithium usually comes in 300-mg tablets. Therapeutic effects are not reached for 2 to 3 weeks after therapy is started. The therapeutic level range is 0.6 to 1.2 mEq/l. Levels greater than 2 mEq/l are considered toxic. Peak blood levels occur in about 2 to 4 hours after ingestion. Lithium is not protein bound, and the volume of distribution is about 0.6 to 1/kg, about the same as total body water. The serum half-life of lithium is 14 to 24 hours, depending on the functional level of the kidneys. In a patient with chronic lithium use, the half-life can be up to 57 hours.

Pathology

The exact pathophysiologic function of lithium is yet unknown. It is believed to inhibit the phosphoinositide system, or it may be a second messenger system for neurotransmitters. It also accelerates the reuptake of norepinephrine and blocks the synthesis of the hormonal response to cyclic AMP. Lithium also has anti-adrenergic properties. Lithium is entirely eliminated by the kidneys; thus overdose treatment is directed at excretion of lithium through the kidneys.

Clinical Presentation/Examination

A patient with lithium toxicity presents with an acute onset of neuromuscular and CNS changes. Neuromuscular system changes include muscle jerking, tremors, lethargy, lip smacking, and confusion. These symptoms progress to seizures, stupor, and coma. Nausea, vomiting, and diarrhea also occur. In severe toxicity, cardiac changes such as bradycardia, conduction defects, and ST and T wave changes can occur. Severe hypertension has also occurred.

In the patient who is on chronic lithium therapy, who is toxic and who presents to the ED, an attempt should be made to determine what caused the toxicity. Factors that increase the level of lithium are: dehydration, impaired renal functions, decreased salt intake, a disturbance in the sodium balance, or a drug interaction with drugs such as methyldopa, thiazide, spironolactone, ibuprofen, indomethacin, or the acetylcholinesterase inhibitors.

Other signs of lithium toxicity are polyuria, polydipsia, fine hand tremors, tearing, blurring of vision, exophthalmos, scotomatas, and pseudotumor cerebri. When urine osmolarity is present, nephrotic syndrome, or nephrogenic diabetes insipidus can occur.

Long-term use of lithium can cause acne, cutaneous ulcers, edema, aplastic anemia, and neutrophilia. In pregnancy, lithium crosses the placenta and is excreted in breast milk. Lithium is teratogenic. It can also cause hyperparathyroidism and nontoxic goiter.

Diagnosis

A diagnosis is made by a history of acute or chronic ingestion of lithium, lithium serum levels, and physical examination of the patient.

Laboratory Findings

A CBC, electrolytes, BUN, creatinine, LFTs, ABG, ECG, and chest x-ray should be performed on all patients on lithium. A lithium blood level should be performed, but it is not reliable for severity of toxicity. There will be a reduced anion gap in acute lithium toxicity. Remember that the patient on a chronic maintenance dose of lithium will usually be more toxic than the patient who acutely ingests lithium in a suicidal attempt. Mild hyperkalemia is often present, and thyroid function tests should also be drawn secondary to lithium's affinity to the thyroid gland.

Treatment

Any patient who presents to the ED with a possible lithium overdose should have two large-gauge IV lines placed with normal saline. The patient should be placed on a cardiac monitor, and the aforementioned laboratory values drawn. An ABG should be taken, and if a gag reflex is present, perform a gastric lavage. If the lithium is a long-acting preparation, gastric lavage should be repeated in 2 to 4 hours. An ECG should be performed and will often show the opposite of hyperkalemia, flattened T waves such as those found in hypokalemia. The use of activated charcoal is not effective in binding of lithium; however, charcoal should be used when co-ingestion is suspected or if the history of other medication ingestion is uncertain.

The use of normal saline is of key importance in the treatment of lithium toxicity. A saline solution ensures a good supply of sodium ions to the proximal renal tubules and thus increased excretion of lithium.

The mainstay of lithium toxicity is the alkalinization of the urine and osmotic diuresis. Some suggest sodium bicarbonate or carbonic anhydrase inhibitors to increase alkalinization of the urine and promote osmotic diuresis, but there are no good clinical studies at this time. Aminophylline, mannitol, and urea have also been advocated to increase the speed of lithium excretion.

In severe toxicity, hemodialysis has been used. The goal of hemodialysis is a lithium level of 1 mEq/l 6 to 8 hours after dialysis. Indications for hemodialysis are:

1. Clinical signs of severe poisoning
2. Deteriorating clinical conditions, such as seizures, ventricular arrhythmias, or coma
3. Renal failure or decreasing urine output
4. Lack of an expected drop in lithium level of 20% in 6 hours
5. Lithium level between 3.5 and 4.0 or toxic looking with a lithium level between 2 and 3.5 mEq/l

There is also a rebound phenomenon postdialysis secondary to lithium being liberated from the tissues and thus an elevated serum level. Lithium levels should be followed closely after dialysis.

MERCURY

Definition

Mercury occurs in inorganic and organic forms, and all forms of mercury are toxic. Organic mercury forms are short- and long-chained alkyl and aryl compounds. Inorganic compounds are divided into elemental mercury, mercurous salts, and mercuric salts. The short-chained alkyls are methyl mercury and ethyl mercury and are the most toxic to humans.

Epidemiology

Exposure to mercury is usually from occupational exposure or accidental exposure to mercury salts. The mercury used in glass thermometers is not absorbed by the GI tract unless the GI tract is damaged or fistulas are present.

Pathology

Elemental mercury crosses the blood-brain barrier and is ionized in brain tissue and is then trapped in the CNS. Elemental mercury is absorbed by inhalation of vapors and dermally. There is usually very little absorption by the GI tract of elemental mercury.

Mercuric salts are deposited in the ionized form in the kidney, liver, and spleen. Mercuric mercury salts and organic mercury are absorbed by the GI tract. The short-chained alkyl organic compounds are more readily absorbed than are the aryl organic compounds.

Organic short-chained mercury compounds are more lipid soluble and easily cross membranes; thus toxicity is usually from exposure to short-chained mercury compounds. They affect the liver, kidneys, CNS, RBCs, and the fetus.

Long-chained mercury compounds are biotransformed into inorganic mercuric ions in the body; thus they are less toxic than are short-chained mercury compounds. Short-chained compounds are primarily excreted in the bile and undergo significant enterohepatic circulation. Aryl organic mercurials and inorganic mercury compounds are primarily eliminated in the feces and urine.

Acute or chronic mercury poisoning is caused by the diverse number of enzyme and protein systems that mercury affects. Mercury binds with sulfhydryl groups and forms methyl mercury, which inhibits choline acetyl transferase. Choline acetyl transferase is the final step in the production of acetylcholine and can produce an acute acetylcholine deficiency.

Clinical Presentation/Examination

A patient with acute mercury poisoning can present with neurologic, renal, pulmonary, dermal, or GI symptoms based on the type of mercury ingested: elemental, mercury salt form, short-chained alkyls, or long-chained alkyls or aryls. All types of mercury poisoning cause mild nausea and vomiting.

Any type of mercury poisoning can present with neuropsychiatric or CNS complaints, including: depression, mania, irritability, anxiety, sleep disturbances, memory loss, and excessive shyness. Tremor is a frequently noted physical finding.

Elemental mercury poisoning will cause stomatitis, excessive salivation, and gingivitis. Short-chained alkyls can produce visual and auditory changes, ataxia, paresthesias, muscular rigidity, or spasm and CNS teratogenic effects. Chronic exposure to elemental and organic forms of mercury can cause renal glomerular and tubular necrosis.

Mercury salts have little or no effect on the CNS system. They do affect the GI tract and can cause corrosive gastroenteritis with severe abdominal pain followed by cardiovascular collapse in a very short time. Mercury salts can cause acute tubular necrosis within 24 hours.

Children present with a generalized rash, acrodynia, fever, splenomegaly, irritability, and generalized hypotonia with specific weakness of the pectoral muscles and pelvic muscles.

Diagnosis

A diagnosis is made by a history of occupational exposure, physical examination, and laboratory tests. A diagnosis is made by performing a 24-hour urine test. A normal level of mercury for unexposed individuals is equal to or less than 10 to 15 µg/l. A level greater than 100 µg/l connotes significant exposure. Serum mercury levels are less reliable. Seafood acutely ingested can elevate serum mercury levels to the toxic range.

Laboratory Findings

A CBC, electrolytes, amylase, lipase, BUN, creatinine, serum mercury level, 24-hour urine, urinalysis, and liver and cardiac enzymes should be performed on all patients with suspected mercury poisoning. Normal serum mercury levels are less than 1.5 µg/dl. Thyroid function tests should be performed. Thyroid disease can mimic heavy metal poisoning.

Treatment

A patient with suspected mercury poisoning should be placed on a cardiac monitor and have a large-gauge IV line of normal saline placed. The patient should also be placed on 2 liters of oxygen and have the aforementioned laboratory tests performed. A toxic drug screen should also be performed. X-rays of the chest and abdomen should be performed.

The mainstay of acute ingestion is gastric decontamination. Gastric lavage should be performed, and activated charcoal should be given at 1 g/kg. Mercury salts also bind readily with milk, egg whites, and activated charcoal. Diarrhea is often present; thus cathartics are often not needed.

Treatment of mercury poisoning with chelation therapy with dimercaprol and D-penicillamine is the mainstay of pharmacologic therapy. Neostigmine has been used to treat methyl mercury–induced motor dysfunction by improving acetylcholine levels.

Use dimercaprol for mercury salt poisoning, 3 to 5 mg/kg per dose IM every 4 hours for 2 days, then the same dose every 6 hours for 2 days, then every 12 hours for 7 days. Do not use dimercaprol in methyl mercury poisoning, because it can exacerbate CNS symptoms. If renal failure is present and dimercaprol is used, consider hemodialysis to increase removal of mercury from the body.

Use D-penicillamine for elemental mercury poisoning and mild mercury salt poisonings. Give 100 mg/day to a maximum dose of 1 g in four divided doses for 3 to 10 days. DMSA is under investigational use for mercury poisoning.

Hospitalize all patients with suspected mercury salt ingestion, inhaled elemental mercury vapor, or patients who require dimercaprol therapy.

METHANOL ALCOHOL

Definition

Methanol alcohol, which is commonly called "wood alcohol," is distilled from wood and is synthesized from carbon oxides and hydrogen. Methanol is found in paint solvents, antifreeze, duplicating fluids, windshield washer fluid, window cleaner, carburetor fluid, gasoline additives, canned fuels (Sterno), and home heating fuels. Methanol ingestion can cause blindness and death.

Epidemiology

There have been epidemics of methanol ingestion secondary to "bootleggers" who substitute methanol for ethanol in "moonshine." Most ingestions are from accidental oral ingestion.

Pathology

Methanol is 90 to 95% metabolized in the liver. The volume of distribution of methanol is 0.6 l/kg. The toxic dose of methanol varies. Methanol is converted in the liver by alcohol dehydrogenase to formaldehyde. Formaldehyde is then converted to formate by aldehyde dehydrogenase. Formate accumulates in the blood; formaldehyde rapidly metabolizes to formate; thus formaldehyde is not considered in discussion. Formate inhibits mitochondrial respiration and cytochrome oxidase, both of which lead to diffuse cellular hypoxia. Cellular hypoxia causes a severe anion gap. When formate is metabolized in great quantities, there can be no, or zero level, plasma bicarbonate function; thus severe acidemia occurs.

The ocular symptoms are secondary to the high formate concentrations in the vitreous humor and optic nerve of the eyes. Blindness is caused by the interruption of the cytochrome oxidase, Na^+, K^+, -ATPase processes in the optic nerve.

Clinical Presentation/Examination

A patient with methanol toxicity presents with photophobia, hyperpnea, anorexia, CNS depression, and severe metabolic acidosis. The patient is often confused, lethargic, or comatose. A patient can also present with toxic levels of methanol and show no evidence of intoxication.

Generalized seizures are common. Cerebral edema and putamen infarcts are common in methanol intoxication. A residual parkinsonism is commonly reported with methanol intoxication.

The patient commonly presents with nausea, vomiting, and abdominal pain, secondary to gastritis or acute pancreatitis. The patient will often present with symptoms of snow blindness as the presenting eye complaint. The patient's pupils can be dilated sluggishly to light or can be unreactive to light. Papilledema may be present.

Diagnosis

The toxic dose of methanol is quite variable. A potentially lethal dose of methanol is 0.4 ml/kg of a 40% methanol solution. A 30-ml dose of 100% methanol in an adult is regarded as a lethal dose. A 10-ml dose has caused blindness. The hallmark of methanol intoxications is severe anion gap acidosis.

The toxic dose of methanol can be determined by the following formula:

$$C = \frac{dose}{V_d}$$

Volume of distribution (V_d) = 0.6 l/kg for methanol

Specific gravity of methanol = 0.8 g/ml

$$C = \frac{(dose)(SG)}{(V_d)(patient's\ weight)}$$

Serum osmolarity:

$$Osm\ cal = 2[Na] + \frac{glucose\ (mg/dl)}{18} + \frac{BUN\ (mg/dl)}{2.8}$$

To correct for the presence of ethanol: Add $\dfrac{ethanol\ level\ (mg/dl)}{4.6}$

Laboratory Findings

A CBC, PT, PTT, electrolytes, BUN, creatinine, calcium, amylase, lipase, AST, ALT, GGT, LDH, urinalysis, serum osmolarity, and ABG should be performed. Alcohol levels, including ethanol and methanol, should be drawn. There will be a severe anion gap acidosis and a high osmolal gap.

An osmolal gap is the difference between the measured osmolarity (mOsm/kg) and the calculated osmolarity (mOsm/l). An osmolal gap of greater than 10 mOsm/1 is considered abnormal. An elevated osmolal gap is predictive of the presence of another osmotically active substance in the serum, such as an alcohol. Mannitol, glycerol, urea, isopropyl, ethanol, and ethylene glycol can all cause osmolal gaps. A normal osmolal gap does not exclude a toxic ingestion of methanol.

Treatment

Any patient with suspected methanol ingestion should be placed on a cardiac monitor and placed on oxygen. The patient should have at least one large-gauge IV line of normal saline placed and should be put on pulse oximetry. An ECG and a chest x-ray should be performed along with the aforementioned laboratory tests drawn and an ABG performed. If the patient is unconscious, give glucose 1 ampule, thiamine 100 mg IV or IM, and naloxone 0.4 to 2 mg IV. Treatment of acute methanol toxicity is directed at correction of metabolic acidosis, prevention of conversion of methanol to formate, and elimination of methanol and formate.

If the patient presents within 1 to 2 hours of ingestion or if co-ingestion is suspected, perform a gastric lavage. Activated charcoal should be given in case of a suspected secondary ingestion but is of little benefit in methanol ingestion. Methanol is poorly absorbed by charcoal. Acidosis should be corrected by sodium bicarbonate, and hypoglycemia should be corrected with glucose.

The indicated therapy for methanol toxicity is ethanol. Ethanol, like methanol, is a substrate of alcohol dehydrogenase; however, ethanol has an affinity 10 times greater to alcohol dehydrogenase than does methanol. The goal of ethanol administration is a serum ethanol level of 100 to 150 mg/dl. At this level, methanol will be prevented from metabolizing to formate. The serum glucose of any patient who is given ethanol IV should be watched very closely, secondary to the occurrence of hypoglycemia. Treat hypoglycemia as needed.

The loading dose of ethanol is 0.8 g/kg, which is equal to 1 ml of 100% ethanol, which is equal to 10 ml/kg of 10% ethanol. When ethanol is given IV it should be given in a solution equal to or less than 10%. Then give a maintenance dose of ethanol at 130 mg/kg/hr to 0.15 ml/kg/hr of 100% ethanol, which is 1.5 ml/kg/hr of 10% ethanol for nontolerant patients. In tolerant patients, double the maintenance dose to a serum level of 100 to 150 mg/dl.

Bottle spirits can also be given. A loading dose is (200/proof)ml/kg. A maintenance dose is (30/proof)ml/kg/hr.

Folinic acid, 1mg/kg IV, is recommended also in the treatment of methanol intoxication. Folinic acid is an active co-enzyme of folate. Folate, 1 mg/kg, should also be given every 4 hours for 24 hours.

If the patient is severely intoxicated, the methanol level is greater than 25 mg/dl; visual impairment is present or visual symptoms are occurring; renal failure or severe acidosis is present; and hemodialysis should be considered. Hemodialysis can remove formaldehyde, formate, and methanol and helps to correct acidosis.

Any patient with methanol intoxication should be admitted to the ICU.

NARCOTICS

Definition

Currently the term narcotic is reserved for opioids that are primarily used for analgesia. Narcotics include morphine, heroin, codeine, meperidine hydromorphine, and oxycodone. Heroin is often altered for street use with quinine, baking soda, lactose, sucrose, magnesium silicate (talc), and procaine; thus co-toxicity or complications of ingesting or injecting these co-drugs or compounds must always be assumed. Narcotic substances are used in antidiarrheal medications, cough medications, and analgesics.

Epidemiology

Five percent of acute intoxications involve narcotics. There is a high mortality rate for narcotic intoxication in the United States and Canada. Morphine, codeine, and propoxyphene are the primary agents of intoxication.

Pathology

Narcotics are readily absorbed nasally, from the GI tract, parenterally, and from the respiratory mucosa. They are usually absorbed parenterally in 10 minutes, in 30 minutes with an IM injection, and within 90 minutes with PO or subcutaneous administration.

Heroin, codeine, methadone, and meperidine all cross the blood-brain barrier and can affect newborn children if the mother has injected, ingested, or was administered a narcotic around the time of delivery. Ninety percent of narcotics are excreted in the urine within 24 hours of ingestion or injection.

Narcotics work on opioid receptors in the nervous system, with increased concentrations in areas that involve pain perception and appreciation, mostly in the spinothalamic, limbic, and extrapyramidal systems.

Clinical Presentation

A patient who is intoxicated with narcotics presents with euphoria, drowsiness, miosis (pinpoint pupils), slowed respirations, and conjunctival redness. The CNS respiratory center is affected, and patients can present with hypoxia secondary to decreased minute and tidal volume. A patient often complains of pruritus, nausea, and vomiting.

The classic picture of narcotic intoxication is one of lacrimation, piloerection, rhinorrhea, yawning, nasal stuffiness, sweating, vomiting, diarrhea, abdominal cramping, and myalgia.

A patient who presents with an acute narcotic overdose will present with pinpoint pupils and hypoventilation. If the patient is hypoxic, the pupils can be midrange in size or dilated secondary to CNS hypoxia.

A patient can present with abscesses, cellulitis, or thrombophlebitis secondary to the chronic injection of narcotics. Those who inject narcotics run the risk of infection with HIV or hepatitis. Complications of injection include septicemia and endocarditis. The causative organisms of septicemia and endocarditis are usually penicillinase-producing staphylococci organisms.

If the hand or fingers are infected with gangrene, immediate surgical drainage is required. Mycotic aneurysms should be considered in abscesses in the groin or neck and should be drained by a surgeon. All masses in the groin or neck should be carefully evaluated for a bruit or pulsations before a scalpel is used to drain what is a suspected abscess.

The legs and thighs are susceptible to septic thrombophlebitis in the IV heroin user. Septic thrombophlebitis presents with a very painful, warm extremity.

Pulmonary effects of narcotic abuse include noncardiogenic pulmonary edema and pneumonia. The cause of noncardiogenic pulmonary edema in the heroin addict is not well understood. Pulmonary edema from heroin use usually clears in 24 to 36 hours with oxygen therapy alone. Aspiration pneumonia is very common in narcotic abusers secondary to the decreased tidal volume and a shallow respiratory rate, secondary to intoxication.

Cardiac effects of narcotic use most commonly include endocarditis with right-sided infections. The most common ECG finding is atrial fibrillation or P waves suggestive of cor pulmonale. The tricuspid valve is the most common valve involved. A patient may present with or without a murmur. The infecting organism is almost always *Staphylococcus aureus.* A patient with a septic valve will often present as a patient with symptoms of pneumonia with staphylococcal septicemia. Round wedge-shaped lesions may appear successively on the lung periphery. If pulmonary infarcts occur, they may progress to empyema, cavitation, or abscesses.

If pre-existing disease of the aortic or mitral valve is present, there is an increased risk of infection of these valves. If left-sided endocarditis is present, the organisms of infection are usually *Escherichia coli, Klebsiella, Pseudomonas, Streptococcus,* and *Candida albicans. C. albicans* never affects a previously normal valve. Septic pulmonary emboli can go systemic and cause embolization of the extremities, viscera, and brain. Emboli to the heart can cause an acute myocardial infarction. Acute mitral valve rupture is characterized by sudden severe pulmonary edema in the presence of a loud mitral insufficiency murmur.

Two other complications of narcotic use are tetanus and malaria. Malaria is not seen very much in the United States but is associated with heroin use in lesser developed countries. Tetanus is seen more in subcutaneous injectors and in women. All drug abusers should be asked about their tetanus status.

Examination

The patient should be completely undressed. The skin should be inspected for "tracks" or sites of injection, including the web spaces of the fingers and toes, the popliteal area behind the knees, and the axilla. The eyes should be pinpointed. If they are dilated, suspect a co-ingestion or another type drug or a co-overdose. Meperidine can cause dilated pupils also; therefore, don't rule in or out a narcotic overdose based on pupil size. The heart should be examined for signs of mitral valve pathology. The lungs should be auscultated for rales or wheezes. Obtain a complete history of all drugs ingested. Drug abusers are usually polydrug abusers. Often alcohol, tobacco, glue, or paint sniffing is used as a substitute when narcotics cannot be obtained.

Bones and joints should be evaluated for signs and symptoms of septic arthritis or osteomyelitis. Septic arthritis is usually caused by *Pseudomonas aeruginosa* and *Serratia marcescens.*

Always determine the pregnancy status of a female in child-bearing years, because there is a high incidence of toxemia and premature delivery of females who abuse drugs. If this is an emergent delivery of a child born to a drug-using mother, be prepared for respiratory depression, arrest, or neonatal withdrawal.

Diagnosis

A diagnosis is made by history, clinical presentation, and positive drug screen.

Laboratory Findings

A CBC, electrolytes, BUN, creatinine, LFTs, hepatitis (type B, serum) panel, amylase, lipase, blood cultures, urinalysis, and urine culture should be drawn. A serum or urine drug screen should be performed along with an alcohol level. Discussion of HIV status should take place, and a HIV test should be drawn if the patient consents to the test.

Treatment

Any patient with an acute narcotic overdose should be placed on a cardiac monitor, and two large-gauge IV lines should be placed with normal saline. The patient should be placed on oxygen, and naloxone should be administered along with glucose and thiamine in an unconscious or comatose patient. A chest x-ray and an ECG should be performed.

Remember that most drug abusers are polydrug abusers. They can be going through narcotic and alcohol withdrawal at the same time. Give thiamine if alcohol abuse is suspected. Perform a dextrose stick to evaluate glucose level in an unconscious or comatose patient.

Heroin withdrawal generally occurs 12 to 14 hours after the last dose. Methadone withdrawal symptoms occur 24 to 36 hours after the last dose. Acute withdrawal of heroin in an adult is not life threatening. A patient will often look like he or she is suffering from an acute febrile illness. There is no treatment for symptomatic withdrawal from heroin or methadone. Clonidine can be used to decrease the chills, lacrimation, rhinorrhea, sweating, myalgia, and arthralgias associated with withdrawal from heroin or methadone. Clonidine inhibits the adrenergic activity at the α_2-adrenergic receptors. Clonidine can cause hypotension, drowsiness, and dry mouth.

Treatment of an acute narcotic overdose consists of airway and ventilation support and giving naloxone, which is a pure narcotic antagonist, 0.4 to 2 mg in an adult and 0.01 mg/kg in children and neonates. Naloxone can be given intratracheally, subcutaneously, IV, or transmuscularly. In severe overdoses, naloxone can be given as a continuous infusion and titrated to clinical response. Put 2 mg of naloxone in 500 mg of normal saline or 5% dextrose for a concentration of 0.004 mg/ml or 0.4 mg/100 ml. The usual continuous infusion rate is 400 μg (0.4 mg)/hr. The serum half-life of naloxone is 1 hour with a duration of 2 to 3 hours. Methadone patients should be watched closely for 72 hours secondary to methadone's long half-life.

NEUROLEPTICS

Definition

The neuroleptics comprise five classes of drugs that all share a three-ring structure. This group of antipsychotic drugs includes lithium, oxidase inhibitors, the phenothiazines, the butyrophenones (including haloperidol), the thioxanthines (including thiothixene), and the dibenzoxapines (including loxapine). These antipsychotic drugs are used as major tranquilizers to treat schizophrenia, mania, major depression with psychotic features, schizoaffective disorders, paranoid disorders, atypical psychoses, and other functional psychoses.

The neuroleptics are also used to treat nonpsychiatric disorders such as Huntington's chorea, chorea in rheumatic fever, Gilles de la Tourette syndrome, and Meige's syndrome. They are also used to treat hiccoughs, chlorpromazine, and tension and vascular headaches. The phenothiazine class of neuroleptics is also used to treat nausea and vomiting. The phenothiazines block the dopaminergic chemoreceptor trigger zone in the medulla and stop vomiting. Promethazine and chlorperazine should not be used in pregnancy, because they are both class C agents and are at risk for causing fetal abnormalities. A patient who has neuroleptic side effects will present with akathisia, dystonias, parkinsonism symptoms, tardive dyskinesia, and neuroleptic malignant syndrome (NMS).

Neuroleptics include:

Phenothiazines
    Aliphatics: chlorpromazines, promethazine
    Piperidines: mesoridazine, thioridazine
    Piperazines: prochlorperazine, fluphenazine
Thioxanthenes: thiothixene
Dibenzoxazepines: loxapine

Butyrophenone: haloperidol
Dihydroindolene: molindone

Pathology

From the toxicologic standpoint, the neuroleptics are very safe and have an extremely wide toxic-therapeutic range. All neuroleptics share a basic three-ring structure. They work by blocking dopaminergic (D_1 and D_2), adrenergic (α_1 and α_2), muscarinic and histaminic (H_1 and H_2) neurotransmission at the receptor sites. The blockage of the D_2-dopamine receptors causes behavior modification but can also cause extrapyramidal symptoms. When the α-adrenergic receptors are blocked, orthostatic hypotension and vasodilatation can occur. The muscarinic receptor blockage will cause parasympathetic nervous system symptoms such as tachycardia, hyperthermia, mydriasis, flushing, urinary retention, dry mouth, and constipation. CNS symptoms can occur either as CNS stimulation or sedation.

Neuroleptics lower the seizure threshold and have a prolonged duration of action. They should not be used in patients who are agitated, who have overdosed on other medications, are in acute alcohol-intoxication with DTs, or are in sedative-hypnotic withdrawal. They should not be used in the very young pediatric population to treat nausea or vomiting, secondary to their effect in lowering the seizure threshold in this patient group. Cocaine, phencyclidine, and amphetamines can all cause seizure activity on their own. Neuroleptics will lower the seizure threshold even lower in these overdoses and thus should be avoided.

Clinical Presentation/Examination

A patient with neuroleptic toxicity will present with an acute dystonic reaction, which is generally not dose related but is an idiosyncratic reaction that usually occurs in the early stages of treatment with neuroleptics.

A patient can present with dystonias, which are idiosyncratic drug reactions that cause acute involuntary muscle movement and spasm. Dystonias are not dose dependent; therefore prophylactic therapy to prevent dystonias is of little help.

Akathisia is a condition that describes motor restlessness. Akathisia is often treated incorrectly. The symptoms of akathisia are often falsely ascribed to worsening psychosis. The health care provider increases the dose of antipsychotic medication only to worsen the akathisia. Often decreased dosing of the current neuroleptic or a change to a less potent neuroleptic will relieve akathisia.

Tardive dyskinesia is a repetitive movement disorder with rhythmic motions of the limbs, fingers, or facial muscles. The nigrostriatal pathway is affected by the increased dopaminergic stimulation, thus causing tardive dyskinesia.

Parkinsonian symptoms can also occur secondary to dopamine blockade in the nigrostriatal brain pathways. Like akathisia, parkinsonian symptoms can be relieved by reducing the neuroleptic dose or by changing to a less potent neuroleptic drug.

The most life-threatening side effect of neuroleptics is the acute onset of *neuroleptic malignant syndrome* (NMS). This life-threatening reaction can occur any time during therapy. The patient presents with muscular rigidity, hyperthermia, autonomic nervous system instability, and altered level of consciousness. Haloperidol has the greatest association of any neuroleptic drug with NMS. The incidence of NMS is 0.05 to 1% of all treated patients.

The proposed cause of NMS is the effect that neuroleptics have on the dopamine antagonism response in the nigrostriatal pathway. This response causes muscular rigidity. The neuroleptics then cause the blockade of hypothalamic thermoregulation, thus causing hyperthermia. A patient can present in NMS after an abrupt withdrawal of neuroleptics. The second therapy that may cause NMS is that endorphins have a role via the modulation of dopaminergic neurotransmission. When dopamine transmission is interfered with, NMS occurs.

A patient with NMS will present with a temperature higher than 41° C (106° F), with altered mental status, tachycardia, labile blood pressure, muscular hypertonicity, and lead-pipe rigidity. The patient is often in a coma. NMS can be confused with heat stroke, tetanus, strychnine poisons, vascular CNS events, and fatal catatonic and malignant hyperthermia. Patients who go into NMS have a 5 to 20% mortality rate. Pulmonary embolism, pulmonary edema, acute respiratory failure secondary to chest muscle wall restriction, secondary to rigid chest muscles, cardiac arrhythmias, seizures, and disseminated intravascular coagulation (DIC) are major causes of death in NMS.

A patient who overdoses on phenothiazine can have pinpoint pupils. Any neuroleptic overdose can present from mild sedation to frank coma with respiratory depression.

Mesoridazine and thioridazine have a quinidine-like effect that can prolong the PR or QT intervals with a widening of the QRS complex. Torsades de pointes and ventricular arrhythmias have also occurred with mesoridazine and thioridazine overdoses. Hypotension, reflex tachycardia, superventricular tachycardia, and AV dissociation have also been reported.

Diagnosis

A diagnosis is made by a history of neuroleptic use and physical examination.

Laboratory Findings

A patient should have a CBC, electrolytes, BUN, creatinine, calcium, magnesium, phosphorus, CPK, CPK-MB, LFTs, and serum or urine myoglobin drawn. An ECG should be performed. CPK is usually elevated in NMS along with the AST and ALT. If rhabdomyolysis is present, urine myoglobinuria will be present. An ABG should be performed to determine acid-base balance. A drug screen should also be done to rule out salicylate overdose, which can cause hyperthermia. An ethanol and acetaminophen level should be performed also.

Treatment

Dystonias can be treated with diphenhydramine 12.5 to 50 mg or benztropine 2 mg IV. Acute dystonias should resolve in 15 to 20 minutes. Oral therapy should be given for 2 to 3 days after resolution of dystonias with IV medications.

A patient with tardive dyskinesia is very difficult to treat. There is no known beneficial treatment for tardive dyskinesia.

Akathisia can be treated with benztropine, propranolol, or amantadine. Parkinsonian symptoms can be treated with amantadine and benztropine.

Any patient who presents with what is believed to be NMS should have their airway, breathing, and circulation evaluated (including vital signs). The patient should be placed on a cardiac monitor, given oxygen, and have two large-gauge IV lines started of normal saline or lactated Ringer's solution for pressure support. The patient should be given naloxone, dextrose, and thiamine if he or she presents in coma and the history is uncertain. If the patient presents in hypotension and fluids do not support hypotension, start an IV drip of epinephrine or norepinephrine. A chest x-ray and an abdominal flat plate should be performed to rule out an ileus and to look for phenothiazine pills. Phenothiazine pills are radiopaque.

A patient with NMS should be admitted to the ICU for ventilation support, relief of muscle rigidity, rehydration, and reversal of hyperthermia. A patient with suspected NMS should have his or her neuroleptic medication discontinued at once.

The treatment of muscle rigidity can be achieved by giving large doses of diazepam. If, however, the rigidity is not relieved in 15 to 20 minutes with diazepam, rapid-sequence intubation should be performed with neuromuscular paralytic agents. Pancuronium is the drug of choice for continued paralysis. Dantrolene and bromocriptine have also been used to relieve and control muscular rigidity.

If ventricular arrhythmias are present, give bicarbonate 1 to 3 mEq/kg IV followed by a continuous bicarbonate drip to keep the pH between 7.45 and 7.5. Bicarbonate restores the activity of the sodium channels in the phase O depolarization of myocardial conducting tissue. Do not give class IA antiarrhythmics, such as quinidine, disopyramide, or procainamide, because they can exacerbate cardiac toxicity of neuroleptics. Ventricular rhythms can be treated with lidocaine or phenytoin. Torsades de pointes should be treated with magnesium, isoproterenol, or overdrive pacing.

All overdose patients with an intact gag reflex should have a gastric lavage followed by activated charcoal 1 g/kg, followed by 0.5 g/kg every 4 hours. If the patient is intubated, still perform gastric lavage and give activated charcoal.

Cool the patient with rectal Tylenol and cooling blankets. Treat seizures with benzodiazepines, phenobarbital, or phenytoin.

ORGANOPHOSPHATE, CARBAMATE, AND PESTICIDE POISONING

Definition

Pesticides include herbicides, insecticides, rodenticides, fumigants, and fungicides. These pesticides are divided into two groups: the organophosphates and the carbamates. Eighty percent of all pesticide poisonings occur secondary to organophosphates. Organophosphates include the now banned forms of DDT, heptachlor, Kepone, and chlordane. These pesticides are still used in Third World countries where there is less regulation.

Epidemiology

There were more than 200,000 pesticide poisonings between 1988 and 1990 in the United States. There is on average 20 fatalities annually secondary to pesticide poisonings. There are over 25,000 brand name pesticides in the United States and over 1 billion pounds of pesticides are produced in the United States annually. More than 900 different chemical compounds are present in these 25,000 different commercial pesticides. Organophosphates were used as "nerve gas" during World War I with great morbidity and mortality, but these chemicals are now outlawed by the Geneva Convention for use in warfare on humans.

Pathology

Organophosphates and carbamate are popular pesticides used in agriculture, secondary to their rapid hydrolysis into harmless compounds with very little accumulation in the environment. Organophosphates are highly lipid soluble and are readily absorbed by the skin, respiratory tract, and GI tract. Because of their high lipid solubility, organophosphates can rapidly accumulate in the body fat and can create a toxic level that can cause symptoms of organophosphate poisoning.

Organophosphates rapidly bind irreversibly to cholinesterase molecules. Carbamates form a reversible bond with cholinesterase. Cholinesterase (acetylcholinesterase) and serum cholinesterase (pseudocholinesterase) rapidly hydrolyze acetylcholine into inactive fragments of acetic acid and choline after completion of neurotransmission. Organophosphates cause an irreversible cholinesterase inhibition secondary to the covalent binding of phosphate radicals to active sites of cholinesterase, causing the cholinesterase to form enzymatically inert proteins.

This organophosphate-cholinesterase bond is permanent if it is not reversed pharmacologically within 24 to 48 hours of binding when the cholinesterase is destroyed. The carbamate-cholinesterase bond spontaneously reverses in 4 to 6 hours without destroying the cholinesterase molecule with or without pharmacologic intervention.

Acetylcholine accumulates at the synapse after cholinesterase is inhibited. The accumulation of acetycholine causes overstimulation and disruption of the peripheral nervous system and CNS. Muscarinic neuroeffector junctions (postganglionic parasympathetic nerve endings) and the nicotinic receptors (autonomic ganglia and skeletal myoneural junctions) are both affected by cholinesterase inhibition.

Clinical Presentation/Examination

A patient can become toxic by dermal contact, oral exposure, contact with the conjunctiva, inhalation, and GI exposure. The most common exposure is through agricultural use, but suicidal and homicidal intent have been reported. Pet groomers who flea-dip animals can be exposed to organophosphates by direct or indirect contact.

A patient can present with the mnemonic symptoms of SLUD for *s*alivation, *l*acrimation, *u*rination, and *d*efecation secondary to acetylcholinesterase inhibition. Bradycardia is also mentioned as a "classic" sign of organophosphate poisoning; however, often there is an increased release of norepinephrine from the postganglionic sympathetic neurons precipitated by excess cholinergic activity at the sympathetic ganglia. This causes a normal or elevated heart rate or tachycardia. When the sympathetic nervous system is stimulated, hyperactivity and diaphoresis can occur secondary to stimulation of the preganglionic (nicotinic) and postganglionic (muscarinic) sites.

Muscarinic overstimulation causes hyperactivity of the parasympathetic nervous system, leading to hypersecretion of the salivary, lacrimal, and bronchial glands; miosis; nausea; vomiting; diarrhea; bronchoconstriction; muscle fasciculations; cramping; and weakness. Nicotinic effects include cramping, fasciculations, and weakness. Any patient who presents with miosis and muscle fasciculations should be considered to have pesticide poisoning until proven otherwise. In mild exposure, the patient will be alert and oriented and will present with blurred vision, headache, dizziness, weakness, tremor, wheezing, chest tightness, muscle fasciculations, incoordination, abdominal cramping, and often a cough. The key to recognizing severe poisoning is to recognize the symptoms of incontinence, a history of unconsciousness, or unconsciousness or convulsions as symptoms of severe poisoning. A patient who has been chronically exposed can present with vague symptoms of fatigue, weakness, anorexia, and malaise.

Diagnosis

A diagnosis is made by confirming the presence of reduced levels of cholinesterase activity in the blood, clinical presentation, physical examination, and response to atropine.

Always ask if the patient has ingested mushrooms of the *Amanita muscaria* species. This species of mushrooms can produce cholinergic-like symptoms.

Laboratory Findings

A CBC, electrolytes, BUN, creatinine, amylase, lipase, LFTs, urinalysis, and an ABG should be performed. Both RBC and plasma cholinesterase levels should be ordered. Often a nonketotic hyperglycemia, hypokalemia, and elevated serum amylase will be present. Leukocytosis with a shift to the left is often present. On urinalysis, proteinuria and glycosuria are often present.

Treatment

The first rule of treating a patient with suspected pesticide poisoning is to protect yourself and other staff members from contamination with the pesticide. Initial stabilization and decontamination should take place simultaneously. Remove all exposed clothes and wash the skin vigorously with soap and water. Ensure that you and your staff wear protective clothing at all times to prevent accidental contamination.

Any patient with a suspected organophosphate or carbamate poisoning with miosis, muscle fasciculations, bradycardia, and respiratory distress should have two large-gauge IV lines of normal saline placed. The person should receive oxygen therapy and should be placed on a cardiac monitor. The aforementioned laboratory examinations should be performed. A chest x-ray and an ECG should be performed. Early after ingestion, an intense sympathetic tone will cause sinus tachycardia. Later, there is an increased parasympathetic tone that will cause sinus bradycardia with ST and T wave abnormalities and often an AV block. The QT interval is often prolonged.

If the pesticide has been ingested, gastric lavage should be performed. Activated charcoal should be placed down the lavage tube but always ensure adequate airway protection when a lavage is performed.

Treatment is divided into latent, mild, moderate, and severe poisoning. Establishment of an adequate airway and ventilation should be the first priority. In moderate and severe poisoning, there will often be copious secretions of the oropharynx. If the secretions are too much to be adequately suctioned, then tracheal intubation and mechanical ventilation are required. Succinylcholine is the depolarizing neuromuscular blocking agent of choice. The effects of succinylcholine can be prolonged secondary to inhibition of pseudocholinesterase.

The mainstay of treatment for organophosphate or carbamate poisoning is atropine and pralidoxime. Atropine is a physiologic antidote for acetylcholine excess. Atropine competitively blocks the action of acetylcholine at the muscarinic receptors, stopping excessive parasympathetic stimulation.

Atropine causes flushing, tachycardia, anhidrosis, and xerostomia. Pupils will dilate, but this is an unsensitive predictor of adequate therapy. The starting dose for moderate to severe poisoning is 2 mg IV every 5 to 15 minutes until an adequate level has been reached. Give 0.05 mg/kg every 15 minutes for the poisoned pediatric patient. Enormous amounts of atropine may be required to counteract organophosphate or carbamate poisoning. The usual cause of death is that an inadequate atropine dose was given. Give glycopyrrolate (Robinul) to decrease the CNS side effects of atropine.

Pralidoxime (Protopam, 2-PAM chloride) reverses the cholinergic nicotinic effects that are not reversed by the sites that are unaffected by atropine. Pralidoxime corrects the nicotinic effects of fasciculations and muscle weakness by direct reaction and detoxification of unbound organophosphate molecules, reactivation of cholinesterase by cleavage of phosphorylated active sites, and by its endogenous anticholinergic effect in normal doses.

The initial dose of pralidoxime is 1 g IV over 15 to 30 minutes. In pediatric doses, give 20 to 50 mg/kg over 15 to 30 minutes. This dose should be repeated every 1 to 2 hours for 10 to 12 hours. Pralidoxime can be given in a continuous IV infusion at 0.5 g/hr for adults and 10 to 20 mg/kg in children.

If seizures occur, use IV diazepam or lorazepam. If a ventricular arrhythmia occurs and does not respond to lidocaine, you could try bretylium, cardioversion, IV isoproterenol, or overdrive pacing.

PHENYTOIN

Definition

Phenytoin (Dilantin) is an antiepileptic and antiarrhythmic medication that stabilizes excitable membranes through the sodium and calcium channels by blocking their effects and through facilitation of potassium and chloride conductance. The majority of deaths from phenytoin are not from overdoses, but rather from rapid IV administration in digoxin-intoxicated patients, patients with hypersensitivity reactions, co-ingestion of other drugs, or complications of extravasation of infusions. *IV infusion of phenytoin should not exceed 30 mg/min.*

Pathology

Phenytoin is highly protein bound and its volume of distribution is 0.6 l/kg. Phenytoin works by enhancing activity at the GABA receptors at neurotransmitter sites in the cerebral cortex, which limits repetitive firing and propagation of seizure activity. GABA has excitatory effects in the cerebellum. This effect on the cerebellum acts to suppress cortical seizure formation at therapeutic phenytoin levels in the inhibitory cerebellar pathways. This same pathway causes cerebellar-vestibular symptoms at toxic levels.

Peak levels of IV phenytoin are usually seen in 10 minutes, and oral phenytoin peak levels are seen in 3 to 10 hours (8 hours) after ingestion. Phenytoin is poorly absorbed in the gut; therefore, gastric absorption can be prolonged in large doses.

Phenytoin has class IB antiarrhythmic effects on the heart, which are similar to that of lidocaine. Phenytoin can cause AV blocks and prolongation of the PR and QRS intervals at toxic levels. As negative inotropic effects increase on the myocardium, there is more and more depression of the pacemaker and Purkinje cell automaticity. Phenytoin can also cause peripheral vasodilation, which can lead to hypotension. The prolongation of the PR interval and QRS complex, bradycardia, hypotension, and even cardiac arrest are usually caused by the negative inotropic effects secondary to rapid IV administration of phenytoin.

Phenytoin is usually diluted with 40% propylene glycol and 10% ethanol with a corrected pH of 12 with sodium hydroxide (Dilantin). Glycol can cause circulatory collapse, coma, seizures, ventricular arrhythmia, hypotension, and cardiac nodal depression. Propylene is a vasodilator and a mycocardial depressant. Toxic effects of propylene are also associated with rapid infusion rates. Propylene glycol can induce lactate-associated metabolic acidosis, hemolysis, and hyperosmolality.

Phenytoin is metabolized almost entirely by the liver, which metabolizes it to an inactive metabolite. Only 1 to 4% of phenytoin is excreted in the urine unchanged. Elimination is by first-order kinetics at low levels. As phenytoin levels rise and toxicity occurs, metabolism changes to a fixed-rate, zero-order or saturation kinetics. Thus, plasma concentration levels increase disproportionately to the dose of the drug given.

Toxic symptoms of phenytoin are related to free fractions of phenytoin in the plasma. As these free drug fractions rise, uremia, hypoalbuminemia, liver disease, and acidosis can be seen, especially in patients who are on valproic acid or if they have viral hepatitis.

Clinical Presentation/Examination

A patient with acute phenytoin toxicity can present with hypotension, bradyarrhythmias, new heart blocks, seizures, and extravasation of IV phenytoin, which can be limb-threatening, after rapid IV administration. Patients who are taking cimetidine, valproic acid, dicoumarol, isoniazid, disulfiram, and propoxyphene are at increased risk for toxicity because of the inhibiting effect of phenytoin on the microsomal enzyme activity of the liver.

Signs and symptoms of toxicity are from the effect that phenytoin has on the inhibitory cortical and excitatory cerebellar-vestibular areas of the brain. Nystagmus is usually the first sign of toxicity. The nystagmus of phenytoin toxicity is an upward-beating, bidirectional, or alternating nystagmus but may only occur in severe toxicity. Nystagmus disappears at levels higher than 35 to 55 μg/ml along with the loss of the corneal reflex and complete ophthalmoplegia.

Patients can present in any progression of symptoms, including ataxic gait, lethargy, dysarthria, apnea, or coma. If the patient presents with frank seizures, these seizures are usually brief in duration. Acute dystonias, opisthotonos, or choreoathetosis can occur secondary to cerebellar stimulation. Deep tendon reflexes can either be hypoactive or hyperactive depending on the phenytoin level.

A patient can present with altered mental status, including agitation, irritability, auditory hallucinations, euphoria, and combativeness.

A very serious complication of phenytoin administration is vascular extravasation and soft tissue injury and toxicity. An IM injection is still recommended by the manufacturer but can have serious side effects, such as hematoma, sterile abscess, and myonecrosis at the injection site. IV extravasation has led to compartment syndrome, gangrene, soft tissue necrosis, amputation, and death. Bluish discoloration of the affected extremity, erythema, edema, bullae, vesicles, and local tissue ischemia are described in the literature as a separate syndrome.

Signs of cardiovascular toxicity include hypotension, AV nodal blocks, ventricular tachycardia, bradycardia, ventricular fibrillation, and asystole. A patient often presents with syncope as the original cardiac complaint. On an ECG, the PR interval can be prolonged, the QRS interval can be widened, and the ST and T waves can be altered.

A patient can present with hyperglycemia as a reaction to phenytoin therapy secondary to inhibition of insulin release. This can cause nonketotic hyperosmolar coma or diabetic ketoacidosis.

A delayed hypersensitivity reaction has also been described. It occurs 1 to 6 weeks after the onset of phenytoin therapy. The most common hypersensitivity reaction is an erythematous morbilliform rash, which occurs more frequently in the summer. These hypersensitivity reactions can include fever, erythema multiforme, systemic lupus erythematosus, Stevens-Johnson syndrome, rhabdomyolysis, toxic epidermal necrolysis, lymphadenopathy, DIC, leukopenia, and renal failure.

Phenytoin is teratogenic and can lead to fetal hydantoin. A pregnant woman should not be started on phenytoin therapy. If the patient is taking phenytoin, she should have close follow-up with her obstetrician and neurologist.

Nystagmus begins at levels greater than 20 μg/ml. Ataxia usually occurs at levels above 30 μg/ml and lethargy at levels greater than 40 μg/ml. Death usually occurs at levels greater than 90 μg/ml. Deaths have been reported at levels of 50 μg/ml, and children have survived levels greater than 100 μg/ml.

Diagnosis

A diagnosis is made by a history of acute or chronic ingestion, presenting symptoms, physical examination, serum phenytoin levels, and an ECG.

Laboratory Findings

A CBC, electrolytes, BUN, creatinine, LFTs, amylase, lipase, albumin, and urinalysis should be drawn and performed on each patient with suspected phenytoin toxicity. Serum phenytoin levels should be drawn. The therapeutic phenytoin range for treatment of seizures and arrhythmias is 10 to 20 μg/ml. Many patients, especially those with brain injury, can become toxic at much lower blood levels.

Free phenytoin concentrations are more useful in predicting toxicity than are serum levels. Corrected serum phenytoin levels can be calculated in hypoproteinemic patients with a known albumin level. The normal serum albumin level is:

$$C_{normal} = \frac{C_{measured} \times 4.4}{\text{albumin concentration}}$$

The free phenytoin fraction (FPF) for hypoalbuminemic patients is:

$$FPF = \frac{1}{1 + (2.1 \times \text{albumin})}$$

Treatment

Any patient who presents with a history of an acute or chronic ingestion of phenytoin should be placed on a cardiac monitor, and two large-gauge IV lines of normal saline should be started. The aforementioned laboratory levels should be drawn. If metabolic acidosis is suspected, an ABG should be performed and the patient should be monitored very closely. Respiratory acidosis should be treated with oxygen and ventilatory support. All acute ingestions should be treated with activated charcoal 1 g/kg with multiple doses at least three times in the first 24 hours. Cathartics are not recommended in phenytoin overdose.

Hemoperfusion and hemodialysis are of no clinical benefit in phenytoin toxicity. Seizures are often of short duration, and usually no treatment is required. If treatment is necessary, give benzodiazepines or phenobarbital.

Symptomatic bradycardia is treated with atropine or temporary pacing. If extravasation of IV phenytoin occurs, a general surgeon or an orthopedic surgeon should be consulted.

All patients who have acute phenytoin toxicity should be admitted to the ICU secondary to the erratic absorption and long half-life of phenytoin.

SALICYLATES

Definition

Salicylate or aspirin (acetylsalicylic acid [ASA]) is found in over 200 over-the-counter medications and prescription drugs. Fiorinal,

Percodan, and Darvon all contain ASA. Methyl salicylate is found in oil of wintergreen, and sodium salicylate is used as a ketolytic agent. ASA is also found in over-the-counter medications such as Excedrin, Pepto-Bismol, Bayer Decongestant, Dristan, Coricidin, BC Cold Powder, Sine-Off, and 4-Way Cold tablets.

Epidemiology

There are two distinct patterns in those persons who become poisoned with ASA. The first group includes the young adult who has prior psychiatric history and who intentionally overdoses on ASA products. The second group includes the chronic unintentional overdose by the elderly person. In a chronic salicylate overdose in the elderly, there is a 25% mortality rate and a 30% morbidity rate. The mortality rate for acute ASA poisoning is 1%. ASA poisoning is the most common poisoning in children younger than 5 years of age. One teaspoon of oil of wintergreen is potentially fatal in a 2 year old. Fifty percent of suicide attempts involve ingestion of ASA. The elderly use large doses of salicylate-containing products secondary to arthritis, stomach upset, and home remedies. The diagnosis of salicylate poisoning is often missed at the time of admission in the elderly patient secondary to the health care provider not inquiring about the size of the dose or the duration of ingestion of the ASA product.

Pathology

After oral ingestion of salicylic acid, it is rapidly absorbed in the GI tract in 60 minutes, with peak blood levels in 4 to 6 hours. In large doses, concretions can occur. After salicylates are absorbed, they are rapidly hydrolyzed to free salicylic acid, which is then protein bound to albumin. When the albumin-binding sites are saturated, the unbound fraction of salicylate increases. This unbound salicylate in the plasma then enters the body cells. Once all albumin-binding sites are saturated, any increase in salicylate dose increases the levels of unbound salicylate.

ASA also inhibits the synthesis of prostaglandins, which stimulate platelet aggregation and vasoconstriction. Nephrotoxicity has been associated with prolonged large doses of ASA.

At low doses, salicylates are eliminated by first-order kinetics. In higher doses, salicylates are eliminated by zero-order kinetics. The salicylate half-life is from 15 to 30 hours in large doses. Salicylic acid has a blood pH of 7.4. The level of pH is very important in ASA poisoning. A drop in pH from 7.4 to 7.2 will double the amount of un-ionized ASA that is able to diffuse out of the plasma. This increase in un-ionized salicylic acid will change the volume of distribution. Patients with chronic ASA ingestions will have a larger volume of distribution. Because of this change in volume of distribution, interpretation of salicylate levels can only be interpreted by the salicylate nomogram for single-dose ingestions. Thus, a pH of greater than 7.5 will increase trapping of salicylate in the urine and thus excretion.

Commercial products can have variable rates of absorption secondary to their co-compounds or their enteric coating. If the ASA product is enteric-coated, the absorption rate can be as long as 6 to 9 hours.

The metabolic acidosis of an acute ASA ingestion is caused by the enhanced lipolysis, uncoupled oxidative phosphorylation, and the inhibition of various enzymes involved in energy production and amino acid metabolism. Acute salicylate poisoning causes an increase in oxygen consumption. However, in very high doses, it causes a decreased oxygen consumption. Oxidative phosphorylation is a major buffer of hydrogen ions; thus when ASA uncouples the oxidative phosphorylation action, acute metabolic acidosis results. Salicylic acid also increases glycolytic activity, which causes an elevation in circulating lactate. Ketoacids are elevated secondary to enhanced lipolysis. Very high doses of ASA will cause respiratory depression.

A large ingestion of ASA will cause an increased mobilization of glycogen stores and thus hyperglycemia. A salicylate is also a potent inhibitor of gluconeogenesis; thus an acute ingestion can cause normoglycemia, hypoglycemia, or hyperglycemia. Children usually develop hypoglycemia.

Clinical Presentation

A patient with salicylate poisoning presents with a mixed metabolic acidosis and respiratory alkalosis. A patient will present with acute gastric upset, vomiting, and GI bleeding. Renal failure is a rarely reported consequence of an acute poisoning.

CNS complaints consist of lethargy, convulsions, respiratory arrest, coma, and brain death. The decreased production of ATP causes uncoupling of oxidative phosphorylation and acute brain failure and cerebral edema. Often patients will present with altered mental status as if they have bacterial meningitis. This mental status change is secondary to the low glucose concentrations in the cerebrospinal fluid. The glucose levels in the cerebrospinal fluid are often much lower than serum glucose; thus serum glucose levels are a poor determination of actual glucose levels in the brain.

Pulmonary complaints include noncardiogenic pulmonary edema or ARDS. Pulmonary edema or ARDS is more common in adults than in children.

Cardiac effects of an acute ASA poisoning include arrhythmias, ventricular premature beats, ventricular fibrillation, and ventricular tachycardia. Cardiac toxicity is secondary to the impairment of ATP production, electrolyte abnormalities, acidosis, and hyperthermia.

Examination

All patients should be given a complete examination, including cranial nerves I to XII and a rectal examination to rule out an acute GI bleed.

Diagnosis

A diagnosis is made based on the history of chronic or acute ingestion of ASA products, physical examination, and presenting symptoms. An acute aspirin ingestion of 150 mg/kg or less is not toxic. An acute ingestion of 150 to 300 mg/kg will produce mild symptoms of vomiting, diaphoresis, tinnitus, hyperpnea, and mild acid-base changes. Any acute ingestion greater than 300 mg/kg is considered to be severely toxic. A dose over 500 mg/kg is considered lethal.

The Done nomogram is used to determine the likelihood of ASA toxicity. It can be used only for a single acute ingestion. It cannot be used for chronic ingestion, enteric-coated aspirin ingestion, or if a second dose of ASA has been taken within the previous 24 hours. The nomogram is based on serum salicylate in milligrams percent and on the time since ingestion. It is divided into asymptomatic, mild, moderate, and severe toxicity levels.

A simple test for salicylate overdose is the ferric chloride test. Place a few drops of 10% ferric chloride solution on the patient's urine. If salicylic acid is present in the urine, a violet-to-purple color develops. Reagent sticks (Phenistix) can also react to salicylate acid by turning brown to purple.

If the first level is in the normal or safe range, a second level should be drawn in 2 hours. If the second level is greater than the first level, then serial levels should be drawn until the levels are decreasing instead of increasing.

Laboratory Findings

A CBC, PT, PTT, electrolytes, BUN, creatinine, and salicylate and acetaminophen levels should be drawn. An ABG should be performed to rule out metabolic acidosis. Vomiting can cause an acute loss of potassium and acidosis. Normoglycemia, hypoglycemia, or hyperglycemia can be present.

Treatment

Any patient with a suspected salicylate overdose should have two large-gauge IV lines of normal saline placed. The patient should be placed on 2 liters of oxygen via nasal cannula and should also be placed on a cardiac monitor. The aforementioned laboratory tests should be performed, and an ABG should be drawn. A baseline chest x-ray should be performed to rule out acute pulmonary edema.

GI decontamination can be lifesaving. Activated charcoal should be given after gastric lavage. Always protect the patient's airway when lavaging. Give 1 g/kg of activated charcoal.

Most patients who have acutely ingested salicylates are dehydrated. They will usually need several liters of IV normal saline to correct dehydration. Be careful with forced diuresis in the treatment of salicylate poisoning, because this can lead to pulmonary edema, which is a major cause of mortality. In children, a fluid overload in those with inappropriate secretion of antidiuretic hormone can predispose these children to pulmonary edema.

Every effort should be made to keep the arterial pH above 7.5. Remember that even a small decrease in pH will cause a greater concentration in un-ionized salicylate. Give sodium bicarbonate in a 1 mEq/kg bolus to make the urine alkaline and keep the serum pH above 7.5. Start a continuous IV infusion of 1 liter of 5% dextrose in water with 50 to 100 mmol of sodium bicarbonate and 40 mEq of potassium chloride at three times the normal maintenance rate. Monitor the serum pH and urine pH to prevent hyperkalemia, hypokalemia, or hyponatremia. A very large dose of bicarbonate and potassium may be needed to alkalinize the urine. Up to 110 mEq of potassium every 4 hours may be necessary to alkalinize the urine. If a fluid overload does develop, give furosemide (Lasix). Do not give anhydrase inhibitors (e.g., acetazolamide) because they increase mortality.

Dialysis should be considered in any patient:

1. With a deteriorating condition despite alkaline urine and diuresis
2. With acidic urine despite alkalemic blood and hyperkalemia
3. Patient in acute renal failure
4. Cardiac toxicity
5. Comatose patient
6. Patient in ARDS in whom the salicylate levels are not following

Peritoneal dialysis is effective, and 5% albumin should be placed in the peritoneal solution to enhance salicylate clearance through protein binding. Peritoneal dialysis is not as effective as hemodialysis.

Any patient with continued mental deterioration despite supportive care should have immediate dialysis for treatment of cerebral edema.

If the ASA poisoning has caused a prolonged PT, parenteral vitamin K_1 will be required to stop the bleeding. Serum electrolytes should be re-evaluated every 2 to 3 hours, and an ABG should be performed every 2 to 3 hours to monitor blood pH.

All patients with altered mental status, salicylate levels in the mild or greater range, or GI bleeding or in patients who are in metabolic acidosis or respiratory alkalosis should be admitted to the ICU. All infants should be admitted to the hospital.

THEOPHYLLINE

Definition

Theophylline relaxes bronchial smooth muscles and has some prophylactic anti-inflammatory effects. It is used in the treatment of chronic asthmatics and COPD patients. Its bronchial dilatation effects are dose dependent. The response to theophylline therapy varies among patients. It has a very narrow therapeutic range of 5 to 15 μg/ml. Toxicity is also complicated by many drugs and social habits (tobacco use) that interact with theophylline levels. Serum concentrations greater than 20 μg/ml are considered toxic. Death has been associated with rapid infusion and serum levels as low as 25 μg/ml.

Cardiac, neurologic, and metabolic abnormalities can occur with a toxic ingestion of theophylline. Three common forms of theophylline are used: aminophylline, oxytriphylline, and dyphylline. Aminophylline contains 80 to 85% theophylline. Oxytriphylline contains 65% theophylline, and dyphylline contains 50% theophylline. IV aminophylline will raise the theophylline level by 2 μg/ml for every milligram per kilogram given.

Epidemiology

There are approximately 6000 toxic ingestions of theophylline each year with approximately 30 deaths per year.

Pathology

The action of theophylline is probably due to its inhibition of phosphodiesterase. It is also suggested that it affects prostaglandin action, cyclic AMP, intracellular calcium, catecholamine release, and adenosine. It is eliminated by first-order kinetics and is 60% protein bound with a volume of distribution of 0.3 to 0.7 l/kg. The serum half-life is 4 to 8 hours, and the half-life is affected by smoking, cardiac disease, liver metabolism, diet, and medications.

Theophylline is absorbed both orally and IV. Its peak serum level after oral dosing is approximately 90 to 120 minutes. With enteric-coated tablets, peak levels are not reached for 6 to 8 hours after dosing. After IV administration, serum levels peak after 30 minutes.

Drugs that decrease the half-life of theophylline are phenytoin, phenobarbital, rifampin, and carbamazepine. Drugs that increase the half-life of theophylline are cimetidine, erythromycin, allopurinol, quinolone antibiotics, troleandomycin, and possibly oral contraceptives. Cigarette smoking and charcoal-broiled foods also decrease the half-life of theophylline. Children also have a decreased half-life metabolism of theophylline; however, neonates have an increased half-life of theophylline. Obese persons also have an increased half-life of theophylline.

Clinical Presentation/Examination

Because of the narrow therapeutic range of theophylline, toxicity can occur at normal or very low serum levels. Common cardiovascular effects such as sinus tachycardia, atrial tachycardia, multifocal atrial tachycardia, atrial fibrillation, and ventricular arrhythmias can all occur. In the elderly, sustained ventricular tachycardia can occur at serum levels of 40 to 60 μg/ml. Hypotension can occur at any serum level. Young persons can usually tolerate higher serum levels than the elderly before signs of toxicity occur.

Patients often present with GI symptoms of nausea, vomiting, and abdominal pain. Usually nausea and vomiting are present with serum levels greater than 25 μg/ml. A patient can present with only a history of esophageal reflux as the presenting complaint. GI bleeding has been reported.

A patient with a toxic serum level can present with neurologic complaints of headache, irritability, tremors, sleeplessness, and muscular twitching. Psychosis and hallucinations have both been reported with moderate elevations. In mildly elevated serum levels, patients can present with tonic-clonic or focal motor seizures. Seizures do not correlate with serum levels or the prognosis. If the patient has a prior history of epilepsy, he or she is at an increased risk of seizures while on theophylline therapy.

Diagnosis

A diagnosis is made by a history of acute or chronic ingestion of theophylline, serum level of theophylline, presenting complaints, and physical examination.

Laboratory Findings

A CBC, electrolytes, calcium, magnesium, phosphorus, BUN, creatinine, urinalysis, LFTs, serum theophylline level, and an ABG should all be performed. Hypokalemia can occur in acute ingestion or chronic toxicity. β-Agonists can also exacerbate hypokalemia. Ketosis and lactic acidosis can occur with toxicity. Hyperglycemia is often present secondary to increased circulating catecholamines of toxicity.

Treatment

Any patient with suspected theophylline toxicity should have at least one large-gauge IV line of normal saline placed. The patient should be placed on a cardiac monitor and on oxygen therapy. Pulse oximetry should be performed, and an ECG and a chest x-ray should be done. The aforementioned laboratory levels should be drawn, and an ABG should be performed. Treatment is directed at decontamination in acute ingestion and cardiac and metabolic stabilization in chronic ingestions. In acute ingestion, gastric emptying is achieved by gastric lavage and cathartics. Syrup of ipecac is of little use secondary to the vomiting that is usually already present. Activated charcoal should be given. Activated charcoal significantly decreases the half-life of theophylline and should be given in multiple doses every 2 to 4 hours. If severe nausea and vomiting are present, give ranitidine 50 mg IV to reduce the vomiting while activated charcoal is being given.

If seizures are present, diazepam, phenytoin, and phenobarbital can be used. Theophylline-induced status epilepticus is often resistant to diazepam, phenytoin, and phenobarbital. If seizures cannot be stopped with these drugs, then general anesthesia should be performed.

If severe hypotension or life-threatening arrhythmias are present, give propranolol 1 mg IV up to a total of 10 mg. β-Blockers can exacerbate cardiac depression and airway obstruction but can also be lifesaving. Esmolol or labetalol can also be used. Hypokalemia should be treated with potassium. Treat ventricular arrhythmias as usual with lidocaine, phenytoin, or digoxin therapy.

Hemoperfusion and hemodialysis can be used. The clearance rate for hemodialysis is approximately 25 μg/ml/hr. Hemoperfusion should be used in acute life-threatening toxicity, seizures, tachyarrhythmias, and in acute overdose with serum levels greater than 100 μg/ml in patients who are symptomatic. Hemoperfusion should be used in chronic overdoses when levels are higher than 60 μg/ml, and in the elderly, when underlying disease prolongs half-life, in severe cardiac or liver disease, and with levels between 40 and 60 μg/ml.

Patients with serum levels below 25 μg/ml who are asymptomatic and have a normal ECG and normal potassium level can be discharged to home with a 48-hour follow-up. Any patient who has a toxic level and is symptomatic, especially the very old or the very young, or patients with underlying cardiac or liver disease should be admitted to the hospital.

BIBLIOGRAPHY

Auerbach PS: Clinical therapy of marine envenomation and poisoning. In Tu AT (ed): Handbook of Natural Toxins. Vol 3: Marine Toxins and Venoms. New York, Dekker, 1988

Auerbach PS, Halstead BW: Hazardous aquatic life. In Auerbach PS, Geehr ED (eds): Management of Wilderness and Environmental Emergencies, 2nd ed. St Louis, CV Mosby, 1989

Braunwald E, Isselbacher KJ, Petersdorf RG, et al (eds): Harrison's Principles of Internal Medicine, 11th ed. New York, McGraw-Hill, 1987

Bryson PD: Comprehensive Review in Toxicology, 2nd ed. Rockville, MD, Aspen Publishing, 1989

Ellenhorn MJ, Barceloux DG: Medical Toxicology, Diagnosis and Treatment of Human Poisoning. New York, Elsevier Science Publishing Company, 1988

Gosselin RE, Smith RP, Hodge HC (eds): Clinical Toxicology of Commercial Products, 5th ed. Baltimore, Williams & Wilkins, 1984

Haddad JF, Winchester JF: Clinical Management of Poisoning and Drug Overdose, 2nd ed. Philadelphia, WB Saunders, 1990

Hamilton GC, Sanders AB, Strange GR, et al (eds): Emergency Medicine: An Approach to Clinical Problem-Solving. Philadelphia, WB Saunders, 1991

May HL, Aghababian RV, Fleisher GR (eds): Emergency Medicine, 2nd ed. Boston, Little, Brown, 1992

Rosen P, Barkin RM (eds): Emergency Medicine: Concepts and Clinical Practice, 3rd ed. St Louis, Mosby-Year Book, 1992

Schwartz GR, Cayten CG, Mangelsen MA, et al (eds): Principles and Practice of Emergency Medicine. Philadelphia, Lea & Febiger, 1992

Temple AR (ed): Medical Toxicology: Emerg Clin North Am (2) Feb 1989

Tierney LM, McPhee SJ, Papadakis MA (eds): Current Medical Diagnosis and Treatment, 33rd ed. Norwalk, CT, Appleton & Lange, 1994

Tintinalli JE, Krone RL, Ruiz E (eds): Emergency Medicine: A Comprehensive Study Guide, 4th ed. New York, McGraw-Hill, 1996

Chapter 18

Care of the Multiple Trauma Patient

TRAUMA OVERVIEW

Definition

The multiple trauma patient is a complex patient who above all deserves the "team" approach. When a multiple trauma patient arrives in the trauma room, that patient needs to be "attacked" by the trauma team. Seconds often count. Treatment of trauma requires multiple tasks being performed by numerous people simultaneously. Trauma requires a broad-based knowledge, technical skills, sound judgment, and leadership capabilities. Above all, "one" person, the team leader, must be in charge.

Epidemiology

The leading cause of traumatic death in the United States is motor vehicle accidents (MVA). The leading cause of death for those younger than 44 years of age in the United States is trauma. The major cause of death for a black male between 5 and 35 years of age in the United States is gunshot wounds.

With regard to motor vehicle accidents, 70% occur in rural areas. Fifty percent of those deaths are secondary to head trauma, spinal cord injuries, or blunt trauma. The mortality rate from head trauma approaches 40% in the United States, and total recovery only approaches 40 to 50% of those who survive a head injury.

Patients with chest trauma have a high mortality rate. If a patient requires intubation and is in shock at the time of arrival to the emergency department (ED), there is approximately 73% mortality rate. Penetrating chest wounds are very common from low- or high-velocity projectiles. Of those patients who reach the ED alive, the survival rate for gunshot wounds is between 70% and 85% for stab wounds, when both are aggressively treated in the ED and operating room. The problem is that less than one quarter of patients with penetrating chest wall injuries reach the ED alive.

Patients with penetrating chest injuries, who are clinically dead upon arrival at the ED but who have a pulse during transportation and who received a thoracotomy upon arrival to the ED, have a 32% survival rate. Patients with no vital signs or signs of life at the accident scene have a 100% mortality rate.

Almost all trauma deaths can be prevented through use of seat belts, speed limits, and limited sale and availability of guns. The use of helmets by motorcyclists and bikers can significantly decrease the number of head injuries among the younger population. There has been a significant decrease in the number of deaths due to drunk driving in the past 10 years secondary to enforcement of new laws and stiffer penalties for those who drive drunk. Also national public awareness programs have made the public aware of the significant number of deaths caused each year by drunk drivers. Drug abuse and use has a major impact on the use of firearms in the inner city among the black and Hispanic male population. Trauma is truly an epidemic in 1996 in the United States. It must be addressed as an epidemic by our local, state, and national legislators.

Pathology

The treatment of acute trauma is the treatment of shock. An understanding of the pathophysiology of shock is very important when treating a multiple trauma patient. Shock is usually secondary to hemorrhagic hypovolemia in the trauma patient. Shock can also be secondary to neurogenic or cardiogenic shock.

Laboratory Findings

For the trauma patient, laboratory tests include a complete blood count (CBC), prothrombin time (PT), partial thromboplastin time (PTT), electrolytes, blood urea nitrogen (BUN), creatinine, glucose, amylase, lipase, calcium, alkaline phosphatase, magnesium, phosphate, serum glutamic-oxaloacetic transaminase (SGOT), serum glutamic-pyruvic transaminase (SGPT), total bilirubin, creatine kinase (CK), CK-MB, and blood type. Six to 8 units of blood typed and crossed should be the normal treatment for any trauma patient.

X-ray Findings

If there is a severe head injury, there can also be a cervical spine injury. The cervical spine should always be x-rayed to rule out a fracture in any high-speed trauma or fall. Only 5% of patients with severe head injury will have a spinal fracture. Skull fractures can be obtained to rule out depressed or linear skull fractures. The Towne view can be used to look for occiput fractures extending down into the foramen magnum. An x-ray of the chest, abdomen, and pelvis should be performed routinely on all trauma patients. Associated x-rays of the extremities should be taken as needed.

Clinical Presentation/Examination/Treatment

Any trauma patient, including patients with cardiac injury, should have a "safety net" established to include two large-gauge intravenous (IV) lines of normal saline or lactated Ringer's solution. The patient should be placed on 100% oxygen and on a cardiac monitor. The aforementioned laboratory measures should be drawn. The patient should have the normal trauma x-rays taken, including ones of the cervical spine if necessitated by injury, the anteroposterior (AP) chest, abdomen, and pelvis. X-rays of the extremities should be performed as required. An electrocardiogram (ECG) should be performed to rule out an acute myocardial infarction or new bundle branch or atrioventricular (AV) blocks. The most important part of the history is the event that leads up to the traumatic event. The mechanism of injury is very important in directing the evaluation and potential diagnosis.

Upon arrival to the trauma room, the ABCDEs of basic life support should be the first items performed.

A—Airways: establish the airway, remember always to protect the cervical spine.

B—Breathing: auscultate the lungs, look for symmetry and asymmetry in breaths and breath sounds, and note the number of respirations per minute.

C—Circulation: evaluate the pulses, cardiac intensity, blood pressure, and pulse.

D—Disability: do a quick neurologic check and also do the Glasgow Coma Scale (GCS).

E—Exposure: undress the patient completely, and examine the entire patient, including the patient's back.

Basic life support measures and the primary survey should be performed simultaneously. Airway, breathing, and circulation problems are addressed as found. The entire patient should be palpated after the patient's airway, breathing, and circulation have been established to determine the likelihood of abdominal, bony, chest, renal, neck, back, or extremity trauma. The patient should be "log-rolled" to view the back and buttocks. The secret of running a successful trauma team is a constant re-evaluation of the patient on a continuous basis for the entire duration of the trauma period until definitive stabilization of the patient has occurred.

If the patient's airway is compromised, then the patient should be immediately intubated after sedation and paralyzation. If a head injury is present, a quick neurologic examination should be performed prior to intubation for future reference for the neurosurgeon. If the patient cannot be intubated, then a cricothyrotomy should be performed as a last resort.

The old saying "tube and finger in every orifice" still holds true. During the secondary survey, the ears, nose, throat, eyes, urethra, vagina, and rectum should be examined. A rectal examination should be performed on a male to look for a high-riding prostate. A Foley catheter should be placed only after a rectal examination is performed on the patient. A bimanual examination should be performed on any female patient to check for disruption of the pelvic ring or vaginal lacerations. A nasogastric (NG) tube should be placed if there is no facial trauma. If facial trauma is present, then an orogastric tube should be placed.

Shock is treated with crystalloid fluid and blood. Blood should almost always be typed and crossed, if possible, prior to administration. If blood is needed immediately, O-negative blood should be given. Autotransfusion is also a practical way of giving blood at many institutions and will give you time until blood can be typed and crossed. If the patient receives 2 to 3 liters of crystalloid fluid and the patient is still hypotensive or the patient's condition is deteriorating, then that patient should receive blood.

Impending herniation should be treated as per the head injury section with elevation of the head by 30 degrees, mannitol, and hyperventilation. An immediate neurosurgical consultation should be made for decompression.

One of the most dangerous patients to arrive in the trauma room is the intoxicated patient. No intoxicated patient can be discharged from the hospital until he or she is sober, no matter how trivial or minor the patient's complaints are. Another good rule is that if the patient can't walk, the patient can't go home.

After the primary and secondary survey and the patient has been stabilized, each patient requires a complete neurologic, abdominal, cardiac, musculoskeletal, urologic, and gynecologic examination prior to their final disposition. Often this examination can take place in the trauma room, but it is often performed hours or days after the initial trauma in the surgical intensive care unit or on the ward floor. A complete examination should never take precedence over the patient going to the operating room to stop bleeding or herniation.

The pregnant patient presents special problems in the management of trauma. The best rule for a successful trauma resuscitation for a fetus and mother is aggressive treatment of the mother and maintenance of good oxygenation of the mother. Good oxygenation of the mother means good oxygenation of the fetus. After 20 weeks of pregnancy, the mother should be transported on her left side. If the patient is on a backboard, the board should be elevated to a 15-degree angle. Tilting the pelvis to the right removes the uterus from the inferior vena cava and thus increases oxygen supply to the fetus.

Always listen and talk to the patient. The patient will tell you what is wrong in most cases. Always tell a patient what you are going to do to him or her. Remember that the patient has experienced a traumatic event, and the patient does not usually remember the event. The patient is strapped down to a backboard, naked, and is surrounded by numerous strangers, who are all putting a finger or tube in every orifice and no one is telling the patient why! A calming voice and a little reassurance can go a long way in the trauma room!

The two best rules to live by in the trauma room are: "a little oxygen can go a long way," and "if you think about it, you had better do it!" You can never take too many x-rays, do too much laboratory testing, or overexamine or overstabilize any patient in the trauma room. Remember that more patients die from not going to the operating room than do!

Packed red blood cells = 10 ml/kg will increase hematocrit by 5%.
Platelets = 0.1 unit/kg will increase platelet count by 25,000.
Factor VII = 1 unit/kg will increase factor VII by 2%.
Factor II = 1 unit/kg will increase factor II by 1%.

ABDOMINAL TRAUMA

Definition

Abdominal trauma can be caused by penetrating or blunt trauma with many different mechanisms. Often there will be a combination of both blunt and penetrating injuries.

Pathology

Blunt trauma is usually secondary to a motor vehicle accident. The type of injury and the severity of the injury are dependent on the location of the injury in the abdomen. Injuries are divided into extraperitoneal injuries and peritoneal injuries. Extraperitoneal injuries include the retroperitoneum and the extraperitoneal pelvis. The examination of the retroperitoneum and the extraperitoneal pelvis is quite difficult. A diagnostic peritoneal lavage (DPL) is a poor diagnostic tool for diagnosing bleeding in these two areas of the abdomen. These areas have to be evaluated by upper gastrointestinal contrast studies, intravenous pyelogram (IVP), angiography, cystography, or contrast computed tomography (CT) scan.

Penetrating trauma usually occurs from gunshot wounds or stab wounds. All gunshot wounds should probably be explored and débrided in the operating room. Peritoneal lavage is especially helpful in deciding which wounds need to be explored. Remember that gunshot wounds to the superior chest can also injure the diaphragm or lungs.

Stab wounds are usually managed more conservatively than are gunshot wounds. Patients with peritoneal irritation, evisceration, or persistent hypotension and tachycardia should go immediately to the operating room. A positive wound exploration is the finding of a penetration of the superficial fascia.

Examination/Clinical Presentation

The evaluation of a patient with abdominal trauma must be in the context of the entire patient. Maintenance of the airway, breathing, and circulation always come first. A patient with abdominal trauma can present with rigidity, guarding, rebound tenderness, or a palpable mass. Flank pain and ecchymosis are signs of injury. The DPL is still the "gold standard" for diagnosing abdominal trauma in the ED. It is a simple and very noninvasive procedure to perform; however, retroperitoneal injuries are not readily diagnosed by DPL. The diagnosis of an abdominal trauma at many centers has replaced the DPL with a contrast CT scan, but good clinical judgment far outweighs either test. All patients with abdominal trauma require a rectal examination before a Foley catheter is placed. All female patients with abdominal trauma require at least a bimanual pelvic examination. If a hip or pelvic fracture or bleeding from the rectum or vagina is present, then the vagina needs to be visualized with a speculum examination.

The entire abdomen must be visualized. The patient must be log-rolled, and the patient's entire back must be examined. Any patient with a pelvic fracture requires a DPL or a contrast CT scan to evaluate the internal organs. The DPL should be performed through a supra-umbilical incision if a pelvic fracture is present to avoid entering the pelvis and striking a pelvic hematoma. If there is a urethral tear or a high-riding prostate in a male, a urethrogram should be performed prior to a Foley catheter being placed. If there is gross hematuria an IVP or a cystogram must be performed to evaluate the urologic anatomy.

A patient with a spleen injury will present with Kehr's sign, left shoulder-strap pain, tachycardia, hypotension, and syncope. Any right or left lower rib fracture requires an evaluation for liver or spleen injury.

Diagnosis

The goal of diagnosis of abdominal trauma is not to diagnose specific lesions but to recognize a surgical abdomen and to know when to take the patient to the operating room.

The DPL test is 98% sensitive for bleeding in the abdomen. It is a fast test and is very noninvasive. There is, however, a high false-positive incidence secondary to how the procedure is performed. Indications for a DPL are blunt or penetrating trauma with a significant history of abdominal trauma when physical examination is equivocal. The DPL test can be used in intoxicated patients, in head or spinal trauma patients, or in patients with unreliable abdominal examination findings.

There are no absolute contraindications to peritoneal lavage, only relative contraindications. Relative contraindications include a gravid uterus and in patients who have had previous abdominal surgery. If there has been prior abdominal surgery, the DPL incision should be made away from the prior surgical incision.

There are three types of DPL techniques: open, closed, and semi-closed. To perform a DPL, the patient should first have a Foley catheter and an NG tube placed. The skin should be prepared and draped, and a local anesthetic with epinephrine 1:1000 should be used.

The incision is made paramedianly or supraumbilically. In the closed technique, the skin is nicked and a needle is placed in the peritoneum. The Seldinger technique utilizes placement of a large catheter. In the semiclosed technique, the incision is carried down to the fascia, thus the fascia is visualized prior to peritoneal puncture.

After catheter placement, fluid is aspirated. If more than 5 ml of gross blood is returned, the result of the test is positive. If no blood is aspirated, then 20 ml/kg, up to 1000 ml, of lactated Ringer's solution is placed through the catheter into the abdomen. The patient is encouraged to change positions if possible so that the fluid is distributed throughout the entire abdomen. Once the fluid is in the abdomen, the bag is then lowered below the patient and the fluid is drained. The result of the examination is positive if the red blood cell count is greater than 100,000 cells/mm³, the white blood cell count is greater than 500 cells/mm³, the amylase level is greater than 200 units/100 ml, or if bile, bacteria, or vegetable matter is present.

Laboratory Findings

A CBC, electrolytes, glucose, amylase, lipase, SGOT, SGPT, total bilirubin, gamma glutamyl transferase (GGT), calcium, magnesium, alkaline phosphatase, a pregnancy test in a female, and a urinalysis should be performed on all abdominal trauma patients. The patient should be typed and crossed for 6 to 8 units of blood. Toxicology tests should be performed as necessitated.

Treatment

Any patient who presents with trauma to the abdomen should have two large-gauge IV lines of normal saline 0.9% or lactated Ringer's solution placed, and the patient should be placed on 100% oxygen. The patient should also be placed on a cardinal monitor and have the aforementioned laboratory tests performed. The normal trauma x-rays should be performed, including those of the cervical spine, chest, abdomen (both upright and supine or lateral decubitus), pelvis, and extremities, as necessitated.

All patients should have an NG tube placed, if there is no facial trauma, and a Foley catheter should be placed after a rectal examination. Any patient with penetrating trauma or suspicion of a bowel injury should receive antibiotics for both aerobes and anaerobes. Usually triple antibiotic therapy with ampicillin, gentamicin, and clindamycin is the proven, cost-effective regimen. Consult the trauma surgeon at your institution as to his or her preference. The biggest mistake in the treatment of any abdominal trauma is delayed surgical intervention. Most deaths result from delayed intervention.

No patient who is intoxicated or has abnormal mental status can be discharged home. If intoxicated or if the patient has altered mental status, the patient must be admitted to the hospital. Consult a surgeon early and often in the case of a patient with abdominal trauma.

ABDOMINAL TRAUMA IN PREGNANCY

The pregnant patient who is involved in any trauma is at higher risk for morbidity and mortality. There are significant differences in the pregnant patient from the nonpregnant patient. There are changes in every organ system of the pregnant patient. An understanding of these changes is essential to the treatment and resuscitation of the pregnant patient who suffers trauma.

Uterine Differences

The uterus grows about 1 cm for each week of pregnancy. At 20 weeks, the fundus of the uterus should be at the umbilicus. The blood flow increases from 60 ml/min to 600 ml/min at term. The uterus grows from a 70-g organ to a 1000-g organ.

Urinary Tract Changes

The bladder of the pregnant female is displaced anteriorly and superiorly. These changes move the bladder from the pelvis to the abdomen. The bladder loses its protection of the pelvis as it rises out of the pelvis into the abdomen. The ureters and renal pelvis dilate from 10 weeks to 6 weeks postpartum, from right to left.

Hematologic Differences

The biggest change in the pregnant patient is the change in the volume of blood at term. Blood volume is increased by 45% in the term patient. The pregnant woman will have "dilutional anemia." The increased volume of plasma will allow greater red blood cell loss before hypovolemia occurs. The normal erythrocyte sedimentation rate (ESR) is 78 mm/hr in the pregnant patient.

A leukocytosis of 18,000 to 25,000 is normal during pregnancy. Fibrinogen and factors VII, VIII, IX, and X are all increased in the normal pregnancy. The PT and PTT are unchanged. The pregnant patient is at increased risk for venous thrombosis, and the release of thromboplastic materials in the traumatized patient can lead to disseminated intravascular coagulation (DIC).

Gastrointestinal Differences

When examining the pregnant patient, the signs of peritoneal irritation are less diagnostic. The pregnant patient has decreased rebound tenderness, and rigidity is decreased or delayed in the pregnant patient. There is decreased gastric motility and gastric emptying in the pregnant patient. This increases the likelihood of aspiration in the traumatized pregnant patient.

As the uterus grows, the intra-abdominal contents are displaced cephalad. In penetrating trauma, there is almost always intestinal injury.

Cardiovascular Differences

On an electrocardiogram there will be a left-axis deviation of 15° secondary to the displacement of the abdominal contents into the chest, in late pregnancy, secondary to the enlarging uterus. The T wave in lead III can be inverted and flattened.

The normal heart rate for the pregnant patient is increased by 15 to 20 beats/min in the third trimester. The patient's blood pressure falls by 10 to 15 mm Hg in the second trimester only to increase to normal by the end of the third trimester. The pregnant woman's cardiac output increases in the first 10 to 12 weeks by 1 to 1.5 l/min, and is maintained until term. In the third-trimester patient, the enlarged uterus can occlude the flow of blood in the inferior vena cava. This occlusion of the vena cava causes the preload to decrease, and the cardiac output falls. All pregnant patients should be placed in the left lateral decubitus position. This is performed by elevating the right side of the patient by 6 inches under the right hip. If this cannot be performed, the uterus should be manually displaced.

Pulmonary Differences

Respiratory rate changes little during pregnancy. PCO_2 averages 30 mm Hg during pregnancy. Tital volume is increased by 40%, and residual volume decreases by 25%. The pH does not change.

Treatment of the Pregnant Traumatized Patient

The three main causes of injury during pregnancy are penetrating objects, accidents, and falls. *The injured pregnant patient is treated in the same way, with the same resuscitation protocols, as a nonpregnant patient is.* Airway, breathing, and circulation (ABCs), oxygen, two large-gauge IV lines, same trauma laboratory values, same cervical spine x-rays, and a urinary catheter and rectal examination are performed. The best care that a fetus can obtain, and the best chance for survival of the fetus, is the administration of good care to the mother. Do not get focused on the fetus inside the mother. Take care of the mother, and the chances of a normal term pregnancy are increased. Keep the mother well oxygenated, and keep good cardiopulmonary circulation in the mother. This will ensure good oxygenation of the fetus.

Position the mother on her left side, if she presents after 20 weeks of pregnancy. Realize that the pregnant female has increased plasma volume and can lose 30 to 35% of her blood volume before the normal signs of hypovolemia (tachycardia and hypotension) will occur. Fluid replacement and resuscitation should be increased by 50% in a shocky pregnant patient.

After the mother has been stabilized and your primary and secondary surveys have been performed, examine the fetus. Note the fetal heart tones with a Doppler. Fetal heart tones should be heard with a Doppler after 10 weeks' gestation. Note the fundal height in centimeters. Perform a pelvic examination. Note the external genitalia and the vagina for hematomas, abrasions, or lacerations. Always get a history of herpes from the mother, and examine the genitals for herpes lesions in case an emergent delivery is necessitated. Note the presence of dilatation or effacement of the cervix, tenderness of the cervix, and if any blood or products of conception are present. Take a small sample of vaginal fluid and note the pH with nitrazine paper. Look for "ferning" on microscopic examination. Ferning is dried amniotic fluid which, when dried, presents a fern-like pattern. If ferning is present, then you have ruptured membranes.

Note the number of uterine contractions per hour. Perlman and associates found that if the patient had more than eight uterine contractions per hour in the first 4 hours after trauma occurred, 10% of the pregnancies suffered adverse outcomes. In his study when contractions were not felt in the first 4 hours, *no* immediate adverse outcomes were noted. All pregnant women who have suffered even minor trauma should be observed for 4 hours. This 4-hour monitoring period is highly sensitive to prediction of a bad outcome in women who are at 20 weeks' gestation.

FETOMATERNAL HEMORRHAGE

Fetomaternal hemorrhage (FMH) is a condition in which the fetal blood and the maternal blood are mixed in the maternal circulation. The placenta is a hemochorial system. Normally the fetal and maternal blood usually do not mix. The danger of a mixture of fetal and maternal blood is the chance of isoimmunization of maternal antibodies against Rho (D) antigen on the surface of Rh-positive fetal cells. If this cross-over takes place, the maternal IgG antibodies cross the placenta and can cause fetal red blood cell hemolysis in the current and future pregnancies. The Rh status of the mother should be routine on all trauma laboratory measures.

The amount of FMH following trauma in pregnancy is important when calculating the correct dose of Rho (D) immune globulin: The normal dose is 300 μg IM. This dose, however, in the presence of FMH, may not be enough to protect the patient and the fetus from isoimmunization. The proper dose of Rho (D) immune globulin can be calculated by performing the Kleihauser-Betke assay, which identifies and quantitates FMH.

Do not use vasopressors unless they are absolutely necessary, because they reduce uterine blood flow; however, do not withhold vasopressors if they are needed to save the mother's life. If excessive bleeding occurs from trauma to the uterus and the uterus is empty give oxytocin or ergonovine.

TYPES OF INJURIES SPECIFIC TO A PREGNANT PATIENT

Abruptio Placentae

Abruptio placentae is a common presenting complication of a pregnant patient who has been in an MVA. It is usually secondary to a decelerative injury or a hyperflexion of the torso over the pregnant uterus. Abruptio placentae is when the placenta separates from the uterine wall. A patient will present to the trauma room with vaginal bleeding, abdominal pain, uterine irritability, tetanic uterine contractions, and in frank fetal death.

The mechanism of injury is a shearing force of the placenta away from the decidua basalis. This is secondary to the compression of the elastic uterus around the inelastic placenta, with a simultaneous increase in abdominal pressure, thus creating a shearing effect.

When this shearing effect occurs, there is bleeding from the uteroplacental site. If there is release of thromboplastic material into the maternal circulation, the patient is predisposed to DIC.

Pelvic Fractures

Pelvic fractures in any patient, pregnant or nonpregnant, have a high mortality and morbidity. Pelvic fractures cause hemorrhage, fat embolisms, vaginal and uterine lacerations, bladder, urethral and ureteral lacerations, fetal skull fractures, and lumbar plexus injuries. Hypovolemic shock is secondary to retroperitoneal hemorrhage. The retroperitoneum can hold 4 liters of blood.

Uterine Rupture

Uterine rupture occurs after the 12th week of pregnancy. Up to the 12th week, the uterus is protected by the bony pelvis. Uterine ruptures occur in rapid deceleration events such as an MVA when the uterus is propelled into the anterior abdominal wall, causing the uterus to elongate and rupture.

TREATMENT OF THE TRAUMATIZED PREGNANT PATIENT

1. ABCs.
2. Cervical spine control with a cervical collar and backboard; clear cervical spine with an x-ray.
3. If pregnancy is over 20 weeks or uteral height is to the umbilicus, place the patient in the left lateral decubitus position.
4. Two large-gauge IV lines with normal saline or lactated Ringer's solution should be established.
5. Give oxygen 100% by facemask.
6. Take the patient's vital signs, and re-evaluate the vital signs every 5 minutes. Remember that the pregnant patient has a 40% increase in plasma and can lose 30 to 35% of blood volume before signs of hypovolemia occur. Have a high index of suspicion of intra-abdominal bleeding!
7. Perform a primary and secondary survey.
8. Perform other x-rays, including a pelvic x-ray if you suspect a pelvic fracture. Attempt to shield the fetus when performing the chest and cervical spine x-rays.
9. Examine the fetus. Note fetal heart tone, fundal height, and the presence of vaginal bleeding. Perform a pelvic examination and a rectal examination. Note the vaginal pH and check for ferning.

10. Trauma laboratory values should include a CBC, electrolytes, liver function tests, amylase, lipase, PT, PTT, type and crossmatch of blood, with special attention to the Rh factor. A uterine artery (UA) with culture should be performed.
11. A Foley catheter should be placed in all traumatized patients. Urine output should be noted. No or decreased urine output is a sure sign of intra-abdominal trauma.
12. Early abdominal ultrasound should be performed to look for abruptio placentae, a ruptured uterus, or retroperitoneal bleeding.
13. All traumatized patients should be monitored for at least 4 hours after injury. Note fetal movement and contractions greater than eight per hour, increased abdominal pain, or vaginal bleeding. An early obstetric consultation should be scheduled. All patients with fetal bradycardia, tachycardia, fetal beat-to-beat variability, or uterine contractions should merit an immediate referral to an obstetrician.

POST MORTEM CESAREAN AND CARDIAC ARREST

If the mother arrives at the ED within 15 minutes in full arrest and no signs of life (i.e., pulseless, no cardiac rhythm, and fixed and dilated pupils) and the fetus is past 28 weeks' gestation, a post mortem cesarean should be considered. Early thoracotomy and open-chest massage may improve both maternal and fetal outcome. Post mortem cesarean section is a very successful procedure if performed in the first 10 to 15 minutes. The best chance of fetal survival is when:

1. Gestational age is greater than 28 weeks or fetal weight is greater than 100 g
2. Cesarean section is performed:
    a. <5 minutes—excellent
    b. 5–10 minutes—good
    c. 10–15 minutes—fair
    d. 15–20 minutes—poor
    e. >20 minutes—unlikely

The classic vertical uterine incision should be performed. After delivery, a neonatologic consultation is scheduled.

BURN INJURIES

Definition

Thermal burns are divided into first-, second-, and third-degree burns, or they are classified by the depth of the burn by full thickness or partial thickness.

Epidemiology

It is estimated that 2 million thermal burns occur in the United States annually. Only 3 to 5% of all burns are life threatening. Two-hundred thousand of these burns are associated with clothing fires, and 20,000 persons die each year from burns or fires. For children younger than 12 years of age, burn injuries are the second leading cause of death. Hot tap water is a major cause of burns in children younger than 5 years of age.

Pathology

Of all the organs of the body, the skin is by far the largest. It has numerous functions, from thermal regulation to acting as a barrier against infection.

The outer layer of the skin is the epidermis and consists of five layers. The second layer of skin is the stratum corneum and is important for the passive holding of water. The third layer of the skin is the stratum germinativum from which new skin is formed. It is also where the pigment of the skin is stored.

The skin contains nerve fibers for pressure and pain sensation and a vascular supply that is responsible for heat regulation and control of radiation, and this layer also contains hair follicle and sweat glands.

Heat regulation is maintained by the stratum corneum, and any breach of the stratum corneum will result in evaporative heat loss, secondary to the distortion and derangement of the lipid-water barrier that is contained in this layer. Water loss can be 19 times greater than usual after an acute burn when the stratum corneum has been injured. This increased loss will continue for the next 18 hours. After 18 hours, the water loss is reduced to four times the normal rate.

When the skin is burned, it immediately undergoes coagulation necrosis, which leaves a pabulum composed of a warm, moist protein medium, which is an excellent site for bacterial growth. In the central zone of coagulation, thermal coagulation and irreversible cellular death occur. Leukocyte immigration is inhibited but is not completely blocked. Around the zone of coagulation lies the zone of stasis. In the zone of stasis, formed blood elements clot within a short period of time. This increases vasoconstriction, which decreases blood flow to the injured areas. If not treated, the zone of stasis will revert to a zone of coagulation. The zone of hyperemia is the area that surrounds the entire wound. It is a transitional zone, which is bright red and has an acute inflammatory process present.

Clinical Presentation

As mentioned, burns are defined by the depth of the burned area as full thickness or partial thickness or first-, second-, or third-degree burns. First-degree burns involve the epidermis and are associated with minimal injury, but these burns can be very painful. No blistering is present.

Second-degree burns or partial-thickness burns can be superficial or deep. Hair follicles, sweat glands, and the stratum germinativum are injured. A portion of the adnexal structures is viable. Blistering will be present.

Third-degree burns or full-thickness burns involve destruction of tissue below the hair follicles and sweat glands. There is no pain sensation, and thrombosed blood vessels will be noted in a firm, translucent exudate. If charring of the skin is present, then a fourth-degree burn is present.

The area of the body that has been burned is defined by the "rule of nines." The head counts as 9%; the trunk and back count as 18%; the chest and abdomen count as 18%; the chest and abdomen count as 18%; the arms count as 9%; and the legs count as 18%. Each percentage is used to document the amount of burned area of the body. Children, because of the larger head and trunk, have a slightly different distribution of burn area percentages. A simple way to gauge the area of burn is to use the patient's palm as approximately 1% of his or her total body surface area.

Laboratory Findings

A CBC, PT, PTT, electrolytes, BUN, creatinine, glucose, magnesium, phosphorus, CPK, SGOT, SGPT, lactate dehydrogenase (LDH), GGT, and urinalysis should also be performed in the ED as baseline tests for any severely burned patient. An arterial blood gas and a carboxy-hemoglobin level should be taken on any patient who was a victim of thermal burns, especially those injured in a burning building. Blood and urine cultures should also be performed. An ethanol test and a drug screen should also be done. Blood and urinary myoglobin tests should be performed to rule out rhabdomyolysis.

Treatment

As with any trauma patient who presents to the ED, basic life support comes first, followed by the primary and secondary surveys. Any burn patient who presents to the ED with a severe thermal burn requires two large-gauge IV lines of lactated Ringer's solution, and the patient should be placed on 100% oxygen. The patient should also be placed on a cardiac monitor. All burning or smoking clothing must be removed. The patient must be kept warm. After the clothes have been removed, the patient should be wrapped in clean sterile sheets. A Foley catheter should be placed to monitor urine output.

Vital signs should be taken every 5 minutes until the patient is determined to be in a stable condition. The immediate threat to any burn patient is hypovolemic shock or respiratory injury secondary to inhaled smoke. Neurogenic shock can also be present if pain is present and severe.

The entire patient must be evaluated. Chest, pelvis, and abdominal x-rays are the minimal x-rays to be taken. In a burn injury that involves a fall or a motor vehicle accident, a cervical spine fracture must be ruled out. Extremities will need to be x-rayed for fractures, as in any other patient.

The nose and oral mucosa must be quickly examined for burns or edema. Remember to intubate early if there are signs of burns or edema of the oral mucosa. The risk of carbon monoxide poisoning must also be addressed in the patient who was in a burning building. Also, if the patient is not responsive to oxygen therapy, and the patient is very red, cyanide poisoning from burning carpets or plastic material must be considered.

All burn victims should receive tetanus prophylaxis. An NG tube should be placed to prevent gastric dilatation and an adynamic ileus, which is very common in burn victims.

Prophylactic antibiotics should not be given until the patient reaches the burn unit because of the high resistance of the residual bacterial population on the patient and in the burn unit. The most common organisms that cause infections in the burn patient are the gram-negative organisms. Streptococci and *Pseudomonas aeruginosa* are the two most common organisms.

If there is a circumferential burn that is compromising the circulation of an extremity and constricting eschar is present, with a decreased pulse or changing neurologic status, then an emergent escharotomy should be performed.

The goal of fluid resuscitation is a urine output of 50 ml/hr in adults and 1 ml/kg/hr in children. The goal is also for the patient to have a clear mental status with the elimination of all signs of shock and the resumption of normal cardiac function within 8 to 10 hours of the burn without metabolic acidosis.

The most widely selected formula for fluid resuscitation is 2 to 4 ml of crystalloid solution/kg/% of total body surface burn. Give one half of the fluid in the first 8 hours; then give one fourth in the next 8 hours; and give the final fourth in the next 8 hours.

After the patient has been admitted to the burn unit, a 0.5% silver nitrate solution or silver sulfadiazine cream is applied after débridement. Today, silver sulfadiazine is the agent of choice because of its lesser side effects. It can still cause rashes and an early leukopenia. Silver sulfadiazine is also painless when applied.

Any burn patient with severe burns should be referred to a burn unit for care. Any patient with inhalation burns will require a bronchoscopy. Patients with minor burns can be released from the ED after the wound is débrided, covered with silver sulfadiazine cream, and dressed. If the burn is circumferential or involves joints, hands, face, or genital area, the patient should have an immediate surgical consultation. All burns should be referred to a general surgeon for follow-up within 48 hours, no matter how trivial, to declare its thickness depth in 1 or 2 days.

THORACIC HEART TRAUMA

Definition

Chest trauma can involve the heart, lungs, bronchi, diaphragm, and great vessels of the chest. The trauma can be either blunt or penetrating.

Heart Trauma

Heart trauma can be either penetrating or blunt. The survival of a patient after penetrating trauma to the heart involves many factors, including the type of weapon used, the velocity of the projectile, the size of the myocardial injury, the part of the heart or chamber injured, the presence of cardiac tamponade, coronary artery damage, the time taken to reach the hospital, and associated noncardiac injuries.

Most deaths from penetrating injuries to the heart are secondary to massive hemorrhage within the chest. If pericardial tamponade is present, it can sometimes give the victim vascular stability—time to reach the hospital—by tamponading off bleeding. Acute tamponade can also kill the patient. The rule is that if there is a penetrating injury between the midclavicular line on the right and the anterior axillary line on the left, a cardiac injury should be considered until proven otherwise.

Beck's triad is distended neck veins, hypotension, and muffled heart sounds, secondary to an acute pericardial tamponade, myocardial infarction, pneumothorax, myocardial contusion, or systemic air embolism. Traumatic cardiac tamponade can also cause increased distention of the neck veins during inspiration and pulsus paradoxus. Pulsus paradoxus is a drop in systolic blood pressure of more than 15 mm Hg during normal inspiration. Both bronchospasm and hypovolemia can cause pulsus paradoxus.

Laboratory Findings

A CBC, electrolytes, glucose, PT, PTT, cardiac enzymes to include a CK and CK-MB, SGOT, SGPT, liver function tests (LFTs), and a urinalysis should be performed on all trauma patients. Type and crossmatch of 6 to 8 units of blood should be the standard procedure for any trauma patient. An arterial blood gas should be drawn.

Treatment

Any trauma patient, including patients with cardiac injury, should have a "safety net" established, including two large-gauge IV lines of normal saline or lactated Ringer's solution. The patient should be placed on 100% oxygen and should be placed on a cardiac monitor. The aforementioned laboratory examinations should be drawn. The patient should have the standard trauma x-rays done, including the cervical spine if necessitated by injury and x-rays of the AP chest, abdomen, and pelvis. X-rays of the extremities should be performed as required. An ECG should be performed to rule out an acute myocardial infarction, new bundle branch, or AV blocks.

The treatment for acute cardiac tamponade is pericardiocentesis. An 18-gauge, 10-cm spinal needle with an attached stopcock with a 20-ml syringe is utilized to perform this procedure. If possible, this procedure is performed with continuous ECG monitoring with one of the V leads attached to the needle. The needle is passed at a 45-degree angle for 4 to 5 cm slowly, as the syringe is being aspirated, toward the left scapula tip. As little as 5 to 10 ml of pericardial blood removed by pericardiocentesis can be lifesaving and can increase stroke volume by 25 to 50%. If no blood is aspirated, normal saline can be injected to clear the needle of blood clots. No air should be injected at any time. If more than 20 ml of nonclotting blood is removed, then the needle is probably too far in and blood is being aspirated from the right ventricle. If the result of the pericardiocentesis is positive, and an immediate thoracotomy cannot be performed, then a plastic catheter (inserted over a needle or a Seldinger wire) should be placed so that continuous aspiration of blood can be performed until the patient can go to the operating room.

Complications of pericardiocentesis are perforations of the right or left ventricle or coronary artery, any of which could produce a tamponade by itself.

Pericardial tamponade can also be diagnosed by performing a subxiphoid pericardial window under local anesthesia. If blood is present in the pericardium, the patient is placed under general anesthesia and an incision can be extended up as a midsternotomy to repair the cardiac injury. This procedure is more dangerous than pericardiocentesis and has no real advantage in the ED over pericardiocentesis.

An emergency thoracotomy can be lifesaving in the ED, in a few highly selected patients with penetrating cardiac injuries, when the injury can be surgically repaired. The survival rate of a patient who receives a thoracotomy in the ED is determined by the site of injury, mechanism of injury, signs of life at the scene and at the time of arrival in the ED, and the availability of a cardiothoracic surgeon.

An open thoracotomy is performed on an intubated patient by making an incision at the left fifth intercostal space, which is the space just below the horizontal nipple line. The incision should be as long as possible from the sternum to the midaxillary line in the axilla. The incision is extended through the intercostal muscles just above the sixth rib into the pleural cavity, ensuring not to cut the lung or heart. The ribs are then spread by a rib spreader as wide as possible so that two hands can fit into the chest cavity. If you are having trouble opening the chest, the intercostal cartilages above and below the incision can be cut to increase exposure. If the internal mammary artery or vein is cut, it should be clamped or suture-ligated. If the penetrating injury is on the right side, a right thoracotomy should be performed just like the left thoracotomy, which has been described. A right and left thoracotomy can be connected transversely by dividing the sternum with a Gigli saw or a rib cutter.

Once the chest is opened, a pericardiotomy should be performed. This is performed by grasping the pericardium with a forceps or by hooking the pericardium with a scissor blade. A scissor or a knife blade can be utilized to open the pericardium. If a scalpel is used, make sure that the underlying myocardium or the left anterior descending coronary artery is not injured. After the pericardium is grabbed, it should be opened with a longitudinal incision anterior to the left or right phrenic nerve, about 1 to 2 cm. This procedure should be performed with a pair of scissors. The entire pericardial incision should be extended from the apex of the heart or the diaphragm to the superior great vessels. If the pericardium is still tight around the heart, a transverse incision can be performed. The pericardium should then be evacuated of all liquid or clotted blood products, and open cardiac massage should be performed.

After the blood has been evacuated from the pericardial sac and open cardiac massage is being performed, the descending aorta should be clamped if severe hypotension or cardiac arrest is present. Clamping the descending aorta will increase coronary and cerebral arterial blood flow. The right ventricle and right atrium are the most commonly injured, so that the heart should be swung to the left to visualize the right side of the heart for injuries.

The descending aorta is exposed by lifting the left lung almost out of the hemithorax. The descending aorta is then bluntly dissected out, and the pleura and the fascia in the front of the aorta are opened. The posterior fascia is then undermined so that a finger can fit behind the aorta. A vascular clamp is then hooked around the aorta and closed. The time when the clamp is applied to the aorta is noted, and the lung is placed back into the hemithorax. The aorta above the clamp should have pulsations from the heart beating or from the cardiac massage compressions, but no pulsations should be present below the clamp.

If there is a wound to the heart, the examiner should place his or her finger over or in the wound until a Satinsky vascular clamp or a running 3–0 or 4–0 polypropylene suture can be applied. Ventricular wounds can be closed with a pledget and a horizontal mattress suture of 2–0 silk or Prolene. If the cardiac wound is near or around a major coronary artery, the suture is placed underneath the artery to avoid ligation of a coronary artery. Large wounds can be tamponaded off by placing a 5- to 30-ml Foley balloon catheter in the hole until a pursestring suture can be applied.

If a large defect is present and cannot be sutured while the heart is beating and cardiopulmonary bypass is not readily available, occlusion of the superior vena cava and the inferior vena cava by vascular tapes or clamps can slow the heart and finally stop it. The wound can be quickly repaired with wide horizontal mattress sutures. The heart is then restarted with 20 to 40 watts-second (ws) of electricity.

If coronary arteries have been injured, small ones can be ligated.

Larger main coronary arteries should have a saphenous vein graft performed by a cardiothoracic surgeon. Valve injuries and ventricular septal defects can also occur with penetrating trauma. These will need to be evaluated and repaired by a cardiothoracic surgeon.

If open cardiac massage is being performed, warm saline at a temperature of 40 to 42.2° C (104 to 108° F) should be poured over the heart to prevent ventricular fibrillation and hypothermia. If ventricular fibrillation does occur, the patient's heart should be defibrillated with internal paddles at 20 to 40 ws. Lidocaine should be given after cardioversion.

If the lung is also injured, a vascular clamp can be placed proximal to the wound to prevent a systemic air embolism and to stop bleeding. If there is a very large or central injury to the lung, then the clamp can be placed across the hilum. If a hilar clamp does not stop the bleeding, then the clamp is applied too close to the heart so that an individual pulmonary vessel should be clamped.

There is also a possibility of an acute air embolism occurring during intubation or while opening the patient's chest. If sudden cardiac arrest occurs during either one of these procedures, the cardiac chambers should be immediately aspirated for air. This procedure can be lifesaving though rare in occurrence.

Blunt chest trauma is usually secondary to a high-speed automobile accident. Blunt trauma to the chest can be caused by blast injuries, athletic trauma, football, soccer, falls, crush injuries, and seat belt injuries. Trauma can cause valvular injuries, rupture of an outer chamber of the heart causing bleeding and tamponade, aortic valve injury, myocardial contusion, pericardial injuries, and laceration or thrombosis of major coronary arteries. These injuries are caused by the "hydraulic ram effect" that compresses the abdomen forcibly, displacing the abdominal viscera against the heart with a sudden great force, direct compression of the heart and great vessels between the sternum and the spinal column, sudden acceleration or deceleration injuries causing a shearing force of great vessels, or strenuous prolonged cardiac massage.

Cardiac rupture is usually diagnosed at time of autopsy and usually involves the anterior right ventricle and anterior interventricular septum near the apex. It should be considered in any patient with persistent shock despite adequate hemorrhage control. If cardiac rupture is suspected, an immediate anterior thoracotomy or median sternotomy should be performed with cardiopulmonary bypass.

Myocardial contusions are quite common secondary to motor vehicle accidents (MVA). During a motor vehicle accident, there is rapid deceleration and the heart can be slammed against the sternum or spine. This causes subendocardial hemorrhage, focal myocardial edema, interstitial hemorrhage, and myofibrillar degeneration, which leads to myocytolysis with polymorphonuclear leukocytic infiltrates. The anterior right ventricular wall is the part of the heart that is most commonly involved with an acute cardiac contusion.

Cardiac contusion can also involve not only the heart wall but also the coronary arteries that can cause spasm, intimal tear, and compression, which can lead to myocardial injury and acute ischemia. Rarely, a severe transmural ventricular aneurysm can occur. A myocardial contusion can also impair myocardial function, especially in patients with pre-existing cardiac problems. These patients are at a greater risk for an arrhythmia such as atrial fibrillation, premature ventricular contractions (PVCs), or conduction defects.

Any patient who is in a motor vehicle accident at a speed greater than 35 mph at the time of impact and who was struck in the chest should be considered to have a cardiac injury. Signs of cardiac contusion are tachycardia out of proportion to other injuries or prolonged tachycardia, friction rub, or abnormal heart sounds.

A chest x-ray should be performed on all trauma patients. The greatest consistent findings on x-ray for a cardiac contusion are a fractured sternum, fractures of the first two ribs, or fractures of the clavicle. The most significant finding for a cardiac contusion is a fractured sternum. Acute cardiac decompensation can be diagnosed on x-ray by evidence of acute pulmonary edema associated with a normal heart size. A widened azygous vein is suggestive of cardiac tamponade.

Serial ECGs should be performed at 24, 48, and 72 hours in the presence of a possible cardiac contusion. New onset atrial fibrillation, new presence of multiple PVCs, or new conduction disturbances are diagnostic for acute cardiac contusion. If Q waves develop, this is a sign of a severe transmural injury.

Any patient who is believed to have an acute cardiac contusion should have a two-dimensional echocardiogram performed. It is a very noninvasive test and can evaluate the heart for cardiac tamponade, intracardiac thrombus or shunts, wall motion abnormalities, and the status of the cardiac chambers. It can also differentiate between right and left ventricular contusions by showing impaired regional systolic function, increased echo brightness of damaged or contused heart muscle, and increased end-diastolic wall thickness. The most common findings of cardiac contusion on an echocardiogram are right ventricular free wall dyskinesia and mural thrombi attached to the contused myocardium.

A technetium pyrophosphate scan can be useful in diagnosing an acute cardiac contusion. When myocardial cells die, there is an inflow of calcium ions that bind to crystalline lattice or hydroxyapatite within the mitochondria. This can be helpful in the diagnosis of an acute cardiac contusion, but it is not very sensitive. Radionuclide angiography and single photon emission computed tomography (SPECT) can also be used in the diagnosis of an acute cardiac contusion.

The treatment of a contused heart involves stabilization of any arrhythmias and treatment of electrolyte abnormalities and underlying cardiac disease if present. There is usually little treatment required other than rest for the contused heart. Oxygen should be given to keep the Po_2 greater than 80 mm Hg. Coronary vasodilators should not be used unless the patient has a pre-existing cardiac condition requiring their use. Good fluid volume should be maintained. Fluid volume can be determined by following the patient's pulmonary artery wedge pressure (PAWP). Good pain management with morphine is a necessity. Anticoagulation should not be used because of the possibility of increasing intramural bleeding or the possibility of causing an acute cardiac tamponade.

Penetrating trauma to the great vessels can involve simple or severe lacerations causing severe exsanguination, hemothorax, air embolism, or tamponade. Arteriovenous fistulas or false aneurysms can also occur. The severity of the injury is determined by the type of weapon used, the length of the weapon, the force of the weapon, and the area of the injury.

One rule when looking at a chest x-ray of a patient who has suffered a penetrating gunshot wound is not to assume that a "fuzzy" foreign body (i.e., a bullet) is secondary to poor radiologic technique. If a bullet is lodged against a large pulsating vessel, this can cause a "fuzzy" looking foreign object.

An arteriogram, venogram, contrast Gastrografin or barium swallow, or CT scan should be performed immediately on all penetrating chest wounds if the patient is in stable condition based on the physical examination. Gastrografin is the medium of choice at most trauma centers. If the patient is unstable, he or she should be taken immediately to the operating room for an open thoracotomy.

Blunt trauma to the great vessels can be life threatening and can cause death in a matter of minutes. The most common injury is at the isthmus of the descending aorta, secondary to bending stress, shear forces, and torsion stress. The majority of aortic injuries occur between the left subclavian artery and the ligamentum arteriosum. The second most common site of injury is the innominate artery at its origin. The majority of these patients die before reaching the hospital.

To diagnose an acute rupture is to have a very high index of suspicion. If the patient is alive and conscious upon arrival at the ED, he or she will complain of severe exacerbations of pain with a rise in blood pressure.

On examination, the patient may present with an acute onset of upper extremity hypertension, with a difference in pulse pressure from the upper and lower extremities, and a harsh systolic murmur over the pericardium or posterior intrascapular area.

The most-used tool in the ED for the diagnosis of an acute aortic rupture is a chest x-ray. If an acute aortic rupture is present, a widening superior mediastinum will be present. The normal mediastinum should be between 8 and 8.5 cm. A patient with a mediastinum wider than 8.5 cm with a history of trauma should be considered to have an acute aortic rupture until proven otherwise. The widening is usually caused by a subadventitial or periadventitial hematoma. However, the most accurate sign on AP x-ray for an acute ruptured aorta is the deviation of the esophagus by more than 1 to 2 cm to the right of the spinous process at T4. A deviated esophagus greater than 2 cm to the right is frequently due to a ruptured aorta bleeding. Also, blurring or obscuration of the aortic knob or descending aorta is indicative of a ruptured aorta. The easiest way to evaluate for a deviated esophagus is the placing of an NG tube, performing an AP chest x-ray, and then looking for the NG tube's position. Also, if the left apical cap is displaced from the left main stem bronchus by more than 40 degrees below the horizontal with obliteration of the usually clear space between the aortic knob and the left pulmonary artery, with widening of the right paratracheal stripe, and with displacement of the right paraspinous interface, an aortic isthmus tear should be considered. Paratracheal striping is a linear structure to the right of the tracheal air column.

If the patient is stable, a transesophageal ultrasound, CT scan, magnetic resonance imaging (MRI), or an aortogram should be performed. On an aortogram, the most common finding is a pseudoaneurysm at the isthmus of the aorta.

The mainstay of treatment in the ED for a ruptured aorta is good blood pressure control and stabilization. If hypertensive, the patient's blood pressure should be maintained at a diastolic pressure that does not go over 110 to 120 mm Hg. Fluid administration should be used sparingly. The patient should not perform any Valsalva maneuvers. Blood pressure control (the goal of systolic pressure is 110 to 120 mm Hg) can be achieved by giving:

1. Sodium nitroprusside, starting at 0.5 to 3 μg/min until the desired pressure is reached
2. Propranolol (β-blocker) for heart rate control, starting at 1 mg IV every 5 minutes, to reduce heart rate to 60 to 80 beats/min; can give 3 to 6 mg every 4 to 6 hours for rate control
3. Esmolol can be given as a continuous infusion, 500 μg/kg loading dose over 1 minute, then 50 μg/min over 4 minutes. If no response occurs, give another loading dose over 1 minute, then titrate up to 200 μg/min, for the desired heart rate.

An immediate surgical consultation is necessitated for any patient with a suspected aortic rupture.

Subclavian artery injuries are usually secondary to blunt trauma from motor vehicle accidents. These injuries almost always also damage the brachial plexus, thus a complete neurologic examination should also be performed. Horner's syndrome can also be present, which is indicative of avulsion of nerve roots from the spinal cord. The patient presents with an absence of a radial pulse or a decreased radial pulse and a partial tear of the subclavian artery. A patient can develop a subclavian steal syndrome. Subclavian artery injuries can be diagnosed by finding a pulsatile mass or bruit in the root of the neck. On chest x-ray, a widened mediastinum without obscuration of the aortic knob shadow will be noted. The diagnosis is made by angiogram. There is an association of other major vessel or cardiac injury in 10% of patients with subclavian artery injuries. Immediate repair is indicated to save the limb.

An injury to the innominate artery is second only to an aortic isthmus rupture. It is seen in patients with rib fractures, flailed chest, hemopneumothorax, head injuries, abdominal injuries, and fractured extremities. On chest x-ray, there will be a widened mediastinum. An aortogram should be performed. If a tear in the innominate artery is present, the aortogram will show bulbous dilatation of the vessel just distal to its origin, associated with a crescentic line across its base, representing retraction of the torn intima into the lumen of the vessels. There is an associated brachycephalic vessel injury or aorta injury in 10% of patients with an innominate artery injury.

GENITOURINARY TRACT TRAUMA

Definition

If urinary tract trauma is present, there is often other severe trauma present also. Urologic trauma should be treated only after the patient's airway, breathing, and circulation have been treated and other more severe trauma is addressed.

Clinical Presentation

A patient will present with five types of genitourinary trauma: trauma to the kidney, ureter, bladder, urethra, or genital area. Any patient with microscopic hematuria, fractures of the transverse processes of the lumbar spine or bony pelvis, a palpable mass in the flank or side of the abdomen, was involved in a high-speed accident, or has been injured by a high-velocity projectile should be considered to have an injury to the genitourinary tract until proven otherwise.

A patient will present with renal contusions, lacerations, ruptures, renal pelvic ruptures, and pedicle injuries. Most penetrating renal injuries are secondary to gunshot wounds. Gunshot wounds often have other associated injuries. Stab wounds to the kidney are usually not associated with other organ injuries. Blunt trauma to the kidney is usually secondary to a MVA or a fall.

Renal contusions are secondary to blunt trauma, which causes minor tears of renal tissue and bruises, but the renal capsule is left intact. Ninety-two percent of all renal injuries are renal contusions. Occasionally, there can be a subcapsular hematoma.

Renal lacerations account for 5% of all renal injuries. Lacerations cause disruption if the parenchyma with damage to the renal capsule with or without calyceal disruption. Lacerations cause perirenal hematomas and can fill and displace the Gerota fascia, which can act to tamponade the spread of blood within the flank.

There is controversy as to how to treat renal lacerations. Some authors treat lacerations to the kidney conservatively with bed rest and monitoring of the vital signs and hematocrit for signs of hematuria. Other authors suggest surgical intervention as the treatment of choice.

Ruptures of the renal pelvis involve extravasation of urine into the perirenal space along the psoas muscle. A patient will present with a high fever and increased abdominal pain. A rupture of the renal pelvis is often mistaken for a renal laceration. The diagnosis is confirmed by a retrograde pyelogram.

Renal ruptures are rare and account for fewer than 1% of all renal injuries. The kidney is fragmented or shattered, and this creates a large perirenal hematoma. The patient becomes clinically unstable within hours. An IVP will show extravasation of contrast in the abdomen. Open surgical treatment is the treatment of choice often with nephrectomy.

Renal pedicle injury is the tearing or occlusion of the renal vein or artery or its branches, which is usually secondary to a deceleration, a high-velocity injury, or a penetration injury. An IVP will show nonfunction of the kidney, and an arteriogram will show renal artery occlusion or bleeding. These injuries require surgical intervention.

Injury to the ureter can occur from both blunt or penetrating trauma. An injury can be easily diagnosed by an IVP, which will show a normal functioning kidney, but there will be extravasation of contrast into the abdomen. If not diagnosed early, these patients will present with an increasing fever, toxic appearance, and abdominal pain. The diagnosis is confirmed by a retrograde pyelogram.

Bladder injuries can also be caused by blunt trauma, penetrating trauma, and pelvic fractures. The bladder is an intra-abdominal organ in the child but not in the adult. In the adult the bladder lies in the bony pelvis, which gives it some protection.

Bladder contusions are very common in blunt trauma and are defined as bruising of the bladder wall with hematuria. Bladder contusion is treated conservatively with bed rest.

If there is a bony pelvic fracture, a large hematoma is usually present that will cause the displacement of the bladder either superiorly or laterally. Intraperitoneal bladder ruptures are usually a result of a deceleration injury to the abdomen when the bladder is full of urine. There is usually a very large amount of urine spilled into the pelvis. A cystogram will show intraperitoneal extravasation of contrast into the abdomen. The treatment is surgical repair.

Urethral injuries can occur to the anterior, bulbous, and penile areas or to the posterior area, the posteromembranous area. If a rupture of the urethra is suspected, a urethrogram should be performed. If a rupture is present, there will be extravasation of contrast at the site of the injury and no contrast will pass into the bladder. In a partial urethral rupture, contrast may pass into the bladder slowly. Partial ruptures are managed by passing a catheter into the bladder, and then the partial ruptures are allowed to heal. Complete ruptures will require surgical repair.

Posterior urethral injuries are associated with pelvic fractures. Anterior urethral injuries are associated with a direct blow to the pelvis (e.g., kicks). On the digital rectal examination, in a posterior urethral injury, the prostate will be riding high or detached. If detached, then the urethra is completely disrupted. The perineum should be visualized. If there is a posterior urethral injury with bleeding, the classic "butterfly rash" will be present, secondary to a perineal hematoma, limited by the attachments of the fascia lata.

Genital injuries can also be caused by penetrating or blunt trauma. The testes should be examined for tenderness, blue scrotal masses, cremaster muscle contraction, hematocele, or hydrocele. A scrotal ultrasound can be utilized to evaluate the testicle for tunica albuginea or tunica vaginalis injury, testicular rupture, or scrotal hematomas. Hematomas must be evacuated because of their high rate of infection and testicular atrophy. All penetrating injuries to the scrotum should be explored to rule out tunica vaginalis perforation.

The penis can suffer many injuries, including self-inflicted injuries, such as vacuum cleaner injuries or blunt trauma. Traumatic rupture of the corpus cavernosum of the penis or a fracture of the penis occurs when the penis is in an erect state. Usually the penis is forcibly impacted on a hard object, often the sexual partner's pubis bone or the floor. The patient will state that he heard a "cracking" sound with immediate pain, detumescence, rapid swelling, discoloration, and distortion. Surgical evacuation of the blood clot and repair of the tunica albuginea of the corpus cavernosum is required.

Examination

The entire abdomen must be visualized and examined. The patient must be "log-rolled" to examine the back of the patient. The external meatus should be examined for blood. If present, a retrograde urethrogram should be performed with contrast solution, with 10 ml of radiocontrast solution being injected into the urethral meatus. While this is taking place traction is maintained on the penis, and oblique x-rays of the pelvis are taken.

A cystogram is performed after the bladder has been catheterized. Five-hundred milliliters (5 ml/kg in children) of contrast is placed into the bladder through the catheter and AP x-rays are taken. The bladder is then washed out with saline solution, and another AP "washout" film is taken.

An IVP is utilized to examine the kidneys and ureters. One hundred milliliters of a 60% iodine-containing solution is injected IV, if the patient has no allergies to iodine. Films are taken at 5, 10, and 20 minutes. If extravasation, incomplete filling, or delayed visualization is noted, then a CT scan should be obtained of the abdomen.

A renal ultrasound can be utilized to examine the kidney's anatomy for hematomas, rupture of the capsule, or lacerations and enlargement of the kidney.

Diagnosis

The simple and most inexpensive test for trauma to the genitourinary tract is a dip stick test of the urine. A positive blood test requires further evaluation. A positive dip stick for blood and negative on microscopic examination for red blood cells is suggestive of myoglobinuria.

Laboratory Findings

A CBC, electrolytes, glucose, LFTs, amylase, lipase, and a complete urinalysis should be performed on any patient with any abdominal or genitourinary trauma. If bleeding is suspected, 6 to 8 units of blood should be typed and crossmatched. Blood and urine cultures should also be obtained if urine extravasation has occurred.

Treatment

As with any trauma patient, a "safety net" should be made. Two large-gauge IV lines should be placed with normal saline 0.9% or lactated Ringer's solution. The patient should be placed on 100% oxygen and on a cardiac monitor. The aforementioned laboratory examinations should be performed. The normal trauma x-rays should be performed, including x-rays of the cervical spine, chest, and pelvis. Remember that basic life support takes precedence over all other evaluations and treatment. Evaluation of trauma to the genitourinary tract is performed by urethrograms, cystograms, IVPs, contrast CT scans, and renal ultrasound. Early and frequent consultation with a urologist should be standard procedure.

HEAD TRAUMA

Definition

Head injuries can be classified as open or closed and primary or secondary. Closed-head injuries are further defined as diffuse or focal injuries.

Epidemiology

The leading cause of death for those younger than 44 years of age in the United States is trauma, and 50% of those who die, die of head trauma. The mortality rate for head trauma is approximately 40% in the United States, and total recovery only approaches 40 to 50% of those who survive a head injury. Mortality rates for patients with head injuries with a GCS score of less than 10 is higher than for those with a GCS score above 10. The mortality rate for patients with a GCS score of 3 to 5 is three times greater than for those with a score of 6 to 8 (60% versus 20%).

Pathology

The brain is enclosed in the skull for protection. However, this protection, which is rigid and inflexible, maintains the intracranial pressure (ICP) at a constant pressure. Head injuries are divided into primary and secondary brain injuries. When the brain receives a primary injury, there are axonal injuries and there is mechanical neuronal damage that is untreatable. Secondary brain injury is caused by hypoxia, ischemia, hemorrhage, hypercarbia, and increased ICP.

ICP is fairly constant. Elastance is the increase in pressure given and the increase in intracranial volume. Compliance is the reciprocal of elastance. The skull contains brain, blood, and cerebrospinal fluid (CSF). If there is an increased volume in any one—brain, blood, or CSF—then there must be a reciprocal decrease in one of the other two; if not, there is increased ICP. For a time, CSF will be displaced into the spinal cord, but when this space becomes full, there is a risk of brain herniation. Increased ICP is defined as a CSF pressure greater than 15 mm Hg; uncontrolled ICP involves a CSF pressure greater than 20 mm Hg.

As ICP increases, there is an acute vasodilatation and autoregulation is lost. As autoregulation is lost, there is a failure of resistant vessels to constrict normally, and systemic pressure is communicated to the capillaries and veins. When this occurs, there is an outpouring of fluid from the intravascular space to the extracellular space (vasogenic edema).

Anatomy and Physiology of the Head

The head is made up of the scalp, skull, and brain. The scalp has five layers: the skin, subcutaneous tissue, galea, areolar tissue, and the pericardium.

The skull is a bony container that provides protection to the brain. The inside of the skull is not smooth. It has sphenoid wings, orbital roofs, and a petrous apex, all of which with contrecoup injuries can cause tearing or shearing injuries to the brain.

The brain is compartmentalized and is attached to the dura. The midline divides the brain into left and right hemispheres at the falx cerebri. The brain weighs approximately 1300 to 1500 g and is approximately 1900 ml in volume in the average adult. The superior and inferior parts of the brain are divided by the tentorium cerebelli, brain stem, and cerebellum in the inferior part of the brain. The cerebral hemispheres connect the posterior fossa contents to the midbrain, which contains the tentorial hiatus. The white matter of the brain consists of axons and myelin sheaths. The gray matter contains nerve cells and the connecting dendrites and axons of the cells that form myriad synapses.

Cerebral blood flow to the brain remains fairly constant. It averages 3 to 4 ml/100 g of brain tissue with an average cerebral blood flow of 50 to 100 ml/g/min with 25 ml/100 g/min going to the gray matter and 75 ml/min going to the white matter. The brain receives approximately 15% of all daily cardiac output, and 20% of all oxygen for the entire body is consumed by the brain. Oxygen demand for the brain is driven by the PCO_2 level. Hypocapnia causes cerebral vasoconstriction, and hypercapnia causes cerebral vasodilatation. The brain will maintain constant blood flow even with total body perfusion changes.

CSF is formed in the choroid plexuses at a rate of 0.35 ml/min or 500 ml over a 24-hour period. There is at any one time approximately 150 ml of CSF in the brain and approximately 25 to 30 ml in the ventricles. CSF bathes the brain; acts as a cushion; and buffers the brain against injury. It also provides a medium for chemical substances to travel to intercellular spaces of the brain and for metabolites to be returned to the venous system. The path of the CSF is from the lateral ventricles through the foramen of Monro into the third ventricle and then via the aqueduct of Sylvius into the fourth ventricle, out through the foramina of Luschka and Magendi, through the basal cistern, to be absorbed in the arachnoid villi along the sagittal sinus and lateral sinus.

Clinical Presentation

Herniation is the great fear connected with any head injury. Herniation can occur at several locations. The most important herniation is a transtentorial or uncal herniation. The least important herniation is a cingulate or subfalcial herniation. Cingulate or subfalcial herniations occur when one of the cerebral hemispheres is displaced underneath the falx cerebri into the opposite supratentorial space.

A transtentorial or uncal herniation is usually caused by a head injury, which causes a subdural or temporal lobe mass that forces the ipsilateral uncus of the temporal lobe through the tentorial hiatus into the space between the cerebral peduncle and the tentorium. This is often noted in the trauma room as a fixed and dilated pupil on the ipsilateral side of the injury. The uncus herniates down and compresses the oculomotor nerve, causing parasympathetic paralysis of the ipsilateral pupil, along with compression of the cerebral peduncle, which causes contralateral hemiparesis. On rare occasions the contralateral cerebral peduncle will be forced against the free edge of the tentorium on the opposite side, which will result in ipsilateral paralysis, thus causing a dilated pupil and paralysis on the same side. This is a false localizing sign.

As the ICP increases, the patient loses consciousness. Sometimes as the ICP rises, the posterior cerebral artery will become compressed against the free edge of the tentorium causing an infarction of the occipital lobe. As the ICP rises and the herniation continues, there will be continued brain stem deterioration, which will lead to hyperventilation, extensor response (decerebrate posturing), apnea, and death.

Uncal herniation can also occur bilaterally, thus both pupils will be dilated with decerebrate posturing. Cerebellar tonsillar herniation occurs through the foramen magnum, but this is rare in head trauma. If this does occur, the patient will present with onset of bradycardia, respiratory arrest, and death secondary to medullary compression.

Closed-head injuries are defined as focal or diffuse head injuries. Focal closed-head injuries include contusion, skull fractures, epidural hematoma, subdural hematoma, intracerebral hemorrhage, penetrating injuries, and brain lacerations.

Contusions occur when the crest of gyri is injured. When injured, the area is surrounded by edema and the effects of hemorrhage, with overlying subarachnoid hemorrhage most frequently present. Contusions can occur at the site of impact or on the contralateral side, a contrecoup lesion. Contusions can occur anywhere on the brain but are most common at the subfrontal cortex, frontal poles, and anterior temporal lobes. The cortical gyri move over the rough surfaces of the internal skull and cause tears and bleeding.

Skull fractures can be mild or life threatening. Nondepressed linear skull fractures with the scalp intact do not require treatment. Depressed skull fractures are life threatening, especially if they are over the middle meningeal artery or a major dural sinus. They are classified as open or closed.

Fractures of the petrous portion of the temporal bone or any part of the base of the skull are called basilar skull fractures and are life threatening. Transverse fractures, which are rare, longitudinal fractures into the vault of the petrous bone, are most common. Basilar skull fractures can be identified on clinical evaluation by the findings of otorrhea, hemotympanum, disarticulation of the ossicles, and ecchymosis in the mastoid region (Battle's sign). If a transverse fracture of the petrous bone is present, it is usually in association with a severe head injury secondary to a blow to the occiput, with seventh or eighth nerve transection.

Epidural hematoma is secondary to arterial bleeding, usually secondary to a skull fracture, which tears the middle meningeal artery in 80% of the cases. The skull fracture usually does not cause severe brain damage in and of itself. Epidural hematomas can also occur if the fracture is through a large venous lake or through a major dural sinus. Epidural hematomas are rare in the elderly because of the close attachment of the dura to the periosteum of the inner table of the skull in the elderly.

Subdural hematomas are primary venous bleeding beneath the dura overlying the arachnoid and the brain. This injury is usually secondary to an acute acceleration-deceleration injury. The venous bleeding is usually secondary to a tear of the bridging veins that extend from the subarachnoid space to the dural venous sinuses or from tears in the pial arteries. As the bleeding increases, the blood dissects over the cerebral convexities from the sagittal sinus to the floor of the temporal fossa or from the frontal region back to the parietal and occipital lobes.

Patients at risk for subdural hematomas are the elderly and patients with atrophy of the brain secondary to alcoholism. These patients can present with subacute subdural hematoma, which will take 24 hours to 2 weeks before symptoms of injury can develop. Chronic subdural hematoma can occur after 2 weeks of an injury. Chronic subdurals are secondary to liquefaction of a blood clot.

Penetrating injuries secondary to gunshot wounds or penetrating sharp objects can affect brain tissue secondary to the energy exerted on the brain, causing shear force and direct damage to the brain. The degree of damage is determined by what type of object penetrated the skull, the velocity of the object, and the location of the penetration. Acute hemorrhage and increased ICP are acute concerns in the trauma room. All penetrating head wounds should receive antibiotics.

Brain lacerations are secondary to crude penetrating injuries that tear the parenchyma of the brain. Brain lacerations cause hemorrhage and necrosis to brain tissue.

Prolonged traumatic coma and *concussion syndromes* are diffuse injuries. Concussion is defined as a transient loss of consciousness that occurs immediately after a nonpenetrating blunt impact to the head. The loss of consciousness lasts only a few seconds to minutes, rarely hours. All loss of consciousness is secondary to impairment of the reticular activating system. This is usually caused by rotation of the cerebral hemispheres on the brain stem. Diffuse axonal injury is a tearing or shearing of nerve fibers that occurs at the time of impact. Coma lasting longer than 6 hours is considered diffuse axonal injury, usually secondary to an accelerating or decelerating injury. Diffuse axonal injury and recovery are dependent on the site and degree of axonal injury. This type of injury results in functional or physiologic changes rather than in grossly demonstrable or anatomic abnormalities.

Patients usually recover from concussion without sequelae, but rarely patients will complain of memory loss, persistent headache, insomnia, anxiety, and dizziness that can last for weeks or months.

Examination

The examination of a patient with a head injury begins with the history of the event that caused the injury (e.g., automobile accident, gunshot, fall). Vital signs should then be taken every 5 minutes until the extent of the patient's injury is determined. Cushing reflex, hypertension with bradycardia, is a sign of rising ICP and is often a terminal event. Remember that hypotension is usually not caused by a head injury. If the patient is hypotensive, look for another source of hypotension other than the head injury. In infants and small children, profound blood loss can cause hypotension along with increased ICP.

Every patient needs a neurologic examination that is as complete as possible, hopefully before the patient is paralyzed and intubated. Like vital signs, this is a baseline value that has to be followed to determine if the patient is improving or deteriorating.

The most common, and quickest way to determine neurologic status is the GCS. If a person can speak, the central nervous system

(CNS) is relatively intact. If a patient obeys commands, he or she has a fairly intact CNS.

Eyes		Score
Open:	Spontaneously	4
	To verbal command	3
	To pain	2
No response:		1

Best Verbal Response		
	Oriented and converses	5
	Disoriented and converses	4
	Inappropriate words	3
	Incomprehensible sounds	2
	No response	1

Best Motor Response		
To verbal command:	Obeys	6
To painful stimulus:	Localizes pain	5
	Flexion-withdrawal	4
	Abnormal flexion (decorticate rigidity)	3
	Extension (decerebrate rigidity)	2
	No response	1
		3–15

Diagnosis

A diagnosis is made by history, physical examination, neurologic examination, MRI or CT scan, and laboratory tests.

Laboratory Findings

A CBC, electrolytes, arterial blood gas, urinalysis, ethanol level if the patient is intoxicated, and toxicologic analysis if drug ingestion is suspected should be performed on all patients who have a head injury. A PT and PTT should be obtained if the patient is on coumadin or warfarin therapy. Fibrinogen levels should be also drawn in the ED if DIC is suspected.

X-ray Findings

If there is a severe head injury, there can also be a cervical spine injury. The cervical spine should be x-rayed to rule out a fracture. Only 5% of patients with severe head injury will have a spinal fracture. Skull fractures can be obtained to rule out depressed or linear skull fractures. The Towne view can be used to look at the occiput for fractures extending down into the foramen magnum. X-rays of the chest, abdomen, and pelvis should be performed routinely on all trauma patients.

The indications for a CT scan of the head are clinical neurologic deterioration, persistent decreased level of consciousness, persistent focal neurologic deficit, or a skull fracture in the vicinity of the middle meningeal artery or major vessels.

If there are no generalized or focal neurologic changes, if the patient is not intoxicated and has not lost consciousness, and there is no evidence of a depressed or linear skull fracture or a basilar skull fracture, then a CT scan series of the skull is probably not required.

Treatment

Any patient who presents to the ED with a history of a head injury should be evaluated immediately. Any patient who has had a loss of consciousness, deteriorating neurologic examination, obvious skull fracture, or altered mental status should have a "safety net" placed, consisting of two IV lines of normal saline or lactated Ringer's solution to keep the vein open; 100% oxygen via nasal cannula; and cardiac monitoring. The aforementioned laboratory tests should be drawn. If a trauma patient, the patient should have the usual trauma x-rays performed, including x-rays of the cervical spine, chest, abdomen, and pelvis. Patients who have not lost consciousness and who have no open or closed skull fracture, normal neurologic examination, no memory loss or other complaints can be discharged home with appropriate observation by family or friends. Those who cannot be safely monitored at home should be admitted to the hospital.

If the patient presents with a seizure after a head injury, give phenytoin 18 mg/kg at 25 mg/min with cardiac and blood pressure monitoring for hypotension. Any patient who has had a loss of consciousness, unequal or lateralized motor deficit, possible mass effect, or expanding mass lesion should have an immediate CT scan of the head with a neurosurgical consult. Any patient with a persistent decreased level of consciousness, depressed skull fracture, bleed on CT scan, basilar skull fracture, deterioration of neurologic status, or lateralized extremity weakness should also have a neurosurgical consultation.

If the head injury is severe, remember that basic life support should always take precedence over any other treatment, including a head injury. If a head injury is present, an adequate airway should be established and hyperventilation should be performed to decrease brain swelling. The P_{CO_2} should be maintained at 25 to 30 mm Hg. This should be performed in the gentlest manner with sedation and paralyzation. If a cervical spine injury is suspected, then nasotracheal intubation is preferred if there is no facial trauma.

Vital signs, blood pressure, and pulse should be monitored every 5 minutes. Hypotension can greatly reduce cerebral perfusion. Treat hypertension with increased ICP very carefully. Attempts to decrease blood pressure can lead to inadequate cerebral perfusion and death. Treatment of hypertension in a head-injured patient can lead to wide swings in blood pressure and cerebral perfusion.

If ICP is suspected and the patient has lateralizing motor findings, pupil inequality, and neurologic deterioration or a GCS score of less than 6, give 1 g/kg of IV mannitol as a solution of 500 ml of 20% mannitol (Osmitrol), rapidly. Mannitol creates an osmotic gradient and draws water out of the brain, thus decreasing ICP. The head of the patient's bed should be elevated to 30 degrees. This will also decrease ICP.

There is controversy as to whether to give dexamethasone to patients who have a head injury. It is good to know the policy of the neurosurgeon who services your institution. The dose of dexamethasone is 1 mg/kg IV, then 10 mg every 6 hours for 2 to 3 days.

If the patient is herniating in spite of the head of the bed being elevated to 30 degrees, mannitol, dexamethasone, hyperventilation, and immediate decompression should be considered by the most experienced individual present. If no neurosurgeon is available, an emergency burr hole over the temporal fossa on the side of the dilated pupil can be lifesaving.

The treatment goal of increased ICP is to keep the pressure under 20 mm Hg. If ICP is above 20 mm Hg, the patient should be hyperventilated to a P_{CO_2} of less than 20 mm Hg, and mannitol should be given at 1 g/kg. The patient should be paralyzed with pancuronium (Pavulon), and placed in a barbiturate coma, with an immediate neurosurgical referral.

NECK TRAUMA

Definition

The neck can be injured by blunt or penetrating trauma. The concern with any injured neck are spinal cord injury, airway control, and hemorrhage.

Pathology/Anatomy

The neck is divided into two triangles. The sternocleidomastoid (SCM) divides the neck into the anterior and posterior triangles. The SCM inserts on the mastoid and extends to the superior sternum and clavicle. This is the anterior triangle. The posterior triangle is bounded by the sternomastoid muscle, the trapezius, and the clavicle. The anterior triangle contains most of the visceral structures and the major vessels of the neck. The posterior triangle has few dangerous structures except at its base, which contains the spinal accessory nerve (cranial nerve [CN] XI), which divides the posterior triangle further into the careful and the carefree regions of the neck.

The platysma muscle is invested in fascia originating along the entire length of the clavicle. This is important because it can tamponade off bleeding from a neck injury and make direct evaluation difficult.

The anatomy of the anterior triangle includes the great vessels of the neck, the jugular veins, the carotid arteries, and the thyrocervical trunk. The vertebral arteries are protected by the bones of the neck. The subclavian artery is located in the base of the posterior triangle.

The neurologic structures can be injured by either blunt or penetrating trauma. The spinal accessory nerve, located in the posterior triangle, can be injured with posterior triangle injuries. The sympathetic chain ganglia lies posterior to the carotid sheath and is provided some protection by the sheath.

Clinical Presentation

A patient can present to the ED with low-velocity (e.g., stab wounds) or high-velocity (e.g., gunshot wounds) penetrating neck wounds. Vascular injuries are by far the most common type of neck injuries from penetrating neck wounds. Blunt trauma can also cause injuries to the larynx, trachea, or cervical spine along with vascular or neurologic injury. Patients who are accidentally or intentionally hanged present with airway, vascular, or cervical spine injuries. The carotid arteries can be avulsed after a hanging accident. Cerebrovascular infarcts can also occur secondary to blunt trauma injuries to the neck.

Examination

The most important part of the initial examination is a history of the event that caused the injury. Examine the patient for respiratory compromise. Determine if there is new hoarseness, pain on speaking, dysphagia, odynophagia, or hematemesis.

Always listen to the lungs to determine if there is a hemothorax or pneumothorax secondary to the close proximation of the neck to the superior lung. Ensure that the trachea is midline and nontender. Evaluate the cranial nerves especially CN XI. Feel for crepitus over the spine, mandible, trachea, and larynx. Determine if the platysma has been penetrated; if so, there can be a major source of bleeding. Do not probe wounds, because this can start uncontrollable hemorrhage. Wounds should be explored in the operating room by an ear, nose, throat (ENT) specialist.

Treatment

The major causes of death in neck injuries are airway compromise, exsanguination, and CNS injury. Airway compromise and exsanguination can be treated by the emergency health provider. CNS injuries occurring at the time of injury are usually fatal.

The mainstay of any trauma patient's treatment, whether a neck injury or not, is basic life support. A "safety net" should be placed consisting of two large-gauge IV lines of normal saline or lactated Ringer's solution. The patient should be placed on a cardiac monitor and on 100% oxygen. A Foley catheter should be placed. The patient should be immediately intubated if there is any sign of airway compromise. Remember that the neck is a closed space, and any injury to the neck can cause airway compromise; therefore, if there is any doubt about airway compromise, intubate early. As bleeding occurs around the platysma, the airway is decreasingly compromised, and intubation may become impossible in only a few minutes. Try to avoid a cricothyrotomy if at all possible, thus intubate early.

A cervical spine x-ray should be obtained to rule out a fracture. If an esophageal injury is considered, a barium or Gastrografin esophogram should be performed to rule out perforation. Fiberoptic endoscopy can be performed to visualize the gastrointestinal or respiratory tract. If there is penetrating trauma and vascular injury is considered, an arteriogram should be performed. The neck is divided into three zones when evaluating the vascular areas of the neck. Zone I is from the clavicles to the cricoid; zone II is from the cricoid to the angle of the mandible; and zone III is any part of the neck superior to the angle of the mandible. There is controversy as to if, and in what zone, a penetrating wound should be explored. Some authors believe that all penetrating wounds should be explored. Some believe that an arteriogram should be performed first. Some believe that only zone II and zone III should be explored. Currently, a CT or an MRI scan is much easier to obtain and is much less evasive. Prior consultation with the ENT surgeon who covers the trauma service should be made in advance as to how the surgeon likes to evaluate penetrating or blunt neck injuries.

Blunt trauma is treated much like penetrating trauma. If bleeding, airway obstruction, and neurologic changes are present, these patients need early intubation and an ENT surgical referral.

PEDIATRIC TRAUMA

The priorities of assessment and management for the pediatric population are the same as for adults, but there are specific differences in the management of children. The most common cause of trauma in the pediatric population is from motor vehicle accidents. Aggressive management of the airway and cardiopulmonary systems should be the norm. Assume the most serious diagnosis and treat the patient based on clinical findings. Consider the nature of the accident in relation to the child's different anatomy, initial appearance, initial vital signs, and changing vital signs and mental status.

Airway Management

The biggest difference in the pediatric population versus the adult population is airway management secondary to the child's anatomy. The child's airway is smaller. The smaller radius of the nasopharynx causes an increased workload to breathe. If edema or a foreign body is present in the smaller airway of the child versus an adult's airway, the child will have a larger percentage of obstruction than does an adult. The child's tongue occupies a larger percentage of oropharynx than an adult's tongue. The glottis is higher in the neck. The shape of the epiglottis is different in the child than in the adult. The child has more lymphoid tissue than does the adult in the oropharynx.

The chest of the child is also different from that of the adult. It is made up of more cartilage than bone and is more compliant. Therefore, direct trauma will cause fewer fractures in a child than in an adult. A child is also a diaphragmatic breather. The child's ribs are more horizontal than are those of an adult. This limits the child's respiratory compensation. The child also has a higher oxygen demand than does an adult. A child rarely dies from cardiac arrest; he or she dies secondary to pulmonary arrest. Pediatric trauma victims need 100% oxygen by a bag-and-mask device if they are not intubated. The child's airway is also much more compliant than is the adult's airway; therefore, by utilizing good airway control and a good bag-mouth-mask technique, you can ventilate a child effectively with an airway obstruction secondary to epiglottitis or foreign bodies in many cases.

If it is impossible to intubate the child, the Seldinger technique can be used in a small child to utilize transtracheal catheter ventilation:

1. Make a small incision over the cricothyroid membrane.
2. Attach a needle to a syringe, and insert the needle at a 60-degree angle caudad until air is aspirated.
3. Remove the syringe, and place a flexible guidewire into the needle, then remove the needle.
4. Place an 18- to 20-gauge end-hole catheter over the guidewire, withdraw the guidewire, attach the catheter to a syringe, and check to see if air can be aspirated.
5. Ventilate with 100% oxygen from the wall and an in-line pressure-reducing valve. (Wall oxygen is usually 50 psi.) The reducing valve should be set at the lowest effective ventilating pressure.

There is an increased risk of barotrauma as time goes on using this ventilation system.

Cricothyrotomy can be utilized in a child but is highly discouraged because of the danger of a major surgical error because of the child's smaller anatomy.

Induction and intubation of a child are also different from that of the adult trauma victim. A dose of lidocaine 1 mg/kg before intubation can relieve increased ICP.

Cardiovascular Management

To assess the circulatory status of a child, evaluate the skin temperature and capillary refill (<2 seconds). Capillary refill of 1 to more than 5 seconds over the forehead or trunk will require rapid volume replacement. Check the quality of peripheral pulses, because good peripheral pulses mean good peripheral circulation. Persistent tachycardia is a sign of hypovolemia. Tachycardia secondary to fear will fluctuate, whereas tachycardia secondary to hypovolemia will stay the same or increase as hypovolemia increases. Evaluate all of the patient's vital signs, knowing the correct pulse rate and blood pressure for the child's age.

As in any trauma patient, multiple IV accesses should be obtained via peripheral vein, intraosseous, femoral vessel access, or subclavian vein. Studies have shown that peripheral vein access delivers the greatest amount of fluid over time.

The initial fluid should be isotonic crystalloid fluids, either normal saline or lactated Ringer's solution. The fluid should be given in a 20 ml/kg bolus and then the patient's vital signs, pulse, capillary refill, skin color, and blood pressure should be reassessed after each bolus. If, after several crystalloid boluses (total of 40 to 50 ml/kg) have been given and no response to these fluid boluses has been obtained, and shock is persistent, then packed red blood cells should be given as type specific and crossmatched. If crossmatched or type specific blood is not available, give O negative blood.

Renal Perfusion Assessment

Urine output is the best monitor for renal status. In children, an output of 0.5 ml/kg/hr is acceptable. No urine output is secondary to intra-abdominal injury or hypovolemia secondary to a lack of renal perfusion.

Neurologic Evaluation

The neurologic status is evaluated by assessing the child's pupillary response, verbal response, eye opening, and motor activity. Use the modified pediatric GCS. Only one person should speak to the child, in a soft calm voice, to reassure the child, calm the child's fears, and tell the child what is going on around him or her. Do not lie to a child, because you will violate the child's trust and he or she will never trust another medical health care provider again.

Look in the ears and nose for CSF leakage. In an infant, evaluate the fontanelles for bulging.

In the head-injured child, a mild head injury can cause transient or no loss of consciousness. The child can have pallor, vomiting, breath holding, lethargy, or increased irritability. The incidence of hematomas on a CT scan in children also differs from that in adults. Space-occupying lesions are fewer (25 to 30) in children than in adults (40 to 50). There is an increased incidence of shearing forces in children with high-speed injuries.

In treating the child with a head injury, hyperventilation is the most effective method to decrease ICP. The goal of hyperventilation is to keep the P_{CO_2} between 25 and 30 mm Hg. The head should be elevated to 30 degrees to facilitate venous drainage from the head.

Mannitol should be given at 1 g/kg IV, rapidly. Mannitol will initially increase intercranial blood flow. Furosemide 1 mg/kg can also be given IV to reduce brain edema without increasing blood flow to the brain.

Any child with a suspected head injury should have a CT scan performed. The child's skull has a thinner calvarium, and the child is subject to leptomeningeal cysts or "growing skull fractures" after head trauma.

The child's cervical spine must also be evaluated differently from that of an adult. On the child's lateral cervical spine, the anterior placement of C2 in relationship to C3 can give a false appearance of traumatic subluxation. You can use the Swischuk technique to evaluate this pseudosubluxation. Draw a line from the anterior aspect of the spinous process of C1 to the anterior aspect of the spinous process of C3. If the posterior cervical line misses the anterior aspect of C2 spinous process by greater than or equal to 2 mm (1.5 mm is borderline), this finding is suggestive of a hangman's fracture. Only use this technique in situations in which C2 is displaced anteriorly on C3. On normal pediatric x-rays that do not exhibit C2 on C3 displacement, the posterior aspect of C2 spinous process may be 2 mm or more.

There is also normal anterior wedging of the vertebral bodies. There can also be an increased distance between the odontoid process and the anterior arch of the atlas (predental space). A prevertebral soft tissue mass can vary with the infant's inspiration. Lordosis is absent in the child's cervical spine up to the age of 16 years. There is less cervical cord injury in children than in adults (3 to 5%). This is secondary to the laxity of the transverse ligament. In children younger than 8 years of age, this space is more than 3 mm in 20% of children. In adults, a distance greater than 2.5 to 3 mm is evidence of a torn transverse ligament or a subluxation of C1 on C2. In children younger than 8 years of age, a predental space greater than 3.5 mm is considered abnormal. However, a predental space of 5 mm may be normal in some children.

The prevertebral soft tissue space in children also differs from that in adults. This space can increase secondary to soft tissue widening due to edema or hemorrhage. In the pediatric population, the soft tissue density of less than 7 mm anterior to C2 or less than three quarters of the adjacent vertebral body is suggestive of normal. However, these numbers become more unreliable the younger the child is because of the flexibility of the neck, causing increased flexion. Furthermore, inspiration and expiration can cause a change in prevertebral soft tissue space.

Chest Evaluation

The child's chest is more compliant than that of an adult. A child is also a diaphragmatic breather. A child suffers fewer fractured ribs than does an adult. A child suffers underlying visceral injury without fracture of the bony thorax. Because of the anatomy of the child's chest, a tension pneumothorax produces more of a lung shift and more respiratory and cardiovascular compromise; thus, hypoxia will be greater in children than in adults. Children need 100% oxygen secondary to their higher oxygen demand. There is also an increase in aerophagia secondary to increased crying. This causes increased gastric distention and a tense, distended abdomen, which can increase the chances of vomiting an aspiration. Early NG tube placement should be standard procedure.

Abdomen Evaluation

Injuries to the liver, spleen, and kidneys are the most common intra-abdominal injuries in the pediatric population. A Foley catheter should be placed to evaluate urine output. A decreased urine output is indicative of an intra-abdominal injury. Look for a pelvic fracture and get an abdominal CT scan if injury is suspected.

EVALUATION AND STABILIZATION OF THE PEDIATRIC TRAUMA PATIENT

- For airway evaluation and stabilization, give 100% oxygen by facemask or bag-valve-mask; and intubate if indicated by using a rapid sequence of induction.
- Immobilize the cervical spine with a rigid cervical collar.
- Assess breathing; treat a pneumothorax; and remember that a pneumothorax is a clinical diagnosis not a radiologic diagnosis.
- Perform a primary survey.
- Evaluate the patient's mental status by using the revised pediatric GCS.
- Assess circulation, capillary refill, skin color, pulse rate, and blood pressure.
- Obtain a vascular access and a minimum of two IV lines; use lactated Ringer's solution or normal saline as IV fluid via peripheral vein, intraosseous, or femoral vein access. Once 40 to 50 ml/kg is given and vital signs are still deteriorating, consider giving the patient blood.
- Obtain blood for laboratory tests, and type and crossmatch the patient's blood.
- Monitor the patient's vital signs and keep reassessing the patient.
- Do a rectal examination and check for blood.
- Place a Foley catheter; evaluate the meatus or urethra for blood before placement of the Foley catheter.
- Place an NG tube.
- Place the patient on a cardiac monitor.
- Splint fractures.
- Keep re-evaluating the five key factors of life-threatening conditions: airway, ventilation, spine, shock, and level of consciousness.
- Obtain x-rays of the cervical spine, abdomen, pelvis, chest, and extremities for suspected fractures.

- If hypovolemia is suspected, give a 20 ml/kg bolus. (Remember that if the patient has stable vital signs that are not deteriorating and the patient is going to the operating room, do not give IV fluids.)
- Consult a surgeon as soon as possible.

PEDIATRIC INDUCTION AND INTUBATION

Give 100% oxygen by facemask for 3 minutes.
Give lidocaine 1 mg/kg.
Give a small dose of nondepolarizing relaxant, such as pancuronium 0.01 mg/kg.
Give atropine 0.02 mg/kg.
Give thiopental 1 to 4 mg/kg or ketamine 1 to 2 mg/kg.
Give succinylcholine 2 mg/kg IV.
Utilize the Sellick maneuver on the tracheal area.
Intubate orotracheally using the proper size of endotracheal tube.
Utilize pancuronium 0.1 mg/kg to keep child paralyzed.

Pediatric Resuscitation Formulas

Weights

Weights in Children Younger Than 1 Year of Age

Full-term newborn	3.5 kg / 7.7 lb
6 months	7 kg / 15.4 lb
1 year	10 kg / 22 lb

Weight in Children Over 1 Year of Age

Weight in kg = 10 + (age − 1)2 (over 1 year of age)

Pediatric Endotracheal Tube Size

Tube size = $\dfrac{\text{age of child in years} + 16}{4}$

Uncuffed endotracheal tube up to 8 years old
The distance to the midtrachea in centimeters from the front teeth is three times the size of the tube.
(Example: tube size 3.5 mm × 7.5 cm = 10.5 cm or 10.5 cm from the front teeth to the midtrachea)
Endotracheal tube size = size of a small finger
Endotracheal tube size = size of the nasal passage
Preterm infant 2.5 to 3.0
Term infant 3 to 3.5
3-month-old infant to 1 year 4.0
2-year-old infant 4.5

Pediatric Chest Tube Size

Chest tube size = 3 × endotracheal tube size (French)

Foley Catheter Size

Foley catheter size = 5 + age in years

Table continued on following page

Pediatric Resuscitation Formulas *Continued*

Nasogastric Tube Size

Nasogastric tube size = 2 × endotracheal tube size

Blood Pressure

Normal for Over 1 Year of Age

Systolic blood pressure = 80 + 2 (age)
The diastolic blood pressure will be 60% of the systolic blood pressure.

Fluid Resuscitation

Crystalloid solution 20 ml/kg
Lactated Ringer's solution or normal saline
Do not use dextrose fluids unless hypoglycemia is documented.
Hypoglycemia can cause osmotic diuresis.

Infant and Child Resuscitation Scoring

Score	Infant	Child
	Eye Opening	
4	Opens eyes spontaneously	Opens eyes spontaneously
3	Opens eyes to speech	Open eyes to speech
2	Opens eyes to pain	Opens eyes to pain
1	No response	No response
	Verbal Response	
5	Coos, babbles, or cries appropriately	Oriented with appropriate use of words
4	Irritable crying	Confused
3	Cries only to pain	Inappropriate use of words
2	Moans to pain	Incomprehensible use of words
1	No response	No response
	Motor Response	
6	Spontaneous movements	Obeys commands
5	Withdraws from touch	Localizes (purposeful movement)
4	Withdraws from pain	Withdraws from pain
3	Abnormal flexion	Abnormal flexion
2	Abnormal extension	Abnormal extension
1	No response	No response

Fluid Requirements

Newborn   Day 1: 3 ml/kg/hr D10W
Newborn   Day 2: 4 ml/kg/hr D10/.25% normal saline
Older children:
4 ml/kg for 1st 10 kg/hr
2 ml/kg for next 10 kg/hr
1 ml/kg for each kg over 20 kg/hr
Maintenance fluid: ¼ normal saline + 20 mEq KCl/l
Urine output: 0.5 ml/hr

Pediatric Vital Signs				
Age	Pulse	Average Blood Pressure	Respiration Rate	Wt (kg)
NB	70–170	80/45	40–90	3
1 Yr	80–160	95/65	20–40	10
2 Yr	80–130	99/65	20–30	12
4 Yr	80–120	99/65	20–25	16
6 Yr	75–115	100/56	20–25	20
8 Yr	70–110	105/56	15–20	26
10 Yr	70–110	110/58	15–20	32

Countershocks

Atrial arrhythmias = 1 J/kg
Defibrillation for ventricular tachycardia or ventricular fibrillation =
  2 to 4 J/kg

Pediatric Resuscitation Medications		
Drug	Dose	How Supplied
Atropine sulfate	0.02 mg/kg/dose	0.1 mg/ml
Sodium bicarbonate	1 to 2 mEq/kg/dose or 0.3 × base deficit	1 mEq/ml
Calcium chloride 10%	20 mg/kg/dose	100 mg/ml (10%)
Calcium gluconate 10%	100 mg/kg IV	
Epinephrine	0.1 mg/kg (0.01 mg/kg)	1:10,000 (0.1 mg/ml)
Epinephrine infusion	Start at 0.1 μg/kg/min	(1:1000 1 mg/ml)
Lidocaine	1 mg/kg/dose	10 mg/ml (1%) 20 mg/ml (2%)
Lidocaine infusion	20 to 50 μg/kg/min	40 mg/ml (4%)
Norepinephrine infusion	Start at 0.1 μg/kg/min	1 mg/ml
Isoproterenol hydrochloride	Start at 0.1 μg/kg/min	1 mg/5 ml
Dexamethasone (Decadron)	0.25 mg/kg/dose	4 and 24 mg/ml
Diazepam	0.2 to 0.3 mg/kg/dose every 2 to 5 min PRN IV	5 mg/ml
Dopamine	5 to 20 μg/kg/min IV drip	40, 80, 160 mg/ml
Dobutamine	1 to 15 μg/kg/min IV drip	250-mg vial
Furosemide (Lasix)	1 mg/kg/dose	10 mg/ml
Hydrocortisone (Solu-Cortef)	4 to 5 mg/kg/dose every 6 hours	100-, 250-, 500-, and 1000-mg vials
Mannitol	0.25 to 0.5 g/kg/dose every 3 to 4 hours	200 to 250 mg/ml

Table continued on following page

Pediatric Resuscitation Medications *Continued*		
Drug	**Dose**	**How Supplied**
Methylprednisolone (Solu-Medrol)	1 to 2 mg/kg/dose every 6 hours	40-, 125-, 500-, and 1000-mg vials
Insulin, regular	DKA: 0.1 to 0.2 units/kg/hr IV drip	
Racemic epinephrine	2.25%, 0.05 ml/kg + 2.5 ml NS	
Glucose D25W	0.5 to 1 g/kg = 2 to 4 ml/kg	D25W
Hydralazine	0.1 to 0.5 mg/kg	20 mg/ml
Lorazepam	0.1 mg/kg = 0.1 ml/kg	4 mg/ml
Morphine	0.1 to 0.2 mg/kg 10 mg/ml	

SPINAL CORD INJURIES

Definition

Patients can present with an anterior cord syndrome, posterior cord syndrome, Brown-Séquard syndrome, cervical sprains or fractures, or sacral, coccygeal, or thoracolumbar injuries.

Epidemiology

Motor vehicle accidents account for 41% of all spinal cord injuries; falls account for 13%; recreation injuries account for 5%; and firearms account for 9%. There are approximately 50 spinal cord injuries per 1 million persons in the United States each year.

Clinical Presentation/Pathology

Patients who present with cervical sprains and damage to ligaments can present with spinal cord instability and neurologic loss with or without a fracture. Total ligament disruption can present without a fracture, which can give the examiner a false sense of security when noting that there is no fracture on the lateral cervical spine.

There are several types or classifications of fractures. The hangman's fracture is a bilateral fracture through the pedicles of C2. The Jefferson fracture is a burst fracture of the ring of C1 from a vertical compression force, usually secondary to a diving injury. Teardrop fractures are large triangular fractures from the anterior aspect of a vertebral body. A burst fracture is a vertical compression fracture in which pieces of the comminuted vertebral body are forced posteriorly into the spinal canal. A clay-shoveler's fracture is an avulsion fracture of the spinous process of C6, C7, or T1 caused by mechanical flexion or by a direct blow to the spinous process. Unilateral facet dislocations are caused by a combination of flexion and rotation. It can be considered an unstable fracture if the dislocation is anterior and greater than 50% on the next vertebral body. A bilateral interfacetal dislocation occurs in pure flexion injuries. There is total ligamentous disruption, and the lesion is unstable.

A patient can also present with sacral or coccygeal injuries secondary to trauma. There are rarely neurologic injuries in sacral injuries, but when they do occur damage to sacral nerves can lead to bladder, bowel, or sexual dysfunction, and posterior motor and sensory leg dysfunction.

Coccygeal injuries are secondary to direct blows to the coccyx and usually only cause pain. Sometimes, however, there can be rectal tears, thus a visual rectal examination is always necessary with a coccygeal fracture.

Thoracolumbar injuries involve the T1 to T2 and the L1 to L5 spinal regions. Fracture of the thoracic spine or lumbar spine involves a compression fracture, burst fracture, and a distraction fracture.

Wedge or compression fractures are usually secondary to axial loading and flexion with failure of anterior column support. Wedge fractures are usually stable fractures, except for severe anterior wedge fractures that are greater than 50% of the vertebral body with partial failure of the posterior ligament. Most wedge fractures occur in the L1, L2, and T1 vertebrae. Patients with a wedge fracture of greater than 50% are at a greater risk for an acute ileus and should be admitted to the hospital for pain control and treatment of ileus.

A burst fracture is secondary to axial loading that causes the failure of the anterior and middle columns. The nucleus pulposus is forced into the vertebral body, secondary to a fracture of the vertebral end plates, causing the body to explode. This can cause spinal cord compression and compromise.

Distraction fractures are secondary to axial rotation. These fractures occur when a person is wearing a seat belt. There is posterior ligamentous failure. There are usually additional abdominal injuries associated with a distraction fracture. A "Chance" fracture is a distraction fracture in which the entire vertebral body is split horizontally through the spinous process, pedicles, laminae, and vertebral body.

A patient can also present with partial or complete cord syndrome. Often the final outcome of a cord injury cannot be determined until after the acute spinal shock has resolved. There are three basic types of spinal cord syndromes: anterior spinal cord syndrome, central spinal cord syndrome, and Brown-Séquard syndrome.

The anterior spinal cord syndrome is secondary to a compression of the anterior spinal cord itself or compression of the anterior spinal artery, which causes an ischemic injury to the cord. The posterior column is spared, therefore gross proprioception, motion, light touch, and vibration are all preserved. The patient presents with complete motor paralysis and loss of pain and temperature sensation distal to the cord lesion. This patient needs an immediate MRI or CT scan or myelogram to determine the level and the extent of the injury. The patient requires an immediate neurosurgical referral.

A central spinal cord syndrome, or a partial cord syndrome, is secondary to hyperextension injuries in the elderly who have a history of spinal stenosis or spondylosis. The cause is unknown but is suspected to be secondary to buckling of the ligamentum flavum into the cord during extension. These patients present with a weakness that is greater in the arms than in the legs and is worse in the hands than in the proximal upper extremities. There is very little treatment for this syndrome.

The Brown-Séquard syndrome involves only one side of the spinal cord and is secondary to penetrating wounds, tumors, hematomas, or laterally placed protruding disks. Patients present with paralysis and loss of gross proprioception and vibratory sensation on the side of the lesion and loss of pain and temperature sensation on the contralateral side. Remember that the pain and temperature fibers (dermatomes) are two levels above their point of nerve root entry. The level of decussation of the motor fibers in the medulla and the decussation of pain and temperature explain this phenomenon.

Examination

A complete neurologic examination should be performed, including a rectal examination. Bulbocavernosus reflexes, perirectal sensation and "wink," and priapism should be noted. Diaphragmatic breathing should be noted. The patient should be examined for gross proprioception, vibration, motion, and light touch. Remember that sensation is a product of the posterior column function and, if preserved, the injury is probably an anterior cord syndrome. *Sacral sparing* and sensation around the anus identify the lesion as an incomplete lesion.

All reflexes should be tested. If all reflexes are absent, then spinal shock is present. Part of any neurologic examination involves repetitive vital sign monitoring. Hypotension, paradoxical bradycardia, warm dry skin, and adequate urine output are all signs of spinal shock. Remember that the primary cause of hypotension and tachycardia is not spinal cord injury but hemorrhage, thus always look for other sources of hypotension.

X-ray Findings

In the ED, the normal cross-table lateral, AP, and odontoid views should be taken. When in doubt of an unstable fracture, flexion and extension views should be performed if the patient is neurologically intact. A CT scan, myelogram, or MRI should be performed to establish the true amount of injury. The MRI is currently the state-of-the-art test used for evaluating spinal cord injuries. An MRI or a myelogram should be performed if there has been loss of function, signs of an anterior cord syndrome, or partial cord syndrome that is not improving. Myelograms can identify disks, bone, and hematomas.

The ability to interpret an x-ray of the spine is very important in the evaluation of any trauma victim. Remember that the lateral view will show 90% of all injuries; the odontoid view will show 9% of all injuries; and the AP view will show less than 1% of all injuries.

Reading a Cervical X-Ray

1. On the lateral view, all seven cervical vertebrae must be clearly seen; if not, a swimmer's view must be performed. The superior margin of T1 must also be seen clearly.
2. Next evaluate all soft tissue on the lateral x-ray. The prevertebral space should be less than 5 mm from C3 to C4. If greater than 5 mm, this suggests a hematoma secondary to a fracture.
3. Visualize each vertebra separately for a fracture.
4. The four lordotic curves should be individually visualized. The spinolaminal line, the posterior margin of the vertebral body, the anterior margin of the vertebral body, and the tips of the posterior spinous process must each be viewed separately. In an adult, there can be up to 3.5 mm of anterior subluxation on a lateral cervical spine x-ray. If there is any doubt, a careful flexion and extension view should be performed.
5. Any angulation of the cervical column greater than 11 degrees should arouse suspicion regarding a possible fracture.
6. Look for fanning of the spinous processes. Fanning, if present, is indicative of a posterior ligamentous disruption.
7. Lateral masses suggest facet dislocations.
8. On the odontoid view, check for a fracture of the odontoid or the body of C2. Ensure that there is good alignment of the lateral masses of C1 with C2. Ensure that there is symmetry of the space between C1 and C2.
9. The predental space should be less than 3 mm in adults and 4 mm in children. If this space is larger than 3 to 4 mm, it is suggestive of a disruption of the cruciform ligament holding the dens (odontoid) forward against the body of C1.
10. Check the AP diameter of the canal on the AP film. The normal AP diameter of the canal should be greater than 9.3 mm. It should not be less than 13 mm on an AP film secondary to magnification on plain films. If smaller than 13 mm on a plain film, then there is increased risk of cord compression.

Treatment

Basic life support is the first priority in any patient with a spinal cord injury. The second priority is the preservation of residual cord function and the avoidance of any further injury. Next, treat the spinal cord injury by allowing the injured spinal cord to recover.

Any patient with a spinal cord injury needs immediate stabilization of the spinal cord with a cervical collar and a backboard, but remember that no cervical collar can immobilize the occiput of C1 and C2. The patient should be placed on a rigid backboard. Any patient who has a compromised airway should be intubated. An attempt at a good neurologic examination should be performed prior to intubation to determine the patient's current neurologic status for future reference. The patient can be intubated with good in-line immobilization and the Sellick maneuver usually without problem. The usual trauma x-rays of the cervical spine, chest, abdomen, and pelvis should be performed. The patient should be placed on 100% oxygen. A Foley catheter should be placed to monitor the patient's renal status.

The hypotensive patient presents a problem in the evaluation of a head injury. If the patient is hypotensive after all other sources of hypotension are ruled out, including hemorrhage, then the drug of choice for pressure support is dopamine.

Any patient with a suspected spinal cord lesion should receive methylprednisolone 30 mg/kg over 15 minutes, then 5.4 mg/kg every hour through a continuous infusion for the next 23 hours.

Traction is the key to preserving and regaining cord function and to remove any extrinsic source of pressure on the spinal cord. Cervical injuries are reduced with Gardner-Wells tongs, and thoracolumbar injuries are treated with a rotary bed. This should be performed by a neurosurgeon or an orthopedic surgeon trained in spinal management.

THORACIC TRAUMA

Definition

Trauma to the thoracic spine can be from either penetrating or blunt etiology. It can involve the chest wall, lung, bronchi, or diaphragm.

Clinical Presentation

Patients with thoracic trauma can present with no or minimal symptoms to frank shock. If the patient is making little or no effort to breathe, then the respiratory problem is probably secondary to head or spinal trauma or to CNS dysfunction secondary to drugs. If there is little or no air movement, then an airway obstruction should be considered. The most common upper airway obstruction occurs when a patient's tongue prolapses back into the pharynx. In a comatose patient, vomitus, dentures, or blood can also cause an airway obstruction of the pharynx, larynx, or upper trachea. The larynx can also be directly damaged by trauma. Acute inspiratory stridor is a sign of an acute upper airway obstruction. The upper airway must be at least 70% obstructed before stridor is present. Any airway obstruction requires an endoscopy or bronchoscopy in the operating room to visualize the laryngeal and esophageal anatomy.

A patient who is making a dramatic effort to breathe usually has an injury to the thorax secondary to a pneumothorax, hemopneumothorax, flailed chest, diaphragmatic injury, or parenchymal injury.

Examination

The chest should be palpated, percussed, and auscultated on every patient. Both anterior and posterior chest walls need to be examined. The chest wall should be inspected both as the patient inspires and exhales, looking for asymmetry or floating ribs of a flailed chest. Open "sucking" chest wounds should be immediately occluded with Vaseline or petroleum jelly gauze.

The classic paradoxical motion of a flailed chest can be noted with inspiration and exhalation. Remember to always examine the posterior thorax for paradoxical motion, because 50% of the lung surface lies posteriorly.

The neck should also always be examined for distended neck veins, tracheal deviation secondary to pericardial tamponade, cardiac failure, tension pneumothorax, or air embolism. Always palpate the neck for subcutaneous emphysema from a torn bronchus or from a laceration of the lung.

A patient with a diaphragmatic injury usually presents with a penetrating injury, particularly gunshot wounds or stab wounds to the lower chest. Rupture of the diaphragm is rare. It takes a significant amount of force to rupture a diaphragm. Most (80 to 90%) of all injuries to the diaphragm are on the left posterior lateral side.

Sixty to 70% of all ventilation depends on the proper function of the diaphragm. Trauma to the diaphragm can cause significant ventilatory compromise. The injury is not usually apparent at the time of injury, unless it is a large injury. Over years the viscera gradually tears secondary to the negative pressure. A patient presents with an intrathoracic bowel, which has become obstructed or strangulated secondary to severe compression of the adjacent lung.

A patient with tracheobronchial injuries or lower trachea or major bronchial tears can rapidly proceed to death secondary to bleeding or hypoxia. On examination there will be massive subcutaneous or mediastinal emphysema present in the neck and anterior chest wall. If the patient is treated for an acute pneumothorax and there continues to be a massive air leak, then tracheal or bronchial tears should be considered. Most tracheal injuries occur within 2 cm of the carina or at the origin of the lobar bronchi. The tear is usually a transverse tear in the main bronchi or a disruption at the origin of an upper lobe bronchus. The characteristic injury in the trachea is a vertical tear in the membranous portion nears its attachment to the tracheal cartilages. The patient usually does not survive tracheal or bronchial injuries.

Diagnosis

A tension pneumothorax is a clinical diagnosis not a radiologic diagnosis. All pneumothoraces are treated on clinical presentation. The diagnosis of other thoracic injuries is made by clinical presentation, physical examination, and radiographic views.

Laboratory Findings

A CBC, electrolytes, glucose, PT, PTT, cardiac enzymes, and an arterial blood gas should be performed on all patients who present to the ED with chest trauma. Six to 8 units of blood should also be typed and crossmatched. If abdominal injuries or 9th, 10th, 11th, or 12th rib fractures are present, also obtain LFTs on these patients.

X-ray Findings

Rib fractures may not be seen acutely on x-rays, especially lateral rib fractures. Cartilaginous fractures may not be seen at all. The simple upright posteroranterior (PA) view is the most specific view for acute rib fractures. Pneumothorax is seen better on expiratory films than on inspiratory films. If possible, both expiratory and inspiratory films should be taken. Always examine the first and second ribs for a fracture on the x-ray. There is an increased risk of myocardial contusion, bronchial tears, or major vascular injury with a first or second rib injury.

Always look for fractures of the 9th, 10th, and 11th ribs. These ribs overlie the spleen and liver and, if fractured, can puncture or lacerate these organs. Any patient who is tachycardiac and hypotensive with lower rib fractures must be assumed to have a spleen or liver laceration until proven otherwise.

A patient with a ruptured diaphragm or a tear will present with abnormal lower lung fields on an x-ray. If an NG tube is in place, the tube will be seen going into the abdomen and then up into the chest as the stomach passes through the diaphragmatic tear. The diagnosis of a diaphragmatic tear can be made by an upper gastrointestinal barium or Gastrografin series to look for viscera into the chest. A CT scan with contrast or an intraperitoneal technetium sulfur colloid test can also be performed.

Treatment

Any patient who presents to the ED with shortness of breath or a history of trauma to the chest should have two large-gauge IV lines of normal saline 0.9% or lactated Ringer's solution placed. The patient should also be placed on a cardiac monitor and on 100% oxygen. A portable chest x-ray should be performed, and the aforementioned laboratory tests should be performed. As with any patient with an airway problem, basic life support should be addressed as the airway first, breathing second, and circulation third. If the patient is hypovolemic, then the patient should be treated with fluids. Any patient who is hypovolemic should be ventilated at only a rate of 8 to 10 ml/kg tidal volume at 10 to 14 times a minute until venous return improves. This is important secondary to a hypovolemic patient in whom ventilation with excessive pressures can further reduce venous return and cause cardiac arrest. If the patient also has subpleural blebs, vigorous bagging of a patient can cause an acute tension pneumothorax.

A patient with hemoptysis or a hemopneumothorax is at increased risk of a systemic air embolism and flooding of the alveoli with blood, causing increased hypoxia.

Any patient with the clinical presentation of hemothorax or pneumothorax should immediately have a 14-gauge or large needle placed into the second intercostal space, midclavicular line, to relieve the pressure. A chest tube should then be placed through the fourth or fifth intercostal space anterior axillary line on the affected side of the pneumothorax or hemothorax. Once the chest tube is in place, it should be connected to 20 to 30 cm H_2O.

Pain caused by a flailed chest can be treated with intercostal nerve blocks. If the patient's pain is controlled, ventilation will increase. Long-acting 0.5% bupivacaine hydrochloride (Marcaine) mixed equally with 1% lidocaine with epinephrine can be used to relieve pain for up to 6 to 8 hours.

BIBLIOGRAPHY

Brandenburg RO, Fuster V, Giuliani ER, et al (eds): Cardiology Fundamentals and Practice. Chicago, Year Book Medical Publishers, 1987

Braunwald E, Isselbacher KJ, Petersdorf RG, et al (eds): Harrison's Principles of Internal Medicine, 11th ed. New York, McGraw-Hill, 1987

Connolly JF: The Management of Fractures and Dislocations: An Atlas. Philadelphia, WB Saunders, 1981

Crenshaw AH: Campbell's Operative Orthopedics, 7th ed. St Louis, CV Mosby, 1987

Davis JH, Drucker WR, Foster RS, et al (eds): Clinical Surgery. St Louis, CV Mosby, 1987

Hamilton GC, Sanders AB, Strange GR, et al (eds): Emergency Medicine: An Approach to Clinical Problem-Solving. Philadelphia, WB Saunders, 1991

Hardy JD, Kukora JS, Pass HI (eds): Hardy's Textbook of Surgery. Philadelphia, JB Lippincott, 1983

Kravis TC, Warner CG, Jacobs LM (eds): Emergency Medicine: A Comprehensive Review, 3rd ed. New York, Raven Press, 1993

May HL, Aghababian RV, Fleisher GR (eds): Emergency Medicine, 2nd ed. Boston, Little, Brown, 1992

Rockwood CA, Wilkins KE, King RE (eds): Fractures in Children. Philadelphia, JB Lippincott, 1984

Rosen P, Barkin RM (eds): Emergency Medicine: Concepts and Clinical Practice, 3rd ed. St Louis, Mosby-Year Book, 1992

Schwartz GR, Cayton CG, Manglesen MA, et al (eds): Principles and Practice of Emergency Medicine, 3rd ed. Philadelphia, Lea & Febiger, 1992

Schwartz SI, Shires GT, Spencer FC (eds): Principles of Surgery, 5th ed. New York, McGraw-Hill, 1989

Tintinalli JE, Krone RL, Ruiz E (eds): Emergency Medicine: A Comprehensive Study Guide, 4th ed. New York, McGraw-Hill, 1996

Turek SL: Orthopedic Principles and Their Applications, 4th ed. Philadelphia, JB Lippincott, 1984

Chapter 19

Urology Emergencies

ACUTE RENAL FAILURE

Definition

Acute renal failure is a constellation of disease which leads to the excessive accumulation of nitrogenous waste products in the blood. Acute renal failure can be divided into two types based on the amount of urine produced: (1) oliguric renal failure, with less than 500 ml in a 24-hour period, and (2) nonoliguric renal failure, with more than 500 ml of urine production in a 24-hour period. Acute renal failure is further divided into three causes: (1) renal, (2) prerenal, and (3) postrenal.

Pathology

The kidneys excrete end-product waste material as creatinine, urea, and uric acid. They also control the electrolyte balance of potassium, sodium, chloride, and hydrogen ions. Ninety-nine percent of the plasma glomerulus ultrafiltrate is reabsorbed in the tubules. The remaining 1% is passed into the collecting system of ureters, bladder, and urethra as urine. Small amounts of blood are passed on as filtrate, and 0.5% of the plasma protein is also passed on in the filtrate. The term glomerular filtration rate (GFR) is the normal amount of filtrate per minute that passes through the kidney, approximately 125 ml/min.

Causes of prerenal acute renal failure include:

Acute pulmonary edema
Valvular heart disease
Myocardial dysfunction
Peritonitis
Pancreatitis
Anaphylaxis

Congestive heart failure
Hypovolemia
Pericardial tamponade
Hepatic failure
Septic shock

Causes of acute renal failure include:

Drug-induced renal failure;
  penicillin, sulfonamides, al-
  lopurinol
Radiographic dyes
Pigments
Ethylene glycol poisoning
Myeloma of the kidney
Thrombotic thrombocytopenic
  purpura
Disseminated intravascular co-
  agulation
Glomerulonephritis

Poststreptococcal nephritis
Lupus erythematosus
Anesthetics
Ischemic tubular necrosis
Uric acid nephropathy
Nonsteroidal anti-inflammatory
  drugs (NSAIDs)
Scleroderma
Malignant hypertension
Bacterial endocarditis
Systemic vasculitis

Causes of acute postrenal failure include:

Kidney stones	Prostatic hypertrophy
Urethral stricture	Bladder tumors
Meatal stenosis	Phimosis
Cancer of the prostate	Neurogenic bladder
Calculi	Papillary necrosis
Intrinsic or extrinsic tumors of the collecting system	

Postrenal renal failure is secondary to a mechanical blockage of the collecting system. Prerenal failure is caused by volume depletion or volume overload. Acute renal failure is caused by an ischemic injury or a nephrotoxic injury to the kidney.

Rapidly progressive glomerulonephritis (RPGN) is a syndrome that involves:

1. Oliguria or anuria
2. Hypertension
3. Inflammation of the glomeruli with hematuria with or without red blood cell casts
4. Very rapid decline in renal function due to azotemia
5. Fifty percent of the glomeruli will have circumferential crescents on a histologic biopsy
6. When rapidly progressive anti-glomerular basement membrane (GBM) glomerulonephritis is present, this is called Goodpasture's syndrome.

Clinical Presentation

Patients with acute renal failure can present with acid-base balance disturbances, electrolyte disturbances, hematuria, proteinuria, or azotemia. Azotemia is an increased level of plasma concentrations of creatinine and urea, which are both end products of protein metabolism.

Examination

The patient should be given a complete examination, including a pelvic examination to rule out tumors (obstruction) and a rectal examination to rule out prostate hypertrophy or tumor.

Radiography

An intravenous pyelogram (IVP) should be performed to rule out obstructions causing acute renal failure. This test must be considered to be an additional risk to the patient who is already azotemic. If IVP cannot or should not be performed, an ultrasonograph can be performed to evaluate the patient's anatomy. A computed tomography (CT) of the abdomen can also be utilized to evaluate hydronephrosis and dilated ureters and obstructive tumors or retroperitoneal hemorrhage.

Laboratory Findings

A complete blood count (CBC), electrolytes, including a blood urea nitrogen (BUN) and creatinine, arterial blood gas, and a urinalysis should be performed on all patients in acute renal failure. A 24-hour urine test should also be performed after hospitalization. On urinalysis, heme, protein, ketones, and pH should be checked for on dipstick along with microscopic examination of the urine. Casts are products of tubular epithelial cells formed from proteins that gel at a low urine pH and high concentrations and are formed in the presence of albumin, tubular cells, and red blood cells. Casts are described as granular, fatty, hyaline, red, or white.

Hyaline casts are formed secondary to dehydration or excessive exercise, and these casts have no contents. White blood cell casts connote renal parenchymal inflammation. Red blood cell casts imply glomerular damage. A red blood cell cast suggests vasculitis or glomerulonephritis. Granular casts are casts that contain cellular debris and remnants, and these casts suggest acute tubular necrosis. Fatty casts imply nephrotic syndrome and are present with proteinuria and in some cases in nonglomerular disease. If casts contain eosinophils after staining of sediment, this is indicative of an allergic interstitial nephritis. If uric acid crystals are present, this suggests ethylene glycol ingestion.

The normal kidney filters approximately 12 g of protein in a 24-hour period with only 40 to 80 mg of protein being passed in the urine. Increased protein excretion above 150 mg in a 24-hour period is considered abnormal in adults and 140 mg in a 24-hour period is considered abnormal in children. Protein excretion greater than 2 g in a 24-hour period is indicative of glomerular disease. Less than 2 g in a 24-hour period is indicative of tubular disease. When protein loss exceeds the liver's capacity to synthesize albumin, hypoalbuminemia occurs and is indicative of nephrotic syndrome. Hypoalbuminemia leads to decreased plasma oncotic pressure and thus to an accumulation of edema in the extremities. A new onset of edema is the hallmark of acute nephrotic syndrome. Usually the 24-hour protein will exceed 3.5 g in nephrotic syndrome. Serum creatinine is a very specific gauge of GFR for a 24-hour period. Creatinine is the breakdown of muscle protein. Serum creatinine is a function of the amount of muscle breakdown (protein) that enters the blood, its rate of excretion, and its distribution. The amount of serum creatinine that enters the blood and the volume of distribution are fairly constant; therefore, any change in serum creatinine reflects the GFR or renal function. Acute rhabdomyolysis is an example of an increased level of creatinine entering the blood. Creatinine is filtered by the glomerulus. The normal serum creatinine level is 0.5 mg/dl in thin persons to 1.5 mg/dl in muscular persons.

BUN is a function of protein intake and turnover. Urea clearance is decreased in patients with prerenal azotemia, acute obstruction, or liver failure. BUN will rise with increased protein intake, trauma, gastrointestinal bleeding, infection, or intake of corticosteroids or tetracycline.

Urinary and serum sodium concentration should be about the same. If there is a low urinary concentration, it indicates that the reabsorption system is intact. Also obtain a fractional excretion of sodium (FENa), which will help to differentiate between prerenal azotemia and acute tubular necrosis. The normal urine sodium is 20 mEq/l, and the normal FENa is less than 1% of the total urine sodium. If the urine concentration is less than 20 mEq/l in the oliguric patient, then the patient has prerenal azotemia. If the urine sodium is greater than 40 mEq/l and the FENa is greater than 1%, then the patient has acute tubular necrosis.

Diagnosis

A diagnosis is made by physical examination, history, radiographic studies, 24-hour urine tests, BUN, creatinine, and electrolyte evaluation.

Treatment

A patient with acute postrenal failure should be treated with IV fluids, and the cause of obstruction should be relieved. A Foley catheter should be placed if the cause is from prostatic hypertrophy. A percutaneous nephrostomy tube is required if a ureteral occlusion is present. If no urine is obtained when the Foley catheter is placed, ultrasonography should be performed to evaluate the patient's anatomy.

Prerenal failure, when caused by decreased intravascular volume, should be addressed by giving IV normal saline or lactated Ringer's solution to the patient. If cardiac failure is the cause of prerenal failure (prerenal azotemia), the intravascular volume should be reduced by diuretics. If the cause is related to a surgical pathology, such as bowel infarction or valvular heart disease, these problems should be corrected.

In acute renal failure from acute ischemic injury or nephrotic injury (e.g., acute tubular necrosis), the kidneys can be supported with fluid and electrolyte management along with peritoneal dialysis or hemodialysis until recovery. Acute onset of edema, red and white blood cell casts, proteinuria with hypertension, pulmonary edema, and oliguria are suggestive of acute glomerulonephritis. A history of the use of antibiotics or NSAIDs should always be obtained.

Patients in renal failure are placed on a high-calorie (3000 to 4000), low-protein (40 to 60 g), low-sodium (2 to 3 g), low-potassium (60 to 80 mEq) diet. Fluids should be restricted to urine daily output plus 500 ml of PO or IV solutions.

Patients with nephrotic syndrome are at increased risk for deep venous thrombosis, renal vein thrombosis, and pulmonary embolism. These patients are in a hypercoagulable state secondary to the loss of antithrombin III and fibrinolytic factors. Patients with nephrotic syndrome are often hyperlipidemic.

Dopamine in low renal doses, 1 to 3 μg/kg/min, can improve cortical blood flow in acute renal failure. Drugs such as magnesium, digoxin, and sedatives should be used with caution.

Treatment of rapidly progressive glomerulonephritis and Goodpasture's syndrome is the same as treatment for acute renal failure. Most patients recover renal function spontaneously. Some institutions use plasmapheresis with immunosuppressive drugs to treat anti-GBM failure. Other institutions have used massive IV doses of steroids to treat Goodpasture's syndrome.

The patient should be admitted to the hospital, and a referral should be made to a nephrologist.

COMMON DISORDERS OF THE PENIS

Definition

Balanitis is an acute inflammation of the glans penis. Posthitis is an acute inflammation of the foreskin. Balanoposthitis is inflammation of both the glans penis and the foreskin in combination. Phimosis is the inability to retract the foreskin proximally from the glans penis. Paraphimosis is the inability to reduce the proximal portion of the foreskin over the distal glans penis to its natural lie. Priapism is when the corpora cavernosa is engorged and the blood has stagnated there. Peyronie's disease is a sudden or gradual curvature with erection of the dorsal penis. Fractures of the penis are uncommon but do occur, usually from vigorous sexual activity.

Pathology/Clinical Presentation

Balanoposthitis is usually caused by poor hygiene. When balanoposthitis is recurrent, it can be an early sign of diabetes.

Phimosis is also usually caused by poor hygiene. It can also be caused by preputial injury or scarring from surgery or trauma.

Paraphimosis is caused by venous engorgement and glans penis edema.

Priapism is caused by engorgement of the corpora cavernosa and thus stagnation of venous blood causing urinary retention, infection, and impotence. Causes of priapism are divided into reversible or nonreversible causes. Common reversible causes are sickle cell anemia, iatrogenic injection of prostaglandin E_1 (PGE_1), phentolamine, or papaverine secondary to treatment of impotence. Leukemic infiltration is also a common cause in chemotherapy patients. Nonreversible causes of priapism are high spinal cord lesions, medications such as trazodone (Desyrel) or phenothiazines. Also idiopathic causes can cause priapism.

A fracture of the penis is caused by a rupture of the tunica albuginea. The penis will be tender, swollen, and discolored secondary to bleeding. A loud, sudden "snapping" sound is often heard during sexual intercourse or sexual activity.

Treatment

Treatment of balanoposthitis is warm soapy water and good hygiene. If secondary infection is present, antibiotics should be given.

If phimosis is present with urinary retention secondary to scarring over the meatus of the penis, a hemostat can be used to dilate the preputial ostium to relieve the urinary retention. A urologic consultation should be ensured.

Paraphimosis is a urologic emergency. The foreskin must be reduced secondary to arterial compromise and possible gangrene secondary to venous engorgement. Treatment consists of local infiltration of 1% lidocaine around the foreskin constricting band, and then a vertical incision of the band should be performed to decompress the glans, thus allowing the foreskin to reduce over the glans penis.

Treatment of priapism can be divided into medical and nonmedical treatment based on reversible or nonreversible causes. If priapism does not respond to medical treatment, a urologic consultation is necessary for surgical shunting. If priapism is caused by sickle cell disease, subcutaneous (SQ) terbutaline 0.25 to 0.5 mg every 4 to 6 hours can be used along with a packed red blood cell transfusion. If there is no response, consider hyperbaric oxygenation. If caused by phentolamine, PGE_1, or papaverine, give terbutaline 0.25 to 0.5 mg SQ every 4 to 6 hours and attempt to aspirate 30 to 90 ml of corporal blood, then inject 30 to 90 ml of 10 mg Neo-Synephrine in 500 ml of normal saline. If priapism is secondary to leukemic infiltration, give terbutaline 0.25 to 0.5 mg SQ every 4 to 6 hours. If priapism is caused by phenothiazines or by trazodone, give terbutaline 0.25 to 0.5 mg SQ every 4 to 6 hours along with pseudoephedrine instillation, corporal aspiration, and heparin irrigation with surgical shunting.

Peyronie's disease only requires reassurance and a urologic referral.

Treatment of a fractured penis requires a urologic referral. A retrograde urethogram should be performed to ensure the integrity of the urethra. Hematoma evacuation and suturing of the apposition of the disrupted tunica albuginea is the definitive treatment.

EPIDIDYMITIS

Definition

Epididymitis is an acute intrascrotal inflammatory process that may or may not be caused by a bacterial infection. Epididymitis is often divided into two types: nonbacterial epididymitis, which is not sexually transmitted, and bacterial epididymitis, which is sexually transmitted.

Epidemiology

Epididymitis affects approximately 600,000 men in the United States. It is rare in the prepubertal male and is most common in sexually active males.

Pathology

The most common pathogens include *Chlamydia trachomatis* and *Neisseria gonorrhoeae* in the sexually active male younger than 35 years of age, and *Escherichia coli* in men older than 35 years of age. Syphilis, in the secondary stage, is a rare cause of epididymitis. Tuberculosis is also a rare cause of epididymitis, usually after a subacute or chronic course of tuberculosis. Epididymitis is caused by a retrograde ascent of common infecting organisms into the urethra. This retrograde ascent of organisms causes a cellular inflammation in the vas deferens. The organisms then descend into the lower pole of the epididymis. If this process is bilateral and peritubular fibrosis occurs secondary to the scarring caused by the inflammation and infection, then occlusion of the ductules ensues and sterility may occur.

Clinical Presentation

A patient will complain of flank or groin pain secondary to the vasitis. The epididymis will be swollen and indurated, and the spermatic cord will be thickened. The epididymis will often double in size over a 3- to 4-hour period of time. A urethral discharge may be present along with a fever, and the patient may appear toxic.

On abdominal examination, the lower abdomen, scrotum, and groin area of the affected side may be tender. The scrotal skin will be warm and red.

Examination

The entire abdomen should be examined. The entire genitalia, including the scrotum, testicles, and epididymis should be examined. Examine the groin area to check for swollen lymph nodes. A prostate examination should be performed with caution. Make sure that prostatitis is not present before examining the prostate, secondary to the risk of bacteremia, secondary to vigorous prostate massage.

Diagnosis

A diagnosis is made by physical examination, patient presentation, history, and cultures.

Laboratory Findings

A CBC, electrolytes, and urinalysis should be performed on all patients with suspected epididymitis. Pyuria will only be present in 24% of cases of epididymitis. If penile discharge is present, *Chla-*

mydia and *Neisseria* cultures should be performed. A Gram's stain should be performed to look for gram-negative intracellular diplococci (*Neisseria*).

Treatment

Antibiotic treatment is directed at the most likely cause of the epididymitis based on age and sexual activity. If the patient is younger than 35 years of age and the patient is sexually active, treat the patient with:

1. Ceftriaxone 250 mg intramuscularly (IM), *or*
2. Amoxicillin 3 g by mouth (PO) plus 1 g of probenecid PO, *with*
3. Doxycycline 100 mg PO twice a day (BID) for 10 days

If the patient is older than 35 years of age and if epididymitis is assumed not to be caused by a sexually transmitted organism, treat the patient with:

1. Trimethoprim-sulfamethoxazole (Septra DS) BID for 14 days, *or*
2. Ampicillin 500 mg four times a day (QID) for 14 days

Patients should be encouraged to use sitz baths or ice packs with bed rest for comfort. Patients should be given a scrotal support for comfort. Good analgesic medications are a must. Any patient who cannot keep oral fluids down or looks toxic should be admitted to the hospital, and a urologic consultation should be made. If epididymitis is caused by a sexually transmitted organism, the sexual partner should also be treated.

PROSTATITIS

Definition

Prostatitis is usually an acute bacterial infection of the prostate gland usually secondary to gram-negative organisms.

Epidemiology

Most patients with prostatitis are older than 40 years of age, and the most common organism is *E. coli*. In men with acute prostatitis younger than 40 years of age, *Chlamydia* and *N. gonorrhoeae* should be also considered, especially if the male has a penile discharge and is sexually active.

Pathology

Prostatitis is usually secondary to *E. coli* in 80% of the cases. The remaining organisms that cause prostatitis are *Proteus, Pseudomonas, Klebsiella,* and *Enterobacter.* Rarely tuberculosis is the cause of prostatitis, but prostatitis is usually secondary to renal tuberculosis.

Clinical Presentation

A patient with acute prostatitis will present with an acute febrile-like syndrome or illness with malaise, arthralgias, myalgias, chills, lower lumbar or back pain, and perineal pain. Often symptoms of dysuria, frequency, and urgency are present.

Examination

On examination, the male will present fever, perineal pain, and urethral exudate. Some mild, nonspecific abdominal pain may be present. Do *not* massage the prostate if acutely inflamed, secondary to the possibility of precipitating bacteremia, especially in the very elderly patient in a nursing home.

Diagnosis

A diagnosis is made by history, physician examination, and urine culture for the specific organism.

Laboratory Findings

Any patient with specific signs and symptoms of prostatitis with fever, chills, underlying disease such as diabetes, toxic appearance, or urinary retention should have a CBC, SMA-7, blood culture, and urine culture performed. If urethral discharge is present, a Gram's stain should be done and cultures should be taken for *N. gonorrhoeae* and *Chlamydia.*

Treatment

The afebrile patient, who is taking oral fluids and who does not look toxic or has an underlying disease, can be treated as an outpatient and can be given:

1. Trimethoprim-sulfamethoxazole (Bactrim or Septra DS) PO BID for 30 days, *or*
2. Ampicillin 500 mg PO QID for 30 days, *or*
3. Ciprofloxacin 500 mg PO BID for 14 days, *or*
4. Erythromycin 500 mg PO QID for 14 days

If the patient has fever, chills, or urinary retention or looks toxic or has underlying disease, the patient needs hospitalization. If urinary retention is present, a urethral catheterization should *not* be performed. Suprapubic needle aspiration is the instrumentation of choice to relieve urinary retention in this patient. Catheterization is very painful, and there is an increased risk of bacteremia.

The patient should be given antiemetics, pain medication, and aspirin or acetaminophen for fever control. IV antibiotics of choice are:

1. Ampicillin 2 g IV Q6H, *and*
2. Gentamicin 3 to 5 mg/kg/day, *or*
3. Tobramycin 3 mg/kg/day

An early urology consultation should be the norm. If the patient is treated as an outpatient, he or she should have a 72-hour follow-up or be told to return to the ED if fever, chills, nausea, vomiting, or abdominal pain occurs.

TORSION OF THE TESTICLE

Definition

Torsion of the testicle is usually the medial rotation of the spermatic cord in males younger than 18 years of age.

Epidemiology

Torsion of the testicle occurs most commonly at the age of puberty secondary to the maximal hormonal stimulation of the male. The most common age at presentation is 16 years old, but torsion can occur at any age. Fifty percent of torsional testes have already infarcted at the time of presentation to the ED.

Pathology

The most common abnormality of the testis that causes torsion is secondary to the testis aligning itself to the horizontal axis versus the vertical axis. There is usually a developmental defect between the posterior scrotal wall and the enveloping tunica vaginalis. This deformity, along with unilateral cremaster muscle contraction with horizontal lie of the testis, causes a torsion of the spermatic cord secondary to the deformity of the posterior scrotal wall and the enveloping tunica vaginalis.

Initially, a torsed testicle has only obstruction of venous return. If the torsion is not relieved, venous thrombosis occurs, and then arterial compromise ensues. If this process is not interrupted, necrosis and infarction of the testicle occur. This deformity is often called a "clapper bell" deformity secondary to a redundant spermatic cord, which ia a high-riding capacious tunica vaginalis deformity.

Clinical Presentation

There is often a history of physical exertion or athletic activity prior to the onset of testicular pain. The pain is often of severe, sudden onset, and the pain can often be felt in the lower right or left abdomen, testis, or inguinal canal. There will be rapid scrotal swelling and erythema. The patient will often give a history of a similar episode of pain that resolved spontaneously in a matter of minutes.

Patients will often present with nausea and vomiting. Symptoms of dysuria, polyuria, urgency, or penile discharge are usually absent.

Examination

Examination is often difficult secondary to testicular pain. The scrotum will be tender, swollen, and often firm upon palpation. Often a hydrocele is present on examination. The hydrocele fluid is a reaction to the infarction of the testicle.

Test the cremaster reflex: It will often be absent if torsion is present. The testicle is often high-riding and will lie in the transverse or horizontal position.

Prehn's sign is used to differentiate epididymitis from torsion, but this sign is very unreliable. It is suggested that if epididymitis is present, pain will not be relieved with elevation of the testicle; however, if pain is relieved, torsion is present. This is a very poor indicator of epididymitis or torsion.

Diagnosis

A diagnosis is made by physical examination, Doppler ultrasound, or radionuclide scan. Both Doppler and radionuclide scan will show decreased blood flow to the testicle if torsion is present. Eighty to 100% of torsions can be salvaged if treated within 4 to 6 hours of onset. Pain that lasts longer than 24 hours usually means testicular infarction.

Laboratory Findings

A urinalysis should be performed on all patients who present with any urinary tract complaints.

Treatment

All patients with suspected torsion should have an immediate urologic consultation for immediate evaluation and exploration. Manual detorsion can be attempted in the ED. This is a very simple procedure and can re-establish blood flow to a torsional testicle. The testicle usually is torsional medially; therefore, to correct a testicle, the testicle should be rolled laterally, as if opening the pages of a book. Adequate pain medication should be given prior to a manual attempt of detorsion. If manual detorsion is successful, the patient still needs a urologic consultation for surgical exploration to correct the anatomic defect.

URINARY TRACT INFECTIONS IN ADULTS

Definition

A urinary tract infection (UTI) describes bacteria in the urinary tract that can be acute or chronic. Bacteriuria describes bacteria in the urine. Cystitis describes infection with mucosal invasion. Pyelone-phritis describes an infection in the renal parenchyma and the collecting system. A patient with an underlying neurologic or structural urinary tract problem is said to have a complicated UTI. UTIs are usually divided into upper and lower UTIs.

Epidemiology

It is estimated that as many as 10 to 20% of all women will or have had a UTI. The mortality rate from pyelonephritis is 1 to 3%.

As the male approaches the fifth or sixth decade of life, the incidence of UTIs increases secondary to prostatic hyperplasia. UTIs also increase with age in women. Nosocomial UTIs are the most common nosocomial infections. Black women with sickle cell disease also have a higher incidence of UTIs.

Risk factors for pyelonephritis are diabetes mellitus, pregnancy, three or more UTIs in the past year, or the immunocompromised patient.

Pathology

UTIs can come from occult contamination, obstruction, instrumentation, vesicoureteral reflux, or congenital abnormalities. Bladder overdistention is a common mechanical cause of infection in men with benign prostatic hypertrophy (BPH).

Sexual activity, anal intercourse, and pregnancy can all increase the risk of infection. In men, a UTI is rare before the age of 50.

Urine is normally sterile because of normal complete emptying of the bladder. *E. coli* (90%) is the most common organism that causes bacteriuria. *Staphylococcus saprophyticus* is the second most common organism that causes UTIs. *Proteus, Klebsiella, Streptococcus faecalis, Enterobacter*, and *Providencia* are less common.

Clinical Presentation/Examination

Patients with a lower UTI present with dysuria, polyuria, urgency, frequency, and lower abdominal pressure. Patients with upper UTIs present with a combination of the aforementioned complaints and fever, chills, malaise, nausea, vomiting, back pain, or flank pain and systemic signs of illness. Always obtain a history of vaginal bleeding or discharge from a female patient. If vaginal bleeding or discharge is present, a pelvic examination needs to be performed with the appropriate cultures drawn.

If a male has penile discharge, cultures for *Chlamydia* and gonorrhea should be performed along with a Gram's stain. In the male patient with possible prostatitis, a rectal examination or prostate massage should *not* be performed. This theoretically can cause systemic "seeding" by the organism or bacteremia causing prostatitis.

Diagnosis

A diagnosis is made by history, clinical presentation, urinalysis, and urine culture. A urine culture with 100,000 bacteria per milliliter is considered the "gold standard" for the diagnosis of a UTI.

Laboratory Findings

Some authors suggest that a midstream clean catch is sufficient for a urinalysis and culture. I recommend catheterization to obtain sterile urine for urinalysis and culture in all female patients. Only with catheterization can you ensure noncontamination of the urine in the female patient. A properly collected sample will contain no or very few epithelial cells. All urine must be refrigerated if it is not sent directly for examination. Bacteria in urine doubles every hour at room temperature.

On microscopic examination, the presence of 8 leukocytes or more in uncentrifuged urine or 2 to 5 leukocytes or more in centrifuged urine on a high-power field is diagnostic of pyuria. In men, 1 or more leukocytes on centrifuged urine on a high-power field is diagnostic of pyuria.

Patients with acute pyelonephritis will have white blood cell casts and clumps of bacteria in their urine. A CBC, electrolytes, blood culture, amylase, lipase, liver function tests (LFTs), BUN, and creatinine should be obtained on any patient with suspected pyelonephritis or severe dehydration secondary to vomiting.

Treatment

Lower UTIs can be treated by outpatient therapy if the patient has no underlying disease such as diabetes and can take fluid and food PO. The duration of therapy ranges from a single dose to 3-, 7-, 10-, and 14-day dosing. Trimethoprim-sulfamethoxazole, amoxillin, ciprofloxacin, nitrofurantoin, doxycycline, amoxicillin/clavulanic acid, and co-trimoxazole can all be used successfully to treat uncomplicated UTIs.

Phenazopyridine (Pyridium) 100 mg PO three times a day (TID) with food is an oral bladder analgesic for patients who present with the complaints of dysuria, urgency, or frequency.

Patients with pyelonephritis will present with costovertebral tenderness, flank pain, fever, chills, and nausea but can take fluids PO and have no underlying disease. These patients usually do not need to be admitted to the hospital. A common treatment in the emergency department (ED) in treating uncomplicated pyelonephritis is the "rule of twos." Give 2 liters of IV fluid, two Tylenol No. 3s, and 2 g of ceftriaxone. If the fever drops 2 degrees, and the patient can drink two glasses of water without vomiting, discharge the patient on co-trimoxazole DS, 1 PO BID for 2 weeks with follow-up in 2 days. All patients with pyelonephritis who are treated by outpatient therapy should be told to return to the ED if they are unable to keep oral fluids down or if they have increased fever or increased back or abdominal pain.

Admission to the hospital is based on the underlying disease, the age of the patient, the patient's ability to take oral fluids, dehydration, pain level control, and fever. If the patient is admitted to the hospital, ampicillin and an aminoglycoside is a common IV drug combination until a definitive urine culture is obtained. A third-generation cephalosporin is also acceptable. If the patient is immunocompromised or has sickle cell disease, diabetes mellitus, chronic nephropathy, or a history of recent instrumentation, underlying cancer, or recent chemotherapy, the organism *Pseudomonas* should be covered with broad-spectrum antibiotics.

Any young male with a documented UTI without urethritis should be referred to a urologist for an evaluation. Any older male with prostatic hypertrophy needs a referral for an examination after the prostatitis has resolved to rule out prostate cancer. Any female who has three UTIs or more in a 12-month period should also be referred to a urologist for further evaluation.

BIBLIOGRAPHY

Bushsbaum HJ, Schmidt JD (eds): Gynecologic and Obstetric Urology. Philadelphia, WB Saunders, 1993

Hamilton GC, Sanders AB, Strange GR, et al (eds): Emergency Medicine: An Approach to Clinical Problem-Solving. Philadelphia, WB Saunders, 1991

Kravis TC, Warner CG, Jacobs LM (eds): Emergency Medicine: A Comprehensive Review, 3rd ed. New York, Raven Press, 1993

Kursh ED, McGurie EJ (eds): Female Urology. Philadelphia, JB Lippincott, 1994

May HL, Aghababian RV, Fleisher GR (eds): Emergency Medicine, 2nd ed. Boston, Little, Brown, 1992

Pearson RD, Guerrant RL, Braunwald E, et al (eds): Harrison's Principles of Internal Medicine, 11th ed. New York, McGraw-Hill, 1987

Rosen P, Barkin RM (eds): Emergency Medicine: Concepts and Clinical Practice, 3rd ed. St Louis, Mosby-Year Book, 1992

Schrier RW, Gottschalk CW (eds): Diseases of the Kidney. Boston, Little, Brown, 1988

Schwartz GR, Cayten CG, Mangelsen MA, et al (eds): Principles and Practice of Emergency Medicine. Philadelphia, Lea & Febiger, 1992

Tanagho EA, McAninch JW (eds): Smith's General Urology, 13th ed. Norwalk, CT, Appleton & Lange, 1992

Tierney LM, McPhee SJ, Papadakis MA (eds): Current Medical Diagnosis and Treatment, 33rd ed. Norwalk, CT, Appleton & Lange, 1994

Tintinalli JE, Krone RL, Ruiz E (eds): Emergency Medicine: A Comprehensive Study Guide, 3rd ed. New York, McGraw-Hill, 1992

Index

Note: Page numbers followed by the letter t refer to tabular material.